Food and Nutrition Board, National Academy of Sciences—National Research Council
Recommended Dietary Allowances,[a] Revised 1989

Designed for the maintenance of good nutrition of practically all healthy people in the United States

Category	Age (years) or Condition	Weight[b] (kg)	Weight[b] (lb)	Height[b] (cm)	Height[b] (in)	Protein (g)	Fat-Soluble Vitamins Vitamin A (μg RE)[c]	Vitamin D (μg)[d]	Vitamin E (mg α-TE)[e]	Vitamin K (μg)	Water-Soluble Vitamins Vitamin C (mg)	Thiamin (mg)	Riboflavin (mg)	Niacin (mg NE)[f]	Vitamin B6 (mg)	Folate (μg)	Vitamin B12 (μg)	Minerals Calcium (mg)	Phosphorus (mg)	Magnesium (mg)	Iron (mg)	Zinc (mg)	Iodine (μg)	Selenium (μg)
Infants	0.0–0.5	6	13	60	24	13	375	7.5	3	5	30	0.3	0.4	5	0.3	25	0.3	400	300	40	6	5	40	10
	0.5–1.0	9	20	71	28	14	375	10	4	10	35	0.4	0.5	6	0.6	35	0.5	600	500	60	10	5	50	15
Children	1–3	13	29	90	35	16	400	10	6	15	40	0.7	0.8	9	1.0	50	0.7	800	800	80	10	10	70	20
	4–6	20	44	112	44	24	500	10	7	20	45	0.9	1.1	12	1.1	75	1.0	800	800	120	10	10	90	20
	7–10	28	62	132	52	28	700	10	7	30	45	1.0	1.2	13	1.4	100	1.4	800	800	170	10	10	120	30
Males	11–14	45	99	157	62	45	1,000	10	10	45	50	1.3	1.5	17	1.7	150	2.0	1,200	1,200	270	12	15	150	40
	15–18	66	145	176	69	59	1,000	10	10	65	60	1.5	1.8	20	2.0	200	2.0	1,200	1,200	400	12	15	150	50
	19–24	72	160	177	70	58	1,000	10	10	70	60	1.5	1.7	19	2.0	200	2.0	1,200	1,200	350	10	15	150	70
	25–50	79	174	176	70	63	1,000	5	10	80	60	1.5	1.7	19	2.0	200	2.0	800	800	350	10	15	150	70
	51+	77	170	173	68	63	1,000	5	10	80	60	1.2	1.4	15	2.0	200	2.0	800	800	350	10	15	150	70
Females	11–14	46	101	157	62	46	800	10	8	45	50	1.1	1.3	15	1.4	150	2.0	1,200	1,200	280	15	12	150	45
	15–18	55	120	163	64	44	800	10	8	55	60	1.1	1.3	15	1.5	180	2.0	1,200	1,200	300	15	12	150	50
	19–24	58	128	164	65	46	800	10	8	60	60	1.1	1.3	15	1.6	180	2.0	1,200	1,200	280	15	12	150	55
	25–50	63	138	163	64	50	800	5	8	65	60	1.1	1.3	15	1.6	180	2.0	800	800	280	15	12	150	55
	51+	65	143	160	63	50	800	5	8	65	60	1.0	1.2	13	1.6	180	2.0	800	800	280	10	12	150	55
Pregnant						60	800	10	10	65	70	1.5	1.6	17	2.2	400	2.2	1,200	1,200	320	30	15	175	65
Lactating	1st 6 months					65	1,300	10	12	65	95	1.6	1.8	20	2.1	280	2.6	1,200	1,200	355	15	19	200	75
	2nd 6 months					62	1,200	10	11	65	90	1.6	1.7	20	2.1	260	2.6	1,200	1,200	340	15	16	200	75

[a] The allowances, expressed as average daily intakes over time, are intended to provide for individual variations among most normal persons as they live in the United States under usual environmental stresses. Diets should be based on a variety of common foods in order to provide other nutrients for which human requirements have been less well defined. See text for detailed discussion of allowances and of nutrients not tabulated.

[b] Weights and heights of Reference Adults are actual medians for the U.S. population of the designated age, as reported by NHANES II. The median weights and heights of those under 19 years of age were taken from Hamill et al. (1979) (see pages 16–17). The use of these figures does not imply that the height-to-weight ratios are ideal.

[c] Retinol equivalents. 1 retinol equivalent = 1 μg retinol or 6 μg β-carotene. See text for calculation of vitamin A activity of diets as retinol equivalents.

[d] As cholecalciferol. 10 μg cholecalciferol = 400 IU of vitamin D.

[e] α-Tocopherol equivalents. 1 mg d-α tocopherol = 1 α-TE. See text for variation in allowances and calculation of vitamin E activity of the diet as α-tocopherol equivalents.

[f] 1 NE (niacin equivalent) is equal to 1 mg of niacin or 60 mg of dietary tryptophan.

Nutrition

&

Diet Therapy

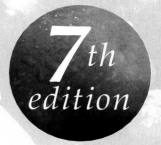

7th edition

Carolynn E. Townsend, BA
Ruth A. Roth, MS, RD

**PARKVIEW HOSPITAL, FORT WAYNE, IN
AND INDIANA/PURDUE UNIVERSITY, FORT WAYNE, IN**

Delmar Publishers

an International Thomson Publishing company

Albany • Bonn • Boston • Cincinnati • Detroit • London • Madrid
Melbourne • Mexico City • New York • Pacific Grove • Paris • San Francisco
Singapore • Tokyo • Toronto • Washington

02-0383

NOTICE TO THE READER

Cover design: Jay Purcell

Delmar Staff:
Publisher: William Brottmiller
Acquisitions Editor: Cathy L. Esperti
Project Editor: Patricia Gillivan
Production Coordinator: James Zayicek
Art and Design Coordinator: Jay Purcell
Editorial Assistant: Darcy M. Scelsi

Printed in the United States of America
3 4 5 6 7 8 9 10 XXX 05 04 03 02 01 00

For more information, contact Delmar, 3 Columbia Circle, PO Box 15015, Albany, NY 12212-0515; or find us on the World Wide Web at http://www.delmar.com

International Division List

Japan:
Thomson Learning
Palaceside Building 5F
1-1-1 Hitotsubashi, Chiyoda-ku
Tokyo 100 0003 Japan
Tel: 813 5218 6544
Fax: 813 5218 6551

Australia/New Zealand
Nelson/Thomson Learning
102 Dodds Street
South Melbourne, Victoria 3205
Australia
Tel: 61 39 685 4111
Fax: 61 39 685 4199

UK/Europe/Middle East:
Thomson Learning
Berkshire House
168-173 High Holborn
London
WC1V 7AA United Kingdom
Tel: 44 171 497 1422
Fax: 44 171 497 1426

Latin America:
Thomson Learning
Seneca, 53
Colonia Polanco
11560 Mexico D.F. Mexico
Tel: 525-281-2906
Fax: 525-281-2656

Canada:
Nelson/Thomson Learning
1120 Birchmount Road
Scarborough, Ontario
Canada M1K 5G4
Tel: 416-752-9100
Fax: 416-752-8102

Asia:
Thomson Learning
60 Albert Street, #15-01
Albert Complex
Singapore 189969
Tel: 65 336 6411
Fax: 65 336 7411

Library of Congress Cataloging-in-Publication Data
Townsend, Carolynn E.
    Nutrition & diet therapy / Carolynn E. Townsend, Ruth A. Roth. —
7th ed.
        p. cm.
    Includes bibliographical references and index.
    ISBN 0-7668-0296-5
    1. Diet therapy. 2. Nutrition. I. Roth, Ruth A. II. Title.
III. Title: Nutrition and diet therapy.
RM216.T738 1999
6.13.2—dc21   99-20354
                                                                CIP

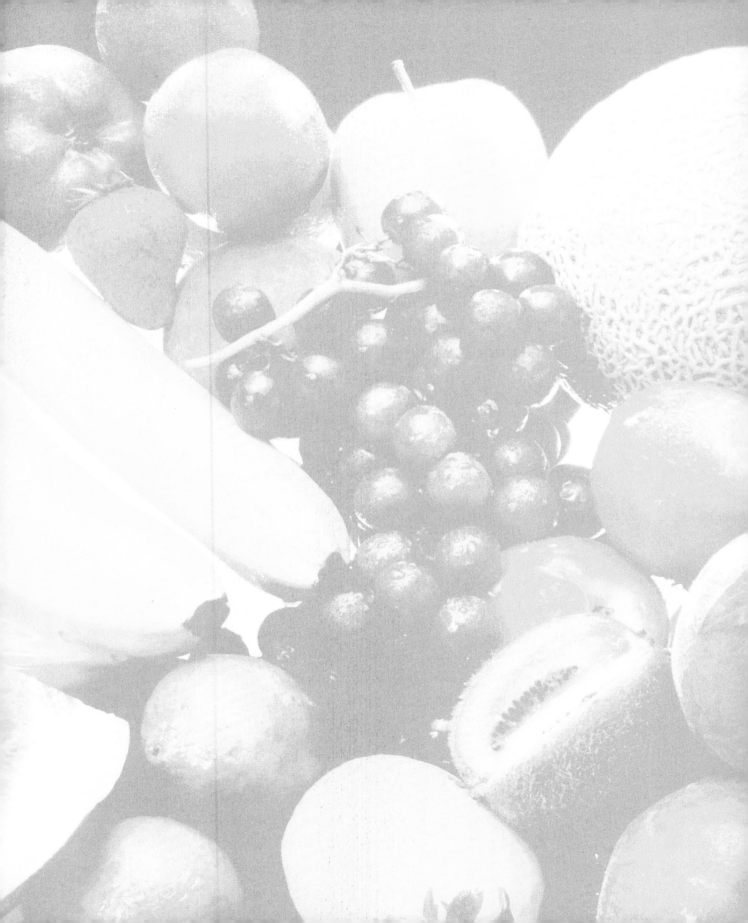

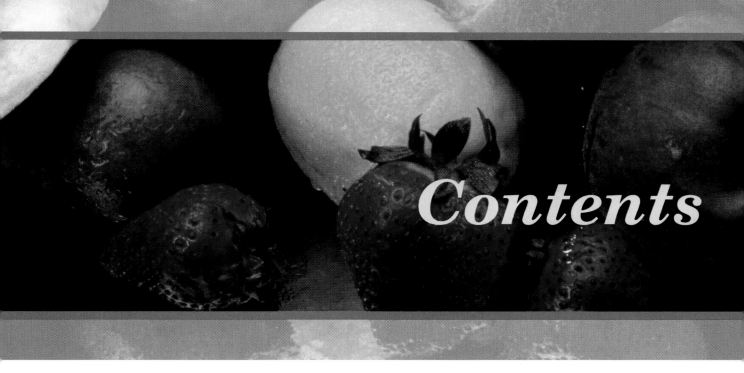

Contents

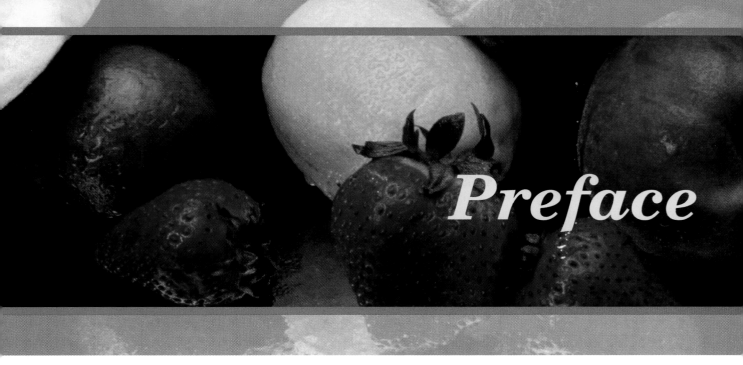

Preface

Just as food should be pleasing to the eye as well as the palate, a text should be visually appealing as well as user-friendly. *Nutrition & Diet Therapy 7th Edition* is now full color! You will certainly notice and appreciate the changes to the new edition. While making certain that the content strengths of its predecessors were maintained, this edition has been revised and updated to include the latest developments in the field, and to stress the importance of good nutrition to good health throughout the life span.

Section 1, **Fundamentals of Nutrition**, includes chapters on the relationship of food and health; planning a healthy diet; digestion, absorption, and metabolism; and chapters on each of the six nutrient groups. Additional tables and figures have been added to reinforce the content of the chapters for the student and enhance learning.

Section 2, **Maintenance of Health Through Good Nutrition**, includes chapters on food related illnesses and allergies, diet planning during the various stages of life from pregnancy and lactation through infancy, childhood, adolescence, young and middle adulthood, and the senior years. This information provides the student with a sound knowledge of the changes in nutritional requirements across the lifespan.

Section 3, **Diet Therapy**, has been expanded. It covers the effects of disease and surgery on nutrition, and the appropriate uses of diet therapy in restoring and maintaining health. It includes chapters with specific nutritional information for patients requiring help with weight control, diabetes mellitus, cardiovascular disease, renal disease, gastrointestinal problems, and cancer. It also discusses the nutritional needs of surgical patients, patients suffering burns and infections including HIV, and patients requiring enteral and parenteral nutrition. There is also a chapter on the general nutritional care of patients.

NEW TO THIS EDITION

- The seventh edition of *Nutrition & Diet Therapy* has a new full color design. We have added more photos, illustrations, and tables to further enhance the reader's comprehension of the content. Students will find the new design to be very user friendly.

- All new case studies at the end of each chapter emphasize the nursing process. These case studies will introduce and reinforce the steps every nurse must learn—assessment, diagnosis, planning, intervention, and evaluation.

- Includes new content on the dietary needs of the patient suffering from HIV/AIDS.

- There are numerous new charts, tables, and photographs throughout the book.

- Each chapter has a section on "Considerations for the Health Care Professional," a number of discussion toics to help develop and nurture critical thinking skills.

SUPPLEMENTAL MATERIALS

Instructor's Guide

This will include the answers to the chapter review questions at the end of each chapter as well as additional suggestions for instructional activities and resources.

Computerized Testbank

This will contain multiple choice questions with answers and text page references

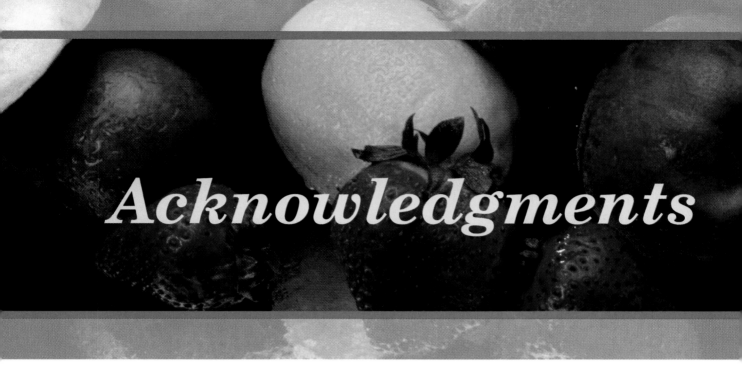

Acknowledgments

The authors wish to express their appreciation to the following people:

Shermane and Magdi Bilal
Rebecca Bender, RN, RD, CDE
Angela Buuck, MS, RD, CNSD
Sue Chubinski, RN, BSN, MA
Kandi Dawson, RD, CDE
Brenda Davis, RD
Tom Donaldson
Cathy L. Esperti
Dawn Gerrain
Patricia Gillivan
Julia Just, RD, CNSD
Rebecca Leichty, LPN
Jay Purcell
Jill Rembetski
Doris Sandker, RD
Dayanne Writtenhouse, RD, CNSD
James Zayicek

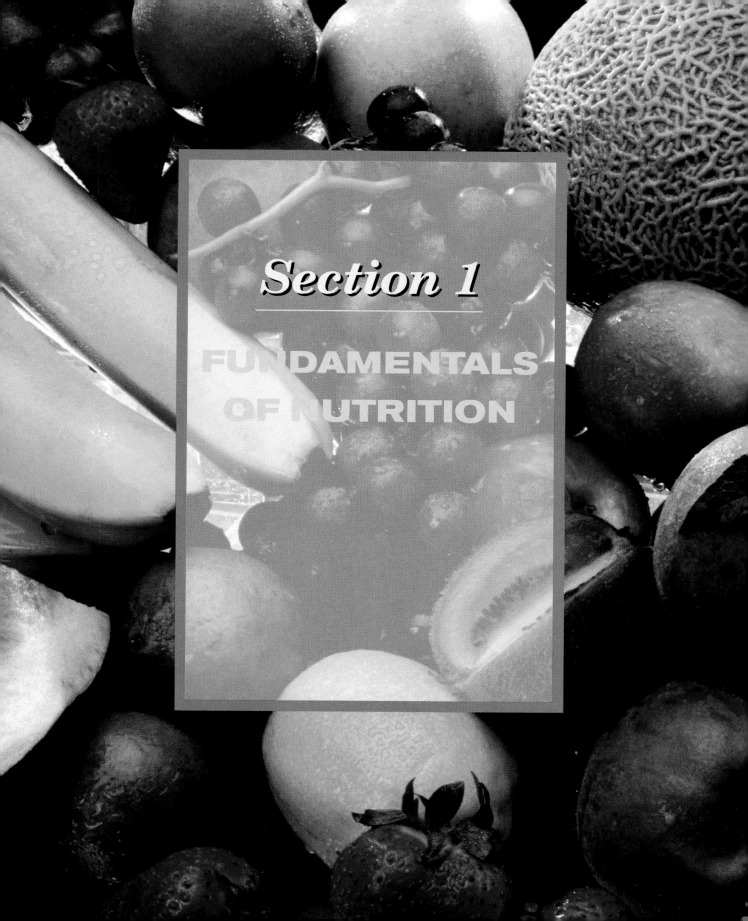

Section 1

FUNDAMENTALS OF NUTRITION

Chapter 1

The Relationship of Food and Health

Key Terms

anthropometric measurements

atherosclerosis

biochemical tests

caliper

carbohydrates (CHO)

circulation

clinical examination

cumulative effects

deficiency diseases

dietary/social history

dietitian

digestion

elimination

fats (lipids)

food diary

goiter

iron deficiency

malnutrition

minerals

nourishing

nutrient density

nutrients

nutrition

nutrition assessment

nutritional status

nutritious

obesity

osteomalacia

osteoporosis

peer pressure

proteins

respiration

rickets

24-hour recall

vitamins

water

Objectives

After studying this chapter, you should be able to:

● Name the six classes of nutrients and their primary functions

● Recognize common characteristics of well-nourished people

● Recognize symptoms of malnutrition

● Describe ways in which food and health are related

● List the four basic steps in nutrition assessment

Most people enjoy food. Although they eat primarily because they are hungry, they also find eating pleasant because of the memories it may invoke and the social climate it promotes and because the taste of the food is pleasing to them. Unfortunately, many people make their food selections only on those bases and are not aware of their bodies' nutritional needs. Hunger is the physiological need for food. Appetite is a psychological desire for food based on pleasant memories of it.

NUTRIENTS AND THEIR FUNCTIONS

nutrients
chemical substances found in food that are necessary for good health

carbohydrates
the nutrient class providing the major source of energy in the average diet

proteins
the only one of the six essential nutrient classes containing nitrogen

fats
highest kcal-value nutrient class

vitamins
organic substances necessary for life although they do not, independently, provide energy

mineral
one of many inorganic substances essential to life and classified generally as minerals

water
major constituent of all living cells; composed of hydrogen and oxygen

circulation
the body process whereby the blood is moved throughout the body

respiration
breathing

digestion
breakdown of food in the body in preparation for absorption

elimination
evacuation of wastes

To function properly, the body must be provided with nutrients. Nutrients are chemical substances that are necessary for life. They are divided into six classes:

- Carbohydrates (CHO)
- Fats (lipids)
- Proteins
- Vitamins
- Minerals
- Water

The body can make small amounts of some nutrients, but most must be obtained from food in order to meet the body's needs. Those available only in food are called essential nutrients. There are about 40 of them, and they are found in all six nutrient classes.

The six nutrient classes are chemically divided into two categories: organic and inorganic (Table 1-1). Organic nutrients contain hydrogen, oxygen, and carbon. (Carbon is an element found in all living things.) Before the body can use organic nutrients, it must break them down into their smallest components. Inorganic nutrients are already in their simplest forms when the body ingests them, except for water.

Each nutrient participates in at least one of the following functions (Table 1-1):

- Providing the body with energy
- Building and repairing body tissue
- Regulating body processes

Carbohydrates, proteins, and fats furnish energy. Proteins are also used to build and repair body tissues with the help of vitamins and minerals. Vitamins, minerals and water help regulate the various body processes such as circulation, respiration, digestion, and elimination.

TABLE 1-1 The Six Essential Nutrients and Their Functions

ORGANIC NUTRIENTS	FUNCTION
Carbohydrates	Provide energy
Fats	Provide energy
Proteins	Build and repair body tissues
	Provide energy
Vitamins	Regulate body processes
INORGANIC NUTRIENTS	**FUNCTION**
Minerals	Regulate body processes
Water	Regulates body processes

Each nutrient is important, but none works alone. For example, carbohydrates, proteins, and fats are necessary for energy but, to provide it, they need the help of vitamins, minerals, and water. Proteins are essential for the building and repair of body tissue, but without vitamins, minerals, and water, they are ineffective. Foods that contain substantial amounts of nutrients are described as nutritious or nourishing. Nutrients are discussed in detail in Chapters 4 through 9.

CHARACTERISTICS OF GOOD NUTRITION

Once foods have been eaten, the body must process them before they can be used. Nutrition is the result of the processes whereby the body takes in and uses food for growth, development, and the maintenance of health. These processes include digestion, absorption, and metabolism. (They are discussed in Chapter 3.) One's physical condition as determined by the diet is called nutritional status.

Nutrition helps determine the height and weight of an individual. Nutrition also can affect the body's ability to resist disease, the length of one's life, and the state of one's physical and mental well-being (Figure 1-1).

Good nutrition enhances appearance and is commonly exemplified by shiny hair, clear skin, clear eyes, erect posture, alert expressions, and firm flesh on well-developed bone structures. Good nutrition aids emotional adjustments, provides stamina, and promotes a healthy appetite. It also helps establish regular sleep and elimination habits (Table 1-2).

nutritious
foods or beverages containing substantial amounts of essential nutrients

nourishing
foods or beverages that provide substantial amounts of essential nutrients

nutrition
the result of those processes whereby the body takes in and uses food for growth, development, and the maintenance of health

nutritional status
one's physical condition as determined by diet

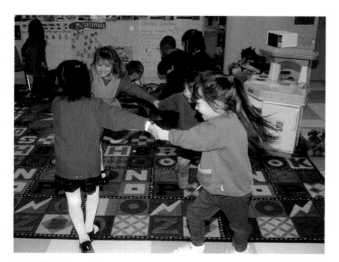 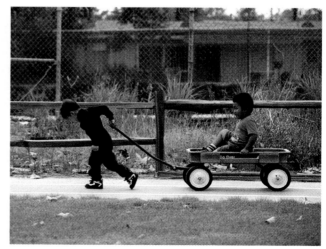

FIGURE 1-1 Good nutrition shows in the happy faces of these children.

TABLE 1-2 Characteristics of Nutritional Status

GOOD	POOR
Alert expression	Apathy
Shiny hair	Dull, lifeless hair
Clear complexion with good color	Greasy, blemished complexion with poor color
Bright, clear eyes	Dull, red-rimmed eyes
Pink, firm gums and well-developed teeth	Red, puffy, receding gums and missing or cavity-prone teeth
Firm abdomen	Swollen abdomen
Firm, well-developed muscles	Underdeveloped, flabby muscles
Well-developed bone structure	Bowed legs, "pigeon" breast
Normal weight for height	Over- or under-weight
Erect posture	Slumped posture
Emotional stability	Easily irritated; depressed; poor attention span
Good stamina; seldom ill	Easily fatigued; frequently ill
Healthy appetite	Excessive or poor appetite
Healthy, normal sleep habits	Insomnia at night; fatigued during day
Normal elimination	Constipation or diarrhea

malnutrition
poor nutrition

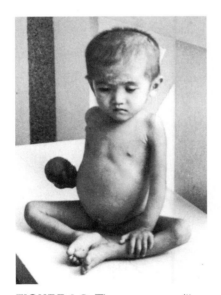

FIGURE 1-2 The poor-quality hair, mottled complexion, dull expression, spindly arms and legs, and bloated abdomen of this baby girl exemplify many signs of malnutrition.

MALNUTRITION

Malnutrition can be caused by overnutrition (excess energy or nutrient intake) or undernutrition (deficient energy or nutrient intake). We usually think of malnutrition as a condition that results when the cells do not receive an adequate supply of the essential nutrients because of poor diet or poor utilization of food. Sometimes it occurs because people do not or cannot eat enough of the foods that provide the essential nutrients to satisfy body needs. At other times people may eat full, well-balanced diets but suffer from diseases that prevent normal usage of the nutrients.

Overnutrition has become a larger problem in the United States than undernutrition. Overeating and the ingestion of megadoses of various vitamins and minerals (without prescription) are two major causes of overnutrition in the United States.

Nutrient Deficiency

A nutrient deficiency occurs when a person lacks one or more nutrients. Nutrient deficiencies are classified as primary or secondary. Primary deficiencies are caused by inadequate dietary intake. Secondary deficiencies are caused by something other than diet, such as a disease condition that may cause malabsorption, accelerated excretion, or destruction of the nutrients. Nutrient deficiencies can result in malnutrition.

INDIVIDUALS AT RISK FROM POOR NUTRITIONAL INTAKE

Persons most prone to malnutrition are infants, preschool children, adolescents, the elderly, and pregnant women (especially if they are adolescents). If mothers do not know about proper nutrition, their children will suffer. Infants and preschool children depend on their mothers' selection of foods. Preschool children may face an additional hazard because they tend to be unusually particular about what they eat.

Adolescents may eat often but at unusual hours. They may miss regularly scheduled meals, become hungry, and satisfy their hunger with foods that have low nutrient density such as potato chips, cakes, soda, and candy. Foods with low nutrient density provide an abundance of calories, but the nutrients are primarily carbohydrates and fats and, except for sodium, very limited amounts of proteins, vitamins, and minerals. Adolescents are subject to peer pressure; that is, they are easily influenced by the opinions of their friends. If friends favor foods with low nutrient density, it is difficult for an adolescent to differ with them. Crash diets, which unfortunately are common among adolescents, sometimes result in a form of malnutrition. This condition occurs because some nutrients are eliminated from the diet when the types of foods eaten are severely restricted.

Pregnancy increases a woman's appetite and the need for certain nutrients, especially proteins, minerals, and vitamins. Pregnancy during adolescence requires extreme care in food selection. The young mother-to-be requires a diet that provides sufficient nutrients for the developing fetus as well as for her own still-growing body.

The elderly are often alone and unwell. Their living conditions are not always conducive to forming a healthy appetite. Part of the joy of eating is sharing one's food in pleasant company. Lack of companionship or illness can make eating unpleasant and difficult.

peer pressure
pressure of one's friends and colleagues of the same age

cumulative effects
results of something done repeatedly over many years

atherosclerosis
a form of arteriosclerosis affecting the intima (inner lining) of the artery walls

obesity
excessive body fat, 20% above average

deficiency disease
disease caused by the lack of a specific nutrient

iron deficiency
intake of iron is adequate, but the body has no extra iron stored

CUMULATIVE EFFECTS OF NUTRITION

There is an increasing concern among health professionals regarding the cumulative effects of nutrition. Cumulative effects are the results of something that is done repeatedly over many years. For example, eating excessive amounts of saturated fats (saturated fats are discussed in Chapter 5) for many years contributes to atherosclerosis, which leads to heart attacks. Years of overeating can cause obesity and may also contribute to hypertension, Type 2 (non-insulin-dependent) diabetes mellitus, gallbladder disease, foot problems, and even personality disorders.

Deficiency Diseases

When nutrients are seriously lacking in the diet for an extended period, deficiency diseases can occur. The most common form of deficiency disease in the United States is iron deficiency, which is caused by a lack of the mineral iron (see Chapter 8). Iron deficiency is particularly common among children and women. Iron is a necessary component of the blood and is lost during each menstrual period. In addition,

rickets

deficiency disease caused by the lack of vitamin D; causes mal-formed bones and pain in infants

osteomalacia

a condition in which bones become soft, usually in adults, because of calcium loss and vitamin D deficiency

osteoporosis

condition in which bones become brittle because there have been insufficient mineral deposits, especially calcium

goiter

enlarged tissue of the thyroid gland due to a deficiency of iodine

nutrition assessment

evaluation of one's nutritional condition

dietitian

professional trained to assess nutrition status and recommend appropriate diet therapy

anthropometric measurements

of height, weight, head, chest, skinfold

clinical examination

physical observation

biochemical tests

laboratory analysis of blood, urine, and feces

dietary/social history

evaluation of food habits, includ-ing patient's ability to buy and prepare food

caliper

mechanical device used to mea-sure percentage of body fat by skinfold measurement

TABLE 1-3 Nutritional Deficiency Diseases and Possible Causes

DEFICIENCY DISEASE	NUTRIENT(S) LACKING
Iron deficiency	Iron
Iron-deficiency anemia	Iron
Beriberi	Thiamin
Night blindness	Vitamin A
Goiter	Iodine
Kwashiorkor	Protein
Marasmus	All nutrients
Osteomalacia	Calcium and vitamin D
Osteoporosis	Calcium and vitamin D
Pellagra	Niacin
Rickets	Calcium and vitamin D
Scurvy	Vitamin C
Xerophthalmia (blindness)	Vitamin A

the amount of iron needed during childhood and pregnancy is greater than normal because of the growth of the child or the fetus.

Rickets is another example of a deficiency disease. It causes poor bone formation in children and is due to insufficient calcium and vita-min D. These same deficiencies in young adults cause osteomalacia and, in older adults, osteoporosis. Osteomalacia is sometimes called "adult rickets." It causes the bones to soften and may cause the spine to bend and the legs to become bowed. Osteoporosis is a condition that causes bones to become porous and excessively brittle. Too little iodine may cause goiter, and a severe shortage of vitamin A can lead to blind-ness.

Examples of other deficiency diseases (and their causes) are included in Table 1-3. Information concerning these conditions can be found in the chapters devoted to the given nutrients.

NUTRITION ASSESSMENT

That old saying "You are what you eat" is true, indeed; but one could change it a bit to read, "You are *and will be* what you eat." Good nutri-tion is essential for the attainment and maintenance of good health. Determining whether a person is at risk requires completion of a nutrition assessment, which should, in fact, become part of a routine exam done by a registered dietitian or other health care professional specifically trained in the diagnosis of at-risk individuals. A proper nutrition assessment includes anthropometric measurements, clin-ical examination, biochemical tests, and dietary/social history.

Anthropometric measurements include height and weight and measurements of the head (for children), upper arm, and skinfold. The skinfold measurements are done with a caliper. They are used to de-termine the percentage of adipose and muscle tissue in the body. Mea-

TABLE 1-4 Clinical Signs of Nutrient Deficiencies

CLINICAL SIGNS	POSSIBLE DEFICIENCIES
Pallor; blue half circles beneath eyes	Iron, copper, zinc, B_{12}, B_6, biotin
Edema	Protein
Bumpy "gooseflesh"	Vitamin A
Lesions at corners of mouth	Riboflavin
Glossitis	Folic acid
Numerous "black and blue" spots and tiny, red "pin prick" hemorrhages under skin	Vitamin C
Emaciation	Carbohydrates, proteins; kcal
Poorly shaped bones or teeth or delayed appearance of teeth in children	Vitamin D or calcium
Slow clotting time of blood	Vitamin K
Unusual nervousness, dermatitis, diarrhea in same patient	Niacin
Tetany	Calcium, potassium, sodium
Goiter	Iodine
Eczema	Fat (linoleic acid)

surements out of line with expectations may reveal failure to thrive in children, wasting (catabolism), edema, or obesity, all of which reflect nutrient deficiencies or excesses.

During the clinical examination, signs of nutrient deficiencies are noted. Some nutrient deficiency diseases, such as scurvy, rickets, iron deficiency, and kwashiorkor, are obvious; other forms of nutrient deficiency can be far more subtle. The clinical examination requires skill because many physical signs may reflect more than one deficiency. Table 1-4 lists some clinical signs and probable causes of nutrient deficiencies.

Biochemical tests include various blood, urine, and stool tests. A deficiency or toxicity can be determined by laboratory analysis of the samples. The tests allow detection of malnutrition before signs appear. The following are some of the most commonly used tests for hospitalized patients.

Serum albumin level measures the main protein in the blood and is used to determine protein status.

Serum transferrin level indicates iron-carrying protein in the blood. The level will be above normal if iron stores are low and below normal if the body lacks protein.

Blood urea nitrogen (BUN) may indicate renal failure, insufficient renal blood supply, or blockage of the urinary tract.

Creatinine excretion indicates amount of creatinine excreted in the urine over a 24-hour period and can be used in estimating body muscle mass. If the muscle mass has been depleted, as in malnutrition, the level will be low.

Serum creatinine indicates the amount of creatinine in the blood and is used for evaluating renal function.

Examples of other blood tests are hemoglobin (Hgb), hematocrit (Hct), red blood cells (RBCs), and white blood cells (WBCs). A low Hgb and Hct can indicate pernicious anemia. Not a routine test, but ordered on many heart patients, is the lipid profile, which includes total serum cholesterol, high-density lipoprotein (HDL), low-density lipoprotein (LDL), and serum triglycerides. Urinalysis also can detect protein and sugar in the urine, which can indicate kidney disease and diabetes mellitus.

The dietary/social history involves evaluation of food habits and is very important in the nutritional assessment of any patient. It can be difficult to obtain an accurate dietary assessment. The most common method is the **24-hour recall**. In this method, the patient is usually interviewed by the dietitian and is asked to give the types, amounts, and preparation used for all food eaten in the 24 hours prior to admission (PTA). Another method is the **food diary**. The patient is asked to list all food eaten in a three- or four-day period. Neither method is totally accurate because patients forget or are not always totally truthful. They are sometimes inclined to say they have eaten certain foods because they know they should have done so. Computer analysis of the diet is the best way to determine if nutrient intake is appropriate. It will reveal any nutrient deficiencies or toxicities.

The social history is important to determine whether the patient has the financial resources to obtain the needed food and the ability to properly store and cook food once home. Food-drug interactions can lead to malnutrition. Patients need to be instructed by a dietitian on possible interactions, if any.

When the preceding steps are evaluated together, and in the context of the patient's medical condition, the dietitian has the best opportunity of making an accurate nutrition assessment of the patient. This assessment can then be used by the entire health care team. The doctor will find it helpful in evaluating the patient's condition and treatment. The dietitian can use the information to plan the patient's dietary treatment and counseling, and other health care professionals will be able to use it in assisting and counseling the patient.

CONSIDERATIONS FOR THE HEALTH CARE PROFESSIONAL

The practice of good nutrition habits would help eliminate many health problems caused by malnutrition. The health professional is obligated to have a sound knowledge of nutrition. One's personal health, as well as that of one's family, depends on it. Parents must have a good, basic knowledge of nutrition for the sake of their personal health and that of their children. Children learn by imitating their parents. Family members and friends who know that the health professional has studied nutrition will ask questions. Anyone, in fact, who plans and prepares meals should value, have knowledge of, and be able to apply the principles of sound nutrition practice.

24-hour recall

listing the types, amounts, and preparation of all foods eaten in past 24 hours

food diary

written record of all food and drink ingested in a specified period

Patients will have questions and complaints about their diets. Their anxieties can be relieved by clear and simple explanations provided by the health professional. Sometimes patients must undergo diet therapy, prescribed by their physicians, which becomes part of their medical treatment. The health professional must be able to check the patient's tray quickly to see that it contains the correct foods for the diet prescribed. In many cases, diet therapy will have to be a lifelong practice for the patient. In such cases, eating habits will have to be changed, and the patient will need advice or instructions from a registered dietitian and support from other health professionals.

Nutrition is currently a popular subject. It is important to recognize that some books and articles concerning nutrition may not be scientifically correct. Also, food ads can be misleading. People with knowledge of sound nutrition practices will not be misled. They will recognize fad and distinguish it from fact.

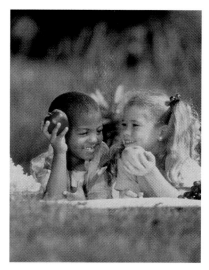

FIGURE 1-3 Good health radiates from these two children. (Courtesy of USDA/ARS #K-48191.)

● SUMMARY

Nutrition is directly related to health, and its effects are cumulative. Good nutrition is normally reflected by good health (Figure 1-3). Poor nutrition can result in poor health and even in disease. Poor nutrition habits contribute to atherosclerosis, osteoporosis, obesity, and some cancers.

To be well nourished, one must eat foods that contain the six essential nutrients: carbohydrates, fats, proteins, minerals, vitamins, and water. These nutrients provide the body with energy, build and repair body tissue, and regulate body processes. When there is a severe lack of specific nutrients, deficiency diseases may develop. The best way to determine deficiencies is to do a nutrition assessment.

With a sound knowledge of nutrition, the health professional will be an effective professional and will also be helpful to family, friends, and self.

● DISCUSSION TOPICS

1. Why is food commonly served at meetings and parties?
2. What relationship might nutrition and heredity have to each of the following?
   a. the development of physique
   b. the ability to resist disease
   c. the lifespan
3. How might nutritional status affect personality?
4. What habits, in addition to good nutrition, contribute to making a person healthy?
5. What are the six classes of nutrients? What are their three basic functions?
6. Why are women under 52 prone to iron deficiency?

7. Why are some foods called low nutrient density foods? Give examples of these foods.

8. Ask anyone in the class who has been on a crash diet to discuss the diet's effects. Discuss possible reasons for those effects.

9. What is meant by the saying "You are what you eat"?

10. Why are people in the following age groups sometimes prone to malnutrition?
    a. young children
    b. adolescents
    c. the elderly

11. What is meant by the phrase "the cumulative effects of nutrition." Describe some.

12. How could someone be overweight and at the same time suffer from malnutrition?

13. If anyone in class has seen someone suffering from malnutrition, ask for a description. Discuss possible reasons for the malnutrition.

14. Discuss why salesclerks in health food stores may not provide customers nutritionally accurate information concerning the store's products.

15. Discuss why health care professionals should be knowledgeable about nutrition.

● SUGGESTED ACTIVITIES

1. List ten signs of good nutrition and ten signs of poor nutrition.

2. List the foods you have eaten in the past 24 hours. Underline those with low nutrient density.

3. Write a brief description of how you feel at the end of a day when you know you have not eaten wisely.

4. Observe television ads for food products. Keep a log of those that are misleading or factually inaccurate.

5. Write the manufacturer of a food product used in your home. Ask for nutrition information on that product.

6. Name the laboratory tests used to determine nutritionally at-risk patients.

7. List and define the key terms at the beginning of the chapter and keep the list in your notebook.

8. Write a brief paragraph discussing nutritional status.

9. Briefly describe rickets, osteomalacia, and osteoporosis. Include their causes.

10. List and include the uses for the biochemical tests described in this chapter. Keep this list in your notebook.

11. Invite a registered dietitian to speak to your class about nutrition problems commonly seen in your area.

● REVIEW

Multiple choice. Select the *letter* that precedes the best answer.

1. The result of those processes whereby the body takes in and uses food for growth, development, and maintenance of health is
   a. respiration
   b. diet therapy
   c. nutrition
   d. digestion

2. Nutritional status is determined by
   a. heredity
   b. employment
   c. personality
   d. diet

3. To nourish the body adequately, one must
   a. avoid all low nutrient density foods
   b. eat foods containing the six classes of nutrients
   c. include fats at every meal
   d. restrict proteins at breakfast

4. Nutrients used primarily to provide energy to the body are
   a. vitamins and water
   b. carbohydrates, proteins, and fats
   c. proteins and vitamins
   d. vitamins and minerals

5. Nutrients used mainly to build and repair body tissues are
   a. proteins, vitamins, and minerals
   b. carbohydrates and fats
   c. fats and water
   d. iron and fats

6. Foods such as potato chips, cakes, sodas, and candy are called
   a. dietetic foods
   b. essential nutrient foods
   c. foods with low nutrient density
   d. nutritious foods

7. An inadequate supply of the six classes of nutrients in the diet may result in
   a. stamina
   b. malnutrition
   c. indigestion
   d. diabetes

8. Iron deficiency is caused by a lack of
   a. proteins
   b. carbohydrates
   c. vitamins
   d. iron

9. The cumulative effect of a high-fat diet could be
   a. iron deficiency
   b. blindness
   c. heart disease
   d. diabetes mellitus

10. Malnutrition could be caused by
   a. poor posture
   b. constipation
   c. disease or drug therapy
   d. hypertension

11. High blood pressure is commonly referred to as
   a. atherosclerosis
   b. non-insulin-dependent diabetes mellitus
   c. osteoporosis
   d. hypertension

12. Iron is a mineral that is a necessary component of
   a. blood
   b. urine
   c. saliva
   d. vitamin A

13. A cumulative condition is one that develops
   a. within a very short period of time
   b. over several years
   c. only in women under 52
   d. in premature infants

14. Low nutrient dense foods
   a. are found only in crash diets
   b. are very helpful to pregnant adolescents
   c. provide very few nutrients
   d. provide good stamina

15. Another term for fats is
   a. CHO
   b. lipids
   c. inorganic nutrient
   d. protein enhancer

16. Another term for carbohydrates is
   a. CHO
   b. lipids
   c. inorganic nutrient
   d. protein enhancer

17. Proteins are
   a. the body's primary source of energy
   b. an excellent substitute for carbohydrates
   c. essential for building and repairing body tissues
   d. inorganic nutrients

18. Vitamins and minerals
   a. help proteins to build and repair body tissues
   b. are both organic nutrients
   c. are the primary providers of energy to the body
   d. should be taken in mega-doses to prevent disease

19. Nutritional status
   a. is determined by heredity
   b. never changes
   c. is not reflected in one's appearance
   d. can affect the body's ability to resist disease

20. Infants, young children, adolescents, pregnant adolescents, and the elderly
   a. are commonly overweight
   b. are among those prone to malnutrition
   c. all commonly suffer from osteomalacia
   d. never suffer from primary nutrient deficiencies

C A S E   S T U D Y

Ryan D. was an energetic five-year-old boy who lived with his mother and his grandfather, Grandpa Joe. Mrs. D. was a secretary who worked all day. Ryan didn't mind because Grandpa Joe took care of him while she was gone. He walked Ryan to and from afternoon kindergarten. They played in the park after school.

Every day on the way to school, the two of them would stop at the corner convenience store and buy Ryan's lunch. His favorite meal was fruit punch, a bag of chips, a banana, and a chocolate bar. One day, the banana got soft and brown, and after that Ryan didn't pick any more fruit.

By late October, his teacher, Miss Stewart, called Mrs. D. and said Ryan was falling asleep in the afternoon and didn't want to play during recess. Miss Stewart asked Mrs. D. to come to school before going to work one morning so they could discuss this problem.

ASSESSMENT

1. What data had the teacher collected about this problem?

2. What did the teacher suspect was the cause of the problem?

3. What could be some other causes of Ryan's sleepiness?

   At the meeting with Miss Stewart, Mrs. D. described Ryan as a happy, energetic child who ate a nutritious breakfast and dinner. After the meeting with the teacher, Mrs. D. talked to Grandpa Joe about Ryan's behavior. Grandpa Joe was also very concerned.

DIAGNOSIS

4. Complete the diagnostic statement. Ryan's deficit in nutrition is caused by _____.

5. What factors have contributed to the problem?

6. Who needs to be involved in the solution?

PLAN/GOAL

7. What change do you want to see in Ryan's diet? State it in one sentence with a measurable reasonable goal.

8. Suggest some alternatives to Ryan's current lunch source and selection of food that would supply Ryan with a healthy lunch.

IMPLEMENTATION

9. How would you present these choices to Grandpa Joe and Ryan?

10. What role would Miss Stewart play?

EVALUATION/OUTCOME CRITERIA

11. What behavior might Ryan demonstrate that will indicate to Mrs. D. and Miss Stewart that the plan was successful?

12. What are some other ways they can tell it was successful?

C A S E   S T U D Y

Charlotte G. was an 89-year-old woman who continued to live in her own home after her husband, Elmer, died a year ago. Charlotte was independent; she drove to the grocery store, church, and the beauty shop. Her children and grandchildren lived more than three hours away. They called frequently and visited for holidays and special occasions. She and her husband had enjoyed entertaining and inviting friends to share meals. Charlotte took pride in being an excellent homemaker and hostess.

For the past four or five months, her close friend and neighbor Vera had thought something was wrong. Charlotte forgot lunch dates. Her clothes were baggy and rumpled. Vera saw Charlotte in the store in such clothes. Charlotte would not normally be seen outside the house in her old cleaning clothes. Vera worried that Charlotte wasn't taking her blood pressure medication. She convinced Charlotte to see her doctor and went with her. Vera explained her concerns to the doctor. After the doctor completed a physical examination and had some blood drawn, he suggested Charlotte consider a nursing home. He was concerned about her 30-pound weight loss since her visit last year. Charlotte refused to consider a nursing home and wanted to stay in her own home! The doctor reluctantly agreed but only if she would agree to have a home health nurse visit her. He gave her a prescription for a daily vitamin and a referral to the home health dietitian. He told Charlotte she had to take better care of herself and gain some weight, and he set up an appointment to see her in three months.

ASSESSMENT

1. What observations prompted Vera to be concerned?

2. What objective data did the doctor have?

DIAGNOSIS

3. Which of the following nursing diagnoses could apply to Charlotte's problems: Alzheimer's disease, dementia, depression, loneliness, lack of proper nutrition, or dehydration?

4. What contributed to the development of the problems?

PLAN/GOAL

5. What changes do you want to see for Charlotte?

IMPLEMENTATION

6. Name at least three methods that could be used to improve Charlotte's nutrition.

7. How could Meals on Wheels help?

8. How could a home health aide who visited three times a week help?

9. How could friends and neighbors help?

10. What could her family do to help?

EVALUATION/OUTCOME CRITERIA

11. What can the doctor measure at the next appointment to see if the plan is working?

12. What observations could Vera offer about the success of the plan?

13. What would the home health aide report?

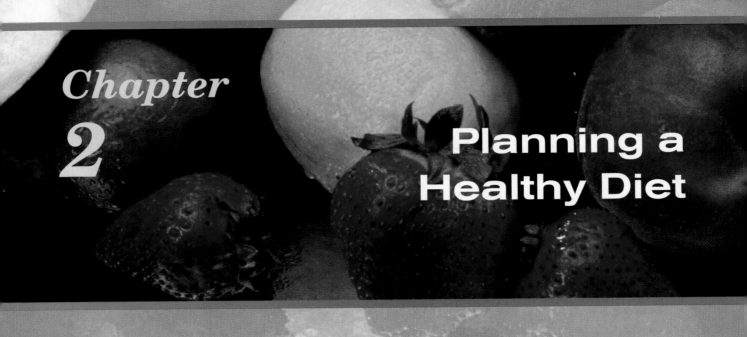

Chapter 2

Planning a Healthy Diet

Key Terms

balanced diet

daily values

descriptors

Dietary Guidelines

dietary laws

food customs

Food Guide Pyramid

hypertension

lacto-vegetarian

lacto-ovo vegetarian

legumes

nutrient density

vegan

Objectives

After studying this chapter, you should be able to:

● Define a balanced diet

● List the U.S. government's Dietary Guidelines for Americans and explain the reasons for each

● Identify the food groups and their placement on the Food Guide Pyramid

● Describe information commonly found on food labels

● List some food customs of various cultural groups

● Describe the development of food customs

A BALANCED DIET

The statement "eat a balanced diet" has been repeated so often that its importance may be overlooked. The value of this statement is so great, however, that it deserves serious consideration by people of all ages. A balanced diet includes all six classes of nutrients and kilocalories in amounts that preserve and promote good health.

Daily review of the Recommended Dietary Allowances (RDA) (see Table A-1 in the appendix) would provide enough information to plan balanced diets. However, ordinary meal planning would be cumbersome and time-consuming if that table had to be consulted each time a meal was planned. Fortunately, the United States Department of Agriculture (USDA) and the U.S. Department of Health and Human Services (DHHS) developed a simple system to help with the selection of healthful diets. It is called the Dietary Guidelines for Americans. In addition, the Food Guide Pyramid was developed by the USDA as an outline for daily food choices based on the Dietary Guidelines.

balanced diet
one that includes all the essential nutrients in appropriate amounts

Dietary Guidelines
general goals for optimal nutrient intake

Food Guide Pyramid
outline for making food selections based on Dietary Guidelines

nutrient density
nutrient value of foods compared with number of kcal

DIETARY GUIDELINES FOR AMERICANS

Dietary guidelines are general goals for nutrient intake. The 1995 revision of these guidelines is as follows:

1. Eat a variety of foods.
2. Balance your food intake with physical activity; maintain or improve your weight.
3. Choose a diet with plenty of grain products, vegetables, and fruit.
4. Choose a diet low in fat, saturated fat, and cholesterol.
5. Choose a diet moderate in sugars.
6. Choose a diet moderate in salt and sodium.
7. If you drink alcoholic beverages, do so in moderation.

Eat a Variety of Foods

There are over 40 nutrients needed by the body. Because no one food contains all of these nutrients, eating a variety of foods is the best way to ensure a healthy diet. In addition, if some foods contain toxins, such as residue of insect repellents or additives that behave as allergens, variety would reduce the amount ingested.

It's important to choose foods with high nutrient density. These are foods that provide many nutrients but few kilocalories. For example, tuna fish salad made with an oil dressing and served with tomatoes and mixed greens has high nutrient density. A meal consisting of a hamburger with french fries has low nutrient density.

Balance Your Food Intake with Physical Activity; Maintain or Improve Your Weight

Overweight increases the risk of developing high blood pressure and diabetes (disorders associated with increased risk of heart attacks and strokes) and possibly some cancers (see Table A-2 in the appendix for acceptable body weights.) Energy needs of people differ, depending on basal metabolism, age, size, sex, physical condition, and activity. (The unit used to measure the amount of energy in food is the kilocalorie [kcal], commonly known as calorie. It represents the amount of heat needed to raise one kilogram of water one degree Celsius.) However, the general rule remains this: the number of kcal taken in must not exceed the number of kcal burned by the body each day if the current weight is to be maintained.

Losing weight should be done on a gradual basis of no more than 1 to 2 pounds a week. That rate may seem slow, but in fact 26 to 52 pounds can be lost in a 6-month period. Gradual weight loss is the most effective method because it is most conducive to effecting genuine change in eating habits, which helps to maintain the reduced weight afterward. It is also the safest method of weight loss. Diets of fewer than 1,000 kcal a day (crash diets) tend to limit the varieties of foods to such an extent that the nutrient intake may be reduced below the recommended daily allowances. This type of diet can damage one's health and, in extreme cases, cause death.

Because 1 pound of body fat contains 3,500 kcal, 3,500 kcal must be burned to lose 1 pound. If, for example, a person takes in 500 calories less than are burned each day, there will be a 1-pound weight loss at the end of the week. One way to speed weight loss is to cause additional calories to be burned by increasing physical activity.

Conversely, it is important that weight loss does not continue beyond the acceptable range. Extreme weight loss can contribute to nutrient deficiencies, menstrual irregularities, infertility, hair loss, skin changes, intolerance to cold, constipation, psychological disturbances, and even death. If there is unexplained weight loss, a physician should be consulted because it can be an indication of underlying disease.

Choose a Diet with Plenty of Grain Products, Vegetables, and Fruits

In this guideline, adults are advised to eat a minimum of three servings of vegetables, two fruits, and six servings of grain products each day. These foods provide numerous vitamins, minerals, complex carbohydrates, and dietary fiber. With the exception of avocado, they are very low in fat. Also, a person who follows this guideline probably will eat fewer fat-rich foods.

Choose a Diet Low in Fat, Saturated Fat, and Cholesterol

Because fats contain slightly more than twice the kcal of carbohydrates or proteins, they contribute to obesity and, thus, heart disease, diabetes, and some forms of cancer. In addition, large amounts of saturated fats also increase the risk of heart disease by raising blood cholesterol levels. It is considered advisable to limit one's total fat intake to 30% or less of total daily kcal intake. Blood cholesterol levels in adults should be kept to 200 mg/dl (milligrams per deciliter) or less. Both goals may be met without sacrificing necessary nutrients or flavor:

- Lean meats, fish, poultry, and legumes (various beans and peas) can be substituted for fatty meats.
- The fat on meats can be trimmed.
- The skin on poultry should not be eaten.
- Fat-free milk can be substituted for whole milk.
- Whenever possible, water-packed instead of oil-packed canned goods should be used.
- Foods should be baked, broiled, or boiled rather than fried.
- Eggs, organ meats, butter, margarine, and cream can be used in moderation.

Choose a Diet Moderate in Sugars

Sugar serves as a preservative and thickener in jellies and jams and adds color and flavor to numerous foods. However, the foods in which it is commonly found, such as desserts and candies, tend to have few other nutrients except for fats. Thus, if one eats sugar-rich foods in place of other foods, the total nutrient intake will be inadequate but the kcal content will be high. In addition, sugar causes tooth decay (dental caries).

Choose a Diet Moderate in Salt and Sodium

Excessive amounts of sodium can contribute to hypertension (blood pressure over 140/90), which is known to increase the risk of coronary heart disease (see Chapter 18). It is recommended that little, if any, salt be added during cooking or at the table. Canned and frozen foods generally have had salt added, so fresh foods are preferred.

If You Drink Alcoholic Beverages, Do So in Moderation

One ounce of gin, rum, vodka, or whiskey contains approximately 80 kcal and only traces of a few nutrients. In moderate drinkers, alcohol tends to increase the appetite and so can contribute to weight gain. Conversely, heavy drinkers can lose their appetites, not eat, and subsequently suffer nutritional deficiencies. The use of alcohol by pregnant women can cause birth defects. Heavy drinking can cause cirrhosis of the liver and brain damage, and it can increase the risk of cancer of the throat and neck. One drink a day for a woman and two for a man is considered moderate drinking. Twelve ounces of beer, 5 ounces of wine, or 1½ ounces of 80-proof liquor all count as *one* drink.

FOOD GUIDE PYRAMID

The Food Guide Pyramid (Figure 2-1), introduced in 1992, is intended as an outline to help the consumer plan meals. It is hoped that the Pyramid will promote healthful food habits among adults and children.

legumes
plant food that is grown in a pod; for example, beans and peas

hypertension
higher than normal blood pressure

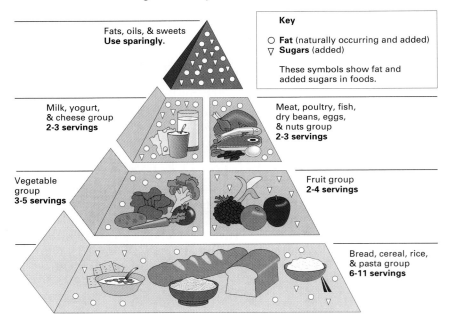

FIGURE 2-1 Food Guide Pyramid. (Courtesy of USDA and DHHS. 1992. The food guide pyramid: A guide to daily food choices. Leaflet no. 572. Washington, D.C.)

The Pyramid consists of six food groups that are presented in proportions appropriate for a healthful diet:

- Bread, cereal, rice, and pasta group
- Vegetable group
- Fruit group
- Milk, yogurt, and cheese group
- Meat, poultry, fish, dry beans, eggs, and nuts group
- Fats, oils, and sweets group

Bread, Cereal, Rice, and Pasta Group

The largest section of the Pyramid is made up of the bread, cereal, rice, and pasta group (Table 2-1). These foods are rich in complex carbohydrates and should make up 50 to 55% of one's diet. In addition, when they are made from whole grains, these foods provide dietary fiber, B vitamins, iron, and magnesium. Enriched products also contain B vitamins and iron, but if they are not made from whole grains, they contain little dietary fiber.

It is recommended that one have from 6 to 11 servings of these foods each day. One serving is considered one slice of bread; one-half an English muffin; one ounce dry cereal; or one-half cup cooked cereal, pasta, or rice.

TABLE 2-1 Bread, Cereal, Rice, and Pasta Group

Breads
    whole wheat
    dark rye
    enriched
    oatmeal bread
Cornmeal, whole grain or enriched
Rolls or biscuits made with whole
    wheat or enriched flour
Flour, enriched
    whole wheat, other whole grain
    grits, enriched
Cereals
    whole wheat
    rolled oats
    other cereals, if whole grain or restored
Rice
    brown rice
    converted rice
Pasta
    noodles, spaghetti, macaroni

(Photo Courtesy of Price Chopper Supermarkets)

Vegetable Group

All vegetables are included in the vegetable group: green and leafy, yellow, starchy, and legumes (Table 2-2). Vegetables provide carbohydrates; dietary fiber; vitamins A, B-complex, C, E, and K; and iron, calcium, phosphorus, potassium, magnesium, copper, manganese, and sometimes, molybdenum.

It is recommended that one have from three to five servings of vegetables each day. One-half cup of cooked or chopped raw vegetables or one cup of uncooked, leafy vegetables is considered one serving.

Fruit Group

All fruits are included in the fruit group. They provide vitamins A and C, potassium, magnesium, iron, and carbohydrates, including dietary fiber (Table 2-3).

It is recommended that two to four servings be included in the diet each day, at least one being an especially rich source of vitamin C. One serving is three-quarters cup fruit juice; a half of a grapefruit; one whole raw apple, orange, peach, pear, or banana; a half cup canned or cooked fruit; and a quarter cup dried fruit.

TABLE 2-2 Vegetable Group

SOURCES OF VITAMIN A	SOURCES OF VITAMIN C
Carrots	Raw or lightly cooked cabbage
Squash	Green peppers
Spinach	Turnip greens
Kale	Broccoli
Other greens	Potatoes
Pumpkin	Brussels sprouts
Sweet potatoes	Tomatoes
Corn	Red peppers
Broccoli	Asparagus
Chard	Spinach

(Photo Courtesy of W. Altee Burpee Company)

TABLE 2-3 Fruit Group

SOURCES OF VITAMIN A	SOURCES OF VITAMIN C	
Bananas	Oranges	Cantaloupe
Cantaloupe	Lemons	Kiwi fruit
Avocados	Grapefruit	Honeydew melon
Apricots	Limes	Watermelon
Mangoes	Raspberries	Mangoes
	Strawberries	Papaya
	Pineapple	

(Photo Courtesy of USDA)

Milk, Yogurt, and Cheese Group

Milk, yogurt, and cheese are excellent sources of carbohydrate (lactose); calcium, phosphorus, and magnesium; proteins; riboflavin, vitamins A, B_{12}, and, if the milk is fortified, vitamin D. Unfortunately, all contain sodium, and whole milk and whole-milk products also contain saturated fats and cholesterol. Fat-free milk has had the fats removed.

It is recommended that two to three servings of these foods be included in one's daily diet. The serving size is one 8-ounce glass of milk or the equivalent in terms of calcium content.

Children	2 servings
Adolescents	3 servings
Adults	2 servings
Pregnant or lactating women	3 servings
Pregnant or lactating teens	4 servings

The following dairy foods contain calcium equal to that found in one 8-ounce cup of milk:

- 1½ ounces of cheddar cheese
- 2 cups "creamed" cottage cheese
- 1¾ cups of ice cream or ice milk
- 1 cup yogurt

Milk used in making cream sauces, gravies, or baked products fulfills part of the calcium requirement. A cheese sandwich would fulfill one of the serving requirements, and a serving of ice cream or milk could fulfill half of one of the serving requirements. Obviously, drinking milk is not the only way to fulfill the calcium requirement.

Some patients suffer from lactose intolerance and cannot digest milk or milk products. If they eat or drink foods containing untreated lactose, they experience abdominal cramps and diarrhea. This condition is caused by a deficiency of lactase (see Chapter 4). In such cases, milk that has been treated with lactase can be used, or commercial lactase can be added to the milk or taken in tablet form before drinking milk or eating dairy products.

Meat, Poultry, Fish, Dry Beans, Eggs, and Nuts Group

All meats, poultry, fish, eggs, soybeans, dry beans and peas, lentils, nuts and seeds are included in this group (Table 2-4). These foods provide proteins, iron, copper, phosphorus, zinc, sodium, iodine, B vitamins, fats, and cholesterol.

Caution must be used so that the foods selected from this group are low in fat and cholesterol. Many meats contain large amounts of fats, and egg yolks and organ meats have very high cholesterol content.

It is recommended that one have two to three servings from this group each day for a daily total of approximately 6 ounces.

TABLE 2-4 Meats, Poultry, Fish, Dry Beans, Eggs, and Nuts

Beef	Dried beans
Lamb	Dried peas
Veal	Lentils
Pork, except bacon	Nuts
Organ meats, such as heart, liver, kidney, brain, tongue, sweetbread	Peanuts
	Peanut butter
Poultry, such as chicken, duck, goose, turkey	Soybean flour
	Soybeans
Fish, shellfish	

(Photo Courtesy of Price Chopper Supermarkets)

Fats, Oils, and Sweets Group

This group contains butter, margarine, cooking oils, mayonnaise and other salad dressings, sugar, syrup, honey, jam, jelly, and sodas. All of these foods have a low nutrient density, meaning they have few nutrients other than fats and carbohydrates and have a high kcal content. There are no serving recommendations except that items from this group should be used sparingly because of their low nutrient content and high kcal content.

FOOD LABELING

As a result of the passage by Congress of the Nutrition Labeling and Education Act (NLEA) in 1990, new nutrition labeling regulations became mandatory in May 1994 for nearly all processed foods. The primary objective of the changes was to ensure that labels would be on most foods and would provide consistent nutrition information. The resulting food labels provide the consumer with more information on the nutrient contents of foods and how those nutrients affect health than former labels provided. Health claims allowed on labels are limited and set by the Food and Drug Administration (FDA). Serving sizes are determined by the FDA and not by the individual food processor. Descriptive terms used for foods are standardized. For example, "low fat" means that each serving contains 3g of fat or less.

Current Label

The nutrition label has a formatted space called *Nutrition Facts* (Figure 2-2) that includes required and optional information.

The items, with amounts per serving, that must be included on the food label are:

- Total calories
- Calories from fat
- Total fat
- Saturated fat
- Cholesterol
- Sodium
- Total carbohydrates
- Dietary fiber
- Sugars
- Protein
- Vitamin A
- Vitamin C
- Calcium
- Iron

The food processor can voluntarily include additional information on food products. If a health claim is made about the food or if the food is enriched or fortified with an optional nutrient, then nutrition infor-

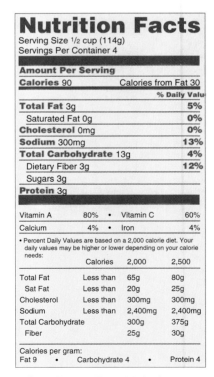

FIGURE 2-2 Food label.
(Courtesy of FDA)

TABLE 2-5 Household and Metric Measures

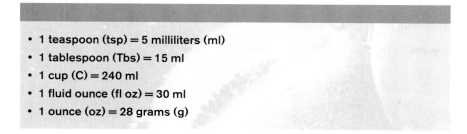

- 1 teaspoon (tsp) = 5 milliliters (ml)
- 1 tablespoon (Tbs) = 15 ml
- 1 cup (C) = 240 ml
- 1 fluid ounce (fl oz) = 30 ml
- 1 ounce (oz) = 28 grams (g)

mation about that nutrient becomes required. The standardized serving size is based on amounts of the specific food commonly eaten, and it is given in both English and metric measurements (Table 2-5).

Daily values on the label give the consumer the percentage per serving of each nutritional item listed, based on a daily diet of 2,000 kcal. For example, Total Fat on Figure 2-2 shows 13g, which represents 20% of the amount of fat someone on a 2,000-kcal diet should have (9 kcal per gram times 13 equals 117 kcal). The label also shows the *maximum* amount of a nutrient that should be eaten (for example, fat) or the *minimum* requirement for specified nutrients (for example, carbohydrates) based on a daily diet of 2,000 kcal and another based on 2,500 kcal. The items included here are the amounts of total fat, saturated fat, cholesterol, sodium, total carbohydrate, and fiber. In addition, the label lists the calories per gram for fats, carbohydrates, and proteins.

daily values
represent percentage per serving of each nutritional item listed on new food labels based on daily intake of 2,000 kcal

Health Claims

Because diet has been implicated as a factor in heart disease, stroke, and cancer, the following *health claims* linking a nutrient to a health-related condition are allowed on labels. They are intended to help consumers both choose foods that are the most healthful for them and avoid being deceived by false advertisements on the label. The allowed claims are for the relationship between:

- Calcium and *osteoporosis*
- Sodium and *hypertension*
- Diets low in saturated fat and cholesterol and high in fruits, vegetables, and grains containing dietary fiber and *coronary heart disease*
- Diets low in fat and high in fruits and vegetables containing dietary fiber and the antioxidants, vitamins A and C, and *cancer*
- Diets low in fat and high in fiber-containing grains, fruits, and vegetables and *cancer*

Two additional criteria must also be met:

1. A food whose label makes a health claim must be a naturally good source (containing at least 10% of the daily value) of at least one of the following nutrients: protein, vitamin A, vitamin C, iron, calcium, or fiber.

2. Health claims cannot be made for a food if a standard serving contains more than 20% of the daily value for total fat, saturated fat, cholesterol, or sodium.

Terminology

The FDA has also standardized descriptors (terms used by manufacturers to describe products) on food labels to help the consumer select the most appropriate and healthful foods. The following are examples:

- *Low calorie* means 40 kcal or less per serving.
- *Calorie free* means less than 5 kcal per serving.
- *Low fat* means a food has no more than 3g of fat per serving or per 100g of the food.
- *Fat free* means a food contains less than 0.5g of fat per serving.
- *Low saturated fat* means 1g or less of saturated fat per serving.
- *Low cholesterol* means 20 mg or less of cholesterol per serving.
- *Cholesterol free* means less than 2 mg of cholesterol per serving.
- *No added sugar* means that no sugar or sweeteners of any kind have been added at any time during the preparation and packaging. When such a term is used, the package must also state that it is not low calorie or calorie reduced (unless it actually is).
- *Low sodium* means less than 140 mg of sodium per serving.
- *Very low sodium* means less than 35 mg of sodium per serving.

Obviously, the information on food labels is useful to all consumers and especially to those who must select foods for therapeutic diets. Health care professionals should become thoroughly knowledgeable about the labeling law. On request, many food manufacturers will provide the consumer with additional detailed information about their products.

FOOD CUSTOMS

The Food Guide Pyramid and Nutrition Facts labels are useful in planning a nutritionally sound diet, but dietary and religious customs must also be taken into consideration. People from each country have favorite foods. Frequently, there are distinctive food customs originating in just a small section of a particular country. People of a particular area favor the foods that are produced in that area because they are available and economical. Some religions have dietary laws that require particular food practices. Because most people prefer the foods they were accustomed to while growing up, food habits are often based on nationality and religion.

One's economic status and social status also contribute to food habits. For example, the poor do not grow up with a taste for caviar, whereas the wealthy may at least be accustomed to it—whether or not they like it. Those in a certain social class will be apt to use the same foods as others in their class. And the foods they choose will probably depend on the work they do. For example, people doing hard, physical labor will require higher-calorie foods than will people in sedentary jobs.

When people move from one country to another, or from one area to another, their economic status may change. They will be introduced to new foods and new food customs. Although their original food customs may have been nutritionally adequate, their new environment may cause them to change their eating habits. For example, if milk was a staple (basic) food in their diet before moving and is unusually expensive in the new environment, milk may be replaced by a cheaper, nutritionally inferior beverage such as soda, coffee, or tea. Candy, possibly a luxury in their former environment, may be inexpensive and popular in their new environment. As a result, a family might increase consumption of soda or candy and reduce purchases of more nutritious foods. Someone who is not familiar with the nutritive values of foods can easily make such mistakes in food selection.

The meal patterns of national and religious groups different from one's own may seem strange. However, the diet may well be nutritionally adequate. When a patient's eating habits need to be corrected, such corrections are most easily made if the food customs of the patient are known and understood. The health care professional can gain this knowledge by talking with the patient and learning about her or his background. A dietitian can use that knowledge to plan nourishing menus consisting of foods that appeal to the patient. The necessary adjustments in the diet can then be made gradually and effectively.

FOOD PATTERNS BASED ON CULTURE

American cuisine (cooking style) is a marvelous composite of countless national, regional, cultural, and religious food customs. Consequently, categorizing a patient's food habits can be difficult. Nevertheless, it is sometimes helpful to be able to do so to a certain extent. People who are ill commonly have little interest in food, and sometimes foods that were familiar to them during their childhood and youth are more apt to tempt them than other types. The following section briefly discusses some food patterns typical of various cultures, regions, and countries. Of course, there can be and usually are enormous variations within any one classification.

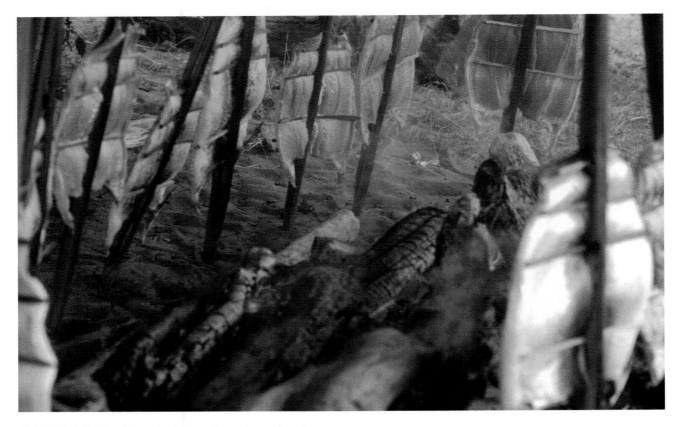

FIGURE 2-3 Traditional Native American food.

Native American

It is thought that approximately half of the edible plants commonly eaten in the United States today originated with the Native Americans. Examples are corn, potatoes, squash, cranberries, pumpkins, peppers, beans, wild rice, and cocoa beans (Figure 2-3). In addition, they used wild fruits, game, and fish. Foods were commonly prepared as soups and stews or were dried. The original Native American diets were probably more nutritionally adequate than are current diets, which frequently consist of too high a proportion of sweet and salty, snack-type low nutrient density foods. Native American diets today may be deficient in calcium, vitamins A, C, and riboflavin.

U.S. Southern

Hot breads such as corn bread and baking powder biscuits are common in the U.S. South because the wheat grown in the area does not make good-quality yeast breads. Grits and rice are also popular carbohydrate foods. Favorite vegetables include sweet potatoes, squash, green beans, and lima beans. Green beans cooked with pork are commonly served. Watermelon, oranges, and peaches are popular fruits. Fried fish is served often, as are barbecued and stewed meats and poultry. These diets have a great deal of carbohydrate and fat and limited amounts of protein in some cases. Iron, calcium, and vitamins A and C may be deficient.

Mexican

Mexican food is a combination of Spanish and Native American foods. Beans, rice, chili peppers, tomatoes, and corn meal are favorites (Figure 2-4). Meat is often cooked with the vegetable, as in chili con carne. Corn meal or flour is used to make tortillas, which serve as bread. The combination of beans and corn makes a complete protein. Corn tortillas filled with cheese (called enchiladas) provide some calcium, but the use of milk should be encouraged. Additional green and yellow vegetables and vitamin C–rich foods would also improve these diets.

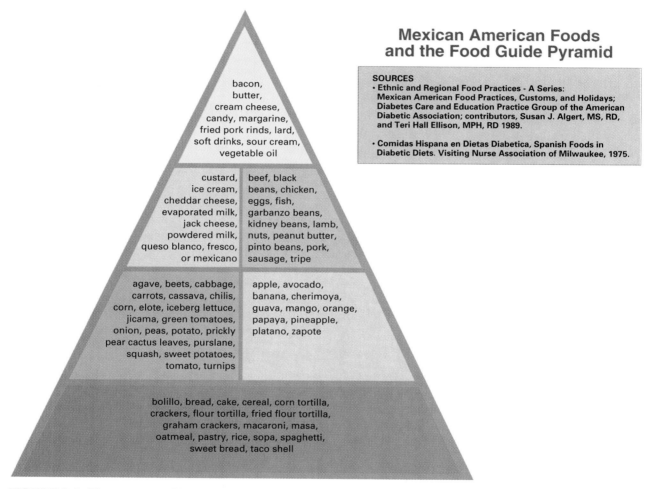

Mexican American Foods and the Food Guide Pyramid

bacon, butter, cream cheese, candy, margarine, fried pork rinds, lard, soft drinks, sour cream, vegetable oil

custard, ice cream, cheddar cheese, evaporated milk, jack cheese, powdered milk, queso blanco, fresco, or mexicano

beef, black beans, chicken, eggs, fish, garbanzo beans, kidney beans, lamb, nuts, peanut butter, pinto beans, pork, sausage, tripe

agave, beets, cabbage, carrots, cassava, chilis, corn, elote, iceberg lettuce, jicama, green tomatoes, onion, peas, potato, prickly pear cactus leaves, purslane, squash, sweet potatoes, tomato, turnips

apple, avocado, banana, cherimoya, guava, mango, orange, papaya, pineapple, platano, zapote

bolillo, bread, cake, cereal, corn tortilla, crackers, flour tortilla, fried flour tortilla, graham crackers, macaroni, masa, oatmeal, pastry, rice, sopa, spaghetti, sweet bread, taco shell

SOURCES
- **Ethnic and Regional Food Practices - A Series: Mexican American Food Practices, Customs, and Holidays; Diabetes Care and Education Practice Group of the American Diabetic Association; contributors, Susan J. Algert, MS, RD, and Teri Hall Ellison, MPH, RD 1989.**
- **Comidas Hispana en Dietas Diabetica, Spanish Foods in Diabetic Diets. Visiting Nurse Association of Milwaukee, 1975.**

FIGURE 2-4 Placement of Mexican American foods on the Food Guide Pyramid. (© 1993 *Pyramid Packet*, Penn State Nutrition Center, 417 East Calder Way, University Park, PA 16801-5633; 814-865-6323)

Puerto Rican

Rice is the basic carbohydrate food in Puerto Rican diets (Figure 2-5). Vegetables commonly used include beans, plantains, tomatoes, and peppers. Bananas, pineapple, mangoes, and papayas are popular fruits. Favorite meats are chicken, beef, and pork. Milk is not used as much as would be desirable from the nutritional point of view.

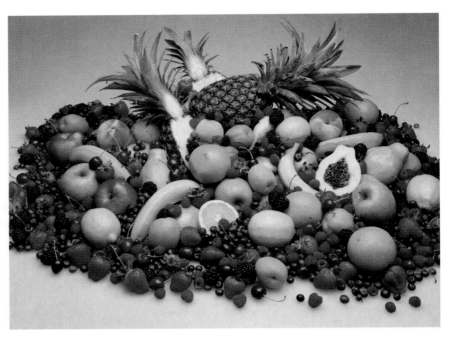

FIGURE 2-5 Traditional Puerto Rican food.

Italian

Pastas with various tomato or fish sauces and cheese are popular Italian foods. Fish and highly seasoned foods are common to southern Italian cuisine; meat and root vegetables are common to northern Italy. The eggs, cheese, tomatoes, green vegetables, and fruits common to Italian diets provide excellent sources of many nutrients, but additional fat-free milk and low-fat meat would improve the diet.

Northern and Western European

Northern and Western European diets are similar to those of the U.S. Midwest, but with a greater use of dark breads, potatoes, and fish and fewer green vegetable salads. Beef and pork are popular, as are various cooked vegetables, breads, cakes, and dairy products. The addition of fresh vegetables and fruits would add vitamins, minerals, and fiber to these diets.

Central European

Citizens of Central Europe obtain the greatest portion of their calories from potatoes and grain, especially rye and buckwheat. Pork is a popular meat. Cabbage cooked in many ways is a popular vegetable, as are carrots, onions, and turnips. Eggs and dairy products are used abundantly. Limiting the number of eggs consumed and using fat-free or low-fat dairy products would reduce the fat content in this diet. Adding fresh vegetables and fruits would increase vitamins, minerals, and fiber.

Middle Eastern

Grains, wheat, and rice provide energy in Middle Eastern diets. Chickpeas in the form of hummus are popular. Lamb and yogurt are commonly used as are cabbage, grape leaves, eggplant, tomatoes, dates, olives, and figs. Black, very sweet coffee is a popular beverage (Figure 2-6). There may be insufficient protein and calcium in this diet, depending on the amounts of meat and calcium-rich foods eaten. Fresh fruits and vegetables should be added to the diet to increase vitamins, minerals, and fiber.

Chinese

The Chinese diet is varied (Figure 2-7). Rice is the primary energy food and is used in place of bread. Foods are generally cut into small pieces. Vegetables are lightly cooked, and the cooking water is saved for future use. Soybeans are used in many ways, and eggs and pork are commonly served. Soy sauce is extensively used, but it is very salty and could present a problem for patients on low-salt diets. Tea is a common beverage, but milk is not. This diet may be low in fat.

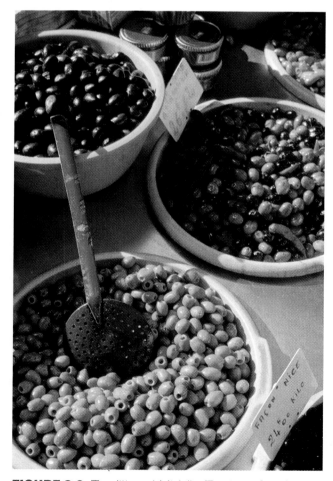

FIGURE 2-6 Traditional Middle Eastern food.

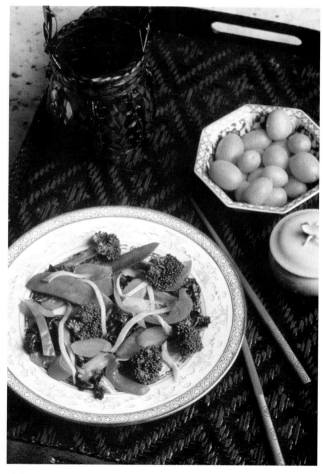

FIGURE 2-7 Traditional Chinese food.

Japanese

Japanese diets include rice, soybean paste and curd, vegetables, fruits, and fish. Food is frequently served tempura style, which means fried. Soy sauce (shoyu) and tea are commonly used. Current Japanese diets have been greatly influenced by Western culture. Japanese diets may be deficient in calcium given the near total lack of milk in the diet. Although fish is eaten with bones, it may not supply sufficient calcium to meet needs. Japanese diets may contain excessive amounts of salt.

Indian

Many Indians are vegetarians who use eggs and dairy products. Rice, peas, and beans are frequently served. Spices, especially curry, are popular. Indian meals are not typically served in courses as Western meals are. They generally consist of one course with many dishes. Eating with one's fingers is considered acceptable.

Thai, Vietnamese, Laotian, and Cambodian

Rice, curries, vegetables, and fruit are popular in Thailand, Vietnam, Laos, and Cambodia (Figure 2-8). Meats and fish are used in small amounts. The wok (a deep, round fry pan) is used for sautéing many foods. A salty sauce made from fermented fish is commonly used. Thai, Vietnamese, Laotian, and Cambodian diets may contain inadequate amounts of protein and calcium.

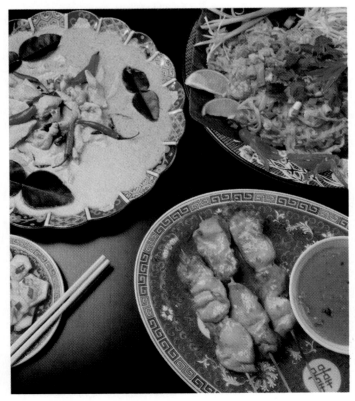

FIGURE 2-8 Traditional Thai food.

FOOD PATTERNS BASED ON RELIGION OR PHILOSOPHY

Jewish

Interpretations of the Jewish dietary laws vary. Persons who adhere to the Orthodox view consider tradition important and always observe the dietary laws. Foods prepared according to these laws are called *kosher* (Figure 2-9). Conservative Jews are inclined to observe the rules only at home. Reform Jews consider their dietary laws to be essentially ceremonial and so minimize their significance. Essentially the laws require the following:

● Slaughtering must be done by a qualified person, in a prescribed manner. The meat or poultry must be drained of blood, first by severing the jugular vein and carotid artery, then by soaking in brine before cooking.

● Meat and meat products may not be prepared with milk or milk products.

● The dishes used in the preparation and serving of meat products must be kept separate from those used for dairy foods.

● Dairy products and meat may not be eaten together. Six hours must elapse after eating meat before eating dairy products, and at least 30 minutes to 1 hour must elapse after eating dairy products before eating meat.

● The mouth must be rinsed after eating fish and before eating meat.

● There are prescribed fast days: Passover Week, Yom Kippur, and Feast of Purim.

● No cooking is done on the Sabbath, from sundown Friday to sundown Saturday.

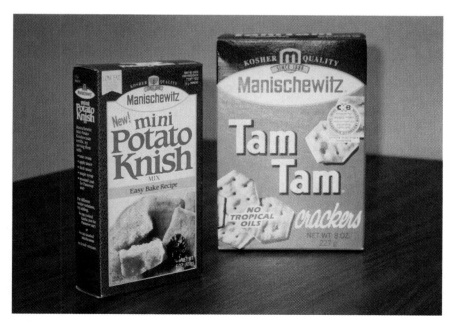

FIGURE 2-9 Kosher food label.

Jewish dietary laws forbid the eating of the following:

- The flesh of animals without cloven (split) hooves or that do not chew their cud
- Hindquarters of any animal
- Shellfish or fish without scales or fins
- Birds of prey
- Creeping things and insects
- Leavened (contains ingredients that cause it to rise) bread during the Passover

In general, the food served is rich. Chicken and fresh smoked and salted fish are popular, as are noodles, eggs, and flour dishes. These diets can be deficient in fresh vegetables and milk.

Roman Catholic

Although the dietary restrictions of the Roman Catholic religion have been liberalized, meat is not allowed its adherents on Ash Wednesday and Fridays during Lent.

Eastern Orthodox

The Eastern Orthodox religion includes Christians from the Middle East, Russia, and Greece. Although interpretations of the dietary laws vary, meat, poultry, fish, and dairy products are restricted on Wednesdays and Fridays and during Lent and Advent.

Seventh Day Adventist

lacto-ovo vegetarians
vegetarians who will eat dairy products and eggs, but no meat, poultry, or fish

In general, Seventh Day Adventists are lacto-ovo vegetarians, which means they use milk products and eggs, but no meat, fish, or poultry. They may also use nuts, legumes, and meat analogues (substitutes), and tofu (made from soybeans). They consider coffee, tea, and alcohol to be harmful.

Mormon (Latter Day Saints)

The only dietary restriction observed by the Mormons is the prohibition of coffee, tea, and alcoholic beverages.

Islamic

Adherents of Islam are called Muslims. Their dietary laws prohibit the use of pork and alcohol, and other meats must be slaughtered according to specific laws. During the month of Ramadan, Muslims do not eat or drink during daylight hours.

Hindu

To the Hindus, all life is sacred, and animals contain the souls of ancestors. Consequently, most Hindus are vegetarians. They do not use eggs because eggs represent life.

OTHER FOOD PATTERNS

Vegetarians

There are several vegetarian diets. The common factor among them is that they do not include red meat. Some include eggs, some fish, some milk, and some even poultry. When carefully planned, these diets can be nutritious. They can even contribute to a reduction of obesity and a reduced risk of high blood pressure, heart disease, some cancers, and possibly diabetes. They must be carefully planned so that they include all the needed nutrients.

    Lacto-ovo vegetarians use dairy products and eggs but no meat, poultry, or fish.

    Lacto-vegetarians use diary products but no meat, poultry, or eggs.

    Vegans avoid all animal foods. They use soybeans, chickpeas, meat analogues, and tofu. It is important that their meals be carefully planned to include appropriate combinations of the essential amino acids. For example, beans served with corn or rice, or peanuts eaten with wheat, are better in such combinations than any of them would be if eaten alone. Vegans can show deficiencies of calcium; vitamins A, D, and B_{12}; and, of course, proteins.

lacto-vegetarians
vegetarians who eat dairy products

vegans
vegetarians who avoid all animal foods

Zen-Macrobiotic Diets

The macrobiotic diet is a system of 10 diet plans, developed from Zen Buddhism. Adherents progress from the lower number diet to the higher, gradually giving up foods in the following order: desserts, salads, fruits, animal foods, soups, and ultimately vegetables, until only cereals—usually brown rice—are consumed. Beverages are kept to a minimum, and only organically grown foods are used. Foods are grouped as Yang (male) or Yin (female). A ratio of 5:1 Yang to Yin is considered important. Most macrobiotic diets are nutritionally inadequate. As the adherents give up foods according to plans, their diets become increasingly inadequate. These diets can be especially dangerous because avid adherents promise medical cures from the diets that cannot be attained, and so medical treatment may be delayed when needed.

CONSIDERATIONS FOR THE HEALTH CARE PROFESSIONAL

Learning and understanding the tools with which to plan a healthy diet are important for all health care professionals so that they can help their patients. All patients should be viewed as individuals whose food customs, which may be different from the health care professional's, must be respected. A registered dietitian will help with a specific diet plan for a hospitalized patient. The dietitian will take into account the patient's likes, dislikes, and food customs.

● SUMMARY

The Food Guide Pyramid emphasizes grains, fruits, and vegetables—all plant foods. It also includes milk, yogurt, and cheese; meat, poultry, fish, dry beans, eggs, and nuts; fats, oils, and sweets. Each group has a recommended number of servings. The recommendations are useful in planning a nutritious diet. The Dietary Guidelines are important tools in the maintenance of good health through good nutrition. Their basic recommendation is to eat a balanced diet.

Food habits have many diverse origins. Nationality, religion, and economic and social status all affect their development. When food customs result in inadequate diets, corrections should be made gradually. Corrections are easier to make and are more effective when the reasons for the food habits are understood.

● DISCUSSION TOPICS

1. Discuss the reasons why health care professionals should practice the rules of good nutrition themselves.

2. How do food habits originate?

3. What effects does environment have on particular food habits? When do the effects of a new environment improve diets, and when do they impair them?

4. From personal experience, explain why certain foods are enjoyed more than others that are commonly available in the local area.

5. Why are hot breads more popular with people from the U.S. South than are yeast breads?

6. Why might Scandinavians like fish more than Hungarians do?

7. Why are Zen-macrobiotic diets dangerous?

8. Discuss vegetarian diets. Are they safe? Explain.

9. Why is it difficult to convince someone to change her or his food habits? Discuss.

10. Define a balanced diet.

11. Describe the Food Guide Pyramid, including number of servings recommended for each group.

12. How does careful use of the Food Guide Pyramid eliminate the need to check menus with a chart of the recommended dietary allowances?

13. How might one include milk in the diet of a four-year-old who refuses to drink it?

14. Why would yogurt be a good snack or dessert for a pregnant woman?

15. List the Dietary Guidelines and state the reasons for them.

16. Alcohol is not considered a food, so why is there a Dietary Guideline devoted to it?

17. Why should "crash" or "fad" reducing diets be avoided? What is a better alternative? Why?

18. What would you advise your best friend if she or he was about to begin an 800-calorie reducing diet? Why would you give such advice?

19. Discuss the sale of foods with low nutrient density in school cafeterias. Is it a good practice? If so, why? If not, why not? What would your position be on this subject if you were principal of an elementary school? Of a junior or senior high school?

20. Discuss how the following family dinner menu might be adapted to the needs of a family member on a reducing diet:

Fried hamburgers
Boiled potatoes with butter
Steamed broccoli
Lettuce with mayonnaise
Rolls with butter
Angel cake with whipped cream
Whole milk

● SUGGESTED ACTIVITIES

1. Give a series of short reports on food customs. Each student should select a different country or area within a country for study. After the reports have been presented, hold a class discussion on whether climate, availability of food, or economic or other factors determine the food customs of the countries studied. Include answers to the following questions: What is the climate of the country? What type of crops are grown there? Are modern methods of agriculture used? Does the country depend on imports for much of its food supply? If so, what foods are imported? Is the majority of the citizenry poor? What types of foods are popular? What types are expensive? Which of these foods are produced in the country? Which are imported? What is the prevalent religion?

2. Plan a Good Friday menu for a patient of the Roman Catholic faith.

3. Role-play a situation in which a diet counselor tries to persuade a patient to use more milk.

4. Buy some fruits and vegetables that are new to you. Bring them to class and sample them. Share ideas as to their potential uses. Perhaps these might be added to home menus.

5. Using a restaurant menu, choose breakfast, lunch, and dinner. Check the selection of foods against the Food Guide Pyramid. Are they balanced meals? Discuss the problems that people who eat all their meals in restaurants might have in maintaining a well-balanced diet.

6. Using the following table, fill in the "Menus" column with the foods eaten in the past two days. In the "Food Groups Used" column list the group to which each food belongs. To evaluate personal dietary habits, fill in the "Food Groups Not Used" column. Compare the table with those of the rest of the class and discuss how your eating habits could be improved.

Menus	Food Groups Used	Food Groups Not Used
Breakfast		
Lunch		
Dinner		
Snacks		

7. Check labels on sour cream and yogurt containers. Which would be preferable for someone on a fat-restricted diet? Why? How does the calcium content compare?

8. Adapt the following menu for a person of the Orthodox Jewish faith.

Baked ham
Scalloped potatoes
Buttered peas
Bread and butter
Fresh fruit
Milk or coffee

● REVIEW

Multiple choice. Select the *letter* that precedes the best answer.

1. Food customs mean one's
   a. food nutrients   c. food requirements
   b. food habits   d. all of the above

2. Food customs
   a. may be based on religion or nationality
   b. are always nutritious
   c. are easily changed
   d. are not affected by one's social status

3. Moving to a new environment or experiencing a change in salary
   a. rarely changes established food habits
   b. usually influences established food habits
   c. always reduces the amount of food eaten
   d. never reduces the quality of food eaten

4. Hot breads are common to diets of people from
   a. Mexico   c. China
   b. the U.S. Midwest   d. the U.S. South

5. Rice is a popular carbohydrate food in
   a. Puerto Rico   c. Northern Europe
   b. Central Europe   d. all of the above

6. In general, the diets of U.S. Southerners, Mexicans, Puerto Ricans, and Italians would be improved by the addition of more
   a. rice   c. milk
   b. corn   d. pasta

7. A diet of dried beans, corn, and chili peppers would most likely be used by a(n)
a. Mexican family   c. Armenian family
b. Italian family   d. Orthodox Jewish family

8. A balanced diet is one that includes
a. equal amounts of carbohydrates and fats
b. no animal products
c. all six classes of nutrients
d. more vegetables than fruits

9. Fruits and vegetables are rich sources of
a. vitamins   c. proteins
b. fats   d. all of the above

10. Teenagers should have a serving of milk (or its substitute)
a. not more than twice a day
b. three times a day
c. not more than four times a week
d. not at all if they are overweight

11. Milk products are made from milk and include
a. butter and margarine
b. yogurt and cottage cheese
c. bean curd and coconut milk
d. all of the above

12. Milk and its products are the best dietary source of
a. proteins and fats   c. carbohydrates
b. calcium   d. all of the above

13. Breads, cereals, rice, and pasta are rich sources of
a. vitamin D   c. carbohydrates
b. fats   d. all of the above

14. Foods from the meat group should be served
a. once a day   c. 6–11 times a day
b. 2–3 times a day   d. 3–5 times a day

15. Foods from the meat group are rich sources of
a. proteins   c. vitamin C
b. carbohydrates   d. all of the above

16. An example of a breakfast with high nutrient density is
a. pancakes and cocoa
b. melon, bran muffin, and cocoa made with fat-free milk
c. fruit-flavored beverage, cinnamon bun, and coffee
d. fried eggs, bacon, and coffee

17. The number of kcal in one pound of body fat is
a. 500   c. 3,500
b. 1,000   d. 7,000

18. To lose one pound of body fat a week, one would have to eliminate the following number of kcal from the diet each day:
a. 500   c. 3,500
b. 1,000   d. 7,000

19. Excessive amounts of salt in the diet
    a. raise cholesterol levels substantially
    b. are thought to contribute to hypertension
    c. cause cirrhosis of the liver
    d. have no relevance to one's nutritional status

20. The Food Guide Pyramid
    a. food groups are nutritionally interchangeable
    b. is an outline for meal planning for adults only
    c. advises that fruits and vegetables be eaten in moderation
    d. recommends that one have 6–11 servings of bread, cereal, rice, and pasta each day

21. The Nutrition Labeling and Education Act of 1990
    a. requires that descriptive words used for foods be standardized
    b. sets maximum amounts of cholesterol allowed for each food serving
    c. permits no health claims on food containers
    d. does not require the food manufacturer or processor to list the total amounts in each serving of kcal, sodium, or dietary fiber

22. Foods rich in complex carbohydrates, such as breads and cereals, are also excellent sources of
    a. calcium and phosphorus
    b. vitamins C and D
    c. dietary fiber and B vitamins
    d. proteins and fats

23. When choosing foods from the meats, poultry, and fish food group, one should be careful to select foods that
    a. are rich in calcium and phosphorus
    b. provide at least one-half of one's daily need for carbohydrates
    c. have limited amounts of protein and iron
    d. are low in saturated fats and cholesterol

24. The two vitamins that the Nutrition Labeling and Education Act of 1990 requires be included as amounts per serving on food labels are
    a. vitamin A and thiamin   c. vitamins A and C
    b. niacin and folic acid   d. vitamins D and K

25. Immoderate use of alcoholic beverages
    a. by pregnant women can cause birth defects
    b. can cause cirrhosis of the liver only in men
    c. has little or no effect on one's nutritional status
    d. has no effect on one's appetite

C A S E S T U D Y

When Roberto got a great job in a factory in Cleveland, he invited his brother George and George's wife, Josie, to move to Cleveland and live with him until they could find a place of their own. George had one son, Juan, and a daughter, Maria. They were fearful and excited about leaving their rural Mexican home. George and the kids spoke some English, but Josie spoke none. George worked 12–14 hours five or six days a week and all of the overtime he could get. Josie was very busy taking care of the children and adapting to life in the United States, and trying to save as much money as possible so they could get their own apartment.

Josie was having trouble getting the children to accept American food, especially vegetables and milk. They had had a goat and a garden in Mexico.

ASSESSMENT

1. Name at least two reasons why Juan and Maria aren't drinking milk and eating vegetables.
2. How significant is the problem?
3. Who might help Josie with this problem?

DIAGNOSIS

4. Complete the nursing diagnosis statement. Juan and Maria have altered nutrition related to _____ as demonstrated by their behavior of _____.

PLAN/GOAL

5. What changes do you want to see in the children's diet? What time frame is reasonable?

IMPLEMENTATION

6. Name three reasonable solutions to the problem.
7. What other dairy products could Josie use?
8. What alternative to American vegetables does Josie have?
9. Who else needs to be involved in executing the plan?

EVALUATION/OUTCOME CRITERIA

10. How will Josie determine the success of the plan?
11. What will the children do if the plan is effective?

CASE STUDY

Ted M. is a 20-year-old engineering major and cross-country runner for State College. Ted's new roommate, Jason, is a vegetarian and loves to cook. He has been preparing vegetarian meals that Ted has enjoyed. Ted is now thinking about becoming a vegetarian, but he is concerned about how it might affect his running. He talked to the coach, who gave him a referral to the Student Health Clinic. He is scheduled for a physical with the nurse practitioner (NP) and a consultation with the dietitian.

ASSESSMENT

1. What objective data does the nurse need about Ted to assess his current state of health?

2. What information would be obtained from a food diary and food history?

3. What potential problems need to be addressed with Ted before he changes to a vegetarian diet?

DIAGNOSIS

4. Complete the following nursing diagnosis. Ted has a potential nutrition problem related to _____ caused by _____.

PLAN/GOAL

5. What changes will there be in Ted's diet? State Ted's goal in measurable terms.

IMPLEMENTATION

6. Which type of vegetarian diet would be best suited for Ted and his running?

7. How would you as the dietitian advise Ted to make the transition to a vegetarian diet?

8. What foods can the dietitian recommend to Ted, who says he is on a limited budget?

EVALUATION/OUTCOME CRITERIA

9. What criteria should be used to determine if the diet change is successful?

10. What would Ted report when the diet change is successful?

Chapter 3

Digestion, Absorption, and Metabolism

Key Terms

adipose tissue

aerobic metabolism

anabolism

anaerobic
  metabolism

basal metabolic
  rate (BMR)

bile

bolus

calorie

calorimeter

capillaries

cardiac sphincter

catabolism

catalyst

chemical digestion

cholecystokinin

chyme

colon

digestion

duodenum

energy balance

energy requirement

enzymes

esophagus

feces

fundus (of stomach)

gastric juices

gastrin

gastrointestinal (GI)
  tract

hormones

hydrolysis

ileum

jejunum

kilocalorie (kcal)

lactase

lacteals

lean body mass

lymphatic system

maltase

mechanical
  digestion

(continued)

Objectives

After studying this chapter, you should be able to:

● Describe the processes of digestion, absorption, and metabolism

● Name the organs in the digestive system and describe their functions

● Name the enzymes or digestive juices secreted by each organ and gland in the digestive system

● Calculate your basal metabolic rate (BMR)

Although the body is infinitely more complex than the automobile engine, it may be compared to the engine because both require fuel to run. The body's fuel is, of course, food. For the body to use its fuel, it must first prepare the food and then distribute it appropriately. It does this through the processes of digestion and absorption. The actual use of the food as fuel, resulting in energy, is called metabolism.

metabolism	peristalsis
pancreas	pylorus
pancreatic amylase	saliva
pancreatic lipase (steapsin)	salivary amylase
pancreatic protease	secretin
pepsin	sucrase
peptidases	villi

metabolism

the use of the food by the body after digestion which results in energy

digestion

breakdown of food in the body in preparation for absorption

gastrointestinal (GI) tract

pertaining to the digestive system

DIGESTION

Digestion is the process whereby food is broken down into smaller parts, chemically changed, and moved through the gastrointestinal system. The gastrointestinal (GI) tract consists of the body structures that participate in digestion. Digestion begins in the mouth and ends at the anus. Along the entire GI tract secretions of mucus lubricate and protect the mucosal tissues. As the process of digestion is discussed, refer to Figure 3-1 and note the locations of the structures that perform the functions of digestion.

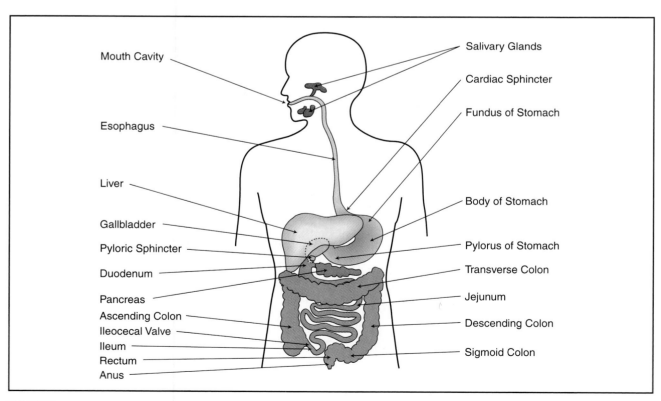

FIGURE 3-1 The digestive system.

Digestion occurs through two types of action—mechanical and chemical. During **mechanical digestion**, food is broken up by the teeth. It is then moved along the gastrointestinal tract through the esophagus, stomach, and intestines. This movement is caused by a rhythmic contraction of the muscular walls of the tract called **peristalsis**. Mechanical digestion helps to prepare food for chemical digestion by breaking it into smaller pieces. Small pieces have more surface area than large ones and thus are more readily changed by digestive juices.

During **chemical digestion**, the composition of carbohydrates, proteins, and fats is changed. Chemical changes occur through the addition of water and the resulting splitting, or breaking down, of the food molecules. This process is called **hydrolysis**. Food is broken down into nutrients that the tissues can absorb and use. Hydrolysis also involves digestive **enzymes**, which are digestive juices that act on food substances, causing them to break down into simple compounds. An enzyme can also act as a **catalyst**, which speeds up the chemical reactions without itself being changed in the process. Digestive enzymes are secreted by the mouth, stomach, **pancreas**, and small intestine (Table 3-1). An enzyme is often named for the substance on which it acts. For example, the enzyme sucrase acts on sucrose, the enzyme maltase acts on maltose, and lactase acts on lactose.

Digestion in the Mouth

Digestion begins in the mouth, where the food is broken up by the teeth and mixed with saliva (Figure 3-2). At this point, each mouthful of food that is ready to be swallowed is called a **bolus**. **Saliva** is a secretion of the salivary glands that contains water, salts, and a digestive enzyme called **salivary amylase** (also called ptyalin), which acts on complex

TABLE 3-1 Enzymes and Foods Acted Upon

SOURCE	ENZYME	FOOD ACTED UPON
Mouth	Salivary amylase	Starch
Stomach	Pepsin	Proteins
	Rennin	Proteins in milk
	Gastric lipase	Emulsified fat
Small intestine	Pancreatic amylase	Starch
	Pancreatic proteases	Proteins
	(trypsin)	
	(chymotrypsin)	
	(carboxypeptidases)	
	Pancreatic lipase	Fats
	(steapsin)	
	Lactase	Lactose
	Maltase	Maltose
	Sucrase	Sucrose
	Peptidases	Proteins

mechanical digestion
the part of digestion that requires certain mechanical movement such as chewing, swallowing, and peristalsis

peristalsis
rhythmical movement of the intestinal tract; moves the chyme along

chemical digestion
chemical changes in foods during digestion caused by hydrolysis

hydrolysis
the addition of water resulting in the breakdown of the molecule

enzyme
organic substance that causes changes in other substances

catalyst
a substance that causes another substance to react

pancreas
gland that secretes enzymes essential for digestion and insulin, which is essential for glucose metabolism

bolus
food in the mouth that is ready to be swallowed

saliva
secretion of the salivary glands

salivary amylase
also called *ptyalin*; the enzyme secreted by the salivary glands to act on starch

carbohydrates (starch). Food is normally held in the mouth for such a short time that only small amounts of carbohydrates are chemically changed there. The salivary glands also secrete a mucus material that lubricates and binds food particles to help in swallowing the bolus. The final chemical digestion of carbohydrates occurs in the small intestine.

The Esophagus

The **esophagus** is a muscular tube through which food travels from the mouth to the stomach. When swallowed, the bolus of food is moved down the esophagus by peristalsis and gravity. At the lower end of the esophagus, the **cardiac sphincter** opens to allow passage of the bolus into the stomach. The cardiac sphincter prevents the acidic content of the stomach from flowing back into the esophagus.

Digestion in the Stomach

The stomach consists of an upper portion known as the **fundus**, a middle area known as the body of the stomach, and the end nearest the small intestine called the **pylorus**. Food enters the fundus and moves to the body of the stomach, where the muscles in the stomach wall gradually knead the food, tear it, mix it with gastric juices, and propel

esophagus
tube leading from the mouth to the stomach; part of the gastrointestinal system

cardiac sphincter
the muscle at the base of the esophagus that prevents gastric reflux from moving into the esophagus

fundus (of the stomach)
upper part of the stomach

pylorus
the end of the stomach nearest the intestine

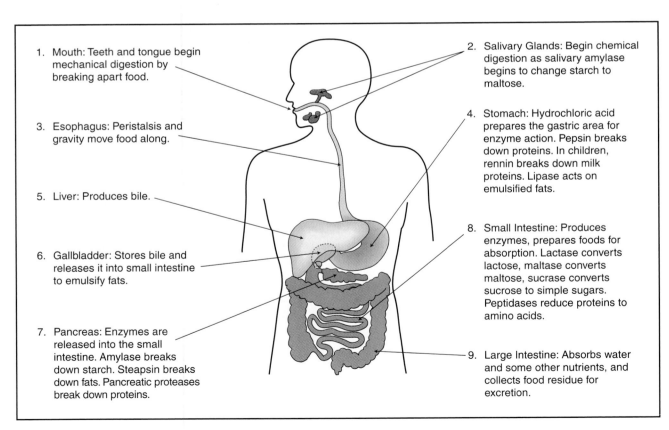

1. Mouth: Teeth and tongue begin mechanical digestion by breaking apart food.

2. Salivary Glands: Begin chemical digestion as salivary amylase begins to change starch to maltose.

3. Esophagus: Peristalsis and gravity move food along.

4. Stomach: Hydrochloric acid prepares the gastric area for enzyme action. Pepsin breaks down proteins. In children, rennin breaks down milk proteins. Lipase acts on emulsified fats.

5. Liver: Produces bile.

6. Gallbladder: Stores bile and releases it into small intestine to emulsify fats.

7. Pancreas: Enzymes are released into the small intestine. Amylase breaks down starch. Steapsin breaks down fats. Pancreatic proteases break down proteins.

8. Small Intestine: Produces enzymes, prepares foods for absorption. Lactase converts lactose, maltase converts maltose, sucrase converts sucrose to simple sugars. Peptidases reduce proteins to amino acids.

9. Large Intestine: Absorbs water and some other nutrients, and collects food residue for excretion.

FIGURE 3-2 Basic functions of the digestive system.

it forward in slow controlled movements. The food becomes a semiliquid mass called **chyme** (pronounced "kime"). When the chyme enters the pylorus, it causes distention and the release of the hormone **gastrin**, which increases the release of gastric juices.

Gastric juices are digestive secretions of the stomach. They contain hydrochloric acid, pepsin, and mucus. Hydrochloric acid activates the enzyme **pepsin**, prepares protein molecules for partial digestion by pepsin, destroys most bacteria in the food ingested, and makes iron and calcium more soluble. As the hydrochloric acid is released, a thick mucus is also secreted to protect the stomach from this harsh acid. In children, there are two additional enzymes: rennin, which acts on milk protein and casein, and gastric lipase, which breaks the butterfat molecules of milk into smaller molecules.

In summary, the functions of the stomach include:

● Temporary storage of food

● Mixing of food with gastric juices

● Regulation of a slow, controlled emptying of food into the intestine

● Secretion of the intrinsic factor for vitamin B_{12} (to be discussed in Chapter 7)

● Destruction of most bacteria inadvertently consumed

Digestion in the Small Intestine

Chyme moves through the pyloric sphincter into the **duodenum**, the first section of the small intestine. Chyme subsequently passes through the **jejunum**, the midsection of the small intestine, and the **ileum**, the last section of the small intestine.

When food reaches the small intestine, the hormone **secretin** causes the pancreas to release sodium bicarbonate to neutralize the acidity of the chyme. The gallbladder is triggered by the hormone **cholecystokinin** (CCK), which is produced by intestinal mucosal glands when fat enters, to release **bile**. Bile is produced in the liver but stored in the gallbladder. Bile emulsifies fat after it is secreted into the small intestine. This action enables the enzymes to digest the fats more easily.

Chyme also triggers the pancreas to secrete its juice into the small intestine. Juice secreted from the pancreas contains the following enzymes:

● Trypsin, chymotrypsin, and carboxypeptidases split proteins into smaller substances. These are called **pancreatic proteases** because they are protein-splitting enzymes produced by the pancreas.

● **Pancreatic amylase** converts starches (polysaccharides) to simple sugars.

● **Pancreatic lipase (steapsin)** reduces fats to fatty acids and glycerol.

The small intestine itself produces an intestinal juice that contains the enzymes **lactase**, **maltase**, and **sucrase**. These enzymes split lactose, maltose, and sucrose, respectively, into simple sugars. The

chyme
the food mass as it has been mixed with gastric juices

gastrin
hormone released by stomach

gastric juices
the digestive secretions of the stomach

pepsin
an enzyme secreted by the stomach that is essential for the digestion of proteins

duodenum
first (and smallest) section of the small intestine

jejunum
the middle section comprising about two-fifths of the small intestine

ileum
last part of the small intestine

secretin
hormone causing pancreas to release sodium bicarbonate to neutralize acidity of the chyme

cholecystokinin
hormone that triggers gallbladder to release bile

bile
secretion of the liver, stored in the gallbladder, essential for the digestion of fats

pancreatic protease
the enzyme secreted by the pancreas that is essential for the digestion of protein

pancreatic amylase
the enzyme secreted by the pancreas that is essential for the digestion of starch

pancreatic lipase (steapsin)
the enzyme secreted by the pancreas that is essential for the digestion of fat

lactase
enzyme secreted by the small intestine for the digestion of lactose

maltase
enzyme secreted by the small intestine essential for the digestion of maltose

sucrase
enzyme secreted by the small intestine to aid in digestion of sucrose

peptidases
enzymes secreted by the small intestine that are essential for the digestion of protein

colon
the large intestine

lymphatic system
transports fat-soluble substances from the small intestine to the vascular system

villi
the tiny, hairlike structures in the small intestines through which nutrients are absorbed

capillaries
tiny blood vessels connecting veins and arteries

lacteals
lymphatic vessels in the small intestine that absorb fatty acids and glycerol

small intestine also produces enzymes called **peptidases** that break down proteins into amino acids.

The Large Intestine

The large intestine, or **colon**, consists of the cecum, colon, and rectum. The cecum is a blind pocket so the digested food bypasses it and enters the ascending colon and then moves through the transverse colon and on to the descending colon, the sigmoid colon, the rectum, and, finally, the anal canal.

ABSORPTION

After digestion, the next major step in the body's use of its food is absorption. Absorption is the passage of nutrients into the blood or **lymphatic system** (the lymphatic vessels carry fat-soluble particles and molecules that are too large to pass through the capillaries into the bloodstream).

To be absorbed, nutrients must be in their simplest forms. Carbohydrates must be broken down to the simple sugars (glucose, fructose, and galactose), proteins to amino acids, and fats to fatty acids and glycerol. Most absorption of nutrients occurs in the small intestine, although some occurs in the large intestine. Water is absorbed in the stomach, small intestine, and large intestine.

Absorption in the Small Intestine

The small intestine is approximately 22 feet long. Its inner surface has mucosal folds, villi, and microvilli to increase the surface area for maximum absorption. The fingerlike projections called **villi** have hundreds of microscopic, hairlike projections called microvilli. The microvilli are very sensitive to the nutrient needs of our bodies (Figure 3-3). Each villus contains numerous blood **capillaries** (tiny blood vessels) and **lacteals** (lymphatic vessels). The villi absorb nutrients from the chyme by way of these blood capillaries and lacteals, which eventually transfer them to the bloodstream. Glucose, fructose, galactose, amino acids, minerals, and water-soluble vitamins are absorbed by the capillaries. Fructose and galactose are subsequently carried to the liver, where they are converted to glucose. Lacteals absorb glycerol and fatty acids (end products of fat digestion), in addition to the fat-soluble vitamins.

Absorption in the Large Intestine

When the chyme reaches the large intestine, most digestion and absorption have already occurred. The colon walls secrete mucus as a protection from the acidic digestive juices in the chyme, which is coming from the small intestine.

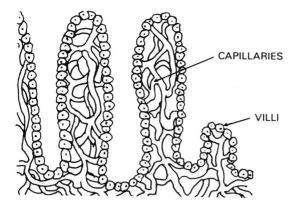

FIGURE 3-3 Wall of the small intestine.

The major tasks of the large intestine are to absorb water, to synthesize some B vitamins and vitamin K (essential for blood clotting), and to collect food residue. Food residue is the part of food that the body's enzyme action cannot digest and consequently the body cannot absorb. Such residue is commonly called dietary fiber. Examples include the outer hulls of corn kernels and grains of wheat, celery strings, and apple skins. It is important that the diet contain adequate fiber because it promotes the health of the large intestine by helping to produce softer stools and more frequent bowel movements (see Chapter 4).

Undigested food is excreted as **feces** by way of the rectum. In healthy people, 99% of carbohydrates, 95% of fat, and 92% of proteins are absorbed.

METABOLISM

After digestion and absorption, nutrients are carried by the blood to the cells of the body. Within the cells, nutrients are changed into energy through a complex process called metabolism. During **aerobic metabolism**, nutrients are combined with oxygen within each cell. This process is known as oxidation. Oxidation ultimately reduces carbohydrates to carbon dioxide and water; proteins are reduced to carbon dioxide, water, and nitrogen. **Anaerobic metabolism** reduces fats without the use of oxygen. The complete oxidation of carbohydrates, proteins, and fats is commonly called the Krebs cycle.

As nutrients are oxidized, energy is released. When this released energy is used to build new substances from simpler ones, the process is called **anabolism**. An example of anabolism is the formation of new body tissues. When released energy is used to reduce substances to simpler ones, the process is called **catabolism**. This building up and breaking down of substances (metabolism) is a continuous process within the body and requires a continuous supply of nutrients.

feces
solid waste from the large intestine

aerobic metabolism
combining nutrients with oxygen within the cell; also called oxidation

anaerobic metabolism
reduces fats without use of oxygen

anabolism
the creation of new compounds during metabolism

catabolism
the breakdown of compounds during metabolism

Metabolism and the Thyroid Gland

Metabolism is governed primarily by the **hormones** secreted by the thyroid gland. These secretions are *triiodothyronine* (T_3) and *thyroxine* (T_4). When the thyroid gland secretes too much of these hormones, a condition known as hyperthyroidism may result. In such a case, the body metabolizes its food too quickly, and weight is lost. When too little T_4 and T_3 are secreted, the condition called hypothyroidism may occur. In this case, the body metabolizes food too slowly and the patient tends to become sluggish and accumulates fat.

ENERGY

Energy is constantly needed for the maintenance of body tissue and temperature and for growth (involuntary activity), as well as for voluntary activity. Examples of voluntary activity include walking, swimming, eating, reading, typing, and so on. The three groups of nutrients that provide energy to the body are carbohydrates, proteins, and fats. Carbohydrates are and should be the primary energy source (see Chapter 4).

Energy Measurement

The unit used to measure the energy value of foods is the **kilocalorie**, or **kcal**, commonly known as the large calorie, or **calorie**. In the metric system it is known as the kilojoule. One kcal is equal to 4.184 kilojoules, but this may be rounded off to 4.2 kilojoules. A kcal is the amount of heat needed to raise the temperature of one kilogram of water one degree Celsius (C).

The number of kcal in a food is its energy value, or caloric density. Energy values of foods vary a great deal because they are determined by the types and amounts of nutrients each food contains.

One gram of carbohydrate yields 4 kcal; one gram of protein yields 4 kcal; and one gram of fat yields 9 kcal. One gram of alcohol yields 7 kcal.

The energy values of foods are determined by a device known as a **calorimeter**. The inner part of a calorimeter holds a measured amount of food and the outer part holds water. The food is burned, and its caloric value is determined by the increase in the temperature of the surrounding water. The number of kcal in average servings of common foods is listed in Table A-4 of the appendix.

Basal Metabolic Rate

One's basal metabolism is the energy necessary to carry on all involuntary vital processes while the body is at rest. These processes are respiration, circulation, regulation of body temperature, and cell activity and maintenance. The rate at which energy is needed only for body maintenance is called the **basal metabolic rate (BMR)**. The BMR may be referred to as the resting energy expenditure (REE).

Medical tests can determine one's BMR (or REE). When such a test is given, the body is at rest and performing only the essential, involuntary functions. Voluntary activity is not measured in a BMR test. Factors that affect one's BMR are lean body mass, body size, sex, age, heredity, physical condition, and climate.

Lean body mass is muscle as opposed to fat tissue. Because there is more metabolic activity in muscle tissue than in fat or bone tissue, muscle tissue requires more kcal than does fat or bone tissue. People with large body frames require more kcal than do people with small frames because the former have more body mass to maintain and move than do those with small frames.

lean body mass
percentage of muscle tissue

Men usually require more energy than women. They tend to be larger and to have more lean body mass than women do.

Children require more kcal per pound of body weight than adults because they are growing. As people age, the lean body mass declines, and the basal metabolic rate declines accordingly. Heredity is also a determining factor. One's BMR may resemble one's parents', just as one's appearance may. One's physical condition also affects the BMR. For example, women require more kcal during pregnancy and lactation than at other times. The basal metabolic rate increases during fever and decreases during periods of starvation or severely reduced kcal intake. People living and working in extremely cold or warm climates require more kcal to maintain normal body temperature than they would in a more temperate climate.

Estimating BMR. Dietitians commonly use the Harris-Benedict equation to determine the BMR (REE) of persons over the age of 18. This equation uses height, weight, and age as factors and results in a more individualized estimate of the REE than some other methods (figure 3-4).

Female: REE = 655 + (9.6 x weight in kg) + (1.8 x height in cm) – (4.7 x age)

Male: REE = 66 + (13.7 x weight in kg) + (5 x height in cm) – (6.8 x age)

W = weight in kilograms (kg) (weight in pounds ÷ 2.2 = kg)
H = height in centimenters (cm) (height in inches x 2.54 = cm)
A = age in years

FIGURE 3-4 Harris-Benedict equation.

Another method used to estimate one's BMR, or REE, is the following.

1. Convert body weight from pounds to kilograms (kg) by dividing pounds by 2.2 (2.2 pounds equal one kilogram).

2. Multiply the kilograms by 24 (hours per day).

3. Multiply the answer obtained in number 2 above by 0.9 for a woman and by 1.0 for a man.

For example, assume that a woman weighs 110 pounds. Divide 110 by 2.2 for an answer of 50 kg. Multiply 50 kg by 24 hours in a day for an answer of 1,200 kcal. Then multiply 1,200 kcal by 0.9 for an answer of 1,080 kcal. This is the estimated basal metabolic energy requirement for that particular woman.

Calculating Total Energy Requirements

energy requirement
number of kcal required by the body each day

An individual's average daily **energy requirement** is the total number of kcal needed in a 24-hour period. Energy requirements of people differ, depending on BMR (REE) and activities. More energy is burned playing soccer than playing the piano.

To determine one's total energy requirement, one must first calculate one's REE, and multiply it by the appropriate multiple of REE, as shown in Table 3-2. An example of this process would be:

1. A 110-lb 51-year-old woman whose REE = 1,080 kcal

2. 1,080 multiplied by 1.5 = 1,620 kcal

However, it is important to remember that such total kcal figures are still estimates.

Energy Balance

adipose tissue
fatty tissue

energy balance
occurs when the kcal value of food ingested equals the kcal expended

A person who takes in fewer nutrients than she or he burns usually loses weight. If someone takes in more nutrients than she or he burns, the body stores them as **adipose tissue** (fat). Some adipose tissue is necessary to protect the body and support its organs. Adipose tissue also helps regulate body temperature, just as insulation helps regulate the temperature of a building. An excess of adipose tissue, however, leads to obesity, which can endanger health because it puts extra burdens on body organs and systems. For the healthy person, the goal is **energy balance**. This means that the number of kcal consumed matches the number of kcal required for body maintenance and activity.

The Food and Nutrition Board of the National Research Council has made recommendations of energy intakes that meet the average needs of people in categories based on age, sex, weight, height, and estimated REE (see Table 3-2).

CONSIDERATIONS FOR THE HEALTH CARE PROFESSIONAL

The health care professional might find that patients have little factual information about digestion and metabolism. At the same time, patients may have very strongly held beliefs about these functions. Some might say, "I can't digest that" regarding specific foods, but will, in fact, not know what occurs during digestion. Some will insist that their metabolism is low and is the cause of their extra weight when, in reality, they simply overeat and don't exercise. Others will say they

TABLE 3-2 Median Heights and Weights and Recommended Energy Intake

CATEGORY	AGE (YEARS) OR CONDITION	WEIGHT (kg)	WEIGHT (lb)	HEIGHT (cm)	HEIGHT (in)	REE (kcal/day)	AVERAGE ENERGY ALLOWANCE (KCAL) Multiple of REE	Per kg	Per day
Infants	0.0–0.5	6	13	60	24	320		108	650
	0.5–1.0	9	20	71	28	500		98	850
Children	1–3	13	29	90	35	740		102	1,300
	4–6	20	44	112	44	950		90	1,800
	7–10	28	62	132	52	1,130		70	2,000
Males	11–14	45	99	157	62	1,440	1.70	55	2,500
	15–18	66	145	176	69	1,760	1.67	45	3,000
	19–24	72	160	177	70	1,780	1.67	40	2,900
	25–50	79	174	176	70	1,800	1.60	37	2,900
	51+	77	170	173	68	1,530	1.50	30	2,300
Females	11–14	46	101	157	62	1,310	1.67	47	2,200
	15–18	55	120	163	64	1,370	1.60	40	2,200
	19–24	58	128	164	65	1,350	1.60	38	2,200
	25–50	63	138	163	64	1,380	1.55	36	2,200
	51+	65	143	160	63	1,280	1.50	30	1,900
Pregnant	1st trimester								+0
	2nd trimester								+300
	3rd trimester								+300
Lactating	1st 6 months								+500
	2nd 6 months								+500

Reprinted with permission from *Recommended Dietary Allowances: 10th Edition.* Copyright 1989 by the National Academy of Sciences. Courtesy of the National Academy Press, Washington, D.C.

"eat" too many kcal and are, thus, overweight. The health care professional can help such patients by educating them about digestion and metabolism. Creative presentation of the information will motivate patients to learn and remember it.

● SUMMARY

The body is comparable to an automobile engine because both require fuel. Food acts as fuel but, to be usable, it must undergo a series of processes that includes digestion, absorption, and metabolism. Digestion is the process whereby food is broken down into smaller parts, chemically changed, and moved along the gastrointestinal tract. Mechanical digestion refers to that part of the process performed by the teeth and muscles of the digestive system. Chemical digestion refers to that part of the process wherein food is broken down to molecules that the blood can absorb. Enzymes are essential for chemical digestion. After digestion, food is absorbed by the blood, primarily in the small intestine, and then carried to all body tissues. After absorption, food is metabolized. During metabolism, carbohydrates and proteins are combined with oxygen in a process called oxidation. Energy released during oxidation is measured by the kcal or kilojoule. Kcal values of foods vary as do people's energy requirements. Requirements depend on age, body size, sex, lean body mass, physical condition, climate, and activity.

● DISCUSSION TOPICS

1. Describe the process of digestion.
2. Of what value are enzymes to digestion? Name five enzymes and the nutrients on which they act.
3. Describe absorption of nutrients.
4. Of what value is fiber in the diet? What are some examples of foods that provide it?
5. Describe metabolism.
6. What is the BMR? If anyone in the class has undergone a BMR test, ask him or her to describe it.
7. Explain why the body requires fuel even during sleep.
8. Why is it incorrect to say "He ate 2,000 kcal today"? What did he eat? What are kcal? What are kilojoules? How are they comparable?
9. Explain the differences between the terms *energy value* and *energy requirement*.
10. What does it mean to be overweight? What is a common cause of overweight? What reasons do people give for being overweight? How can one prevent excessive weight gain? How might overweight people reduce? How might overweight endanger health?

● SUGGESTED ACTIVITIES

1. Using the method given in this chapter, calculate your minimum caloric requirement.
2. Prepare a brief description of the processes of digestion and absorption that could be presented to a fourth grade class.
3. Role-play a situation where the patient asks the nurse to explain *metabolism*.
4. Divide the class into teams and determine the BMR for each team member.

● REVIEW

A. Multiple choice. Select the *letter* that precedes the best answer.
   1. Digestion begins in the
      a. mouth
      b. stomach
      c. liver
      d. small intestine

2. Most of the digestive processes occur in the
   a. mouth
   b. stomach
   c. small intestine
   d. colon

3. The small intestine is divided into three segments. They are, in descending order,
   a. ileum, jejunum, duodenum
   b. jejunum, ileum, duodenum
   c. duodenum, ileum, jejunum
   d. duodenum, jejunum, ileum

4. The fluid mixture that moves from the stomach through the pyloric sphincter is called
   a. bolus
   b. chyme
   c. food
   d. none of the above

5. A muscular movement that moves food down the GI tract is called
   a. a pump
   b. peristalsis
   c. lymphatic circulation
   d. circular propulsion

6. The pyloric sphincter is between the
   a. ileum and colon
   b. stomach and duodenum
   c. small intestine and colon
   d. colon and rectum

7. A word ending in *ase* usually indicates that a substance is
   a. a hormone
   b. a bacterium
   c. an enzyme
   d. an acid

8. Maltase, sucrase, and lactase are produced in the
   a. stomach
   b. small intestine
   c. colon
   d. pancreas

9. Bile is needed to
   a. digest carbohydrates
   b. digest fiber
   c. digest proteins
   d. digest fats

10. When energy intake is greater than energy output, the body weight will
   a. remain the same
   b. decrease
   c. increase and then decrease
   d. increase

B. Label the structures on the following diagram.

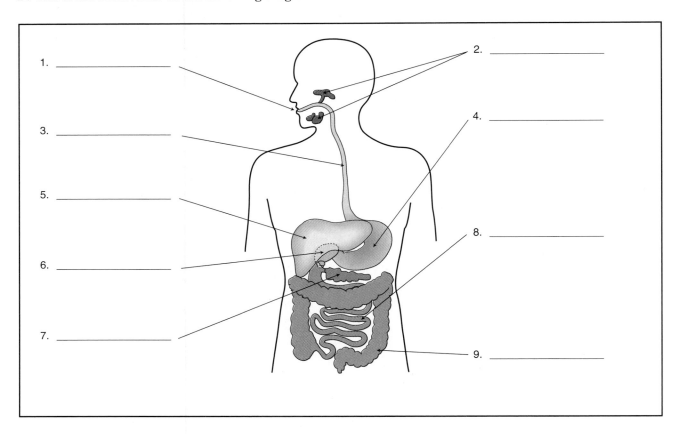

1. _____

2. _____

3. _____

4. _____

5. _____

6. _____

7. _____

8. _____

9. _____

C. Briefly answer the following questions.

  1. Name the three steps in estimating an individual's BMR.

  2. Where does most absorption of nutrients take place?

  3. What is energy balance?

C A S E   S T U D Y

Colletta C. is a 60-year-old legal secretary. She works full-time and thoroughly enjoys her job. Her children are grown. She and her husband walk 1 or 2 miles each evening after work and catch up on each other's day. She enjoys bicycling and Sunday night bowling. She watches her weight and has maintained her weight at about 130 pounds for years. She is 5 foot 4 inches tall.

It has been icy and very cold this winter, and Colletta has skipped many of her walks. Some weekends she has used her exercycle. Colletta has felt tired and lethargic and sometimes falls asleep in the recliner after dinner. She is also upset about her recent weight gain of 8 pounds. Some of her favorite skirts are too snug. Her husband has been urging her to see her doctor.

ASSESSMENT

1. What data do you have?
2. What do you suspect is the medical problem?
3. What lab tests would the doctor order to diagnose the problem?
4. According to Table 3-3, what is the median weight for a female of Colletta's size and age?
5. Using the Harris-Benedict equation, calculate Colletta's REE.

DIAGNOSIS

6. What is the likely cause of Colletta's fatigue?

   A week after her doctor's appointment Colletta started taking Synthroid. Her doctor told her that it will take a while before a therapeutic dose is reached. He also told her that she should feel less lethargic once the medication is at a therapeutic level.

PLAN/GOAL

7. Set two measurable realistic goals for Colletta during this process to prevent further weight gain.
8. How can these goals be modified when her medication is therapeutic?

IMPLEMENTATION

9. What actions would help Colletta carry out those goals?
10. Who can help her?

EVALUATION/OUTCOME CRITERIA

11. What will Colletta do and feel when the plan is successful?
12. What will Colletta be able to measure as evidence of her success?

C A S E   S T U D Y

Carl is a 25-year-old male with Crohn's disease, primarily of the large intestine and colon. He is 5 feet 10 inches tall and weighs 190 pounds. He knows he is prone to flare-ups of malabsorption of carbohydrates, proteins, fats, and folate. He has been having diarrhea on and off for 3 weeks. It has been really bad this last week. He has lost 10 pounds, which he doesn't mind. He would actually like to weigh 175 pounds again. The doctor ordered blood drawn for a CBC, albumin, folate, and B_{12}. The doctor also referred him to the dietitian. On the referral slip, the doctor wrote, "Instruct Carl on a low-lactose, low-fat, high-fiber, high-protein diet."

ASSESSMENT

1. What are the pertinent objective and subjective data related to Carl's problem?

2. Calculate Carl's approximate weight according to Table 3-3.

3. Calculate Carl's REE using the Harris-Benedict equation.

DIAGNOSIS

4. What is the cause of Carl's problem with elimination?

5. Complete the nursing diagnosis statement. Carl's problem with elimination is secondary to _____.

PLAN/GOAL

6. Write a reasonable measurable goal for controlling Carl's diarrhea.

7. Write a goal to help Carl adapt to his new diet. Incorporate Carl's desire to lose weight.

IMPLEMENTATION

8. List at least one action to help Carl meet each goal.

9. List two foods Carl should avoid.

10. List three foods Carl needs to include.

EVALUATION/OUTCOME CRITERIA

11. What will Carl report when your plan for his diarrhea is effective?

12. How will Carl know his new diet is successful?

13. What can the doctor measure when all the goals are successful?

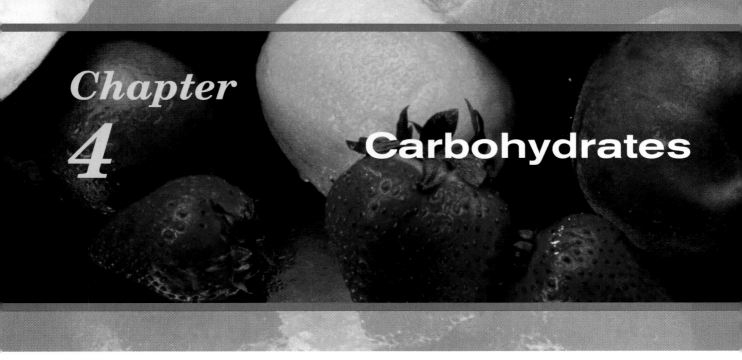

Chapter 4

Carbohydrates

Key Terms

adipose (fatty) tissue	hyperglycemia
bran	hypoglycemia
carbohydrates	insulin
cellulose	islets of Langerhans
dietary fiber	ketones
disaccharides	ketosis
endosperm	lactose
flatulence	lactose intolerance
fructose	lignins
galactose	maltose
germ	monosaccharides
glucagon	polysaccharides
glucose (dextrose)	starch
glycogen	sucrose
hemicellulose	whey

Objectives

After studying this chapter, you should be able to:

- Identify the functions of carbohydrates
- Name the primary sources of carbohydrates
- Describe the classification of carbohydrates

Energy foods are those that can be rapidly oxidized by the body to release energy and its by-product, heat. Carbohydrates, fats, and proteins provide energy for the human body, but carbohydrates are the primary source. They are the least expensive and most abundant of the energy nutrients. Foods rich in carbohydrates grow easily in most climates. They keep well and are generally easy to digest.

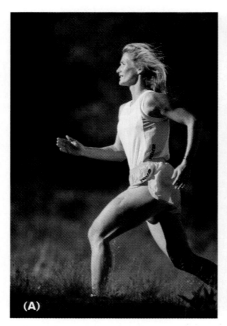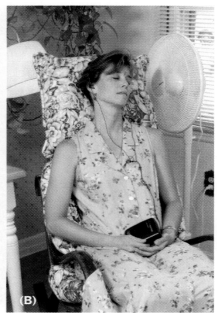

FIGURE 4-1 The need for carbohydrates is constant, whether you are active (A) or at rest (B).

carbohydrate

the nutrient providing the major source of energy in the average diet

Carbohydrates provide the major source of energy for people all over the world (Figure 4-1). They provide approximately half the kcal for people living in the United States. In some areas of the world, where fats and proteins are scarce and expensive, carbohydrates provide as much as 80 to 100% of kcal. Carbohydrates are named for the chemical elements they are composed of—carbon, hydrogen, and oxygen.

FUNCTIONS

Providing energy is the major function of carbohydrates. Each gram of carbohydrate provides 4 kcal. The body needs to maintain a constant supply of energy. Therefore, it stores approximately half a day's supply of carbohydrate in the liver and muscles for use as needed. In this form, it is called glycogen.

Protein-sparing action is also an important function of carbohydrates. When enough carbohydrates (at least 50–100 g/day) are ingested to supply a person's energy needs, they spare proteins for their primary function of building and repairing body tissues.

ketones

substances to which fatty acids are broken down in the liver

ketosis

condition in which ketones collect in the blood; caused by insufficient glucose available for energy

Normal fat metabolism requires an adequate supply of carbohydrates. If there is too little carbohydrate to fulfill the energy requirement, an abnormally large amount of fat is metabolized to help meet it. During such an emergency need for energy, fat oxidization in the cells is not complete and substances called ketones are produced. **Ketones** are acids that accumulate in the blood and urine, upsetting the acid-base balance. Such a condition is called **ketosis**. It can result from IDDM (insulin-dependent diabetes mellitus), also known as Type 1 diabetes (see Chapter 17), from starvation, or from extreme low-carbohydrate diets. It can lead to coma and even death.

When sufficient carbohydrates are eaten, the body is protected against ketones. This is sometimes called the antiketogenic effect of carbohydrates.

Providing fiber in the diet is another important function of carbohydrates. Dietary fiber is found in grains, vegetables, and fruits. Fiber creates a soft, bulky stool that moves quickly through the large intestine.

FOOD SOURCES

The principal sources of carbohydrates are plant foods: cereal grains, vegetables, fruits, nuts, and sugars (Figure 4-2). The only substantial animal sources of carbohydrates is milk.

Cereal grains and their products are dietary staples in nearly every part of the world. Rice is the basic food in Latin America, Africa, Asia, and many sections of the United States. Wheat and the various breads, pastas, and breakfast cereals made from it are basic to American and European diets. Rye and oats are commonly used in breads and cereals in the United States and Europe. Cereals also contain vitamins, minerals, and some proteins. During processing, some of these nutrients are lost. To compensate for this loss, food producers in the United States commonly add four B vitamins—thiamin, riboflavin, folic acid, and niacin—plus the mineral iron to the final product. The product is then called *enriched*.

Vegetables such as potatoes, beets, peas, lima beans, and corn provide substantial amounts of carbohydrates (in the form of starch). Green, leafy vegetables provide dietary fiber. All of them also provide vitamins and minerals.

Fruits provide sugar, fiber, vitamins, and minerals.

Sugars such as table sugar, syrup, and honey and sugar-rich foods such as desserts and candy provide carbohydrates in the form of sugar

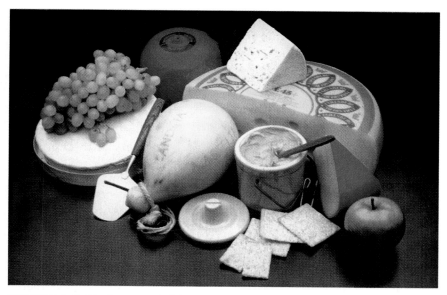

FIGURE 4-2 Fruits, vegetables, grains, and some dairy products are good sources of carbohydrates. (Courtesy of Price Chopper Supermarkets.)

with few other nutrients except for fats. Therefore, the foods in which they predominate are commonly called low nutrient density foods.

CLASSIFICATION

Carbohydrates are divided into three groups: monosaccharides, disaccharides, and polysaccharides (see Table 4-1).

TABLE 4-1 Carbohydrates

TYPE	SOURCE		FUNCTIONS	DEFICIENCY SYMPTOMS
Monosaccharides (Simple Sugars)				
Glucose	Berries	Grapes	Furnish energy	Fatigue
	Sweet corn	Corn syrup	Spare proteins	Weight loss
			Prevent ketosis	
Fructose	Ripe fruits	Soft drinks	Fruits and vegetables provide	
	Honey		vitamins, minerals, and fiber	
Galactose	Lactose			
Disaccharides				
Sucrose	Sugar cane		Furnish energy	Fatigue
	Sugar beets		Spare proteins	Weight loss
	Granulated sugar		Prevent ketosis	
	Confectioner's sugar			
	Brown sugar			
	Molasses			
	Maple syrup			
	Candy			
	Jams and jellies			
Maltose	Digestion of starch			
Lactose	Milk			
Polysaccharides (Complex Carbohydrates)				
Starch	Cereal grains and their products:		Furnish energy	Fatigue
	cereals, breads, rice, flour,		Prevent ketosis	Weight loss
	pasta, crackers		Fruits and vegetables provide	
	Potatoes	Corn	vitamins, minerals, and fiber	
	Lima beans	Yams		
	Navy beans	Green bananas		
	Sweet potatoes			
Dextrins	Starch hydrolysis			
Glycogen	Glucose stored in liver and muscles			
Cellulose	Wheat bran, whole-grain cereals		Provide fiber	Constipation
	green and leafy vegetables,			Colon cancer
	fruits, especially apples, pears,			Diverticulosis
	oranges, grapefruit, grapes			

Monosaccharides

Monosaccharides are the simplest form of carbohydrates. They are sweet, require no digestion, and can be absorbed directly into the bloodstream from the small intestine. They include glucose, fructose, and galactose.

Glucose, also called dextrose, is the form of carbohydrate to which all other forms are converted for eventual metabolism. It is found naturally in corn syrup and some fruits and vegetables. The central nervous system, the red blood cells, and the brain use only glucose as fuel; therefore, a continuous source is needed.

Fructose, also called levulose or fruit sugar, is found with glucose in many fruits and in honey. It is the sweetest of all the monosaccharides.

Galactose is a product of the digestion of milk. It is not found naturally.

Disaccharides

Disaccharides are pairs of the three sugars just discussed. They are sweet and must be changed to simple sugars by hydrolysis before they can be absorbed. Disaccharides include sucrose, maltose, and lactose.

Sucrose is composed of glucose and fructose. It is the form of carbohydrate present in granulated, powdered, and brown sugar and in molasses. It is one of the sweetest and least expensive sugars. Its sources are sugar cane, sugar beets, and the sap from maple trees.

Maltose is a disaccharide that is an intermediary product in the hydrolysis of starch. It is produced by enzyme action during the digestion of starch in the body. It also is created during the fermentation process that produces alcohol. It can be found in some infant formulas, malt beverage products, and beer. It is considerably less sweet than glucose or sucrose.

Lactose is the sugar found in milk. It is distinct from most other sugars because it is not found in plants. It helps the body absorb calcium. Lactose is less sweet than monosaccharides or other disaccharides.

Many adults are unable to digest lactose and suffer from bloating, abdominal cramps, and diarrhea after drinking milk or consuming a milk-based food such as process cheese. This reaction is called **lactose intolerance**. It is caused by insufficient lactase, the enzyme required for digestion of lactose. There are special low-lactose milk products that can be used instead of regular milk. Lactase-containing products are also available.

During the process of making hard cheese, milk separates into curd (solid part from which hard cheese is made) and **whey** (liquid part). Lactose becomes part of the whey and not the curd. Therefore, lactose is not a component of natural cheese. However, manufacturers can add milk or milk solids to process cheese, so it is important that persons who are lactose-intolerant check the labels on cheese products.

There is no test for lactose intolerance. If eating dairy products consistently produces symptoms of flatulence, diarrhea, and abdominal pain, the doctor may recommend eliminating dairy products from the diet and adding them back after a period of time to ascertain the

monosaccharides
simplest carbohydrates; sugars that cannot be further reduced by hydrolysis; examples are glucose, fructose, and galactose

glucose
the simple sugar to which carbohydrate must be broken down for absorption; also known as *dextrose*

fructose
the simple sugar (monosaccharide) found in fruit and honey

galactose
the simple sugar (monosaccharide) to which lactose is broken down during digestion

disaccharides
double sugars that are reduced by hydrolysis to monosaccharides; examples are sucrose, maltose, and lactose

sucrose
a double sugar or disaccharide; examples are granulated, powdered, and brown sugar

maltose
the double sugar (disaccharide) occurring as a result of the digestion of grain

lactose
the sugar in milk; a disaccharide

lactose intolerance
inability to digest lactose because of a lack of the enzyme lactase; causes abdominal cramps and diarrhea

whey
liquid part of milk that separates from the curd (solid part) during making of hard cheese

patient's reaction. If the symptoms persist, the patient is lactose intolerant.

Polysaccharides

polysaccharides
complex carbohydrates containing combinations of monosaccharides; examples include starch, dextrin, cellulose, and glycogen

starch
polysaccharide found in grains and vegetables

endosperm
the inner part of the kernel of grain; contains the carbohydrate

bran
outer covering of grain kernels

germ
embryo or tiny life center of each kernel of grain

Polysaccharides are commonly called *complex carbohydrates* because they are compounds of many monosaccharides (simple sugars). Three polysaccharides are important in nutrition: starch, glycogen, and fiber.

Starch is a polysaccharide found in grains and vegetables. It is the storage form of glucose in plants. Vegetables contain less starch than grains because vegetables have a higher moisture content. Legumes (dried beans and peas) are another important source of starch, as well as of dietary fiber and protein. Starches are more complex than monosaccharides or disaccharides, and it takes the body longer to digest them. Thus, they supply energy over a longer period of time. The starch in grain is found mainly in the **endosperm** (center part of the grain). This is the part from which white flour is made. The tough outer covering of grain kernels is called the **bran** (Figure 4-3). The bran is used in coarse cereals and whole wheat flour. The **germ** is the smallest part of the grain and is a rich source of B vitamins, vitamin E, minerals, and protein. Wheat germ is included in products made of whole wheat. It also can be purchased and used in baked products or as an addition to breakfast cereals.

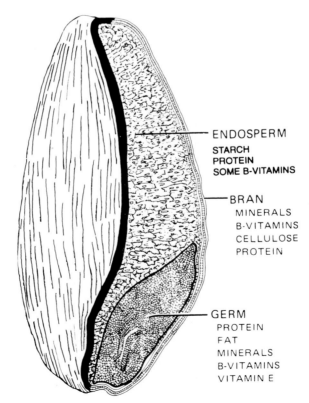

ENDOSPERM
STARCH
PROTEIN
SOME B-VITAMINS

BRAN
MINERALS
B-VITAMINS
CELLULOSE
PROTEIN

GERM
PROTEIN
FAT
MINERALS
B-VITAMINS
VITAMIN E

FIGURE 4-3 A grain of wheat has three parts. All parts are used in whole wheat flour; only the endosperm is used in white flour.

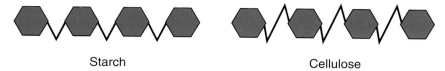

Starch   Cellulose

FIGURE 4-4 The alpha bonds that link glucose molecules together can be broken down during digestion. The beta bonds in cellulose cannot be broken by digestive enzymes and are eliminated without being digested (insoluble fiber).

Before the starch in grain can be used for food, the bran must be broken down. The heat and moisture of cooking break this outer covering, making the food more flavorful and more easily digested. Although bran itself is indigestible, it is important that some be included in the diet because of the fiber it provides.

Glycogen is sometimes called *animal starch* because it is the storage form of glucose in the body. In the healthy adult, approximately one-half day's supply of energy is stored as glycogen in the liver and muscles. The hormone **glucagon** helps the liver convert glycogen to glucose as needed. (See Chapter 13 for information on glycogen loading.)

The Fibers

Dietary fiber, also called roughage, is indigestible because it cannot be broken down by digestive enzymes. Some fiber is insoluble (it does not readily dissolve in water), and some is soluble (it does dissolve in water) (Figure 4-4). Insoluble fibers include cellulose, some hemicellulose, and lignins. Soluble fibers are gums, pectins, some hemicellulose, and mucilages. See Table 4-2 for food sources. **Cellulose** is a primary source of dietary fiber. It is found in the skins of fruits, the leaves and stems of vegetables, and legumes. Highly processed foods such as white bread, macaroni products, and pastries contain little if any cellulose because it is removed during processing. Because humans cannot digest cellulose, it has no energy value. It is useful because it provides bulk for the stool.

glycogen

glucose as stored in the liver and muscles

glucagon

hormone from alpha cells of pancreas; helps cells release energy

dietary fiber

indigestible parts of plants; absorbs water in large intestine, helping to create soft, bulky stool; some is believed to bind cholesterol in the colon, helping to rid cholesterol from the body; some is believed to lower blood glucose levels

cellulose

indigestible carbohydrate; provides fiber in the diet

TABLE 4-2 Sources of Fiber That Are Soluble in Water and Those That Are Insoluble in Water

WATER-SOLUBLE FIBER		WATER-INSOLUBLE FIBER
Fruit (pectin)	**Grains**	All vegetables
Apples	Oats	Fruit
Peaches	Barley	Whole grain bread and cereal
Plums	**Legumes**	Whole grain crackers
Bananas	Dried peas	Brown rice
Vegetables	Beans	Wild rice
Broccoli	Lentils	Wheat bran
Carrots		
Cabbage		

hemicellulose

dietary fiber found in whole grains

lignins

dietary fiber found in woody parts of vegetables

flatulence

gas in the intestinal tract

Hemicellulose is found mainly in whole grain cereal. Some hemicellulose is soluble; some is not. **Lignins** are the woody part of vegetables such as carrots and asparagus or the small seeds of strawberries; they are not a carbohydrate.

Pectins, some hemicellulose, gums, and mucilages are soluble in water and form a gel that helps provide bulk for the intestines. They are useful also because they bind cholesterol, thus reducing the amount the blood can absorb.

Fiber is considered helpful to patients with diabetes mellitus because it lowers blood glucose levels. It may prevent some colon cancers by moving waste materials through the colon faster than would normally be the case, thereby reducing the colon's exposure time to potential carcinogens. Fiber helps prevent constipation, hemorrhoids, and diverticular disease by softening and increasing the size of the stool.

The optimal recommendation for fiber intake is 20–35 g/day. The normal U.S. diet is thought to contain approximately 11 g. In general, Americans do not consume sufficient amounts of fruits and vegetables. They should eat no fewer than five servings of fruits and vegetables each day. Fiber intake should be increased gradually and should be accompanied by an increased intake of water. Eating too much fiber in a short time can produce discomfort, **flatulence** (abdominal gas), and diarrhea. It also could obstruct the GI tract if intake exceeds 50g. Insoluble fiber has binders (phytic acid or phytate), which are found in the outer covering of grains and vegetables. These can prevent the absorption of minerals such as calcium, iron, zinc, and magnesium, so excess intake should be avoided. The type of fiber consumed should be from natural food sources rather than from commercially prepared fiber products because the foods contain vitamins and minerals as well as fiber. Table 4-3 lists the dietary fiber content of selected foods.

DIGESTION AND ABSORPTION

The monosaccharides—glucose, fructose, and galactose—are simple sugars that may be absorbed from the intestine directly into the bloodstream. They are subsequently carried to the liver, where fructose and galactose are changed to glucose. The blood then carries glucose to the cells.

The disaccharides—sucrose, maltose, and lactose—require an additional step of digestion. They must be converted to the simple sugar glucose before they can be absorbed into the bloodstream. This conversion is accomplished by the enzymes sucrase, maltase, and lactase, which were discussed in Chapter 3 (see Table 3-1).

The polysaccharides are more complex, and their digestibility varies. After the cellulose wall is broken down, starch is changed to the intermediate product dextrin; it is then changed to maltose and finally to glucose. Cooking can change starch to dextrin. For example, when bread is toasted, it turns golden brown and tastes sweeter because the starch has been changed to dextrin.

The digestion of starch begins in the mouth, where the enzyme salivary amylase begins to change starch to dextrin. The second step occurs in the stomach, where the food is mixed with gastric juices. The

TABLE 4-3 Dietary Fiber Content of Selected Foods

GRAMS PER SERVING†	0.5 OR LESS	0.5–1.0	1.1–2.0	2.1–3.0	3.0 OR GREATER‡
Fruit†	Banana Cherries Coconut (shredded) Currants (dried) Dates Fruit juice Plums (cooked) Pomegranate Prunes Raisins Rhubarb (raw) Watermelon	Apricots (raw or dried) Apple (peeled or dried) Applesauce Blueberries Cantaloupe Coconut, raw, 1/2 cup Cranberries, relish, 1/2 cup Honeydew Kiwifruit Mango Nectarine Orange Peach (raw or dried) Pear (dried) Pineapple Plums (raw) Prunes Rhubarb, raw (1 cup) and cooked Strawberries Tangerine Watermelon	Apple skin Cranberries, raw (1 cup) Figs Papaya	Blackberries Boysenberries Gooseberries Kumquats Pears	Blackberries (4) Elderberries (5) Guava (5) Raspberries (4)
Vegetables†	Bamboo shoots Bean sprouts (cooked or canned) Cabbage (cooked) Celery Eggplant Endive Lettuce Onions Radishes Summer squash Vegetable juice Water chestnuts Watercress	Artichoke hearts Asparagus Bean sprouts (raw) Beans (string) Beets Broccoli (raw) Cabbage (raw) Carrots Cauliflower Cucumber Green pepper Greens: 　Beet *(continued)*	Artichoke, Jerusalem Broccoli (cooked) Brussels sprouts Chicory Mushrooms Pumpkin Rutabagas Sauerkraut Soybean sprouts (raw) Spaghetti sauce Tomato paste Turnips (raw)		

TABLE 4-3 *continued*

GRAMS PER SERVING*	0.5 OR LESS	0.5–1.0	1.1–2.0	2.1–3.0	3.0 OR GREATER‡
Vegetables†		Collard Dandelion Kale Mustard Spinach Swiss chard Turnip Kohlrabi Mushrooms Okra Parsley Soybean sprouts (cooked) Summer squash (raw) Tomato puree Turnips (cooked)			
Starches	Cornflakes Corn grits Cream of Wheat or Rice Farina Graham crackers Maltomeal Plantain Potato chips Potatoes Puffed cereals Rice, white Rice Krispies Saltines Spaghetti (refined)	Bread, white Cheerios Corn Flour, white Granola Oatmeal (cooked) Roll or bun, white Spaghetti and macaroni from whole wheat flour	Black-eyed peas Bread, whole wheat Flour, whole wheat Grapenuts Green peas Lima beans Popcorn Ralston (cooked cereal) Rice, brown or white Sesame seed kernels Soybeans Squash, winter Sweet potatoes	Beans (dried) 40% Branflakes Bulgur Lentils Parsnips Peas (dried) Pumpkin Raisin Bran Shredded Wheat Wheat germ	All-Bran (9) Bran Buds (8) 100% Bran (6) Bran muffin (3.5) Bulgur (3.5) Rykrisp Wheat bran (9)

Courtesy of Mayo Clinic, Rochester, Minnesota.

Note: Based on the content of one diabetic exchange for each item listed.

* Serving sizes per the Food Guide Pyramid.

† Includes all forms (raw, dried, cooked) for fruits and vegetables except where noted.

‡ Actual dietary fiber content listed in parentheses.

final step occurs in the small intestine, where the digestible carbohydrates are changed to simple sugars by the enzyme action of pancreatic amylase and are subsequently absorbed into the blood.

METABOLISM AND ELIMINATION

All carbohydrates are changed to the simple sugar glucose before metabolism can take place in the cells. After glucose has been carried by the blood to the cells, it can be oxidized. Frequently, the volume of glucose that reaches the cells exceeds the amount the cells can use. In these cases, some glucose is converted to glycogen and is stored in the liver and muscles. (Glycogen is subsequently broken down and released as glucose, which is needed for energy.) When more glucose is ingested than the body can either use immediately or store in the form of glycogen, it is converted to fat and stored as adipose (fatty) tissue.

    The process of glucose metabolism is controlled mainly by the hormone insulin, which is secreted by the islets of Langerhans in the pancreas. When the secretion of insulin is impaired or absent, the glucose level in the blood becomes excessively high. This condition is called hyperglycemia and is usually a symptom of diabetes mellitus. If control by diet is ineffective, insulin injections or an oral hypoglycemic must be used to control blood sugar. When insulin is given, the diabetic patient's intake of carbohydrates must be carefully controlled to balance the prescribed dosage of insulin (see Chapter 17). When blood glucose levels are unusually low, the condition is called hypoglycemia. A mild form of hypoglycemia may occur if one waits too long between meals or if the pancreas secretes too much insulin. Symptoms include fatigue, shaking, sweating, and headache.

    Oxidation of glucose results in energy. With the exception of cellulose, the only waste products of carbohydrate metabolism are carbon dioxide and water. It is a very efficient nutrient.

DIETARY REQUIREMENTS

Although there is no specific daily dietary requirement for carbohydrates, the Food and Nutrition Board of the National Research Council recommends that half of one's energy requirement come from carbohydrates. For example, assume that one's total energy requirement is 2,000 kcal. One half of this is 1,000. Divide 1,000 kcal by 4 (the number of kcal in each gram of carbohydrate), for an estimated carbohydrate requirement of 250 g/day. It is estimated that current U.S. diets contain only 45% of their kcal from carbohydrates.

    A mild deficiency of carbohydrates can result in weight loss and fatigue. A diet seriously deficient in carbohydrates could cause ketosis. To prevent these effects, one needs a minimum of 50–100g of carbohydrates each day.

    Overweight is a major health problem in the United States and eating an excess of carbohydrates is one of the most common causes of obesity. Although some of the surplus carbohydrate is changed to glycogen, the major part of any surplus becomes adipose tissue. Also,

adipose tissue
fatty tissue

insulin
secretion of the islets of Langerhans in the pancreas gland; essential for the proper metabolism of glucose

islets of Langerhans
part of the pancreas from which insulin is secreted

hyperglycemia
excessive amounts of glucose in the blood

hypoglycemia
subnormal levels of blood glucose

an excess of carbohydrate in the form of sugar can spoil an appetite for other nutrients that are more important. Too many carbohydrates may cause tooth decay, irritate the lining of the stomach, or cause flatulence.

CONSIDERATIONS FOR THE HEALTH CARE PROFESSIONAL

The role of the health care professional in teaching about carbohydrates may be complicated. Carbohydrates have been considered "fattening" by many people who have not received nutrition education. Some will have to be taught the nutritional differences between a baked potato and potato chips; between whole wheat toast and Danish pastry; between a fresh peach and canned fruit cocktail. Many will need to learn what dietary fiber is, where it can be found, and why it is needed. Some will need to learn that sugar can be used in moderation; others that it cannot be used in excess. All will require acceptance, understanding, and patience on the part of the health care professional.

● SUMMARY

Energy foods are those that can be rapidly oxidized by the body to release energy. Carbohydrates are and should be the major source of energy. They are composed of carbon, hydrogen, and oxygen. One gram of carbohydrate provides 4 kcal. Carbohydrates are the least expensive and most abundant nutrient. The principal sources of carbohydrates are plant products such as grains and their products, vegetables, fruits, legumes, and sugars. In addition to providing energy, carbohydrates spare proteins, maintain normal fat metabolism, and provide fiber. Digestion of carbohydrates begins in the mouth, continues in the stomach, and is completed in the small intestine. Although they are obviously essential to the health and well-being of the body, eating an excess of carbohydrates can cause dental caries, digestive disturbances, and overweight.

● DISCUSSION TOPICS

1. What are the three basic groups of carbohydrates? Name several foods in each group.

2. Discuss the effects of regularly eating an excess of carbohydrates.

3. Which polysaccharides (starches) may be considered a dietary staple for the following nationalities? Explain why this may be so.
- Italian
- American Indian
- Mexican
- French
- Chinese

4. Why should one's diet contain dietary fiber? Name three sources of dietary fiber.

5. Describe the digestion and metabolism of carbohydrates.

6. What could develop from eating too few carbohydrates?

7. Discuss the following menus. Which foods contain carbohydrates? (Refer to Table A-4 in the appendix.)

Orange juice	Baked chicken	Cheese sandwich on whole
Cereal	Baked potato	wheat bread with
Milk and sugar	Green beans	lettuce and tomato
Toast	Coleslaw	Carrot and celery sticks
Butter and jelly	Bread and butter	Fresh fruit
Milk	Raspberry sherbet	Cookies
Coffee	Milk	Milk

8. Why are complex carbohydrates preferable to simple sugars?

9. Discuss *enrichment*. What does it mean? Why is it done? Which foods are typically enriched in the United States? Would you recommend that one purchase enriched foods? Why?

10. Is it true, as many people say, that "carbos are fattening"? Explain your answer.

● SUGGESTED ACTIVITIES

1. Hold a soda cracker in your mouth until you notice the change in flavor as the starch changes to dextrin.

2. Toast a slice of bread and describe the changes in appearance and flavor that occurred.

3. Make a list of the foods you have eaten in the past 24 hours. Circle the carbohydrate-rich foods and underline the complex carbohydrates. Approximately what percentage of your calories were in the form of carbohydrate? In the form of complex carbos? Could your diet be improved? If so, how?

4. Trace Figure 3-1 in Chapter 3. Use it to explain the digestion of carbohydrates using words and arrows.

5. Role-play a situation between a diet counselor and a teenage girl who has placed herself on an extremely low-kcal diet. She refuses to eat anything that she thinks contains carbohydrates. Explain to her the functions of carbohydrates in the human body.

● REVIEW

Multiple choice. Select the *letter* that precedes the best answer.

1. The three main groups of carbohydrates are
   a. fats, proteins, and minerals
   b. glucose, fructose, and galactose
   c. monosaccharides, disaccharides, and polysaccharides
   d. sucrose, cellulose, and glycogen

2. Galactose is a product of the digestion of
   a. milk
   b. meat
   c. breads
   d. vegetables

3. The simple sugar to which all forms of carbohydrates are ultimately converted is
   a. sucrose
   b. glucose
   c. galactose
   d. maltose

4. Wheat germ is a source of
   a. B vitamins and vitamin D
   b. B vitamins and vitamin C
   c. B vitamins and vitamin E
   d. none of the above

5. A fibrous form of carbohydrate that cannot be digested is
   a. glucose
   b. glycogen
   c. cellulose
   d. fat

6. Glycogen is stored in the
   a. heart and lungs
   b. liver and muscles
   c. pancreas and gallbladder
   d. small and large intestines

7. Glucose is metabolized
   a. by combining it with fat
   b. in all body cells
   c. exclusively in the liver
   d. in the form of glycogen

8. Highly processed foods normally
   a. do not contain cellulose
   b. are excellent sources of fiber
   c. contain large amounts of cellulose
   d. contain no carbohydrates

9. Glucose, fructose, and galactose
   a. are polysaccharides
   b. are disaccharides
   c. are enzymes
   d. are monosaccharides

10. Before carbohydrates can be metabolized by the cells, they must be converted to
    a. glycogen
    b. glucose
    c. polysaccharides
    d. sucrase

11. The only form of carbohydrate that the brain uses for energy is
    a. glycogen
    b. galactose
    c. glucose
    d. glucagon

12. The substance that helps the liver convert glycogen to glucose is
   a. galactose
   b. estrogen
   c. thyroxin
   d. glucagon

13. Lactose intolerance can be caused by
   a. an inadequate supply of galactose
   b. an inadequate supply of lactase
   c. excessive use of milk in the diet
   d. excessive intake of calcium

14. Starch is
   a. the form in which glucose is stored in plants
   b. a monosaccharide
   c. an insoluble form of dietary fiber
   d. found only in grains

15. Dietary fiber
   a. can increase blood glucose
   b. can decrease blood cholesterol
   c. commonly causes diverticular disease
   d. is preferably provided by commercially prepared fiber products

16. The enzyme in the mouth that begins the digestion of starch is
   a. salivary ptyalin
   b. salivary amylase
   c. sucrase
   d. lipase

17. Cellulose
   a. is not digestible by humans
   b. should not be included in the human diet
   c. is a monosaccharide
   d. is an excellent substitute for dextrose

18. Carbohydrates
   a. are rich in fat
   b. are generally expensive
   c. provide approximately half of the kcal in the U.S. diet
   d. frequently are an excellent substitute for proteins in the human diet

19. Glucose metabolism
   a. is controlled mainly by the hormone insulin
   b. is not affected by any secretion of the islets of Langerhans in the pancreas
   c. is managed entirely by glucagon
   d. has no effect on human energy levels

20. Sucrose
   a. is a monosaccharide
   b. is plentiful in fats of all kinds
   c. is a complex carbohydrate
   d. must be converted to glucose before it can be absorbed into the bloodstream

C A S E   S T U D Y

Alma is a 52-year-old black computer programmer who is participating in the company's annual health fair. At the diabetes station, Alma had her fasting blood sugar checked by fingerstick. Her result was 310 mg/dl. She is 5 feet 6 inches tall and weighs 190 pounds. Alma reports that her mother, grandmother, and two aunts have diabetes. Alma has noticed increased fatigue, constant thirst, and nocturia in the last 4–5 months. The nurse measured a blood pressure of 170/98. She suggests Alma see her doctor for further evaluation.

After running a series of tests, her physician confirmed that Alma had Type 2 (non-insulin dependent) diabetes mellitus, put her on an oral agent, and sent her to the Diabetic Education Program. The doctor told Alma she needs to learn how to check her blood sugars, regulate her diet, and lose at least 20 pounds.

ASSESSMENT

1. What does the dietitian need to know about Alma's current meal choices?

2. How could the dietitian get the most accurate information?

3. What else does Alma need to know before she begins the classes?

4. Calculate Alma's ideal weight.

DIAGNOSIS

5. Complete the following statement. Alma has a nutrition problem related to excess calorie intake and _____ caused in part by _____.

6. Complete the following statement. Alma needs more education related to _____.

PLAN/GOAL

7. Name a goal related to weight loss that Alma should achieve at the end of the classes.

8. State two goals for Alma related to her diet and blood sugar.

IMPLEMENTATION

9. List the topics that you would teach Alma to meet the goals set.

10. Who else should be in the class with Alma?

11. What agencies or resources can you provide for Alma's goals?

EVALUATION

12. What can Alma do to show she understands what you have taught?

13. At Alma's next doctor appointment, what should her fasting morning blood sugar be?

C A S E   S T U D Y

William is a 78-year-old newly widowed man. After his wife, Jean, died, William couldn't stand running the farm alone, and he agreed to try living with his daughter, Sarah. He was going to help her in her new delivery business. He was a little concerned about the transition from his small town of 3,000 where he knew everyone to the big city, 4 hours away.

William has been at his daughter's about 3 weeks now. The job is going better than he had expected. He is having some constipation and stomach upset. He's not a picky eater and he thinks all this changing has caused his problems. On the farm he ate fruit right off the trees, raw vegetables right out of the ground, and Jean's homemade bread. He is kind of embarrassed to say anything to his daughter. He thinks she has enough things to worry about.

ASSESSMENT

1. What data do you have about William's diet, bowel function, and the duration of his current problem?

2. What else would you like to know about William?

3. What has contributed to William's problem?

DIAGNOSIS

4. Complete the following sentences. William has a problem with elimination related to _____ as evidenced by _____. William needs more education related to _____.

PLAN/GOAL

5. What changes do you want to see for William?

IMPLEMENTATION

6. Name at least two possible solutions for William's problem.

7. How would a commercially prepared fiber product help William?

8. How would adding apples, raw carrots, and oatmeal help him?

EVALUATION/OUTCOME CRITERIA

9. Two weeks after adding more fiber, what might William report about his bowel function?

10. What might William report that he had learned about his diet?

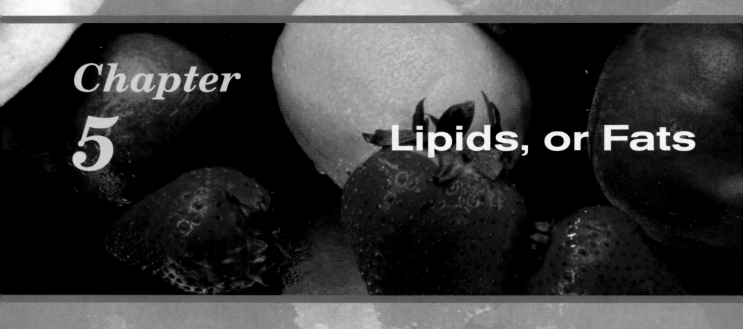

Chapter 5

Lipids, or Fats

Key Terms

adipose tissue
atherosclerosis
cholesterol
chylomicrons
fatty acids
glycerol
high-density lipo-
  proteins (HDLs)
hydrogenation
hypercholester-
  olemia (high serum
  cholesterol)
invisible fats
lecithin
linoleic acid

linolenic acid
lipids
lipoproteins
low-density lipo-
  proteins (LDLs)
monounsaturated fats
omega-3 fatty acids
plaque
polyunsaturated fats
satiety
saturated fats
triglycerides
very-low-density
  lipoproteins (VLDLs)
visible fats

Objectives

After studying this chapter, you should be able to:

● State the functions of fats in the body

● Identify sources of dietary fats

● Explain common classifications of fats

● Describe disease conditions with which excessive use of fats is associated

Fats belong to a group of organic compounds called **lipids**. The word *lipid* is derived from *lipos,* a Greek word for fat. Forms of this word are found in several fat-related health terms such as blood *lipids* (fats in the blood), hyper*lipid*emia (high levels of fat in the blood), and *lipo*proteins (carriers of fat in human blood).

Fats are greasy substances that are not soluble in water. They are soluble in some solvents such as ether, benzene, and chloroform. They provide a more concentrated source of energy than carbohydrates; each gram of fat contains 9 kcal. This is slightly more than twice the kcal content of carbohydrates. Fat-rich foods are generally more expensive than carbohydrate-rich foods. Like carbohydrates, fats are composed of carbon, hydrogen, and oxygen but with a substantially lower proportion of oxygen.

FUNCTIONS

In addition to providing energy, fats are essential for the functioning and structure of body tissues (Table 5-1). Fats are a necessary part of cell membranes (cell walls). They contain essential fatty acids and act as carriers for fat-soluble vitamins. The fat stored in body tissues provides energy when one cannot eat, as may occur during illness. Adipose (fatty) tissue protects organs and bones from injury by serving as protective padding and support. Body fat also serves as insulation from cold. In addition, fats provide a feeling of satiety (satisfaction) after meals. This is due partly to the flavor fats give other foods and partly to their slow rate of digestion, which delays hunger.

lipid
fat

adipose tissue
fatty tissue

satiety
feeling of satisfaction; fullness

FOOD SOURCES

Fats are present in both animal and plant foods. The animal foods that provide the richest sources of fats are meats, especially fatty meats such as bacon, sausage, and luncheon meats; whole, low-fat, and reduced-fat milk; cream; butter; cheeses made with cream, whole, low-fat, or reduced-fat milk; egg yolks (egg white contains no fat; it is almost entirely protein and water); and fatty fish such as tuna and salmon.

The plant foods containing the richest sources of fats are cooking oils made from sunflower, safflower, or sesame seeds, or from corn, peanuts, soybeans, or olives; margarine (which is made from vegetable oils); nuts; avocados; coconut; and cocoa butter.

Visible and Invisible Fats in Food

Sometimes fats are referred to as visible or invisible, depending on their food sources. Fats that are purchased and used as fats such as butter, margarine, lard, and cooking oils are called visible fats. Hidden or invisible fats are those found in other foods such as meats, cream, whole milk, cheese, egg yolk, fried foods, pastries, avocados, and nuts.

It is often the invisible fats that can make it difficult for patients on limited-fat diets to regulate their fat intake. For example, one 3-inch doughnut may contain 12g of fat, whereas one 3-inch bagel contains

visible fats
fats in foods that are purchased and used as fats, such as butter or margarine

invisible fats
fats that are not immediately noticeable such as those in egg yolk, cheese, cream, and salad dressings

TABLE 5-1 Fats

FUNCTIONS	DEFICIENCY SIGNS	SOURCES	
Provide energy	Eczema	Animal	Plant
Carry fat-soluble vitamins	Weight loss	Fatty meats	Vegetable oils
Supply essential fatty acids	Retarded growth	Lard	Nuts
Protect and support organs and bones		Butter	Chocolate
Insulate from cold		Cheese	Avocados
Provide satiety to meals		Cream	Olives
		Whole milk	Margarine
		Egg yolk	

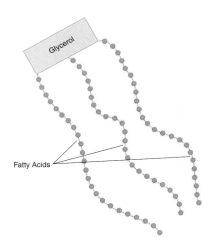

FIGURE 5-1 A triglyceride is composed of three fatty acids attached to a framework of glycerol.

glycerol

a component of fat; derived from a water-soluble carbohydrate

fatty acids

a component of fats that determines the classification of the fat

linoleic acid

fatty acid essential for humans; cannot be synthesized by the body

linolenic acid

one of three fatty acids needed by the body; cannot be synthesized by the body

saturated fats

fats whose carbon atoms contain all of the hydrogen atoms they can; considered a contributory factor in atherosclerosis

monounsaturated fats

fats that are neither saturated nor polyunsaturated and are thought to play little part in atherosclerosis

only 2g of fat. One fried chicken drumstick may contain 11g of fat, whereas one roasted drumstick may contain only 2g of fat.

It is essential that the health care professional confirm that patients on limited-fat diets are carefully educated about sources of hidden fats.

CLASSIFICATION

Triglycerides, phospholipids, and *sterols* are all lipids found in food and the human body. Most lipids in the body (95%) are triglycerides. They are in body cells, and they circulate in the blood.

Triglycerides are composed of three (tri) fatty acids attached to a framework of glycerol, thus their name (Figure 5-1). Glycerol is derived from a water-soluble carbohydrate. Fatty acids are organic compounds of carbon atoms to which hydrogen atoms are attached. They are classified in two ways. One is by the body's need for them. Two fatty acids, linoleic acid and linolenic acid, are considered essential because they cannot be synthesized by the body and must be obtained from the diet. Arachidonic fatty acid, previously thought to be essential, can be synthesized in the body from linoleic fatty acid. Arachidonic acid found in meat and linolenic fatty acid found in fats, oils, nuts, and seeds are stored in the body, so deficiencies are highly unlikely.

The other method of classification of fatty acids is by their degree of saturation with hydrogen atoms. In this method, they are described as *saturated, monounsaturated,* or *polyunsaturated,* depending on their hydrogen content (Figure 5-2).

Saturated Fats

When a fatty acid is saturated, each of its carbon atoms carries all the hydrogen atoms possible. In general, animal foods contain more saturated fatty acids than unsaturated. Examples include meat, poultry, egg yolks, whole milk, whole milk cheeses, cream, ice cream, and butter. Although plant foods generally contain more polyunsaturated fatty acids than saturated fatty acids, chocolate, coconut, palm oil, and palm kernel oils are exceptions. They contain substantial amounts of saturated fatty acids. Foods containing a high proportion of saturated fats are usually solid at room temperature.

Monounsaturated Fats

If a fat is monounsaturated, there is one place among the carbon atoms of its fatty acids where there are fewer hydrogen atoms attached than in saturated fats. Examples of foods containing monounsaturated fats are olive oil, canola oil, avocados, and cashew nuts. Recent research indicates that monounsaturated fats lower the amount of low-density lipoprotein (LDL) ("bad cholesterol") in the blood when they replace saturated fats in one's diet. They do not reduce high-density lipoproteins (HDLs) ("good cholesterol"), which help protect against heart disease. It is recommended that one consume no more than 10% of total daily kcal as monounsaturated fats (Table 5-2).

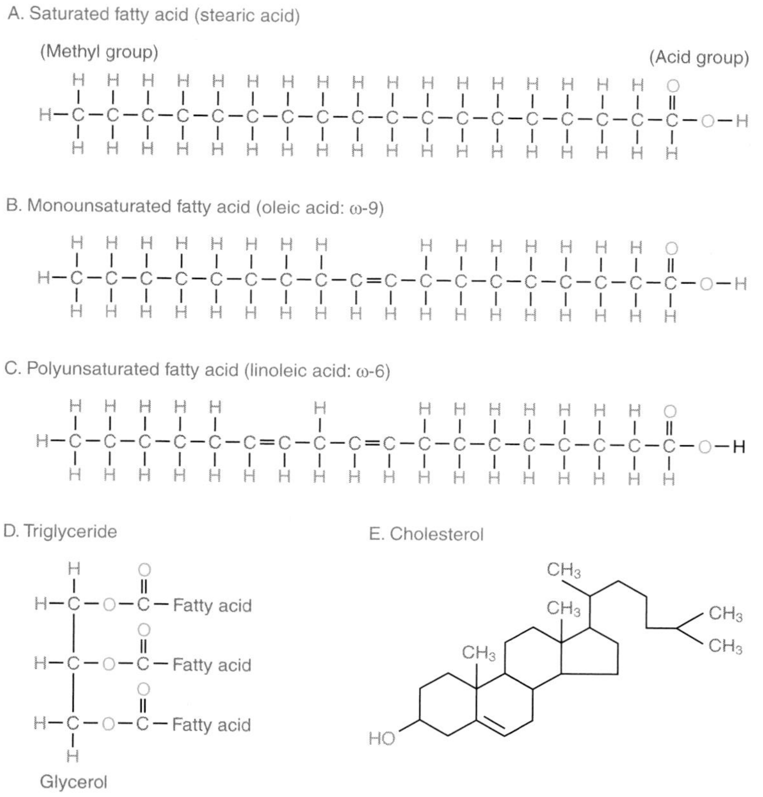

A. Saturated fatty acid (stearic acid)

(Methyl group)   (Acid group)

B. Monounsaturated fatty acid (oleic acid: ω-9)

C. Polyunsaturated fatty acid (linoleic acid: ω-6)

D. Triglyceride

Glycerol

E. Cholesterol

FIGURE 5-2 Chemical formula for (A) saturated fatty acid, (B) monounsaturated fatty acid, (C) polyunsaturated fatty acid, (D) triglyceride, (E) cholesterol.

TABLE 5-2 Sources of Saturated, Monounsaturated, and Polyunsaturated Fatty Acids

SATURATED	MONOUNSATURATED	POLYUNSATURATED
Meats	Canola oil	Safflower oil
Coconut	Olive oil	Soybean oil
Palm oil, palm kernel oil	Peanut oil	Sunflower oil
Butter	Nuts	Soybeans
Egg yolks	Avocados	Tofu
Milk and milk products	Sardines	
(except fat-free)		

Polyunsaturated Fats

If a fat is **polyunsaturated**, there are two or more places among the carbon atoms of its fatty acids where there are fewer hydrogen atoms attached than in saturated fats. The point at which carbon-carbon double bonds occur in a polyunsaturated fatty acid is the determining

polyunsaturated fats
fats whose carbon atoms contain only limited amounts of hydrogen

factor in how the body metabolizes it. The two major fatty acids denoted by the placement of their double bonds are the ω-3 and ω-6 fatty acids. Omega-3 fatty acids have been reported to help lower the risk of heart disease. Because ω-3 fatty acids are found in fish oils, an increased intake of fatty fish is recommended. Omega-6 (linoleic acid) has a cholesterol-lowering effect. The use of supplements of either of these fatty acids is not recommended. Linoleic fatty acid is polyunsaturated. Examples of foods containing polyunsaturated fats include cooking oils made from sunflower, safflower, or sesame seeds or from corn or soybeans; soft margarines whose major ingredient is *liquid* vegetable oil; and fish. Foods containing high proportions of polyunsaturated fats are usually soft or oily. Polyunsaturated fats should not exceed 10% of total daily kcal.

Hydrogenated Fats   Hydrogenated fats are polyunsaturated vegetable oils to which hydrogen has been added commercially to make them solid at room temperature. This process, called **hydrogenation**, turns polyunsaturated vegetable oils into saturated fats. Margarine is made in this way. (Soft margarine contains less saturated fat than firm margarine.)

During hydrogenation, trans fatty acids, commonly called trans-fats, are produced. Their chemical shape differs from the shape of most natural polyunsaturated fatty acids, and it is thought that they may increase LDL and lower HDL. Soft or liquid hydrogenated products contain fewer trans fatty acids than do solid products.

CHOLESTEROL

Cholesterol is a sterol (Figure 5-2). It is not a true fat but a fatlike substance that exists in animal foods and body cells. It does not exist in plant foods. Cholesterol is essential for the synthesis of bile, sex hormones, cortisone, and vitamin D and is needed by every cell in the body. The body manufactures 800–1000 mg of cholesterol a day in the liver.

Cholesterol is a common constituent (part) of one's daily diet because it is found so abundantly in egg yolk, fatty meats, shellfish, butter, cream, cheese, whole milk, and organ meats (liver, kidneys, brains, sweetbreads) (Table 5-3).

Cholesterol is thought to be a contributing factor in heart disease because high serum cholesterol, also called **hypercholesterolemia**, is common in patients with **atherosclerosis**. Atherosclerosis is a cardiovascular disease in which **plaque** (fatty deposits containing cholesterol and other substances) forms on the inside of artery walls, reducing the space for blood flow. When the blood cannot flow through an artery near the heart, a heart attack occurs. When this is the case near the brain, stroke occurs. (See Chapter 18.)

It is considered advisable that blood cholesterol levels not exceed 200 mg/dl (200 milligrams of cholesterol per one deciliter of blood). A reduction in the amount of total fat, saturated fats, and cholesterol and an increase in the amounts of monounsaturated fats in the diet, weight loss, and exercise all help to lower serum cholesterol levels. Soluble dietary fiber also is considered helpful in lowering blood cholesterol

hydrogenation

the combining of fat with hydrogen, thereby making it a saturated fat and solid at room temperature

cholesterol

fatlike substance that is a constituent of body cells; is synthesized in the liver; also available in animal foods

hypercholesterolemia

unusually high levels of cholesterol in blood; also known as *high serum cholesterol*

atherosclerosis

a form of arteriosclerosis affecting the intima (inner lining) of the artery walls

plaque

fatty deposit on interior of artery walls

TABLE 5-3 Fat and Cholesterol Content of Some Common Foods

FOOD	AMOUNT	SATURATED FAT (g)	CHOLESTEROL (Mg)	TOTAL FAT (g)	TOTAL KCAL
Creamed cottage cheese (4% fat)	1 cup	6.4	34	10	235
Uncreamed cottage cheese (0.5% fat)	1 cup	0.4	10	1	125
Cream cheese	1 oz	6.2	31	10	100
Swiss cheese	1 oz	5.0	26	8	105
American processed cheese	1 oz	5.6	27	9	105
Half & half	1 Tbsp.	1.1	6	2	20
Heavy cream	1 Tbsp.	3.5	21	6	54
Nondairy creamer	1 Tbsp.	1.4	0	1	20
Whole milk	1 cup	5.1	33	8	150
Reduced-fat milk	1 cup	2.9	18	5	120
Low-fat milk	1 cup	1.6	10	3	100
Fat-free milk	1 cup	0.3	4	trace	85
Chocolate milk shake	10 oz	4.8	30	8	335
Ice cream (11% fat)	½ cup	8.9	59	14	270
Soft ice milk	1 cup	2.9	13	5	225
Egg	1	1.7	274	6	80
Butter	1 Tbsp.	7.1	31	11	100
Margarine	1 Tbsp.	2.2	0	11	100
Corn oil	1 Tbsp.	1.8	0	14	125
Crabmeat (canned)	1 cup	0.5	135	3	135
Salmon (canned)	3 oz	0.9	34	5	120
Shrimp (canned)	3 oz	0.2	128	1	100
Tuna					
Water-packed	3 oz	0.3	48	1	135
Oil-packed	3 oz	1.4	55	7	165
Avocado	½	2.2	0	15	150
Bagel	1	0.3	0	2	200
Doughnut	1	2.8	20	12	210
English muffin	1	0.3	0	1	140
Peanuts (dry roasted)	1 oz	2.0	0	15	170
Ground beef (lean)	3 oz	6.2	74	16	230
Roast beef (lean)	4.4 oz	7.2	100	18	300
Leg lamb (lean)	5.2 oz	4.8	130	12	280
Leg lamb (lean and fat)	6 oz	11.2	156	26	410
Bacon	3 slices	3.3	16	9	110
Pork chop (lean)	5 oz	5.2	142	16	330
Frankfurter	1.5 oz	4.8	23	13	145
Chicken leg, fried (meat and skin)	5 oz	6.0	124	22	390
Chicken leg, roasted (meat only)	3.2 oz	1.4	82	4	150

Source: Adapted from *Nutritive Value of Foods,* USDA Home & Garden Bulletin No. 72, 1981.

because the cholesterol binds to the fiber and is eliminated via the feces, thus preventing it from being absorbed in the small intestine. In some cases, medication may be prescribed if diet, weight loss, and exercise do not sufficiently lower serum cholesterol.

Because the development of plaque is cumulative, the preferred means of avoiding or at least limiting its development is to limit cholesterol and fat intake throughout life. If children are not fed high-cholesterol foods on a regular basis, their chances of overusing them as adults are reduced. Thus, their risk of heart attack and stroke is also reduced. It is recommended that daily cholesterol intake not exceed 300 mg.

DIGESTION AND ABSORPTION

Although 95% of ingested fats are digested, it is a complex process. The chemical digestion of fats occurs mainly in the small intestine. Fats are not digested in the mouth. They are digested only slightly in the stomach, where gastric lipase acts on emulsified fats such as those found in cream and egg yolk. Fats must be mixed well with the gastric juices before entering the small intestine. In the small intestine, bile emulsifies the fats, and the enzyme pancreatic lipase reduces them to fatty acids and glycerol, which the body subsequently absorbs through villi (Figure 5-3).

Lipoproteins

lipoproteins
carriers of fat in the blood

Fats are insoluble in water, which is the main component of blood. Therefore, special carriers must be provided for the fats to be absorbed and transported by the blood to body cells. In the initial stages of absorption, bile joins with the products of fat digestion to carry fat. Later, protein combines with the final products of fat digestion to form special carriers called **lipoproteins**. The lipoproteins subsequently carry the fats to the body cells by way of the blood.

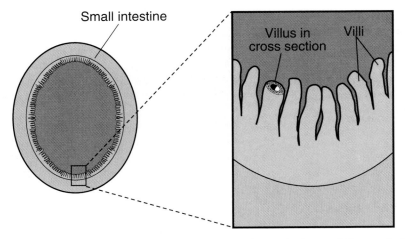

FIGURE 5-3 The body absorbs fatty acids and glycerol through the villi of the small intestine.

Lipoproteins are classified as chylomicrons, very-low-density lipoprotein (VLDL), low-density lipoprotein (LDL), and high-density lipoprotein (HDL), according to their mobility and density. Chylomicrons are the first lipoprotein identified after eating. It is the largest lipoprotein and the lightest in weight. It is composed of 80 to 90% triglycerides. Lipoprotein lipase acts to break down the triglycerides into free fatty acids and glycerol. Without this enzyme, fat could not get into the cells.

Very-low-density lipoproteins are made primarily by the liver cells and are composed of 55 to 65% triglycerides. They carry triglycerides and other lipids to all cells. As the VLDL lose triglycerides, they pick up cholesterol from other lipoproteins in the blood and they then become LDL. Low-density lipoproteins are approximately 45% cholesterol with few triglycerides. They carry most of the blood cholesterol from the liver to the cells. Elevated blood levels greater than 130 mg/dl of LDL are thought to be contributing factors in atherosclerosis. Low-density lipoprotein is sometimes termed *bad cholesterol*.

High-density lipoproteins carry cholesterol from the cells to the liver for eventual excretion. Levels of HDL greater than 35 mg/dl are thought to reduce the risk of heart disease. High-density lipoproteins are sometimes called *good cholesterol*. Exercise, maintaining a desirable weight, and giving up smoking are all ways to increase one's HDL.

chylomicron

largest lipoprotein; transports lipids after digestion into the body

very-low-density lipoproteins (VLDLs)

lipoproteins made by the liver to transport lipids throughout the body

low-density lipoproteins (LDLs)

carry blood cholesterol to the cells

high-density lipoproteins (HDLs)

lipoproteins that carry cholesterol from cells to the liver for eventual excretion

METABOLISM AND ELIMINATION

The liver controls fat metabolism. It hydrolyzes triglycerides and forms new ones from this hydrolysis as needed. Ultimately, the metabolism of fats occurs in the cells, where fatty acids are broken down to carbon dioxide and water, releasing energy. The portion of fat that is not needed for immediate use is stored as adipose tissue. Carbon dioxide and water are waste products that are removed from the body by the circulatory, respiratory, and excretory systems.

FATS AND THE CONSUMER

Fats continue to be of particular interest to the consumer. Most people know that fats are high-calorie foods and that they are related to heart disease. But people who are not in the health field may not know *how* fats affect health. Consequently, they may be easily duped by clever ads for or salespersons of nutritional supplements or new "health food" products.

It is important that the health care professional carefully evaluate any new dietary "supplement" for which a nutrition claim is made. If the item is not included in the Recommended Dietary Allowances, it is safe to assume that medical research has not determined that it is essential. Ingestion of dietary supplements of unknown value could, ironically, be damaging to one's health.

Lecithin

Lecithin is a fatty substance classified as a phospholipid. It is found in both plant and animal foods and is synthesized in the liver. It is a natural emulsifier that helps transport fat in the bloodstream. It is used commercially to make food products smooth.

Lecithin supplements have been promoted by some health food salespersons as being able to prevent cardiovascular disease. To date, this has not been scientifically proven.

Fat Alternatives

Research into fat alternatives has been in progress for decades. Olestra, the newest product on the market, is made from carbohydrates and fat. The Food and Drug Administration (FDA) has approved olestra for use only in snack foods such as potato chips, tortilla chips, and crackers. The government requires that food labels indicate that olestra "inhibits the absorption of some vitamins and other nutrients." Therefore, the fat-soluble vitamins A, D, E, and K have been added to foods containing olestra. Olestra contains no calories, but it can cause cramps and diarrhea. The products manufactured with olestra should be used in moderation.

Simplesse is made from either egg white or milk protein and contains 1.3 kcal/g. Simplesse can be used only in cold foods because it becomes thick or gels when heated. Simplesse is not available for home use.

Oatrim is carbohydrate-based and is derived from oat fiber. Oatrim is heat-stable and can be used in baking but not in frying. Manufacturers have used carbohydrate-based compounds for years as thickeners. Oatrim does provide calories, but significantly less than fat.

The long-term effects these products may have on human health and nutrition are unknown. If they are used in the way the U.S. population uses artificial sweeteners, they probably will not reduce the actual fat content in the diet. They may simply be additions to it. One concern among nutritionists is that they will be used in place of nutritious food that, in addition to fat, also provides vitamins, minerals, proteins, and carbohydrates.

DIETARY REQUIREMENTS

Although no specific dietary requirement for fats is included in the RDAs (see the inside front cover), deficiency symptoms do occur when fats provide less than 10% of the total daily kcal requirement. When gross deficiency occurs, eczema (inflamed and scaly skin condition) can develop. This has been observed in infants who were fed formulas lacking the essential fatty acid linoleic acid and in patients maintained for long periods on intravenous feedings that lack linoleic acid. Also, growth may be retarded, and weight loss can occur when diets are seriously deficient in fats.

On the other hand, excessive fat in the diet can lead to overweight or heart disease. In addition, studies point to an association between high-fat diets and cancers of the colon, breast, uterus, and prostate.

The Food and Nutrition Board's Committee on Diet and Health recommends that people reduce their fat intake to 30% of total kcal. No more than 10% of total kcal should be provided by saturated fats. The National Research Council in its 1989 edition of the RDAs states that 36% of kcal in current U.S. diets are derived from fats.

CONSIDERATIONS FOR THE HEALTH CARE PROFESSIONAL

Because of the attention fats receive in the media and the common concern about heart disease and overweight, many patients have opinions about them. Some are factually correct; many are not. Obviously, it is especially important that the health care professional be able to explain accurately, but simply, the possible damage from too much fat in the diet.

To accomplish dietary change, the health care professional should review patients' usual diets *with* them. Changes then can be introduced clearly, sensitively, and with the patients' active participation. Unless patients understand *why* dietary changes are needed and want to make them, they are unlikely to change their diets.

● SUMMARY

In addition to providing an important source of energy, fats carry essential fatty acids and fat-soluble vitamins, protect organs and bones, insulate from cold, and provide satiety to meals. They are composed of carbon, hydrogen, and oxygen and are found in both animal and plant foods. Each gram of fats provides 9 kcal. Digestion of fats occurs mainly in the small intestine, where they are reduced to fatty acids and glycerol. An excess of fat in the diet can result in obesity and possibly heart disease or cancer.

● DISCUSSION TOPICS

1. Why are fats considered a more concentrated source of energy than carbohydrates?

2. Of what value are fats to the body? List some foods rich in fats. Identify them as animal foods or plant foods. Identify them as saturated or polyunsaturated.

3. Discuss adipose tissue. Is it good? Is it bad? Explain.

4. Describe atherosclerosis. It is said that its effects are cumulative. Explain.

5. Discuss saturated fats and cholesterol. Point out the differences, and explain why patients are often confused by them.

6. What are organ meats? Why might it be unwise to eat them several times a week?

7. Describe the digestion and metabolism of fats. What are the end products of fat digestion?

8. Why might a patient on a low-fat diet complain? How might the health care professional be helpful in such a case?

9. What are hydrogenated fats? Are they polyunsaturated? Explain.

10. Why is there a greater danger of excess fat in the U.S. diet than a deficiency of fat?

11. Discuss invisible fats and their potential impact on low-fat diets.

12. What are the probable reasons that ω-3 fatty acid capsules and lecithin have become so popular with the general public?

● SUGGESTED ACTIVITIES

1. Using Table A-4 in the appendix, make a list of foods containing saturated fats. Make a parallel list of foods containing large amounts of cholesterol. Compare them. Suggest substitutes for those containing large amounts of saturated fats and those containing large amounts of cholesterol.

2. Using no fat, fry an egg in a pan that has been coated to prevent foods from sticking to it. Fry another egg, using fat. Taste and compare them for flavor and appearance.

3. Role-play a situation between a health care professional and a teenage girl who refuses to eat anything she thinks contains fats.

4. List the foods you ate yesterday. Circle those containing visible fats. Underline those containing invisible fats. Explain why some foods are both circled and underlined. Revise it, making it appropriate for someone on a limited-fat diet.

5. Role-play a scene in which a cantankerous patient who is recovering from a heart attack is complaining to the nurse about her or his low-fat diet, saying she or he "can't eat anything good anymore."

6. Visit a health food store and ask for brochures and descriptions of their products intended to prevent heart disease. Evaluate them in class.

7. Using a cookbook, review recipes for baked products and answer the following questions about them.
   a. Why do bagels contain no cholesterol?
   b. Why does angel cake contain no cholesterol?
   c. Why does a doughnut contain cholesterol when an English muffin does not?
   d. Why does French toast contain cholesterol when the white bread it is made from may not?
   e. Why does lemon meringue pie filling contain cholesterol when apple pie filling does not?
   f. Why does a cheeseburger contain more cholesterol than a hamburger?

8. Write down five typical meals in your family's diet—one breakfast, one lunch, one dinner, and two snacks. How could you modify them to reduce the fat content?

● REVIEW

Multiple choice. Select the *letter* that precedes the best answer.

1. Fats provide the most concentrated form of
   a. carbon   c. lipase
   b. oxygen   d. energy

2. Fats are essential because they are carriers of
   a. water-soluble vitamins   c. bile
   b. fatty acids   d. plaque

3. Adipose tissue is useful because it
   a. can synthesize triglycerides
   b. prevents eczema
   c. provides satiety
   d. protects and insulates

4. Atherosclerosis is thought to contribute to
   a. cancer   c. heart attacks
   b. plaque   d. hypercholesterolemia

5. A diet grossly deficient in fats may be deficient in
   a. lipase   c. cholesterol
   b. linoleic acid   d. all of the above

6. Invisible fats can be found in
   a. cake and cookies   c. egg white and skim milk
   b. orange and tomato juice   d. lettuce and tomatoes

7. Plant foods that contain saturated fats are
   a. olives and avocados   c. corn and soybeans
   b. coconut and chocolate   d. none of the above

8. When a polyunsaturated vegetable oil is changed to a saturated fat, the process is called
   a. hydrolysis   c. hydrogenation
   b. hypercholesterolemia   d. none of the above

9. Linoleic acid is one of the fatty acids that is known to be
   a. a triglyceride   c. monounsaturated
   b. saturated   d. essential to the human diet

10. Cholesterol
   a. is not essential to the human diet
   b. is thought to contribute to atherosclerosis
   c. is not found in animal foods
   d. all of the above

11. Another name for fats and fatlike substances is
   a. lipase   c. lipoproteins
   b. lipidemia   d. lipids

12. Three groups of lipids found naturally in the human body and in food are triglycerides, phospholipids, and
   a. cortisone   c. sterols
   b. steroids   d. hydrogenated fats

13. Fatty acids are organic compounds of carbon atoms and
   a. hydrogen atoms   c. triglycerides
   b. arachidonic acids   d. glycerol

14. Classification of fatty acids can be determined by
   a. the number of triglycerides they contain
   b. their degree of saturation with hydrogen atoms
   c. the amount of carbon each contains
   d. the grams of cholesterol in each

15. Cholesterol
   a. is found in both plants and vegetables
   b. is found only in plants
   c. does not contribute in any way to heart disease
   d. is a sterol

16. Lipoproteins
   a. can substitute for other proteins in the diet
   b. carry fats to body cells via the blood
   c. are the same as triglycerides
   d. carry proteins throughout the body

17. HDL (high-density lipoprotein)
   a. is sometimes called good cholesterol
   b. carries lipids to the cells
   c. is the same as lipase
   d. levels should be less than 35 mg/dl of human blood

18. For digestion, fats require the help of gastric lipase,
   a. bile, and fatty acids
   b. bile, and pancreatic lipase
   c. pancreatic lipase, and glycerol
   d. cholesterol, and bile

19. VLDL (very-low-density lipoprotein)
   a. is sometimes called good cholesterol
   b. carries lipids to the cells
   c. is the same as lipase
   d. is interchangeable with cholesterol

20. Fat alternatives
   a. include Oatrim, olestra, and lecithin
   b. are the nutritional equal of margarine
   c. may inhibit the absorption of some vitamins
   d. will definitely reduce the total daily calorie intake of anyone who uses them

C A S E   S T U D Y

Jim B. is a 45-year-old business executive who plays tennis about three times a week on his lunch hour. He is married and has three teenagers. He visited his doctor recently because he had burning in his chest the last two times he played tennis. This scared him.

The doctor did a physical exam and had blood drawn, including a lipid profile. He ran an electrocardiogram. Jim was about 15 pounds overweight. The doctor told him it looked as if he had a mild form of angina pectoris. The doctor explained that this was his heart's way of telling him that it needed more oxygen during exercise. The rest of the test results would be available in about a week. In the meantime, the doctor recommended only walking for Jim. If Jim had any chest pain or shortness of breath while walking, he was to sit down immediately and rest.

The tests revealed that Jim had a cholesterol level of 340 mg/dl, an LDL level of 200 mg/dl, and an HDL level of 22 mg/dl. The doctor referred him to the cardiac education program for diet education and fitness assessment. The doctor wanted Jim to reduce his intake of saturated fats and cholesterol. Jim met with the cardiac dietitian.

ASSESSMENT

1. What data do you have about Jim?
2. As the dietitian, what conclusion can you draw from Jim's lab results?
3. What do you need to know about his current eating habits?
4. What do you need to know about how he learns?

DIAGNOSIS

5. What may have caused Jim's elevated cholesterol and LDL?
6. Complete the statement. Jim's lipid profile can be improved by _____.

PLAN/GOAL

7. What two goals do you have for Jim?

IMPLEMENTATION

8. What topics do you need to cover related to dietary fats?
9. Name three cooking methods that would help decrease saturated fats.
10. Who else should be in the class with Jim?
11. What agencies or resources could you provide to support Jim at home?

After 4 months on the low-fat low-cholesterol diet, Jim has an appointment with his doctor.

EVALUATION/OUTCOME CRITERIA

12. What can the doctor measure to determine the effectiveness of the plan?
13. What can Jim provide to demonstrate his compliance with the plan?

C A S E   S T U D Y

Karen is a 30-year-old female who just had her third child. Alyssa is now 6 months old and weaned from breastfeeding. Karen is anxious to lose the rest of the 30 pounds she gained during this last pregnancy. She soaked up all the weight-loss advice from the other new moms. She tried the liquid weight-loss drinks available in the grocery, but she was always hungry and gained 3 pounds! She tried the grapefruit diet the neighbor raved about, but she got bored with the same food. She saw a TV program that promised quick weight loss with diet pills when combined with a low-fat diet. Karen reasoned that if low fat was the key, she would just cut her fat intake to 10% of her total kcal, and the weight should fall off.

ASSESSMENT

1. What data do you currently have about Karen?

2. What has contributed to her current problem?

3. Is this an unusual problem for a mother of three?

4. What do you know about Karen's personality?

DIAGNOSIS

5. What is the cause of Karen's weight gain?

6. What would be the most nutritious way to lose weight?

PLAN/GOAL

7. What is a reasonable, measurable goal for Karen and her weight-loss problem?

IMPLEMENTATION

8. What is the recommended rate of weight loss?

9. What is the recommended percentage of fat in the diet during weight loss?

10. What else can Karen do besides modify her diet?

11. Given your assessment data, would you recommend that Karen diet alone or in a group?

12. What other resources can be helpful to Karen?

EVALUATION/OUTCOME CRITERIA

13. How often should Karen weigh herself?

14. What other signs will indicate that she is losing weight?

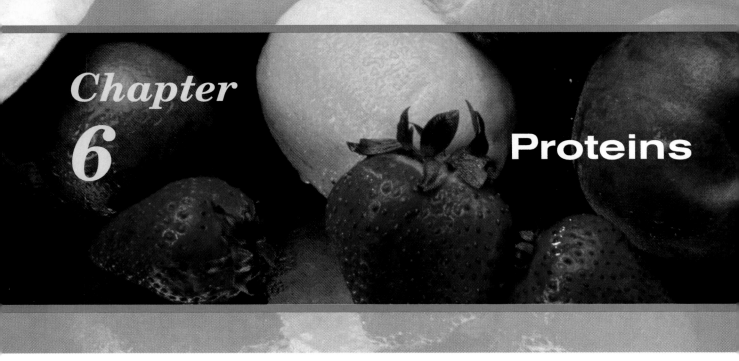

Chapter 6

Proteins

Key Terms

albumin
amino acids
carboxypeptidase
chymotrypsin
complete proteins
incomplete proteins
kwashiorkor
marasmus
mental retardation
negative nitrogen balance
nitrogen
nitrogen balance
pepsin
physical trauma
polypeptides
positive nitrogen balance
protein
protein energy malnutrition (PEM)
trypsin

Objectives

After studying this chapter, you should be able to:

● State the functions of proteins in the body

● Identify the elements of which proteins are composed

● Describe the effects of protein deficiency

● State the energy yield of proteins

● Identify at least six food sources of complete proteins and six food sources of incomplete proteins

Body cells are constantly wearing out. As a result, they are continuously in need of replacement. Of the six nutrient groups, only proteins can make new cells and rebuild tissue.

Proteins are the basic material of every body cell. By the age of 4 years, body protein content reaches the adult level of about 18% of body weight. Obviously, an adequate supply of proteins in the daily diet is essential for normal growth and development and for the maintenance of health. Proteins are appropriately named. The word **protein** is of Greek derivation and means "of first importance."

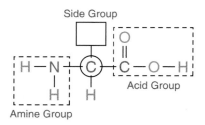

FIGURE 6-1 All amino acids have a chemical backbone of a carbon atom; an amine group, which contains nitrogen; an acid group; and a side group. It is the chemical structure of the side group that gives each amino acid its unique identity.

protein
the only one of six essential nutrients containing nitrogen

nitrogen
chemical element found in protein; essential to life

amino acids
nitrogen-containing chemical compounds of which protein is composed

complete proteins
proteins that contain all nine essential amino acids

incomplete proteins
proteins that do not contain all of the nine essential amino acids

COMPOSITION

Like carbohydrates and fats, proteins contain carbon, hydrogen, and oxygen, but in different proportions. In addition, and most important, they are the only nutrient group that contains **nitrogen**, and some contain sulfur.

Proteins are composed of chemical compounds called **amino acids** (Figure 6-1). Amino acids are sometimes called the building blocks of protein because they are combined to form the thousands of proteins in the human body. Heredity determines the specific types of proteins within each person.

CLASSIFICATION

The quality and classification of a protein depend on the number and types of amino acids it contains. There are 20 amino acids, but only 9 are considered essential to humans (Table 6-1). Essential amino acids are necessary for normal growth and development and must be provided in the diet. Proteins containing all the essential amino acids are of high biologic value and are called **complete proteins** (high quality). The nonessential amino acids can be produced in the body if an adequate supply of amino nitrogen is provided in the diet.

Incomplete proteins (low quality) are those that lack one or more of the essential amino acids. Consequently, incomplete proteins

TABLE 6-1 Amino Acids

ESSENTIAL		NONESSENTIAL	
Histidine	Phenylalanine	Alanine	Glutamine
Isoleucine	Treonine	Arginine	Glycine
Leucine	Tryptophan	Asparagine	Hydroxyproline
Lysine	Valine	Aspartic acid	Proline
Methionine		Cysteine	Serine
		Cystine	Tyrosine
		Glutamic acid	

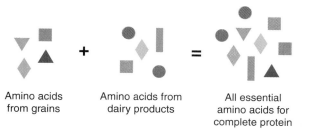

Amino acids from grains + Amino acids from dairy products = All essential amino acids for complete protein

FIGURE 6-2 Two different foods (e.g., grains and dairy products) alone may not provide all the essential amino acids. Combined, however, they form a complete protein and therefore are considered complementary.

TABLE 6-2 Examples of Complementary Protein Foods

Corn	and	Beans
Rice	and	Beans
Bread	and	Peanut butter
Bread	and	Split pea soup
Bread	and	Cheese
Bread	and	Baked beans
Macaroni	and	Cheese
Cereal	and	Milk

cannot build tissue without the help of other proteins. The value of each is increased when it is eaten in combination with another incomplete protein, not necessarily at the same meal, but during the same day. In this way, one incomplete protein food can provide the essential amino acids the other lacks. The combination may thereby provide all nine essential amino acids (Figure 6-2). When this occurs, the proteins are called complementary proteins (Table 6-2). Gelatin is the only protein from an animal source that is an incomplete protein.

FOOD SOURCES

Proteins are found in both animal and plant foods (Table 6-3). The animal food sources provide the highest quality, or complete, proteins. They include meats, fish, poultry, eggs, milk, and cheese.

Despite the high biologic value of proteins from animal food sources, they also provide saturated fats and cholesterol. Consequently, complete proteins should be carefully selected from low-fat animal foods such as fish, lean meats, and low-fat dairy products. Eggs should be limited to two or three a week.

Proteins found in plant foods are incomplete proteins and are of a lower quality than those found in animal foods. Even so, plant foods are important sources of protein. Examples of plant foods containing protein are corn, grains, nuts, sunflower seeds, sesame seeds, and legumes such as soybeans, navy beans, pinto beans, split peas, chickpeas, and peanuts.

TABLE 6-3 Rich Sources of Proteins

COMPLETE PROTEINS		INCOMPLETE PROTEINS	
Meats	Eggs	Corn	Grains
Fish	Milk	Peanuts	Nuts
Poultry	Cheese	Peas	Sunflower seeds
		Navy beans	Sesame seeds
		Soybeans	

Plant proteins can be used to produce textured soy protein and tofu, also called analogues. Meat alternatives (analogues) made from soybeans contain soy protein and other ingredients mixed together to simulate various kinds of meat. Meat alternatives may be canned, dried, or frozen. Analogues are excellent sources of protein, iron, and B vitamins.

Tofu is a soft cheeselike food made from soy milk. Tofu is a bland product that easily absorbs the flavors of other ingredients with which it is cooked. Tofu is rich in high-quality proteins and B vitamins, and it is low in sodium. Textured soy protein and tofu are both economical and nutritious meat replacements.

FUNCTIONS

Proteins build and repair body tissue, play major roles in regulating various body functions, and provide energy if there is insufficient carbohydrate and fat in the diet.

Building and Repairing Body Tissue

The primary function of proteins is to build and repair body tissues. This is made possible by the provision of the correct type and number of amino acids in the diet. Also, as cells are broken down during metabolism (catabolism), some amino acids released into the blood are recycled to build new and repair other tissue (anabolism). The body uses the recycled amino acids as efficiently as those obtained from the diet.

Regulating Body Functions

Proteins are important components of hormones and enzymes that are essential for the regulation of metabolism and digestion. Proteins help maintain fluid and electrolyte balances in the body and thus prevent edema (abnormal retention of body fluids). Proteins also are essential for the development of antibodies and, consequently, for a healthy immune system.

Providing Energy

Proteins can provide energy if and when the supply of carbohydrates and fats in the diet is insufficient. Each gram of protein provides 4 kcal. This is not a good use of proteins, however. In general, they are more expensive than carbohydrates, and most of the complete proteins also contain saturated fats and cholesterol.

pepsin
an enzyme secreted by the stomach that is essential for the digestion of proteins

polypeptides
ten or more amino acids bonded together

DIGESTION AND ABSORPTION

The mechanical digestion of protein begins in the mouth, where the teeth grind the food into small pieces. Chemical digestion begins in the stomach. Hydrochloric acid prepares the stomach so that the enzyme pepsin can begin its task of reducing proteins to polypeptides.

After the polypeptides reach the small intestine, three pancreatic enzymes (**trypsin**, **chymotrypsin**, and **carboxypeptidase**) continue chemical digestion. Intestinal peptidases finally reduce the proteins to amino acids.

After digestion, the amino acids in the small intestine are absorbed by the villi and are carried by the blood to all body tissues. There, they are used to form needed proteins.

METABOLISM AND ELIMINATION

All essential amino acids must be present to build and repair the cells as needed. When amino acids are broken down, the nitrogen-containing amine group is stripped off. This process is called deamination. Deamination produces ammonia, which is released into the bloodstream by the cells. The liver picks up the ammonia, converts it to urea, and returns it to the bloodstream for the kidneys to filter out and excrete. The remaining parts are used for energy or are converted to carbohydrate or fat and stored as glycogen or adipose tissue.

DIETARY REQUIREMENTS

One's protein requirement is determined by size, age, sex, and physical and emotional conditions. A large person has more body cells to maintain than a small person. A growing child, a pregnant woman, or a woman who is breastfeeding needs more protein for each pound of body weight than the average adult. When digestion is inefficient, fewer amino acids are absorbed by the body, consequently the protein requirement is higher. This is sometimes thought to be the case with the elderly. Extra proteins are usually required after surgery, severe burns, or during infections in order to replace lost tissue and to manufacture antibodies. In addition, emotional trauma can cause the body to excrete more nitrogen than it normally does, thus increasing the need for protein foods.

The National Research Council of the National Academy of Sciences considers the average adult's daily requirement to be 0.8g of protein for each kilogram of body weight. To determine your requirement:

1. Divide body weight by 2.2 (the number of pounds per kilogram)

2. Multiply the answer obtained in number 1 by 0.8 (g of protein per kilogram of body weight)

The National Research Council's 1989 chart of Recommended Dietary Allowances (RDAs) of protein for average groups of people is shown in Table 6-4. Table 6-5 provides an idea of the amount of protein in an average day's diet. (For specific amounts of protein in other foods, refer to Table A-3 in the appendix.)

trypsin
pancreatic enzyme; helps digest proteins

chymotrypsin
pancreatic enzyme necessary for the digestion of proteins

carboxypeptidase
pancreatic enzyme necessary for protein digestion

TABLE 6-4 Recommended Dietary Allowances of Protein

CATEGORY	AGE (YEARS) OR CONDITION	WEIGHT (kg)	WEIGHT (lb)	HEIGHT (cm)	HEIGHT (in)	PROTEIN (g)
Infants	0.0–0.5	6	13	60	24	13
	0.5–1.0	9	20	71	28	14
Children	1–3	13	29	90	35	16
	4–6	20	44	112	44	24
	7–10	28	62	132	52	28
Males	11–14	45	99	157	62	45
	15–18	66	145	176	69	59
	19–24	72	160	177	70	58
	25–50	79	174	176	70	63
	51+	77	170	173	68	63
Females	11–14	46	101	157	62	46
	15–18	55	120	163	64	44
	19–24	58	128	164	65	46
	25–50	63	138	163	64	50
	51+	65	143	160	63	50
Pregnant						60
Lactating	1st 6 months					65
	2nd 6 months					62

Reprinted with permission from *Recommended Dietary Allowances: 10th Edition.*
Copyright 1989 by the National Academy of Sciences. Courtesy of the National
Academy Press, Washington, D.C.

Protein Excess

It is easy for people living in the developed parts of the world to ingest more protein than the body requires. There are a number of reasons why this should be avoided. The saturated fats and cholesterol common to complete protein foods may contribute to heart disease and provide more kcal than are desirable. Some studies seem to indicate a connection between long-term high-protein diets and colon cancer and high calcium excretion, which depletes the bones of calcium and may contribute to osteoporosis. People who eat excessive amounts of protein-rich foods may ignore the also essential fruits and vegetables, and excess protein intake may put more demands on the kidneys than they are prepared to handle. Therefore, the National Research Council recommends that protein intake represent no more than 15% to 20% of one's daily kcal intake and not exceed double the amount given in the table of Recommended Dietary Allowances (Table 6-4).

Protein and Amino Acid Supplements

Protein and amino acid supplements are taken for a number of reasons such as "bulking up" by athletes, growing fingernails, and to spare body

TABLE 6-5 Protein in an Average Diet for One Day

	SERVING SIZE	PROTEIN (g)	KCAL
Breakfast			
Orange juice	½ cup	1	45
Cornflakes	¾ cup	1	75
with sugar	2 tsp.		30
Toast	2 slices	4	140
Butter	1 Tbsp.		65
Jelly	1 Tbsp.		60
Fat-free milk	½ cup	4	50
Lunch			
Grapefruit juice	½ cup	1	50
Tuna salad sandwich	⅔ cup tuna salad	20	220
on bread with lettuce	2 slices bread	4	140
Carrot sticks	1 carrot	1	25
Canned pears	½ cup	1	100
Oatmeal cookies	2	1	160
Fat-free milk	1 cup	8	100
Dinner			
Chicken breast	3 oz.	26	160
Baked potato	1	4	145
Asparagus	½ cup		25
Sliced tomato salad	1 tomato	1	25
Roll	1	2	100
with butter	1 Tbsp.		65
Ice cream	⅔ cup	3	200
Fat-free milk	1 cup	8	100
		90	2,080

protein in weight loss. It is weight lifting, not protein bars or protein supplements, that builds muscles. Fingernails have never been affected by extra protein, and dieters need a balanced diet using the guidelines of the Food Guide Pyramid.

High-quality protein foods are more bioavailable than expensive supplements are. Single amino acids can be harmful to the body and never occur naturally in food. The body was designed to handle food, not supplements. If a single amino acid has been recommended, it is very important that a physician be consulted before the amino acid is used.

Nitrogen Balance

Protein requirements may be discussed in terms of **nitrogen balance**. This occurs when nitrogen intake equals the amount of nitrogen ex-

nitrogen balance
when nitrogen intake equals nitrogen excreted

positive nitrogen balance

nitrogen intake exceeds outgo

physical trauma

extreme physical stress

negative nitrogen balance

more nitrogen lost than taken in

albumin

protein that occurs in blood plasma

protein energy malnutrition (PEM)

protein energy malnutrition; marasmus

marasmus

severe wasting caused by lack of protein and all nutrients or faulty absorption; PEM

kwashiorkor

deficiency disease caused by extreme lack of protein

mental retardation

below normal intellectual capacity

creted. Positive nitrogen balance exists when nitrogen intake exceeds the amount excreted. This indicates that new tissue is being formed, and it occurs during pregnancy, during children's growing years, when athletes develop additional muscle tissue, and when tissues are rebuilt after physical trauma such as illness or injury. Negative nitrogen balance indicates that protein is being lost. It may be caused by fevers, injury, surgery, burns, starvation, or immobilization.

Protein Deficiency

When people are unable to obtain an adequate supply of protein for an extended period, muscle wasting will occur, and arms and legs become very thin. At the same time, albumin (protein in blood plasma) deficiency will cause edema, resulting in an extremely swollen appearance. The water is excreted when sufficient protein is eaten. People may lose appetite, strength, and weight, and wounds may heal very slowly. Patients suffering from edema become lethargic and depressed. These signs are seen in grossly neglected children or in the elderly poor or incapacitated. It is essential that people following vegetarian diets carefully calculate the types and amount of protein in their diets so as to avoid protein deficiency.

Protein Energy Malnutrition (PEM)

People suffering from protein energy malnutrition (PEM) lack both protein and energy-rich foods. Such a condition is not uncommon in developing countries where there are long-term shortages of both protein and energy foods. Children who lack sufficient protein do not grow to their potential size. Infants born to mothers eating insufficient protein during pregnancy can have permanently impaired mental capacities.

Two deficiency diseases that affect children are caused by a grossly inadequate supply of protein or energy, or both. Marasmus, a condition resulting from severe malnutrition, afflicts very young children who lack both energy and protein foods as well as vitamins and minerals. The infant with marasmus appears emaciated, but does not have edema. Hair is dull and dry, and the skin is thin and wrinkled (Figure 6-3). The other protein deficiency disease that affects children as well as adults is kwashiorkor (Figure 6-4). Kwashiorkor appears when there is a sudden or recent lack of protein-containing food (such as during a famine). This disease causes fat to accumulate in the liver, and the lack of protein and hormones results in edema, painful skin lesions, and changes in the pigmentation of skin and hair. The mortality rate for kwashiorkor patients is high.

Those who survive these deficiency diseases may suffer from permanent mental retardation. The ultimate cost of food deprivation among young children is high, indeed.

Table 6-6 lists some signs that help distinguish marasmus from kwashiorkor.

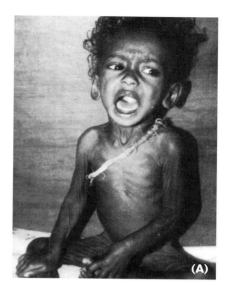
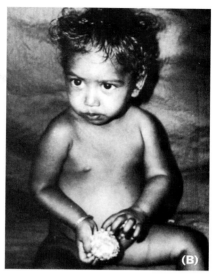

FIGURE 6-3 A child with marasmus may not recover completely but is greatly helped by nutritional therapy. (A) Visible signs of marasmus include extreme wasting, wrinkled skin, and irritability. (B) After 4½ months of nutritional therapy, the same child shows improvement. (Courtesy of the World Health Organization)

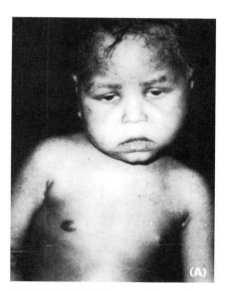
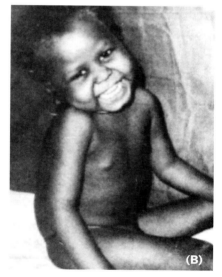

FIGURE 6-4 Effects of kwashiorkor can be partly eliminated by putting protein back into the diet. (A) Edema, skin lesions, and hair changes are common signs of kwashiorkor. (B) Only one month after receiving a proper diet, the child's hunger, discomfort, and visible signs of disease are greatly reduced. (Courtesy of the World Health Organization)

TABLE 6-6 Differentiating Marasmus and Kwashiorkor

MARASMUS	KWASHIORKOR
Total surface fat (TSF)* and midarm circumference (MAC) decreased	TSF and MAC within normal limits
Weight decreased	Weight possibly within normal limits
Visceral proteins (albumin) within normal limits or decreased	Visceral proteins decreased
Immune function within normal limits	Immune function decreased
Dull, dry hair	Reddish color hair
Emaciated, wrinkled appearance	Puffy appearance
Lack of protein and total energy	Edema

* TSF and MAC can be determined by anthropometric measurements (see Chapter 1), which are done by a dietitian. The results are then compared with standard values obtained from measurement of a large number of people.

CONSIDERATIONS FOR THE HEALTH CARE PROFESSIONAL

Proteins have acquired an unfairly high value among the general public in the United States. Also, many people think that proteins are found only in animal food sources. As a result, complete proteins tend to be overused in most diets.

Research about the cumulative effects of the overuse of proteins in the diet is beginning to suggest that excessive use of protein could damage kidneys, and possibly contribute to osteoporosis and cancer, and cause overweight and heart disease.

The health care professional may find that reeducating patients about the need to reduce their protein intake to 15 to 20% of total kcal is a challenging task. Humor and patience combined with suggestions for menus and recipe alterations will all be needed.

● SUMMARY

Proteins contain nitrogen, an element that is necessary for growth and the maintenance of health. In addition to building and repairing body tissues, proteins regulate body processes and can supply energy. Each gram of protein provides 4 kcal. Proteins are composed of amino acids, nine of which are essential for growth and repair of body tissues.

Complete proteins contain all of the essential amino acids and can build tissues. The best sources of complete proteins are animal foods such as meat, fish, poultry, eggs, milk, and cheese. Incomplete proteins do not contain all of the essential amino acids, and two or more of these proteins must be combined in order to build tissues. The best sources of incomplete proteins are legumes, corn, grains, and nuts. The nutritional value of incomplete protein foods can be increased by eating two or more incomplete protein foods during the day. Chemical digestion of proteins occurs in the stomach and small intestine. Proteins are reduced to amino acids and ultimately are absorbed into the blood through the villi in the small intestine.

A severe deficiency of protein in the diet can cause kwashiorkor and can contribute to marasmus in children. Both conditions can result in impaired physical and mental development.

● DISCUSSION TOPICS

1. Why are proteins especially important to children, pregnant women, and people who are ill?

2. Of which elements are proteins composed?

3. What functions do proteins perform in the body?

4. Discuss why it may be unwise to use protein foods as energy foods.

5. Discuss the effects of protein deficiency.

6. Describe the digestion of proteins.

7. Describe the metabolism of proteins.

8. Tell what amino acids are and explain their importance. Tell where they are found.

9. Describe analogue products. If anyone in class has eaten analogue products, ask her or him to describe the taste, color, appearance, and cost of the food.

10. Discuss why foods rich in complete proteins are usually more expensive than foods containing incomplete proteins.

11. Describe complete and incomplete protein foods and name several of each type.

12. Why are complete protein foods also generally rich in saturated fats?

13. What determines protein requirements?

14. Why might someone with a broken hip develop negative nitrogen balance in the hospital?

● SUGGESTED ACTIVITIES

1. Keep a record of the foods you eat in a 24-hour period. Using Table A-4 in the appendix, compute the grams of protein consumed. Did your diet provide the recommended amount of protein as indicated in Table 6-4?

2. Plan a day's menu for yourself. Include foods especially rich in complete proteins.
   a. Alter your planned menu by replacing some of the complete protein foods with those containing incomplete proteins.
   b. Visit a local supermarket and compute the cost of the menu that contains complete proteins. Compute the cost of the menu that contains incomplete proteins. Which is less expensive? Why?

3. Role-play a situation in which a diet counselor attempts to convince a pregnant teenager that she should eat at least two servings of meat, fish, or poultry each day.

4. Write a speech that could be made to a class of 9-year-old children. Explain what proteins are and why foods containing proteins should be eaten every day.

● REVIEW

A. Multiple choice. Select the *letter* that precedes the best answer.

1. The building blocks of proteins are
   a. ascorbic acids   c. nitrogen and sulfur only
   b. amino acids   d. meat and fish

2. Proteins are essential because they are the only nutrient that contains
   a. nitrogen   c. hydrochloric acid
   b. niacin   d. carbon

3. Corn, peas, and beans
   a. are complete protein foods
   b. are incomplete protein foods
   c. contain no protein
   d. lose proteins during cooking

4. A person's daily protein requirement
   a. may be met by use of complementary proteins
   b. can be met only by complete proteins
   c. is not affected by one's age
   d. is difficult to fulfill in the United States

5. Protein deficiency may result in
   a. beriberi   c. edema
   b. goiter   d. leukemia

6. Good sources of complete protein foods are
   a. eggs and ground beef   c. butter and margarine
   b. breads and cereals   d. legumes and nuts

7. One gram of protein provides
   a. 4 kcal   c. 19 kilojoules
   b. 9 kcal   d. 37.8 kilojoules

8. The chemical digestion of protein occurs in
   a. the mouth and stomach
   b. the mouth and small intestine
   c. the stomach and small intestine
   d. all of the above

9. Complete proteins contain all the essential
   a. nutrients   c. amino acids
   b. ascorbic acids   d. kcal

10. The *primary* function of protein is to
   a. build and repair body cells
   b. provide energy
   c. digest minerals and vitamins
   d. none of the above

11. A clinical sign of edema is
   a. severe emaciation
   b. change in hair color
   c. extreme wasting and wrinkled skin
   d. puffy, swollen condition

12. In the stomach, proteins are reduced to
   a. polypeptides   c. analogues
   b. proteases   d. pepsin

13. Once proteins reach the small intestine, chemical digestion continues through the action of
   a. rennin   c. bile
   b. pancreatic enzymes d. hydrochloric acid

14. The process of removing nitrogen from amino acids is called
   a. deamination
   b. creation of negative nitrogen balance
   c. creation of positive nitrogen balance
   d. acidosis

15. It is unwise to regularly ingest excessive amounts of protein because
   a. it can cause positive nitrogen balance
   b. it can contribute to heart disease
   c. it may reduce the work of the kidneys
   d. it may cause uremic poisoning

B. Arrange the following foods into two lists, one containing those that are the best sources of complete proteins and one containing those that are the best sources of incomplete proteins.

   scrambled eggs
   lima beans
   corn on the cob
   hot chocolate milk
   chickpeas and rice
   fat-free milk
   beefburgers
   baked navy beans
   filet of sole
   fried chicken
   peanuts
   Swiss cheese

C A S E   S T U D Y

Edna F. is a 78-year-old female who was in a very serious car accident with her husband, Tom. The emergency medical team had to cut open the car to get them out. Miraculously, Tom had only scrapes and bruises. But Edna suffered bilateral leg fractures, head injury, and internal abdominal injuries. Edna required numerous life-saving surgeries. Although Edna had been seriously injured, the doctors were confident that she would survive.

Initially, Edna was on intravenous feedings of hyperalimentation (see Chapter 20). The hospital dietitian monitored her nutritional status closely. Finally, Edna made the transition to oral nutrition. Edna was going to be hospitalized for at least three more weeks, followed by 6–8 weeks of bed rest for her fractures. She was eating between 40% and 50% of her meals and at times forced herself to eat. The most recent note by the doctor read, "Her wounds are healing but slower than expected." The physical therapist documented, "She can tolerate only 15 minutes of range of motion exercises and complains about being too tired to continue." The dietitian ordered another 48-hour calorie count.

ASSESSMENT

1. What information do you have about Edna and her nutrition?
2. What does the dietitian suspect?
3. What does the doctor suspect?
4. How significant is the problem?
5. If Edna were 5 feet 2 inches tall and weighed 110 pounds before the accident, what would her daily protein requirements be?

DIAGNOSIS

6. What is the cause of Edna's nutrition problem?
7. Write a sentence stating the cause of slow-healing wounds.

PLAN/GOAL

8. What is your goal for Edna?

IMPLEMENTATION

9. What will the calorie count reveal?
10. What do you need to know about Edna's food preferences?
11. What could Tom do to help during meals?
12. What should be the size and frequency of Edna's meals?
13. Should appetite stimulants be used?
14. Should liquid nutritional supplements be used?

EVALUATION/OUTCOME CRITERIA

15. What criteria would the doctor, physical therapist and dietitian use to evaluate the effectiveness of the plan?
16. Would weight gain be an effective criterion? If not, why not?

CASE STUDY

Chad was a football player in middle and high school. He usually played guard or tackle. His coaches had promoted eating more protein during football season, and Chad did. His mom cooked a steak and three or four eggs for breakfast. He ate cheeseburgers and fries almost every day at lunch. Dinner was usually a roast, fried chicken, or a pasta casserole. Occasionally, he ate fish, but it wasn't his favorite. He loved corn on the cob, chili, and baked potatoes. He seldom ate desserts.

During college Chad was injured early in his sophomore season, and he couldn't play football anymore. He retained the same high-protein diet. As a graduating senior planning to seek a job, he was concerned about all the weight he had put on and the loss of energy he felt.

ASSESSMENT

1. What data do you have about Chad's eating habits?

2. What do you know about his ability to develop habits?

3. What's the cause of the problem?

DIAGNOSIS

4. Why is Chad now having problems with healthy eating?

5. What nutrition education does Chad need?

PLAN/GOAL

6. What are two measurable, reasonable goals for Chad?

IMPLEMENTATION

7. After decreasing the percentage of protein, what else does Chad need to decrease?

8. What does he need to add to his diet?

9. Using his preferences, suggest some alternative menus that would help Chad lose weight.

10. What else does Chad need to do to burn calories?

EVALUATION/OUTCOME CRITERIA

11. What criteria would a dietitian use to measure his success?

12. What diseases might Chad avoid by reducing his long-term protein intake?

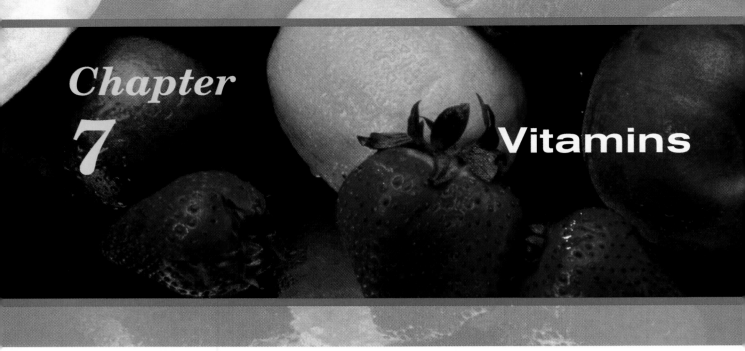

Chapter 7

Vitamins

Key Terms

anencephaly
antioxidant
ascorbic acid
avitaminosis
beriberi
biotin
carotenoid
catalysts
coagulate
cobalamin
coenzymes
collagen
fat-soluble
folate
heme iron
hemolysis
hemorrhage
hormone
hypervitaminosis
International Units
 (IU)

intrinsic factor
megadoses
megaloblastic
 anemia
myelin
neural tube defects
 (NTDs)
niacin
niacin equivalents
 (NE)
nonheme iron
osteomalacia
osteoporosis
pantothenic acid
pellagra
pernicious anemia
precursor
prohormone
provitamin
retinol equivalents
 (RE)

(continued)

Objectives

After studying this chapter, you should be able to:

● State one or more functions of each of the 13 vitamins discussed

● Identify at least two food sources of each of the vitamins discussed

● Identify some symptoms of, or diseases caused by, deficiencies of the vitamins discussed

Vitamins are organic (carbon-containing) compounds that are essential in small amounts for body processes. Vitamins themselves do not provide energy. They enable the body to use the energy provided by fats, carbohydrates, and proteins. The name **vitamin** implies their importance. *Vita* in Latin, means life. They do not, however, represent a panacea (universal remedy) for physical or mental illness or a way to alleviate the stress of modern life. They should not be overused—more is not necessarily better. In fact, **megadoses** can be toxic (poisonous). Normally, a healthy person eating a balanced diet will obtain all the nutrients—including vitamins—needed.

The existence of vitamins has been known since early in the twentieth century. It was discovered that animals fed diets of pure proteins, carbohydrates, fats, and minerals did not thrive as did those fed normal diets that included vitamins.

riboflavin

rickets

scurvy

spina bifida

thiamin

tocopherols

tocotrienols

vitamin

vitamin supplements

water-soluble

xerophthalmia

Vitamins were originally named by letter. Subsequent research has shown that many of the vitamins that were originally thought to be a single substance are actually groups of substances doing similar work in the body. Vitamin B proved to be more than one compound—B_1, B_6, B_{12}, and so on—and consequently is now known as B complex. Many of the 13 known vitamins are currently named according to their chemical composition or function in the body (Table 7-1).

TABLE 7-1 Vitamins

FAT-SOLUBLE (4)	WATER-SOLUBLE (9)	
Vitamin A	Vitamin B complex includes:	
Vitamin D	Thiamin (B_1)	Folate
Vitamin E	Riboflavin (B_2)	Vitamin B_{12} (cobalamin)
Vitamin K	Niacin	Pantothenic acid
	Vitamin B_6	Biotin
	Vitamin C (ascorbic acid)	

Vitamins are found in minute amounts in foods. The specific amounts and types of vitamins in foods vary.

HUMAN REQUIREMENTS

The Food and Nutrition Board of the National Academy of Sciences–National Research Council has prepared a list of RDA (recommended dietary allowances) for those 11 vitamins for which it considers current scientific research adequate for such determinations. (See the table on the inside front cover.) In addition, the board also has prepared a list of estimated safe and adequate daily dietary intakes (ESADDI) of two additional vitamins for which current research is inadequate to allow them to propose RDAs (Table 7-2). Vitamin allowances are given by weight—milligrams (mg) or micrograms (μg or mcg).

Vitamin deficiencies can occur and can result in disease. Persons inclined to vitamin deficiencies because they do not eat balanced diets include alcoholics, the poor and incapacitated elderly, patients with serious diseases that affect appetite, mentally retarded persons, and young children who receive inadequate care. Also, deficiencies of fat-soluble vitamins occur in patients with chronic malabsorption diseases such as cystic fibrosis, celiac disease, and Crohn's disease.

TABLE 7-2 Estimated Safe and Adequate Daily Dietary Intakes of Biotin and Pantothenic Acid

CATEGORY	AGE (YEARS)	BIOTIN (μg)	PANTOTHENIC ACID (mg)
Infants	0–0.5	10	2
	0.5–1.0	15	3
Children and	1–3	20	3
adolescents	4–6	25	3–4
	7–10	30	4–5
	11+	30–100	4–7
Adults		30–100	4–7

Reprinted with permission from *Recommended Dietary Allowances: 10th Edition.* Copyright 1989 by the National Academy of Sciences. Courtesy of the National Academy Press, Washington, D.C.

avitaminosis
without vitamins

hypervitaminosis
condition caused by excessive ingestion of one or more vitamins

vitamin supplements
concentrated forms of vitamins; may be in tablet or liquid form

The term **avitaminosis** means "without vitamins." This word followed by the name of a specific vitamin is used to indicate a serious lack of that particular vitamin. **Hypervitaminosis** is the excess of one or more vitamins. Either a lack or excess of vitamins can be detrimental to a person's health.

Vitamins taken in addition to those received in the diet are called **vitamin supplements**. These are available in concentrated forms in tablets, capsules, and drops. Vitamin concentrates are sometimes termed natural or synthetic (manufactured). Some people believe that a meaningful difference exists between the two types and that the natural are far superior in quality to the synthetic. However, according to the U.S. Food and Drug Administration (FDA), the body cannot distinguish between a vitamin of plant or animal origin and one manufactured in a laboratory, because once they have been dismantled by the digestive system, the two types of the same vitamin are chemically identical.

Synthetic vitamins are frequently added to foods during processing. When this is done, the foods are described as enriched or fortified. Examples of these foods are enriched breads and cereals to which thiamin, niacin, riboflavin, folate, and the mineral iron have been added. Vitamins A and D are added to milk and fortified margarine.

Preserving Vitamin Content in Food

Occasionally, vitamins are lost during food processing. In most cases, food producers can replace these vitamins with synthetic vitamins, making the processed food nutritionally equal to the unprocessed food. Foods in which vitamins have been replaced are called restored foods.

Because some vitamins are easily destroyed by light, air, heat, and water, it is important to know how to preserve the vitamin content of food during its preparation and cooking. Vitamin loss can be avoided by

● Buying the freshest, unbruised vegetables and fruits and using them raw whenever possible

● Preparing fresh vegetables and fruits just before serving

- Heating canned vegetables quickly and in their own liquid
- Following package directions when using frozen vegetables or fruit
- Using as little water as possible when cooking and having it boiling before adding vegetables, or, preferably, steaming them
- Covering the pan (except for the first few minutes when cooking strongly flavored vegetables such as broccoli and cauliflower) and cooking as short a time as possible
- Saving the cooking liquid for later use in soups, stews, and gravies
- Storing fresh vegetables and most fruits in a cool, dark place

CLASSIFICATION

Vitamins are commonly grouped according to solubility. A, D, E, and K are fat-soluble, and B complex and C are water-soluble. In addition, vitamin D is sometimes classified as a hormone and the B-complex group may be classified as catalysts or coenzymes. When a vitamin has different chemical forms but serves the same purpose in the body, these forms are sometimes called vitamers. Vitamin E is an example. Sometimes a precursor, or provitamin, is found in foods. This is a substance from which the body can synthesize (manufacture) a specific vitamin. Carotenoids are examples of precursors of vitamin A, and are referred to as provitamin A.

FAT-SOLUBLE VITAMINS

The fat-soluble vitamins A, D, E, and K are chemically similar. They are not lost easily in cooking, but are lost when mineral oil is ingested. Mineral oil is not absorbed by humans. Consequently, it may be used in salad dressings to avoid the kcal of vegetable oils. It is sometimes used as a laxative by the elderly. Its use should be discouraged because it picks up and carries with it fat-soluble vitamins that are then lost to the body. After absorption, fat-soluble vitamins are transported through the blood by lipoproteins because they are not soluble in water. Excess amounts can be stored in the liver. Therefore, deficiencies of fat-soluble vitamins are slower to appear than are those caused by a lack of water-soluble vitamins. Because of the body's ability to store them, megadoses of fat-soluble vitamins should be avoided as they can reach toxic levels.

Vitamin A

Vitamin A consists of two basic dietary forms: preformed vitamin A, also called retinol, which is the active form of vitamin A; and carotenoids, the inactive form of vitamin A, which are found in plants.

fat-soluble
can be dissolved in fat

water-soluble
can be dissolved in water

hormone
chemical messengers secreted by a variety of glands

catalyst
a substance that causes another substance to react

coenzyme
an active part of an enzyme

precursor
something that comes before something else; in vitamins it is also called a provitamin, something from which the body can synthesize the specific vitamin

provitamin
see precursor

carotenoids
plant pigments, some of which yield vitamin A

Functions. Vitamin A is one of the antioxidant vitamins that protect the cells from destruction by oxygen. Oxygen causes free radicals to form, which damage cell structure and function. Such damage may contribute to some cancers and heart disease. (Free radicals are highly reactive chemical compounds that damage other compounds.)

In addition, Vitamin A is essential for maintaining healthy eyes and skin, for normal growth and reproduction, and for a healthy immune system. It also aids in the prevention of infections by helping to maintain healthy mucous membranes (the lining of the nose and throat, the GI tract, and the genitourinary tract).

Some carotenoids are converted to retinol during absorption in the intestines. Some are converted in the liver after being carried there by the blood, and some are stored in adipose tissue.

Sources. Provitamin A, or beta-carotene, is a particular type of carotenoid that is found in dark green leafy and yellow vegetables and in fruits. Eating "Five-a-Day" of fruits and vegetables is highly recommended. The best sources of beta-carotene are carrots, sweet potatoes, spinach, broccoli, pumpkin, squash (butternut), mango, and cantaloupe.

Research has shown that regular consumption of foods rich in carotenoids decreases the risk of some cancers because of its antioxidant effect. Taking a beta-carotene supplement has not shown the same results.

Preformed vitamin A (retinol) is found in fat-containing animal foods such as liver, butter, cream, whole milk, whole milk cheeses, and egg yolk. It is also found in foods such as low-fat milk products, and cereals that have been fortified with vitamin A, but these are not the best sources.

retinol equivalent (RE)
the equivalent of 3.33 IU of vitamin A

Requirements. A well-balanced diet is the preferred way to obtain the required amounts of vitamin A. Vitamin A values are commonly listed as **retinol equivalents (RE)**. A retinol equivalent is 1 μg retinol or 6 μg beta carotene. Refer to the inside cover of this text for the recommended dietary allowances of vitamin A as prescribed by the Food and Nutrition Board, National Academy of Sciences–National Research Council.

xerophthalmia
serious eye disease characterized by dry mucous membranes of the eye, caused by a deficiency of vitamin A

Hypervitaminosis. The use of vitamin supplements should be discouraged because an excess of vitamin A can have serious consequences. Signs of hypervitaminosis A may include birth defects, hair loss, dry skin, headaches, nausea, dryness of mucous membranes, liver damage, and bone and joint pain. In general, these symptoms tend to disappear when excessive intake is discontinued.

Deficiency. Signs of a deficiency of vitamin A include night blindness (Figure 7-1); dry, rough skin; and increased susceptibility to infections. Avitaminosis A can result in blindness or **xerophthalmia**, a condition characterized by dry, lusterless, mucous membranes of the eye. Lack of vitamin A is the leading cause of blindness in the world (discounting accidents).

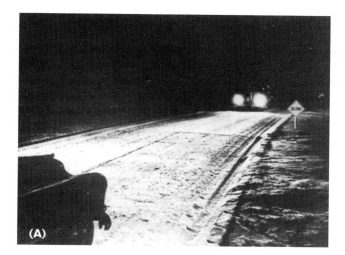
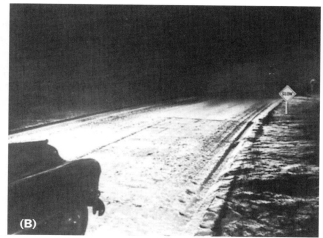
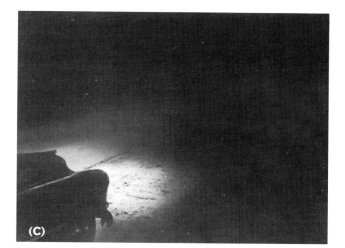

FIGURE 7-1 (A) Both the normal individual and the person suffering from a deficiency of vitamin A see the headlights of the approaching car. (B) After the car has passed, the normal individual sees a wide stretch of road. (C) This reaction to the contrast of light and dark at night is termed night blindness. (Courtesy of the Upjohn Company, Kalamazoo, Michigan)

Vitamin D

Vitamin D exists in two forms—D_2 (ergocalciferol) and D_3 (cholecalciferol). Each is formed from a provitamin when irradiated with (exposed to) ultraviolet light. They are equally effective in human nutrition, but D_3 is the one that is formed in humans from cholesterol in the skin. D_2 is formed in plants. Vitamin D is considered a **prohormone** because it is converted to a hormone in the human body.

Vitamin D is heat-stable and not easily oxidized, so it is not harmed by storage, food processing, or cooking.

Functions.   The major function of vitamin D is the promotion of calcium and phosphorus absorption in the body. By contributing to the absorption of these minerals, it helps to raise their concentration in the blood so that normal bone and tooth mineralization can occur and tetany (involuntary muscle movement) can be prevented. (Tetany can occur when there is too little calcium in the blood. This condition is called hypocalcemia.)

prohormone
substance that precedes the hormone and from which the body can synthesize the hormone

TABLE 7-3 Adequate Intakes for Vitamin D

Newborns through 51 years	5.0 μg (200 IU)
51–70 years	10.0 μg (400 IU)
70+ years	15.0 μg (600 IU)
Pregnant and lactating women	5.0 μg (200 IU)

Source: Dietary Reference Intakes, Food and Nutrition Board, National Academy of Sciences–Institute of Medicine, 1997.

International Units (IU)

units of measurement of some vitamins; 5 μg = 200 IU

rickets

deficiency disease caused by the lack of vitamin D; causes malformed bones and pain in infants

osteomalacia

a condition in which bones become soft, usually in adult women, because of calcium loss

tocopherols

vitamers of vitamin E

tocotrienols

a form of vitamin E

Vitamin D is absorbed in the intestines and is chemically changed in the liver and kidneys. Excess amounts of vitamin D are stored in the liver and in adipose tissue.

Sources. The best source of vitamin D is sunlight, which changes a provitamin to vitamin D_3 in humans. It is sometimes referred to as the sunshine vitamin. The amount of vitamin D that is formed depends on the individual's pigmentation (coloring matter in the skin) and the amount of sunlight available. The best food sources of vitamin D are milk, fish liver oils, egg yolk, butter, and fortified margarine. Because of the rather limited number of food sources of vitamin D and the unpredictability of sunshine, health authorities decided that the vitamin should be added to a common food. Milk was selected. Consequently, most milk available in the United States today has had 10 μg of vitamin D concentrate added per quart.

Requirements. The RDAs (last published in 1989) are being replaced by Dietary Reference Intakes (DRIs). There are several reference values included under the heading DRIs. Vitamin D levels are given as Adequate Intake levels, or AI (Table 7-3).

People who are seldom outdoors, those who use sunscreens, and those who live in areas where there is little sunlight for three to four months a year should be especially careful that their diets provide their Adequate Intake levels of vitamin D. Drinking two cups of vitamin D–fortified fat-free milk each day will provide sufficient vitamin D to those between birth and 50 years of age. Between the ages of 51 and 70, one quart of such milk will be needed each day to fulfill the AI. After 70, 1½ quarts will be needed daily. In this last age group, a vitamin D supplement may be needed.

Vitamin D or, specifically, cholecalciferol values are given in micrograms (μg or mcg.) or in **International Units (IU)**. Five μg equal 200 IU.

Hypervitaminosis. Hypervitaminosis D must be avoided because it can cause deposits of calcium and phosphorus in soft tissues, kidney and heart damage, and bone fragility.

Deficiency. The deficiency of vitamin D inhibits the absorption of calcium and phosphorus in the small intestine and results in poor bone and tooth formation. Young children suffering vitamin D deficiency may develop **rickets** (which causes malformed bones and pain in infants, Figure 7-2), and their teeth may be poorly formed, late in appearing, and particularly subject to decay. Adults lacking sufficient vitamin D may develop **osteomalacia**, softening of bones. It is thought that a deficiency of vitamin D may contribute to osteoporosis (brittle, porous bones).

Vitamin E

Vitamin E consists of two groups of chemical compounds. They are the **tocopherols** and the **tocotrienols**. There are four types of tocopherols: alpha, beta, delta, and gamma. The most biologically active of these is alpha-tocopherol.

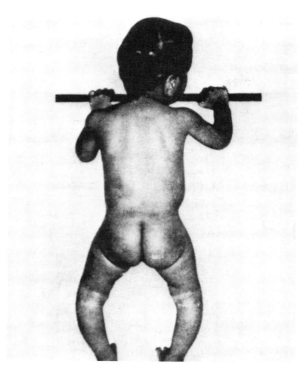

FIGURE 7-2 One of the signs of rickets is bowed legs. It appears after the child has learned to walk. (Courtesy of the Upjohn Company and Dr. R. L. Nemir)

Functions.   Vitamin E is an antioxidant. It is aided in this process by vitamin C and the mineral selenium. It is carried in the blood by lipoproteins. When the amount of vitamin E in the blood is low, the red blood cells become vulnerable to a higher than normal rate of hemolysis. Vitamin E has been found helpful in the prevention of hemolytic anemia among premature infants. It also may enhance the immune system. Because of its antioxidant properties, it is commonly used in commercial food products to retard spoilage.

hemolysis
the destruction of red blood cells

Sources.   Vegetable oils made from corn, soybean, safflower, and cottonseed, and products made from them, such as margarine, are the best sources of vitamin E. Wheat germ, nuts, and green leafy vegetables also are good sources. Animal foods, fruits, and most vegetables are poor sources.

Requirements.   Research indicates that the vitamin E requirement increases if the amount of polyunsaturated fatty acids in the diet increases. In general, however, the U.S. diet is thought to contain sufficient vitamin E. Vitamin E requirements are given as α-TE (alpha-tocopherol equivalents). One milligram of α-TE is the equivalent of 1 IU.

Hypervitaminosis.   Although vitamin E appears to be relatively nontoxic, it is a fat-soluble vitamin and the excess is stored in adipose tissue. Consequently, it would seem advisable to avoid long-term megadoses of vitamin E.

Deficiency. A deficiency of vitamin E has been detected in premature, low-birthweight infants and in patients who are unable to absorb fat normally. Malabsorption can cause serious neurological defects in children, but, in adults, it takes 5 to 10 years before deficiency symptoms occur.

Vitamin K

Vitamin K is made up of several compounds that are essential to blood clotting. Vitamin K_1, commonly called phylloquinone, is found in dietary sources, especially green leafy vegetables such as broccoli and in animal tissue. Vitamin K_2, called menaquinone, is synthesized in the intestine by bacteria and is also found in animal foods. In addition, there is a synthetic vitamin K, called menadione. Vitamin K is destroyed by light and alkalis.

Vitamin K is absorbed like fats, mainly from the small intestine and slightly from the colon. Its absorption requires a normal flow of bile from the liver, and it is improved when there is fat in the diet.

Functions. Vitamin K is essential for the formation of prothrombin, which permits the proper clotting of the blood. It may be given to newborns immediately after birth because human milk contains little vitamin K and the intestines of newborns contain few bacteria. With insufficient vitamin K, newborns may be in danger of intracanial hemorrhage (bleeding within the head).

Vitamin K may be given to patients who suffer from faulty fat absorption; to patients after extensive antibiotic therapy (ingestion of antibiotic drugs to combat infection) because these drugs destroy the bacteria in the intestines; as an antidote for an overdose of anticoagulant (blood thinner such as Warfarin, Coumadin, Warnerin/Canada); or to treat cases of hemorrhage.

Sources. The best dietary sources of vitamin K are green leafy vegetables such as broccoli, cabbage, spinach, and kale. Dairy products, eggs, meats, fruits, and cereals also contain some vitamin K. Cow's milk is a much better source of vitamin K than human milk. The synthesis of vitamin K by bacteria in the small intestine does not provide a sufficient supply by itself. It must be supplemented by dietary sources.

Requirements. Vitamin K is measured in micrograms. The RDA for vitamin K is 80 µg for men and 65 µg for women. This is not increased during pregnancy or lactation. Infants up to 6 months should have 5 µg a day. Those between 6 months and one year should receive 10 µg a day.

Hypervitaminosis. Ingestion of excessive amounts of synthetic vitamin K can be toxic and can cause a form of anemia.

Deficiency. The only major sign of a deficiency of vitamin K is defective blood coagulation. This increases clotting time, making the patient more prone to hemorrhage. Human deficiency may be caused by faulty fat metabolism, antibiotic therapy, inadequate diet, or anticoagulants.

coagulate
to thicken

WATER-SOLUBLE VITAMINS

Water-soluble vitamins include B complex and C. These vitamins dissolve in water and are easily destroyed by air, light, and cooking. They are not stored in the body to the extent that fat-soluble vitamins are stored.

Vitamin B Complex

Beriberi is a disease that affects the nervous, cardiovascular, and gastrointestinal systems. The legs feel heavy, the feet burn, and the muscles degenerate. The patient is irritable and suffers from headaches, depression, anorexia, constipation, tachycardia (rapid heart rate), edema, and heart failure.

Toward the end of the nineteenth century, a doctor in Indonesia discovered that chickens that were fed table scraps of polished rice developed symptoms much like those of his patients suffering from beriberi. When these same chickens were later fed brown (unpolished) rice, they recovered.

Some years later, this mysterious component of unpolished rice was recognized as an essential food substance and was named vitamin B. Subsequently, it was named vitamin *B complex* because the vitamin was found to be composed of several compounds. The B-complex vitamins are listed in Table 7-1.

beriberi
deficiency disease caused by a lack of vitamin B_1 (thiamin)

Thiamin

Thiamin, a coenzyme, was originally named vitamin B_1. It is partially destroyed by heat and alkalies, and it is lost in cooking water.

thiamin
vitamin B_1

Functions.   Thiamin is essential for the metabolism of carbohydrates and some amino acids. It is also essential to nerve and muscle action. It is absorbed in the small intestine.

Sources.   Thiamin is found in many foods, but generally in small quantities. (See Table A-3 in the appendix.) Some of the best natural food sources of thiamin are unrefined and enriched cereals, yeast, wheat germ, lean pork, organ meats, and legumes.

Requirements.   Thiamin is measured in milligrams. The daily thiamin requirement for the average adult female is 1.1 mg a day, and for the average adult male it is 1.5 mg a day. The requirement is not thought to increase with age. In general, however, an increase in kcal increases the need for thiamin.

Most breads and cereals in the United States are enriched with thiamin so that the majority of people can and do easily fulfill their recommended dietary requirements.

Deficiency.   Symptoms of thiamin deficiency include loss of appetite, fatigue, nervous irritability, and constipation. An extreme deficiency causes beriberi. Its deficiency is rare, however, occurring mainly among alcoholics whose diets include reduced amounts of thiamin while their requirements of it are increased and their absorption of it is decreased. Others at risk include renal patients undergoing long-term dialysis; patients fed intravenously for long periods; and patients with chronic fevers.

Because some raw fish contain thiaminase, an enzyme that inhibits the normal action of thiamin, frequent consumption of large amounts of raw fish could cause thiamin deficiency. Eating raw fish is not recommended. Cooking inactivates this enzyme.

There are no know ill effects from excessive oral intake of thiamin, but it may be toxic if excessive amounts are given intravenously.

Riboflavin

riboflavin
the name for vitamin B$_2$

Riboflavin is sometimes called B$_2$. It is destroyed by light and irradiation and is unstable in alkalies.

Functions.   Riboflavin is essential for carbohydrate, fat, and protein metabolism. It is also necessary for tissue maintenance, especially the skin around the mouth, and for healthy eyes. Riboflavin is absorbed in the small intestine.

Sources.   Riboflavin is widely distributed in animal and plant foods but in small amounts. Milk, meats, poultry, fish, and enriched breads and cereals are some of its richest sources. Some green vegetables such as broccoli, spinach, and asparagus are also good sources.

Requirement.   Riboflavin is measured in milligrams. The average adult female daily requirement is thought to be 1.3 mg and the adult male is 1.7 mg. The riboflavin requirement appears to increase with increased energy expenditure. Therefore, the requirement seems to diminish with age.

Deficiency.   Because of the small quantities of riboflavin in foods and its limited storage in the body, deficiencies of riboflavin can develop. The generous use of fat-free milk in the diet is a good way to prevent deficiency of this vitamin. It is important, however, that milk be stored in opaque containers because riboflavin can be destroyed by light. It appears that fiber laxatives can reduce riboflavin absorption, and their use over long periods should be discouraged.

A deficiency of riboflavin can result in cheilosis, a condition characterized by sores on the lips and cracks at the corners of the mouth; glossitis (inflammation of the tongue); dermatitis; and eye strain in the form of itching, burning, and eye fatigue. Its toxicity is unknown.

Niacin

niacin
B vitamin

Niacin is the generic name for nicotinic acid and nicotinamide.

Niacin is fairly stable in foods. It can withstand reasonable amounts of heat and acid and is not destroyed during food storage.

pellagra
deficiency disease caused by a
lack of niacin

Functions.   Niacin serves as a coenzyme in energy metabolism and consequently is essential to every body cell. In addition, niacin is essential for the prevention of **pellagra**. Pellagra is a disease characterized by sores on the skin and by diarrhea, anxiety, confusion, irritability, poor memory, dizziness, and untimely death if left untreated. Niacin, when used as a cholesterol-lowering agent, must be closely supervised by a physician because of possible adverse side effects such as liver damage and peptic ulcers.

Sources. The best sources of niacin are meats, poultry, and fish. Peanuts and other legumes are also good sources. Enriched breads and cereals also contain some. Milk and eggs do not provide niacin per se, but they are good sources of its precursor, tryptophan (an amino acid). Vegetables and fruits contain little niacin.

Requirements. Niacin is measured in **niacin equivalents (NE)**. One NE equals 1 mg of niacin or 60 mg of tryptophan. The general recommendation is a daily intake of 15 mg/NE for adult women and 19 mg/NE for adult men. Because excessive amounts of niacin have caused flushing due to vascular dilation (expansion of blood vessels), self-prescribed doses of niacin concentrate should be discouraged. Other symptoms include gastrointestinal problems and itching. If excessive amounts of niacin are ingested, liver damage may result.

niacin equivalent (NE)
unit of measuring niacin; 1 NE equals 1 mg niacin or 60 mg tryptophan

Deficiency. A deficiency of niacin is apt to appear if there is a deficiency of riboflavin. Symptoms of niacin deficiency include weakness, anorexia, indigestion, anxiety, and irritability. In extreme cases, pellagra may occur.

Vitamin B$_6$

Vitamin B$_6$ is composed of three related forms: pyridoxine, pyridoxal, and pyridoxamine. It is stable to heat but sensitive to light and alkalies.

Functions. Vitamin B$_6$ is essential for protein metabolism and absorption, and it aids in the release of glucose from glycogen. With the help of vitamin B$_6$, amino acids present in excessive amounts can be converted to those in which the body is temporarily deficient. It also serves as a catalyst in the conversion of tryptophan to niacin, and it is helpful in the formation of other substances from amino acids. An example is the synthesis of neurotransmitters such as serotonin and dopamine.

Sources. Some of the nutrient-dense sources of vitamin B$_6$ are poultry, fish, liver, kidney potatoes, bananas, and spinach. Whole grains, especially oats and wheat, are good sources of vitamin B$_6$, but, because this vitamin is lost during milling and is not replaced during the enrichment process, refined grains are not a good source.

Requirements. Vitamin B$_6$ is measured in milligrams, and the need increases as the protein intake increases. For adult females, the daily requirement is 1.6 mg and for males, 2.0 mg. Oral contraceptives interfere with the metabolism of vitamin B$_6$ and can result in a deficiency.

Deficiency. A deficiency of vitamin B_6 is usually found in combination with deficiencies of other B vitamins. Symptoms include irritability, depression, and dermatitis. In infants, its deficiency can cause various neurological symptoms and abdominal problems. Although its toxicity is rare, it can cause temporary neurological problems.

Folate

folate/folic acid

a form of vitamin B, also called folacin; essential for metabolism

Folate, *folacin,* and folic acid are chemically similar compounds. Their names are often used interchangeably.

Functions. Folate is needed for DNA synthesis, protein metabolism, and the formation of hemoglobin.

Sources. Folate is found in many foods, but the best sources are cereals fortified with folate, green leafy vegetables, legumes, sunflower seeds, and fruits such as orange juice and strawberries. Heat, oxidation, and ultraviolet light all destroy folate, and it is estimated that 50 to 90% of folate may be destroyed during food processing and preparation. Consequently, it is advisable that fruits and vegetables be eaten uncooked or lightly cooked whenever possible.

Requirements. Folate is measured in micrograms. The average daily requirement for the adult female is 180 µg, and for the adult male it is 200 µg. There is an increased need for folate during pregnancy and periods of growth because of the increased rate of cell division and the DNA synthesis in the body of the mother and of the fetus. Consequently, it is extremely important that women of childbearing age maintain good folate intake. The recommended amount for a woman one month before conception and through the first 6 weeks of pregnancy is 400 µg a day.

neural tube defects

congenital malformation of brain and/or spinal column due to failure of neural tube to close during embryonic development

spina bifida

spinal cord or spinal fluid bulge through the back

anencephaly

absence of brain

megaloblastic anemia

anemia in which the red blood cells are unusually large and are not completely mature

Deficiency. Folate deficiency has been linked to **neural tube defects (NTDs)** in the fetus such as **spina bifida** (spinal cord or spinal fluid bulge through the back) and **anencephaly** (absence of a brain). Other signs of deficiency are inflammation of the mouth and tongue, poor growth, depression and mental confusion, problems with nerve functions, and **megaloblastic anemia**. Megaloblastic anemia is a condition wherein red blood cells are large and immature and cannot carry oxygen properly.

Hypervitaminosis. The FDA limits the amount of folate in over-the-counter (OTC) supplements to 100 µg for infants, 300 µg for children, and 400 µg for adults because consuming excessive amounts of folate can mask a vitamin B_{12} deficiency and inactivate phenytoin, an anticonvulsant drug used by epileptics.

Vitamin B_{12}

cobalamin

organic compound known as vitamin B_{12}

Vitamin B_{12} (**cobalamin**) is a compound that contains the mineral cobalt. It is slightly soluble in water and fairly stable to heat, but it is damaged by strong acids or alkalies and by light. It can be stored in the human body for 3 to 5 years.

Functions.   Vitamin B_{12} is involved in folate metabolism, maintenance of the myelin sheath, and healthy red blood cells. In order for vitamin B_{12} to be absorbed, it must bind with a glycoprotein (**intrinsic factor**) present in gastric secretions in the stomach and travel to the small intestine, where it combines with pancreatic proteases, then travels to the ileum, where it attaches to special receptor cells to complete the absorption process. A patient who has lost the ability to produce the gastric secretions, pancreatic proteases, intrinsic factor, or the special receptor cells because of disease or surgery will develop **pernicious anemia**.

Sources.   The best food sources of B_{12} are animal foods, especially organ meats, lean meat, seafood, eggs, and dairy products.

Requirements.   Vitamin B_{12} is measured in micrograms. The RDA for adults is 2 μg a day, but it increases during pregnancy and lactation. The amount absorbed will depend on current needs.

Deficiency.   Fortunately, a vitamin B_{12} deficiency is rare and is thought to be caused by congenital problems of absorption, which inhibit the body's ability to absorb or synthesize sufficient amounts of vitamin B_{12}. It may also be due to years of a strict vegetarian diet that contains no animal foods.

When the amount of B_{12} is insufficient, megaloblastic anemia may result. If the intrinsic factor is missing, pernicious anemia develops. Intrinsic factor could be missing because of surgical removal of the stomach, or a large portion of it, or because of disease or surgery affecting the ileum. Dietary treatment will be ineffective; the patient must be given intramuscular injections of B_{12}, usually on a monthly basis.

Vitamin B_{12} deficiency may also result in inadequate myelin synthesis. This deficiency causes damage to the nervous system. Signs of vitamin B_{12} deficiency include anorexia, glossitis, sore mouth and tongue, pallor, neurological upsets such as depression and dizziness, and weight loss.

Pantothenic Acid

Pantothenic acid is appropriately named, because the Greek word *pantothen* means "from many places." It is fairly stable, but it can be damaged by acids and alkalies.

Functions.   Pantothenic acid is involved in metabolism of carbohydrates, fats, and proteins. It is also essential for the synthesis of the neurotransmitter acetylcholine and of steroid hormones.

Sources.   Pantothenic acid is found extensively in foods, especially animal foods such as meats, poultry, fish, and eggs. It is also found in whole grain cereals and legumes. In addition, it is thought to be synthesized by the body.

Requirements.   There is no RDA for pantothenic acid, but the Food and Nutrition Board has provided an estimated intake of 4–7 mg a day for normal adults (see Table 7-2).

myelin
lipoprotein essential for the protection of nerves

intrinsic factor
secretion of stomach mucosa essential for B_{12} absorption

pernicious anemia
severe, chronic anemia caused by a deficiency of vitamin B_{12}; usually due to the body's inability to absorb B_{12}

pantothenic acid
a B vitamin

Deficiency. Natural deficiencies are unknown. However, deficiencies have been produced experimentally. Signs include weakness, fatigue, and a burning sensation in the feet. Toxicity from excessive intake has not been confirmed.

Biotin

biotin
a B vitamin; necessary for metabolism

Function and Sources. Biotin participates as a coenzyme in the synthesis of fatty acids and amino acids. Some of its best dietary sources are liver, egg yolk, soy flour, cereals, and yeast. Biotin is also synthesized in the intestine by microorganisms, but the amount that is available for absorption is unknown.

Requirements. Biotin is measured in micrograms. Although RDAs have not been established, the Food and Nutrition Board has provided suggested daily dietary intakes of 30–100 µg for normal adults (see Table 7-2).

Deficiency. Deficiency symptoms include nausea, anorexia, depression, pallor (paleness of complexion), dermatitis (inflammation of skin), and an increase in serum cholesterol. Toxicity from excessive intake is unknown.

Vitamin C

ascorbic acid
vitamin C

scurvy
a deficiency disease caused by a lack of vitamin C

collagen
protein substance that holds body cells together

nonheme iron
iron from animal foods that is not part of the hemoglobin molecule; and all iron from plant foods

heme iron
part of hemoglobin molecule in animal foods

Vitamin C is also known as ascorbic acid. It has antioxidant properties and protects foods from oxidation. It is readily destroyed by heat, air, and alkalies, and it is easily lost in cooking water.

Functions. Vitamin C is known to prevent scurvy. This is a disease characterized by gingivitis (soft, bleeding gums, and loose teeth); flesh that is easily bruised; tiny, pinpoint hemorrhages of the skin; poor wound healing; sore joints and muscles; and weight loss. In extreme cases, scurvy can result in death. Scurvy used to be common among sailors, who lived for months on bread, fish, and salted meat, with no fresh fruits or vegetables. During the middle of the eighteenth century, it was discovered that the addition of limes or lemons to their diets prevented this disease.

Vitamin C also has an important role in the formation of collagen, a protein substance that holds body cells together, making it necessary for wound healing. Therefore, the requirement for vitamin C is increased during trauma, fever, and periods of growth. Tiny, pinpoint hemorrhages are symptoms of the breakdown of collagen.

Vitamin C aids in the absorption of nonheme iron (from plant and animal sources and less easily absorbed than heme iron—see Chapter 8) in the small intestine when both nutrients are ingested at the same time. Because of this, it is called an iron enhancer.

Vitamin C also appears to have several other functions in the human body that are not well understood. For example, it may be involved with the formation or functioning of norepinephrine (a neurotransmitter and vasoconstrictor that helps the body cope with stressful conditions), some amino acids, folate, leukocytes (white blood cells), the immune system, and allergic reactions.

It is believed to reduce the severity of colds because it is a natural antihistamine and can reduce cancer risk in some cases by reducing nitrites in foods.

Vitamin C is absorbed in the small intestine.

Sources. The best sources of vitamin C are citrus fruits, melon, strawberries, tomatoes, potatoes, red and green peppers, cabbage, and broccoli.

Requirements. Vitamin C is measured in milligrams. The average adult in the United States requires 60 mg a day under normal circumstances. In times of stress, the need is increased. Regular cigarette smokers are advised to ingest 100–200 mg a day.

It is generally considered nontoxic, but this has not been confirmed. An excess can cause diarrhea, nausea, cramps, an excessive absorption of food iron, rebound scurvy (when megadoses are stopped abruptly), and possibly oxalate kidney stones.

Deficiency. Deficiencies of vitamin C are indicated by bleeding gums, loose teeth, tendency to bruise easily, poor wound healing and, ultimately, scurvy.

SUPPLEMENTS

Healthy people who eat a variety of foods using the Food Guide Pyramid (Figure 7-3) should be able to obtain all the vitamins needed to maintain good health. However, some people take supplements because they believe that (1) food no longer contains the right nutri-

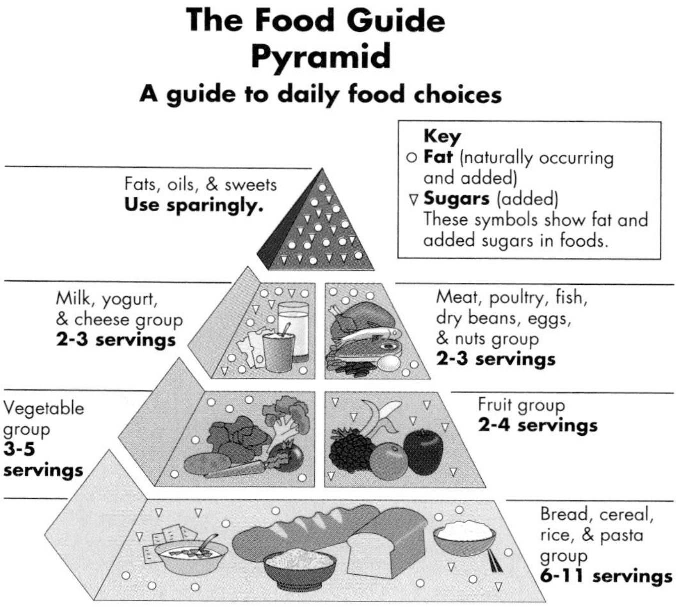

FIGURE 7-3 Food Guide Pyramid. (Courtesy of USDA and DHHS 1992. The food guide pyramid: A guide to daily food choices. Leaflet no. 572. Washington, D.C.)

ents in adequate quantities; (2) supplements can "bulk up" muscles and enhance athletic performance; (3) vitamins provide needed energy; and (4) vitamins and minerals can cure anything, including heart trouble, the common cold, and cancer.

The facts are as follows: (1) A balanced diet *does* provide for the nutritional needs of healthy people. (2) No amount of vitamins will build muscles; only weight lifting will do that. (3) Vitamins do not provide energy themselves. They help to release the energy within the carbohydrates, proteins, and fats that people ingest. (4) Only certain diseases caused by vitamin deficiencies (such as beriberi, scurvy, rickets) can be cured with the help of vitamin supplements. Heart disease, cancer, and the common cold cannot.

Almost everyone can take a daily multivitamin and mineral supplement without fear of toxicity, but a megadose (10 times the RDA) to correct a deficiency or to help prevent disease should be prescribed by a physician. If a multivitamin-mineral is taken as a supplement, it is best not to exceed 100% of the RDA for each vitamin and mineral. An excess of one vitamin or one mineral can negatively affect the absorption or utilization of other vitamins and minerals. One must never prescribe vitamins and minerals for oneself. If vitamin supplements are thought to be necessary, it is essential that a physician or registered dietitian be consulted first.

Herbal products also are included under the heading, "dietary supplements." Some people are interested in herbs because they believe certain ones can improve their health, they require no prescription, and they are often less expensive than prescription drugs.

The U.S. Food and Drug Administration (FDA) requires that manufacturers of prescription and over-the-counter drugs run, monitor, and report results of clinical trials of their products before selling them. Doses are established and side effects and adverse reactions are reported in scientific journals. Also the FDA can inspect drug manufacturing facilities to confirm the purity of ingredients.

The Dietary Supplement Health and Education Act of 1994 exempts dietary supplements from FDA evaluation unless the FDA has evidence that a product is harmful. But before a suspect product can be removed from store shelves, the FDA must prove it is not safe. Manufacturers of supplements cannot claim their products can treat or prevent diseases, but they can make "structure/function" claims. For example, they cannot say vitamin A prevents cancer, but they can say vitamin A is an antioxidant and antioxidants have been linked to reduced rates of cancer.

Misinformation concerning supplements is widely available. Health care professionals must stay well-informed concerning supplements, provide accurate information to their patients, and urge patients to consult with their physicians or registered dietitians before using any supplement. Some herbal products may indeed be helpful, but some may be harmful.

CONSIDERATIONS FOR THE HEALTH CARE PROFESSIONAL

Vitamins are a popular subject about which many people have strong beliefs. Some beliefs are based on fact; many are incorrect. Today's magazines and newspapers frequently contain articles about vitamins, but they are not always factual. Patients who have no other source of nutrition information tend to believe the statements in those articles. It is important that the patient have correct information about vitamins (Figure 7-4). Continuation of a poor diet or continued abuse of vitamin supplements is potentially dangerous to the patient.

Health care professionals will need a solid knowledge of vitamins, a convincing manner, and enormous patience to reeducate patients as may be needed. Some will believe that vitamin E will prevent heart attack; that the only source of vitamin C is orange juice; that megadoses of vitamin A will prevent cancer; that a one-a-day vitamin pill is necessary for nearly everyone. Others will confuse milligrams with grams.

Patient education about vitamins may be difficult until the health care professional gains the confidence of the patient. Simple and clear written materials to reinforce the information will be helpful to the patient.

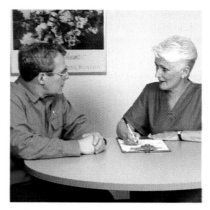

FIGURE 7-4 Patient education about vitamins is important.

● SUMMARY

Vitamins are organic compounds that regulate body functions and promote growth. Each vitamin has a specific function or functions within the body. Food sources of vitamins vary, but generally a well-balanced diet provides sufficient vitamins to fulfill body requirements. Vitamin deficiencies can result from inadequate diets or from the body's inability to utilize vitamins (Table 7-4). Vitamins are available in concentrated forms, but their use should be carefully monitored because overdoses can be detrimental to health. Vitamins A, D, E, and K are fat-soluble. Vitamin B complex and vitamin C are water-soluble. Water-soluble vitamins can be destroyed during food preparation. It is important that care is taken during the preparation of food to preserve its vitamin content.

TABLE 7-4 Fat-Soluble Vitamins and Water-Soluble Vitamins

NAME	FOOD SOURCES	FUNCTIONS	DEFICIENCY/TOXICITY
Fat-soluble vitamins			

Vitamin A (retinol)	Animal
	    Liver
	    Whole milk
	    Butter
	    Cream
	    Cod liver oil
	Plants
	    Dark green leafy vegetables
	    Deep yellow or orange fruit
	    Fortified margarine
		Maintenance of vision in dim light
		Maintenance of mucous membranes and healthy skin
		Growth and development of bones
		Reproduction
		Healthy immune system
			Deficiency
			    Night blindness
			    Xerophthalmia
			    Respiratory infections
			    Bone growth ceases
			Toxicity
			    Birth defects
			    Bone pain
			    Anorexia
			    Enlargement of liver
			                    (*continued*)

TABLE 7-4 *continued*

NAME	FOOD SOURCES	FUNCTIONS	DEFICIENCY/TOXICITY

Vitamin D (calciferol)	Animal
	  Eggs
	  Liver
	  Fortified milk
	  Fortified margarine
	  Oily fish
	Plant
	  None
	Sunlight
		Regulation of absorption of calcium and phosphorus
		Building and maintenance of normal bones and teeth
		Prevention of tetany
			Deficiency
			  Rickets
			  Osteomalacia
			  Osteoporosis
			  Poorly developed teeth and bones
			  Muscle spasms
			Toxicity
			  Kidney stones
			  Calcification of soft tissues

Vitamin E (tocopherol)	Animal
	  None
	Plant
	  Green and leafy vegetables
	  Margarines
	  Salad dressing
	  Wheat germ and wheat germ oils
	  Vegetable oils
	  Nuts
		Antioxidant
		Considered essential for protection of cell structure, especially of red blood cells
			Deficiency
			  Destruction of red blood cells
			Toxicity

Vitamin K	Animal
	  Liver
	  Milk
	Plant
	  Green leafy vegetables
	  Cabbage, broccoli
		Blood clotting	Deficiency
			  Prolonged blood clotting/ hemorrhaging
			Toxicity
			  Hemolytic anemia
			  Interferes with anticlotting medications

Water-soluble vitamins			

Thiamin (vitamin B$_1$)	Animal
	  Lean pork
	  Beef
	  Liver
	  Eggs
	  Fish
	Plant
	  Whole and enriched grains
	  Legumes
	  Brewer's yeast
		Metabolism of carbohydrates and some amino acids
		Maintains normal appetite and functioning of nervous system
			Deficiency
			  Gastrointestinal tract, nervous system, and cardiovascular system problems
			  Beriberi
			Toxicity
			  None

TABLE 7-4 *continued*

NAME	FOOD SOURCES	FUNCTIONS	DEFICIENCY/TOXICITY

Riboflavin (vitamin B$_2$)	**Animal**
	  Liver, kidney, heart
	  Milk
	  Cheese
	Plant
	  Green, leafy vegetables
	  Cereals
	  Enriched bread
		Aids release of energy from food
		Health of the mouth tissue
		Healthy eyes
			Deficiency
			  Cheilosis
			  Eye sensitivity
			  Dermatitis
			  Glossitis
			  Photophobia
			Toxicity
			  None

Niacin (nicotinic acid)	**Animal**
	  Milk
	  Eggs
	  Fish
	  Poultry
	Plant
	  Enriched breads and cereals
		Energy metabolism
		Healthy skin and nervous and digestive systems
			Deficiency
			  Pellagra—dermatitis, dementia, diarrhea
			Toxicity
			  Vasodilation of blood vessels

Pyridoxine (vitamin B$_6$)	**Animal**
	  Pork
	  Fish
	  Poultry
	  Liver, kidney
	  Milk
	  Eggs
	Plant
	  Whole-grain cereals
	  Legumes
		Conversion of tryptophan to niacin
		Release of glucose from glycogen
		Protein metaboplism and synthesis of nonessential amino acids
			Deficiency
			  Cheilosis
			  Glossitis
			  Dermatitis
			  Confusion
			  Depression
			  Irritability
			Toxicity
			  Depression
			  Nerve damage

Vitamin B$_{12}$	**Animal**
	  Seafood
	  Poultry
	  Liver, kidney
	  Muscle meats
	  Eggs
	  Milk
	  Cheese
	Plant
	  None
		Synthesis of red blood cells
		Maintenance of myelin sheaths
		Treatment of pernicious anemia
		Folate metabolism
			Deficiency
			  Degeneration of myelin sheaths
			  Pernicious anemia
			  Sore mouth and tongue
			  Anorexia
			  Neurological disorders
			Toxicity
			  None

(continued)

TABLE 7-4 *continued*

NAME	FOOD SOURCES		FUNCTIONS	DEFICIENCY/TOXICITY

Folate (folic acid)	Animal
	    Liver
	Plant
	    Leafy green vegetables
	    Spinach
	    Legumes
	    Seeds
	    Broccoli
	    Cereal fortified with folate
	    Fruit
			Synthesis of RBCs
			Synthesis of DNA
				Deficiency
				    Anemia
				    Glossitis
				    Neural tube defects such as anencephaly and spina bifida
				Toxicity
				    Could mask a B_{12} deficiency

Biotin	Animal
	    Milk
	    Liver and kidney
	    Egg yolks
	Plant
	    Legumes
	    Brewer's yeast
	    Soy flour
	    Cereals
	    Fruit
			Coenzyme in carbohydrate and amino acid metabolism
			Niacin synthesis from tryptophan
				Deficiency
				    Dermatitis
				    Nausea
				    Anorexia
				    Depression
				    Hair loss
				Toxicity
				    None

Pantothenic acid	Animal
	    Eggs
	    Liver
	    Salmon
	    Poultry
		Plant
		    Mushrooms
		    Cauliflower
		    Peanuts
		    Brewer's yeast
			Metabolism of carbohydrates, lipids, and proteins
			Synthesis of fatty acids, cholesterol, steroid hormones
				Deficiency
				    Rare: burning feet syndrome; vomiting; fatigue
				Toxicity
				    None

Vitamin C (ascorbic acid)	Animal
	    None
	Plants
	    All citrus fruits
	    Broccoli
	    Melons
	    Strawberries
	    Tomatoes
	    Brussel sprouts
	    Potatoes
	    Cabbage
	    Green peppers
			Prevention of scurvy
			Formation of collagen
			Healing of wounds
			Release of stress hormones
			Absorption of iron
			Antioxidant
			Resistance to infection
				Deficiency
				    Scurvy
				    Muscle cramps
				    Ulcerated gums
				    Tendency to bruise easily
				Toxicity
				    Raised uric acid level
				    Hemolytic anemia
				    Kidney stones
				    Rebound scurvy

Source: Courtesy of Delmar Publishers, Albany, NY.

● DISCUSSION TOPICS

1. How do vitamins help to provide energy to the body?

2. Discuss possible times when avitaminosis of one or more vitamins may occur.

3. Discuss any vitamin deficiencies that class members have observed. What treatments were prescribed?

4. Discuss why it may be unwise for anyone but a physician to prescribe vitamin supplements.

5. Discuss the terms *enriched, fortified,* and *restored.* What do they mean in relation to food products? Name foods that are enriched, fortified, or restored.

6. Discuss the proper storage and cooking of foods to retain their vitamin content.

7. If any member of the class has experienced night blindness, ask her or him to describe it. Discuss how this condition occurs and how it can be prevented.

8. Why is it advisable to use liquids left over from vegetable cooking? How might these be used?

9. Explain the role of vitamin C in collagen formation and wound healing.

10. If anyone in the class has taken concentrated vitamin C, ask why. If it was useful, ask how it helped.

11. Why are some vitamins being called prohormones? Coenzymes? Give examples.

12. What is a precursor? Give an example.

13. Discuss appropriate nutritional advice for a young mother who is giving her 4-year-old 50 μg of vitamin D each day.

14. What is beriberi, and how can it be prevented?

15. Why should milk be sold in opaque containers?

● SUGGESTED ACTIVITIES

1. Write a menu for one day that is especially rich in the B-complex vitamins. Underline the foods that are the best sources of these vitamins.

2. List the foods you have eaten in the past 24 hours. Write the names of the vitamins supplied by each food. What percentage of your day's food did *not* contain vitamins? Could this diet be nutritionally improved? How?

3. Plan a day's menu for a person who has been instructed to eat an abundance of foods rich in vitamin A.

● REVIEW

Multiple choice. Select the *letter* that precedes the best answer.

1. The daily vitamin requirement is best supplied by
   a. eating a well-balanced diet
   b. eating one serving of citrus fruit for breakfast
   c. taking one of the many forms of vitamin supplements
   d. eating at least one serving of meat each day

2. All of the following measures preserve the vitamin content of food except
   a. using vegetables and fruits raw
   b. preparing fresh vegetables and fruits just before serving
   c. adding raw, fresh vegetables to a small amount of cold water and heating to boiling
   d. storing fresh vegetables in a cool place

3. Fat-soluble vitamins
   a. cannot be stored in the body
   b. are lost easily during cooking
   c. are dissolved by water
   d. are slower than water-soluble vitamins to exhibit deficiencies

4. Night blindness is caused by a deficiency of
   a. vitamin A   c. niacin
   b. thiamin   d. vitamin C

5. Good sources of thiamin include
   a. citrus fruits and tomatoes
   b. wheat germ and liver
   c. carotene and fish liver oils
   d. nuts and milk

6. Water-soluble vitamins include
   a. A, D, E, and K
   b. A, B_6, and C
   c. thiamin, niacin, and retinol
   d. thiamin, riboflavin, niacin, B_6, B_{12}

7. Injections of B_{12} are given in the treatment of
   a. scurvy   c. pellagra
   b. pernicious anemia   d. beriberi

8. Blindness can result from a severe lack of
   a. vitamin K   c. thiamin
   b. vitamin A   d. vitamin E

9. Organ meats are good sources of the vitamins
   a. thiamin, riboflavin, B_{12} c. vitamins E and K
   b. biotin, vitamin C   d. all of the above

10. Irradiated milk is a good source of
    a. vitamin E   c. vitamin K
    b. vitamin D   d. vitamin C

11. Good sources of vitamin C are
    a. meats   c. breads and cereals
    b. milk and milk products   d. citrus fruits

12. The vitamin that aids in the prevention of rickets is
   a. vitamin A
   b. thiamin
   c. vitamin C
   d. vitamin D

13. The vitamin that is necessary for the proper clotting of the blood is
   a. vitamin A
   b. vitamin K
   c. vitamin D
   d. niacin

14. Vitamins commonly added to breads and cereals are
   a. vitamins A, D, and K
   b. thiamin, riboflavin, niacin, and folate
   c. vitamins E, B_6, and B_{12}
   d. ascorbic acid, pantothenic acid, and folate

15. The vitamin known to prevent scurvy is
   a. vitamin A
   b. vitamin B complex
   c. vitamin C
   d. vitamin D

C A S E   S T U D Y

Chris and Patty were very excited about adopting their Bosnian son, Nicoli. They had been waiting for 2 years for a child. They were told that Nicoli was 3 years old and had been in the orphanage for the 2 years since his parents were killed. When they received a picture of Nicoli, Patty was concerned about his health. She thought he looked very pale, and his skin looked rough. He didn't seem to have as many teeth as other 3-year-olds she saw in the neighborhood.

When Chris and Patty went to bring Nicoli home, they learned more about Nicoli's living conditions. The orphanage was clean but barren and colorless. Electricity and heat were limited. Milk and dairy products were provided intermittently at best. The children seldom went outdoors. All of the children were thin, but they were loved and well cared for, given the circumstances.

Once they got Nicoli back to the United States, they took him to the pediatrician for a complete physical. The doctor was concerned about Nicoli's vision. He gave Patty a prescription for a daily vitamin supplement and a recommendation that she take him to an ophthalmologist.

ASSESSMENT

1. What objective data do you have about Nicoli's health?
2. What did the doctor suspect?
3. What might be lacking in Nicoli's diet?

DIAGNOSIS

4. Complete the following sentence. Nicoli's growth and development problems are related to _____.

PLAN/GOAL

5. What should be the goal for Nicoli's diet?

IMPLEMENTATION

6. What food category is a priority in Nicoli's plan?
7. What else can be done to improve Nicoli's health?

EVALUATION/OUTCOME CRITERIA

8. What criteria should Chris and Patty use to evaluate the success of their actions?
9. What will change in Nicoli when they are successful?

C A S E   S T U D Y

Angela's 5-year-old twin girls started preschool in September. By late November, Angela and the two girls were on their fourth cold. After reading an article in the grocery checkout line about vitamin C, Angela decided to take 1,000 mg of vitamin C daily. After a week and no change in her current cold, she increased the dose to 2,000 mg. Although she did not have a cold in the following 2 months, she began to have flatulence, diarrhea, and ulcerlike symptoms. She visited her doctor because she was very concerned about the symptoms. She failed to mention the vitamin C dur-ing her initial examination. The doctor ordered a battery of tests, which showed only gastritis.

At the follow-up appointment, her doctor was still puzzled about the origin of her symptoms and asked her again about foods, medications, and nonprescription medications. She reported her megadoses of vitamin C. The doctor insisted she stop the vitamin C gradually over the next 2 weeks. The stomach symptoms disappeared about the same time she completely stopped the vitamin C. She caught another cold 2 weeks after she stopped the vitamin C.

ASSESSMENT

1. What data do you have about Angela?
2. Why did Angela take the vitamin C? What does this action demonstrate about her choices?
3. After the tests, what did the doctor suspect was the cause of her stomach problems?
4. What was the real cause of Angela's frequent colds?

DIAGNOSIS

5. What was Angela's health-seeking behavior related to?
6. Where and/or from whom could Angela have obtained better information on supplements?

PLAN/GOAL

7. What is a reasonable measurable goal for Angela and her colds?

IMPLEMENTATION

8. List three strategies to decrease the likelihood of catching a cold.
9. What can she teach the twins about colds?
10. What can she do, once she has a cold, to lessen its impact?

EVALUATION/OUTCOME CRITERIA

11. How will Angela know her actions are successful?

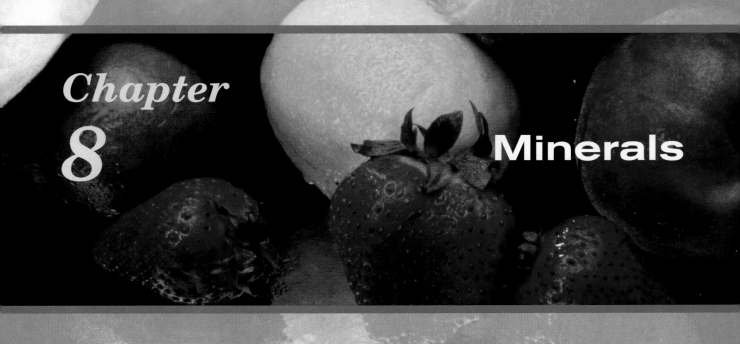

Chapter 8

Minerals

Key Terms

acidosis
alkaline
alkalosis
cardiovascular
dehydration
demineralization
diuretics
edema
electrolytes
enriched foods
etiology
extracellular
goiter
heme iron
hemochromatosis
hyperkalemia

hypertension
hypokalemia
intracellular
iodized salt
ions
iron deficiency
iron deficiency
  anemia
Keshan disease
myoglobin
nonheme iron
osmosis
rickets
tetany
toxicity

Objectives

After studying this chapter, you should be able to:

● List at least two food sources of given minerals

● List one or more functions of given minerals

● Describe the recommended method of avoiding mineral deficiencies

Chemical analysis shows that the human body is made up of specific chemical elements. Four of these elements—oxygen, carbon, hydrogen, and nitrogen—make up 96% of body weight. All the remaining elements are *minerals,* which represent only 4% of body weight. Nevertheless, these minerals are essential for good health.

A mineral is an inorganic (non-carbon-containing) element that is necessary for the body to build tissues, regulate body fluids, or assist in various body functions. Minerals are found in all body tissues. They cannot provide energy by themselves, but in their role as body regulators, they contribute to the production of energy within the body.

Minerals are found in water and in natural (unprocessed) foods, together with proteins, carbohydrates, fats, and vitamins. Minerals in the soil are absorbed by growing plants. Humans obtain minerals by eating plants grown in mineral-rich soil or by eating animals that have eaten such plants. The specific mineral content of food is determined by burning the food and then chemically analyzing the remaining ash.

Highly processed or refined foods such as sugar and white flour contain almost no minerals. Iron, together with the vitamins thiamin, riboflavin, niacin, and folate, are commonly added to some flour and cereals, which are then labeled **enriched**.

Most minerals in food occur as salts, which are soluble in water. Therefore, the minerals leave the food and remain in the cooking water. Foods should be cooked in as little water as possible or, preferably, steamed, and any cooking liquid should be saved to be used in soups, gravies, and white sauces. Using this liquid improves the flavor as well as the nutrient content of foods to which it is added.

enriched foods

foods to which nutrients, usually B vitamins and iron, have been added to improve their nutritional value

CLASSIFICATION

Minerals are divided into two groups. They are the major minerals, so named because each is required in amounts greater than 100 mg a day, and the trace minerals, which are needed in amounts smaller than 100 mg a day (Tables 8-1 and 8-2).

TABLE 8-1 Major Minerals

NAME	FOOD SOURCES	FUNCTIONS	DEFICIENCY/TOXICITY

Calcium (Ca^{++})	Milk, cheese
	Sardines
	Salmon
	Some dark green, leafy vegetables
		Development of bones and teeth
		Transmission of nerve impulses
		Blood clotting
		Normal heart action
		Normal muscle activity
			Deficiency
			  Osteoporosis
			  Osteomalacia
			  Rickets
			  Tetany
			  Retarded growth
			  Poor tooth and bone formation

Phosphorus (P^-)	Milk, cheese
	Lean meat
	Poultry
	Fish
	Whole grain cereals
	Legumes
	Nuts
		Development of bones and teeth
		Maintenance of normal acid-base balance of the blood
		Constituent of all body cells
		Necessary for effectiveness of some vitamins
		Metabolism of carbohydrates, fats, and proteins
			Deficiency
			  Poor tooth and bone formation
			  Weakness
			  Anorexia
			  General malaise

(continued)

TABLE 8-1 *continued*

NAME	FOOD SOURCES	FUNCTIONS	DEFICIENCY/TOXICITY

Potassium (K^+)	Oranges, bananas
	Dried fruits
	Vegetables
	Legumes
	Milk
	Cereals
	Meat
		Contraction of muscles
		Maintenance of fluid balance
		Transmission of nerve impulses
		Osmosis
		Regular heart rhythm
		Cell metabolism
			Deficiency
			  Hypokalemia
			  Muscle weakness
			  Confusion
			  Abnormal heartbeat
			Toxicity
			  Hyperkalemia

Sodium (Na^+)	Table salt
	Beef, eggs
	Poultry
	Milk, cheese
		Maintenance of fluid balance
		Transmission of nerve impulses
		Osmosis
		Acid-base balance
		Regulation of muscle and nerve irritability
			Deficiency
			  Nausea
			  Exhaustion
			  Muscle cramps
			Toxicity
			  Increase in blood pressure
			  Edema

Chloride (Cl^-)	Table salt
	Eggs
	Seafood
	Milk
		Gastric acidity
		Regulation of osmotic pressure
		Osmosis
		Fluid balance
		Acid-base balance
		Formation of hydrochloric acid
			Deficiency
			  Imbalance in gastric acidity
			  Imbalance in blood pH
			  Nausea
			  Exhaustion

Magnesium (Mg^{++})	Green, leafy vegetables Whole grains Avocados Nuts Milk Legumes Bananas	Synthesis of ATP Transmission of nerve impulses Activation of metabolic enzymes Constituent of bones, muscles, and red blood cells Necessary for healthy muscles and nerves	Deficiency Normally unknown Mental, emotional, and muscle disorders
Sulfur (S)	Eggs Poultry Fish	Maintenance of protein structure For building hair, nails, and all body tissues Constituent of all body cells	Unknown

Source: Courtesy of Delmar Publishers, Albany, NY.

TABLE 8-2 Trace Minerals

NAME	FOOD SOURCES	FUNCTIONS	DEFICIENCY/TOXICITY

Iron (Fe$^+$)	Muscle meats
	Poultry
	Shellfish
	Liver
	Legumes
	Dried fruits
	Whole grain or enriched breads and cereals
	Dark green and leafy vegetables
	Molasses
		Transports oxygen and carbon dioxide
		Component of hemoglobin and myoglobin
		Component of cellular enzymes essential for energy production
			Deficiency
			    Iron deficiency anemia characterized by weakness, dizziness, loss of weight, and pallor
			Toxicity
			    Hemochromatosis (genetic)
			    Can be fatal to children
			    May contribute to heart disease
			    Injure liver

Iodine (I$^-$)	Iodized salt
	Seafood
		Regulation of basal metabolic rate	Deficiency
			    Goiter
			    Cretinism
			    Myxedema

Zinc (Zn$^+$)	Seafood, especially oysters
	Liver
	Eggs
	Milk
	Wheat bran
	Legumes
		Formation of collagen
		Component of insulin
		Component of many vital enzymes
		Wound healing
		Taste acuity
		Essential for growth
		Immune reactions
			Deficiency
			    Dwarfism, hypogonadism, anemia
			    Loss of appetite
			    Skin changes
			    Impaired wound healing
			    Decreased taste acuity

Selenium (Se$^-$)	Seafood
	Kidney
	Liver
	Muscle meats
	Grains
		Constituent of most body tissue
		Needed for fat metabolism
		Antioxidant functions
			Deficiency
			    Unclear, but related to Keshan disease
			    Muscle weakness
			Toxicity
			    Vomiting
			    Loss of hair and nails
			    Skin lesions

Copper (Cu$^+$)	Liver
	Shellfish, oysters
	Legumes
	Nuts
	Whole grains
		Essential for formation of hemoglobin and red blood cells
		Component of enzymes
		Wound healing
		Needed metabolically for the release of energy
			Deficiency
			    Anemia
			    Bone disease
			    Disturbed growth and metabolism
			Toxicity
			    Vomiting; diarrhea
			    Wilson's Disease (Genetic)

(continued)

TABLE 8-2 *continued*

NAME	FOOD SOURCES	FUNCTIONS	DEFICIENCY/TOXICITY

Manganese (Mn$^+$)	Whole grains
	Nuts
	Fruits
	Tea
		Component of enzymes
		Bone formation
		Metabolic processes
			Deficiency
			  Unknown
			Toxicity
			  Possible brain disease

Fluoride (F$^-$)	Fluoridated water
	Seafood
		Increases resistance to tooth decay
		Component of bones and teeth
			Deficiency
			  Tooth decay
			  Possibly osteoporosis
			Toxicity
			  Discoloration of teeth (mottling)

Chromium (Cr)	Meat Vegetable oil Whole grain cereal and nuts Yeast	Associated with glucose and lipid metabolism	Deficiency Possibly disturbances of glucose metabolism

Molybdenum (Mo)	Dark green, leafy vegetables
	Liver
	Cereal
	Legumes
		Enzyme functioning
		Metabolism
			Deficiency
			  Unknown
			Toxicity
			  Inhibition of copper absorption

Source: Courtesy of Delmar Publishers, Albany, NY.

ions
electrically charged atoms resulting from chemical reactions

electrolyte
chemical compound that in water breaks up into electrically charged atoms called ions

As mineral salts dissolve in water, they break into separate, electrically charged particles called **ions**. Ions, if positively charged, are called cations. When negatively charged, they are anions. The cations and anions must be balanced within the body fluids to maintain electroneutrality. For example, if body fluid contains 200 positive (+) charges, it must also contain 200 negative (−) charges. These ions are known as **electrolytes**.

Electrolytes are essential in maintaining the body's fluid balance, and they contribute to its electrical balance, assist in its transmission of nerve impulses and contraction of muscles, and help regulate its acid-base balance (see Chapter 9).

Normally, a balanced diet will maintain electrolyte balance. However, in cases of severe diarrhea, vomiting, high fever, or burns, electrolytes are lost and the electrolyte balance can be upset. Medical intervention will be necessary to replace the lost electrolytes.

Scientists lack exact information on some of the trace elements, although they do know that trace elements are essential to good health. The study of these elements continues to reveal their specific relationships to human nutrition. A balanced diet is the only safe way of including minerals in the amounts necessary to maintain health.

The Food and Nutrition Board of the National Academy of Sciences–National Research Council (hereafter NRC) has recommended dietary allowances for minerals where research indicates knowledge is adequate to do so.

For those minerals where there remains some uncertainty as to amounts of specific human requirements, the NRC has provided a table of estimated safe and adequate daily dietary intakes of selected minerals (Table 8-3). The NRC recommends that the upper levels of listed amounts not be habitually exceeded. (Tables 8-1 and 8-2 list the best sources, functions, and deficiency symptoms of minerals.)

In addition, the Institute of Medicine has developed Daily Reference Intakes (DRI) for calcium, fluoride, phosphorus, and magnesium. The DRI incorporates Estimated Average Requirements (EAR), the RDA, and Tolerable Upper Intake Levels.

TABLE 8-3 Estimated Safe and Adequate Daily Dietary Intakes for Selected Trace Minerals

CATEGORY	AGE (years)	COPPER (mg)	MANGANESE (mg)	CHROMIUM (μg)	MOLYBDENUM (μg)
Infants	0–0.5	0.4–0.6	0.3–0.6	10–40	15–30
	0.5–1.0	0.6–0.7	0.6–1.0	20–60	20–40
Children and adolescents	1–3	0.7–1.0	1.0–1.5	20–80	25–50
	4–6	1.0–1.5	1.5–2.0	30–120	30–75
	7–10	1.0–2.0	2.0–3.0	50–200	50–150
	11+	1.5–2.5	2.0–5.0	50–200	75–250
Adults		1.5–3.0	2.0–5.0	50–200	75–250

Reprinted with permission from *Recommended Dietary Allowances: 10th Edition.* Copyright 1989 by the National Academy of Sciences. Courtesy of the National Academy Press, Washington, D.C.

TOXICITY

Because it is known that minerals are essential to good health, some would-be nutritionists will make claims that "more is better." Ironically, more can be hazardous to one's health when it comes to minerals. In a healthy individual eating a balanced diet, there will be some normal mineral loss through perspiration and saliva, and amounts in excess of body needs will be excreted in urine and feces. However, when concentrated forms of minerals are taken on a regular basis, over a period of time, they become more than the body can handle, and toxicity develops. An excessive amount of one mineral can sometimes cause a deficiency of another mineral. In addition, excessive amounts of minerals can cause hair loss and changes in the blood, hormones, bones, muscles, blood vessels, and nearly all tissues. Concentrated forms of minerals should be used only on the advice of a physician.

toxicity
state of being poisonous

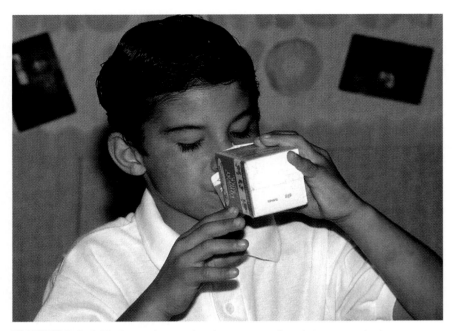

FIGURE 8-1 Milk is an important source of calcium and phosphorus. These minerals are essential for the normal growth and development of bones and teeth.

MAJOR MINERALS

Calcium (Ca)

The human body contains more calcium than any other mineral. The body of a 154-pound person contains approximately 4 pounds of calcium. Ninety-nine percent of that calcium is found in the skeleton and teeth. The remaining 1% is found in the blood.

Functions.   Calcium, in combination with phosphorus, is a component of bones and teeth, giving them strength and hardness. Bones, in turn, provide storage for calcium. Calcium is needed for normal nerve and muscle action, blood clotting, heart function, and cell metabolism.

Regulation of Blood Calcium.   Each cell requires calcium. It is carried throughout the body by the blood, and its delivery to the cells is regulated by the hormonal system. Normal blood calcium levels are maintained even if intake is poor.

When blood calcium levels are low, the parathyroid glands release a hormone that tells the kidneys to retrieve calcium before it is excreted. In addition, this hormone, working with calcitriol (the active hormone form of vitamin D), causes increased release of calcium from the bones by stimulating the activity of the osteoclasts (cells that break down bones). Both of these actions increase blood calcium levels. If calcium intake is low for a period of years, the amount withdrawn from the bones will cause them to become increasingly fragile. Osteoporosis may result.

If the blood calcium level is high, osteoblasts (cells that make bones) will increase bone mass. During growth, osteoblasts will make more bone mass than will be broken down. Bone mass is acquired until one is approximately 30–35 years old. With adequate consumption of calcium, phosphorus, and vitamin D, bone mass will remain stable in women until menopause. After menopause, bones will begin to weaken owing to the lack of the hormone estrogen. A special X-ray can be taken to determine bone density. If a person is at risk for injury due to decreased bone density, the physician will decide the best course of action. Drugs that help prevent further loss of bone mass are available.

Sources. The best sources of calcium are milk and milk products. They provide large quantities of calcium in small servings. For example, one cup of milk provides 300 mg of calcium (Figure 8-1). One ounce of cheddar cheese provides 250 mg of calcium.

Calcium is also found in some dark green, leafy vegetables. However, when the vegetable contains oxalic acid, as spinach and Swiss chard do, the calcium remains unavailable because the oxalic acid binds it and prevents it from being absorbed. When the intake of fiber exceeds 35g a day, calcium will also bind with phytates (phosphorus compounds found in some high-fiber cereal), which also limits its absorption.

Factors that are believed to enhance the absorption of calcium include adequate vitamin D, a calcium-to-phosphorus ratio that includes no more phosphorus than calcium, and the presence of lactose. A lack of weight-bearing exercise reduces the amount of calcium absorbed.

Requirements. The estimated requirement for calcium is now given as an Adequate Intake Level (AI). Calcium is measured in milligrams (mg). The AIs for calcium at different ages and conditions are shown in Table 8-4. The recommendations were made to achieve optimal bone health and to reduce the probability of fractures in later life.

TABLE 8-4 Adequate Intakes for Calcium

0–6 months	210 mg
6–12 months	270 mg
1–3 years	500 mg
4–8 years	800 mg
9–18 years	1,300 mg
19–50 years	1,000 mg
51–70+ years	1,200 mg
Pregnant women, 14–18 years	1,300 mg
Pregnant women, 19–50 years	1,000 mg
Lactating women	Same as for nonlactating women of same age

Source: Dietary Reference Intakes, Food and Nutrition Board, National Academy of Sciences–Institute of Medicine, 1997.

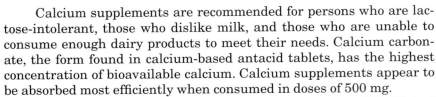

FIGURE 8-2 Always look for the USP seal of approval when purchasing supplements.

Calcium supplements are recommended for persons who are lactose-intolerant, those who dislike milk, and those who are unable to consume enough dairy products to meet their needs. Calcium carbonate, the form found in calcium-based antacid tablets, has the highest concentration of bioavailable calcium. Calcium supplements appear to be absorbed most efficiently when consumed in doses of 500 mg.

When purchasing calcium supplements, check for the USP (United States Pharmacopeia) seal of approval on the product you select (Figure 8-2). USP-approved products are unlikely to contain lead or other toxins. Avoid bone meal products, because they may contain lead.

Deficiency.   Calcium deficiency may result in **rickets**. This is a disease that occurs in early childhood and results in poorly formed bone structure (see Figure 7-2). It causes bowed legs, "pigeon breast," and enlarged wrists or ankles. Severe cases can result in stunted growth. Insufficient calcium can also cause "adult rickets" (osteomalacia), a condition in which bones become soft. And, although the precise **etiology** of osteoporosis is not known, it is thought that long-term calcium deficiency is a contributing factor. Other factors contributing to osteoporosis include deficiency of vitamin D and certain hormones.

Insufficient calcium in the blood can cause a condition characterized by involuntary muscle movement, known as **tetany**. Excessive intake may cause constipation or kidney stones, or it may inhibit the absorption of iron and zinc.

Phosphorus (P)

Phosphorus, together with calcium, is necessary for the formation of strong, rigid bones and teeth. Phosphorus is also important in the metabolism of carbohydrates, fats, and proteins. Phosphorus is a constituent of all body cells. It is necessary for a proper acid-base balance of the blood and is essential for the effective action of several B vitamins. Like calcium, phosphorus is stored in bones, and its absorption is increased in the presence of vitamin D.

Sources.   Although phosphorus is widely distributed in foods, its best sources are protein-rich foods such as milk, cheese, meats, poultry, and fish. Cereals, legumes, nuts, and soft drinks also contain substantial amounts of this mineral.

Requirements.   The requirement for phosphorus is provided as AI (Adequate Intake) for the first 12 months and as EAR (Estimated Average Requirements) after that (Table 8-5). Phosphorus is measured in milligrams.

Deficiency.   Because phosphorus is found in so many foods, its deficiency is rare. Excessive use of antacids can cause it, however, because they affect its absorption. Symptoms of phosphorus deficiency include bone **demineralization** (loss of minerals), fatigue, and anorexia.

rickets

deficiency disease caused by the lack of vitamin D; causes malformed bones and pain in infants

etiology

cause

tetany

involuntary muscle movement

demineralization

loss of mineral or minerals

TABLE 8-5 Adequate Intakes and Estimated Average
Requirements for Phosphorus

AI for phosphorus	
0–6 months	100 mg
6–12 months	275 mg
EAR for phosphorus	
1–3 years	380 mg
4–8 years	405 mg
9–18 years	1,055 mg
19–70+ years	580 mg
Pregnant and lactating women	Same as for nonpregnant and nonlactating women of same age

Source: Dietary Reference Intakes, Food and Nutrition Board, National Academy
of Sciences–Institute of Medicine, 1997.

Potassium (K)

Potassium is an electrolyte found primarily in **intracellular** fluid.
Like sodium, it is essential for fluid balance and osmosis. Potassium
maintains the fluid level within the cell, and sodium maintains the
fluid level *outside* the cell. **Osmosis** moves the fluid into and out of
cells as needed to maintain electrolyte (and fluid) balance. There is normally more potassium than sodium inside the cell and more sodium
than potassium outside the cell. If this balance is upset, and the
sodium inside the cell increases, the fluid within the cell also increases,
swelling it and causing edema. If the sodium level outside the cell
drops, fluid enters the cell to dilute the potassium level thereby causing
a reduction in **extracellular** fluid. With the loss of sodium and reduction of extracellular fluid, a decrease in blood pressure and dehydration can result.

Potassium is also necessary for transmitting nerve impulses, and
for muscle contractions.

Sources. Potassium is found in many foods. Fruits—especially
melons, oranges, bananas, and peaches—and vegetables—notably
mushrooms, Brussels sprouts, potatoes, tomatoes, winter squash, lima
beans, and carrots—are particularly rich sources of it.

Deficiency or Excess. Potassium deficiency (**hypokalemia**)
can be caused by diarrhea, vomiting, diabetic acidosis, severe malnutrition, or excessive use of laxatives or **diuretics**. Nausea, anorexia,
fatigue, muscle weakness, and heart abnormalities (tachycardia) are
symptoms of its deficiency. **Hyperkalemia** (high blood levels of potassium) can be caused by dehydration, renal failure, or excessive intake.
Cardiac failure can result.

intracellular
within the cell

osmosis
movement of a substance
through a semipermeable
membrane

extracellular
outside the cell

hypokalemia
low level of potassium in the
blood

diuretics
substances used to increase the
amount of urine excreted

hyperkalemia
excessive amounts of potassium
in the blood

Sodium (Na)

Sodium is an electrolyte whose primary function is the control of fluid balance in the body. It controls the extracellular fluid and is essential for osmosis. Sodium is also necessary to maintain the acid-base balance in the body. In addition, it participates in the transmission of nerve impulses essential for normal muscle function.

Sources. The primary dietary source of sodium is table salt (sodium chloride), which is 40% sodium. (One teaspoon of table salt contains 2,000 mg sodium.) It is also naturally available in animal foods. Salt is typically added to commercially prepared foods because it enhances flavor and helps to preserve some foods by controlling growth of microorganisms. Fruits and vegetables contain little or no sodium. Drinking water contains sodium but in varying amounts. "Softened" water has a much higher sodium content than "hard," or unsoftened, water.

Requirements. Although no RDA has been established for sodium, the NRC has suggested an estimated minimum requirement for adults of 500 mg a day (Table 8-6). However, studies indicate that dietary intake of sodium in the United States runs from 1,800 to 5,000 mg (about 2–5g) a day.

Deficiency or Excess. Either deficiency or excess of sodium can cause upsets in the body's fluid balance. Although rare, a deficiency of sodium can occur after severe vomiting, diarrhea, or heavy perspiration. In such cases, **dehydration** can result. A sodium deficiency also can upset the acid-base balance in the body. Cells function best in a neutral or slightly **alkaline** medium. If too much acid is lost (which can happen during severe vomiting), tetany due to **alkalosis** may

dehydration
loss of water

alkaline
base; capable of neutralizing acids

alkalosis
condition in which excess base accumulates in, or acids are lost from, the body

TABLE 8-6 Estimated Sodium, Chloride, and Potassium Minimum Requirements

AGE	WEIGHT (kg)	SODIUM (mg)	CHLORIDE (mg)	POTASSIUM (mg)
Months				
0–5	4.5	120	180	500
6–11	8.9	200	300	700
Years				
1	11.0	225	350	1,000
2–5	16.0	300	500	1,400
6–9	25.0	400	600	1,600
10–18	50.0	500	750	2,000
> 18	70.0	500	750	2,000

Reprinted with permission from *Recommended Dietary Allowances: 10th Edition.* Copyright 1989 by the National Academy of Sciences. Courtesy of the National Academy Press, Washington, D.C.

develop. If the alkaline reserve is deficient as a result of starvation or faulty metabolism, as in the case of diabetes, **acidosis** (too much acid) may develop.

An excess of sodium is a more common problem and may cause **edema**. This edema adds pressure to artery walls that can cause **hypertension**. Thus, an excess of sodium is frequently associated with **cardiovascular** conditions such as hypertension and congestive heart failure. In such cases, sodium-restricted diets are prescribed. Depending on the diagnosis, a physician will prescribe either a 3–4g (also called no-added salt, or NAS) or a 1–2g sodium-restricted diet. A physician rarely prescribes a diet of less than 1g sodium because compliance is difficult.

Chloride (Cl)

Chloride is an electrolyte that is essential for maintenance of fluid, electrolyte, and acid-base balance in the body. Like sodium, it is a constituent of extracellular fluid. It is also a component of gastric juices, where, in combination with hydrogen, it is found in hydrochloric acid; cerebrospinal (of the brain and spinal cord) fluid; and muscle and nerve tissue. It helps the blood carry carbon dioxide to the lungs and is necessary during immune responses when white blood cells attack foreign cells.

Sources. Chloride is found almost exclusively in table salt (sodium chloride) or in foods containing sodium chloride.

Requirements. Although there is no RDA for chloride, the estimated minimum requirement for normal adults is 750 mg a day.

Deficiency. Because chloride is found in salt, deficiency is rare. It can occur, however, with severe vomiting, diarrhea, or excessive use of diuretics, and alkalosis can result. Also, it could occur in patients who must follow long-term sodium-restricted diets. In such cases, patients can be provided with an alternative source of chloride.

Magnesium (Mg)

Magnesium is vital to both hard and soft body tissues. It is essential for metabolism and regulates nerve and muscle function, including the heart, and plays a role in the blood-clotting process.

Sources. Like phosphorus, magnesium is widely distributed in foods, but it is found primarily in plant foods. The nutrient-dense foods are green leafy vegetables, legumes, nuts, whole grains, and some fruits such as avocados and bananas. Milk is also a good source if taken in sufficient quantity. For example, 2 cups of fat-free milk provide about 60 mg of magnesium.

Magnesium is lost during commercial food processing and in cooking water, so it is preferable to use vegetables and fruits raw rather than cooked.

acidosis
condition in which excess acids accumulate or there is a loss of base in the body

edema
the abnormal retention of fluid by the body

hypertension
higher than normal blood pressure

cardiovascular
pertaining to the heart and entire circulatory system

TABLE 8-7 Adequate Intakes and Estimated Average Requirements for Magnesium

AI for magnesium		
	0–6 months	30 mg
	6–12 months	75 mg
EAR for magnesium		
Boys and girls	1–3 years	65 mg
	4–8 years	110 mg
	9–13 years	200 mg
Boys	14–18 years	340 mg
Girls	14–18 years	300 mg
Men	19–30 years	330 mg
Women	19–30 years	255 mg
Men	31–70+ years	350 mg
Women	31–70+ years	265 mg
Pregnant women	14–18 years	335 mg
	19–30 years	290 mg
	31–50 years	300 mg
Lactating women	14–18 years	300 mg
	19–30 years	255 mg
	31–50 years	265 mg

Source: Dietary Reference Intakes, Food and Nutrition Board, National Academy of Sciences–Institute of Medicine, 1997.

Requirements. The requirement for magnesium is provided as AI (Adequate Intakes) for the first 12 months and as EAR (Estimated Average Requirements) after that (Table 8-7). Magnesium is measured in milligrams.

Deficiency. Because of the wide availability of magnesium, its deficiency among people on normal diets is unknown. When deficiency was experimentally induced, the symptoms included nausea and mental, emotional, and muscular disorders.

Sulfur (S)

Sulfur is necessary to all body tissue and is found in all body cells. It contributes to the characteristic odor of burning hair and tissue. It is necessary for metabolism.

Sources. Sulfur is a component of some amino acids and consequently is found in protein-rich foods.

Requirements or Deficiency. Neither the amount of sulfur required by the human body nor its deficiency is known.

TRACE MINERALS

Iron (Fe)

The principal role of iron is to deliver oxygen to body tissues. It is a component of hemoglobin, the coloring matter of red blood cells (erythrocytes). Hemoglobin allows red blood cells to combine with oxygen in the lungs and carry it to body tissues.

Iron is also a component of **myoglobin**, a protein compound in muscles that provides oxygen to cells, and it is a constituent of other body compounds involved in oxygen transport. Iron is utilized by enzymes that are involved in the making of amino acids, hormones, and neurotransmitters.

Sources. Meat, poultry, and fish are the best sources of iron because only the flesh of animals contains **heme iron**. Heme iron is absorbed more than twice as efficiently as nonheme iron. **Nonheme iron** is found in whole grain cereals, enriched grain products, vegetables, fruit, eggs, meat, fish, and poultry. The rate of absorption of nonheme iron is strongly influenced by dietary factors and body iron stores. Factors affecting the absorption of both heme and nonheme iron are listed on Table 8-8.

For iron to be absorbed, it must be chemically changed from ferric to ferrous iron. This change is accomplished by the hydrochloric acid in the stomach. Absorption of nonheme iron can be enhanced by consuming a vitamin C–rich food and a nonheme iron–rich food at the same meal. Vitamin C holds onto and keeps the iron in its ferrous form, which facilitates absorption. Meat protein factor (MPF) is a substance in meat, poultry, and fish that aids in the absorption of nonheme iron.

Phytic acid and oxalic acid can bind iron and reduce the body's absorption of it. Polyphenols, such as tannins in tea and related substances in coffee, also reduce the absorption of iron. Antacids containing calcium and calcium supplements should be taken several hours before or after a meal high in iron because calcium also interferes with iron absorption.

myoglobin

protein compound in muscle that provides oxygen to cells

heme iron

part of hemoglobin molecule in animal foods

nonheme iron

iron from animal foods that is not part of the hemoglobin molecule; and all iron from plant foods

TABLE 8-8 Factors That Affect Iron Absorption

INCREASE	DECREASE
Acid in the stomach	Phytic acid (in fiber)
Heme iron	Oxalic acid
High body demand for red blood cells (blood loss, pregnancy)	Polyphenols in tea and coffee
Low body stores of iron	Full body stores of iron
Meat protein factor (MPF)	Excess of other minerals (Zn, Mn, Ca) (especially when taken as supplements)
Vitamin C	Some antacids

Requirements.   The NRC has determined that men lose approximately 1 mg of iron a day and that women lose 1.5 mg a day. On the assumption that only 10% of ingested iron is absorbed, the RDA for men has been set at 10 mg and for women from the age of 11 through the childbearing years at 15 mg. This is doubled during pregnancy and is difficult to meet by diet alone. Consequently, an iron supplement is commonly prescribed during pregnancy. Women should make a special effort to include iron-rich foods in their diets at all times. The rapid growth periods of infancy and adolescence also produce a heavy need for iron.

iron deficiency

intake of iron is adequate, but the body has no extra iron stored

iron-deficiency anemia

condition resulting from inadequate amount of iron in the diet, reducing the amount of oxygen carried by the blood to the cells

Deficiency or Toxicity.   Iron deficiency continues to be a problem, especially for women. **Iron deficiency** can be caused by insufficient intake, malabsorption, lack of sufficient stomach acid, or excessive blood loss, any or all of which can deplete iron stores in the body. Decreased stores of iron prevent hemoglobin synthesis. The result is an insufficient number of red blood cells to carry needed oxygen. What begins as iron deficiency can become **iron-deficiency anemia**. Iron deficiency anemia takes a long time to develop, but it is the most common nutrient deficiency worldwide. Symptoms include fatigue, weakness, irritability, and shortness of breath. Clinical signs include pale skin and spoon-shaped fingernails.

Some people suffer from *hemochromatosis*. This is a condition due to an inborn error of metabolism and causes excessive absorption of iron. Unless treated, this condition can damage the liver, spleen, and heart. To control the buildup of iron, patients with this condition must give blood on a regular basis.

Iodine (I)

Iodine is a component of the thyroid hormones, thyroxine (T_4) and triiodothyronine (T_3). It is necessary for the normal functioning of the thyroid gland, which determines the rate of metabolism.

iodized salt

salt that has had the mineral iodine added for the prevention of goiter

Sources.   The primary sources of iodine are **iodized salt**, seafood, and some plant foods grown in soil bordering the sea. Iodized salt is common table salt to which iodine has been added in an amount that, if used in normal cooking, provides sufficient iodine.

goiter

enlarged tissue of the thyroid gland due to a deficiency of iodine

Requirements.   The RDA for adults is 150 μg a day. Additional amounts are needed during pregnancy and lactation.

Deficiency.   When the thyroid gland lacks sufficient iodine, the manufacture of thyroxine and triiodothyronine is retarded. In its attempt to take up more iodine, the gland grows, forming a lump on the neck called a **goiter** (Figure 8-3). Goiter appears to be more common among women than among men. A thyroid gland that doesn't function properly causes myxedema (hypothyroidism) in adults. The children of mothers lacking sufficient iodine may suffer from cretinism (retarded physical and mental development).

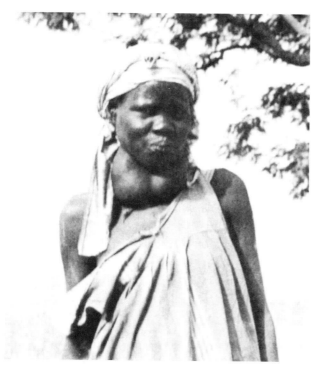

FIGURE 8-3 A goiter, which results primarily from iodine deficiency, is an enlargement of the thyroid gland. (Courtesy of the Food and Agriculture Organization of the United Nations)

Zinc (Zn)

Zinc is a cofactor for more than 300 enzymes. Consequently, it affects many body tissues. It appears to be essential for growth, wound healing, taste acuity, glucose tolerance, and the mobilization of vitamin A within the body.

Sources.   The best sources of zinc are protein foods, especially meat, fish, eggs, and dairy products, and wheat germ and legumes.

Requirements.   The RDA for zinc in normal adult males is 15 mg and for adult females, 12 mg, with increased requirements during pregnancy and further increases during lactation.

Deficiency.   Decreased appetite and taste acuity, delayed growth, dwarfism, hypogonadism (subnormal development of male sex organs), poor wound healing, anemia, acne-like rash, and impaired immune response are all symptoms of zinc deficiency.

Selenium (Se)

Selenium is a constituent of most body tissues, but the heaviest concentration of the mineral is in the liver, kidneys, and heart.

Functions. Selenium is a component of an enzyme that acts as an antioxid.ant. In this way, it protects cells against oxidation and spares vitamin E.

Sources. The best sources of selenium are seafood, kidney, liver, and musc.le meats.

Requirements. The RDA for selenium for an adult male is 70 μg and for an adult female, 55 μg.

Deficiency or Toxicity. Symptoms of selenium deficiency are unclear, but selenium supplements appear to be effective in treating Keshan disease. High doses (1 mg or more daily) are toxic and can cause vomiting, loss of hair and nails, and skin lesions.

Keshan disease
condition causing abnormalities in the heart muscle

Copper (Cu)

Copper is found in all tissues, but its heaviest concentration is in the liver, kidneys, muscles, and brain. As an essential component of several enzymes, it helps in the formation of hemoglobin; aids in the transport of iron to bone marrow (soft tissue in bone center) for the formation of red blood cells; and participates in energy production.

Sources. Copper is available in many foods, but its best sources include organ meats, shellfish, legumes, nuts, cocoa, and whole grain cereals. Human milk is a good source of copper, but cow's milk is not.

Requirements. Although there is no RDA for copper, the NRC's estimated safe intake for adults is 1.5 to 3 mg a day.

Deficiency or Toxicity. Copper deficiency is extremely rare among adults, occurring only in people with malabsorption conditions and in cases of gross protein deficiency, such as kwashiorkor. It is apparent sometimes in premature infants and in people on long-term parenteral nutrition (feeding via a vein) programs lacking copper. A copper deficiency can be caused by taking excess zinc supplements. Anemia, bone demineralization, and impaired growth may result.

Excess copper can be highly toxic. A single dose of 10–15 mg can cause vomiting. Wilson's disease is an inherited condition resulting in accumulation of copper in the liver, brain, kidneys, and cornea. It can cause damage to liver cells and neurons. If the excess is detected early, copper-binding agents can be used to bind copper in the bloodstream and increase excretion.

Manganese (Mn)

Manganese is a constituent of several enzymes involved in metabolism. It is also important in bone formation.

Sources. The best sources of manganese are whole grains and tea. Vegetables and fruits also contain moderate amounts.

Requirements. The estimated safe and adequate daily dietary intake for adults is 2.0 to 5.0 mg.

Deficiency and Toxicity. Its deficiency has not been documented. Toxicity from excessive ingestion of manganese is unknown. However, people who have inhaled high concentrations of manganese dust have developed neurological problems.

Fluoride (F)

Fluoride increases one's resistance to dental caries. It appears to strengthen bones and teeth by making the bone mineral less soluble and thus less inclined to being reabsorbed.

Sources. The principal source of fluoride is fluoridated water (water to which fluoride has been added). In addition, fish and tea contain fluoride. Commercially prepared foods in which fluoridated water has been used during the preparation process also contain fluoride.

Requirements. The requirement for fluoride is given as AI (Adequate Intake) levels (Table 8-9). Fluoride is measured in milligrams (mg).

TABLE 8-9 Adequate Intakes for Fluoride

	0–6 months	0.01 mg
	6–12 months	0.5 mg
	1–3 years	0.7 mg
	4–8 years	1.1 mg
	9–13 years	2.0 mg
Boys	14–18 years	3.2 mg
Girls	14–18 years	2.9 mg
Males	19+ years	3.8 mg
Females	19+ years	3.1 mg
Pregnant and lactating women	Same as for nonpregnant and nonlactating women of same age	

Source: Dietary Reference Intakes, Food and Nutrition Board, National Academy of Sciences–Institute of Medicine, 1997.

Deficiency or Toxicity. The deficiency of fluoride can result in increased tooth decay. Excessive amounts of fluoride in drinking water have been known to cause discoloration or mottling of children's teeth.

Chromium (Cr)

Chromium is associated with glucose and lipid metabolism. Chromium levels decrease with age except in the lungs, where chromium accumulates.

Sources. The best sources of chromium include meat, mushrooms, nuts, yeast, organ meats, and wheat germ.

Requirements.   Although there is as yet no RDA for chromium, the estimated safe and adequate daily intake for adults is 50 to 200 μg. There appears to be no difficulty fulfilling this requirement when one has a balanced diet.

Deficiency.   Chromium deficiency appears to be related to disturbances in glucose metabolism.

 ## Molybdenum (Mo)

Molybdenum is a constituent of enzymes and is thought to play a role in metabolism.

Sources.   The best sources of molybdenum include milk, liver, legumes, and cereals.

Requirements.   The estimated safe and adequate daily intake for adults is 75 to 250 μg. This is normally fulfilled with a balanced diet.

Deficiency or Toxicity.   No deficiencies have been noted in people who consume a normal diet. Excessive intake can inhibit copper absorption.

CONSIDERATIONS FOR THE HEALTH CARE PROFESSIONAL

Second to vitamins, minerals are of great interest to the general public. They often are given mythic powers in current articles.

It is imperative that the health care professional be aware of the dangers of megadoses of minerals and be able to transmit this information in a meaningful way to the patients.

● SUMMARY

Minerals are necessary to promote growth and regulate body processes. They originate in soil and water and are ingested via food and drink. Deficiencies can result in conditions such as anemia, rickets, and goiter. A well-balanced diet can prevent mineral deficiencies. Concentrated forms of minerals should be taken only on the advice of a physician. Excessive amounts of minerals can be toxic, causing hair loss and changes in nearly all body tissues.

● DISCUSSION TOPICS

1. Discuss the special importance of calcium and phosphorus to children and to pregnant women.

2. List ways of supplying an adequate amount of calcium in the diet of an adult who dislikes milk. Plan a day's menu for this adult.

3. Ask if any member of the class has suffered from anemia. If anyone has, ask the class member to describe the symptoms and treatment. What kind of anemia was it? If it's preventable, what measures are being taken to prevent a recurrence of the condition?

4. If a person is to decrease sodium in her or his diet, should animal foods be increased or decreased?

5. Why does the NRC recommend that the upper limits of RDAs for minerals not be habitually exceeded?

6. If anyone in class knows someone with osteoporosis, ask for a description of the patient, including sex, age, physical appearance, physical complaints, life-long dietary habits, and medical treatment.

7. Explain the relationship of sodium and edema.

8. Why is it recommended that patients on sodium-restricted diets have the mineral content of their local water supply evaluated?

9. Explain the relationship of sodium and potassium.

10. Why would a doctor prescribe potassium at the same time a diuretic is prescribed?

11. Although rare, why does chloride deficiency sometimes occur in patients on long-term sodium-restricted diets?

12. Discuss the differences between heme and nonheme iron.

13. Why is iron commonly prescribed for pregnant women?

14. Why is selenium said to spare vitamin E?

● SUGGESTED ACTIVITIES

1. Using outside sources, prepare a report on how sodium and potassium regulate the body's fluid balance.

2. Using other sources, write a report on at least one of the following:
   Rickets
   Goiter
   Hypothyroidism and hyperthyroidism
   Edema
   Osteoporosis
   Osteomalacia

3. Check four or five varieties of bread at the local supermarket. Using the labels on the breads, evaluate their mineral content.

4. List five good sources of heme iron and five sources of nonheme iron.

5. Spend five or ten minutes observing customers at a drugstore display of various vitamin and mineral compounds. Write a short report on which minerals were most frequently purchased. Include your opinion as to why this was the case.

6. Write a short essay on why iodized salt is a better choice than plain salt.

● REVIEW

Multiple choice. Select the *letter* that precedes the best answer.

1. Minerals are inorganic elements that
   a. help to build and repair tissues
   b. are found only in bones
   c. provide energy when carbohydrates are lacking
   d. can substitute for proteins

2. The trace minerals in the human body are defined as
   a. those minerals that cannot be detected in laboratory tests
   b. those essential minerals found in very small amounts
   c. those minerals that are not essential to health
   d. only those minerals that are found in the blood

3. Calcium is necessary for
   a. healthy bones and teeth
   b. normal red blood cells
   c. preventing goiter
   d. energy

4. Phosphorus is found in
   a. poultry
   b. common table salt
   c. vegetable oils
   d. leafy vegetables

5. The coloring matter of the blood is
   a. hemoglobin
   b. lymph
   c. marrow
   d. plasma

6. Some of the common signs of iron deficiency anemia are
   a. muscle spasms and pain in the liver
   b. bowed legs and an enlarged thyroid gland
   c. edema and loss of vision
   d. dizziness and weakness

7. Iodine is essential to health because it
   a. is necessary for red blood cells
   b. strengthens bones and teeth
   c. helps the blood to carry oxygen to the cells
   d. affects the rate of metabolism

8. Sodium is often restricted in cardiovascular conditions because it
   a. causes the heart to beat slowly
   b. encourages the growth of the heart
   c. contributes to edema
   d. raises the blood sugar

9. Iron is known to be a necessary component of
   a. thyroxine
   b. adipose tissue
   c. hemoglobin
   d. amino acids

10. Liquid from cooking vegetables should be used in preparing other dishes because
    a. mineral salts are soluble in water
    b. the hydrogen and oxygen in water aid the digestion of minerals
    c. the amino acids are soluble in water
    d. none of the above

11. Goiter can result from a deficiency of
    a. manganese
    b. magnesium
    c. copper
    d. iodine

12. A deficiency of calcium can cause
   a. lactose intolerance
   b. severe nausea
   c. tetany
   d. hypertension

13. Sodium is especially important in
   a. the blood-clotting process
   b. curing osteoporosis
   c. the prevention of osteomalacia
   d. osmosis

14. Sulfur
   a. is found only in bones and teeth
   b. is richly supplied in carbohydrates
   c. is found in all body cells
   d. deficiency is very common

15. Hypokalemia is
   a. caused by an abnormal heartbeat
   b. caused by potassium deficiency
   c. often a precursor of hyperkalemia
   d. a common result of chronic overeating

C A S E   S T U D Y

Jerry is a 50-year-old divorced man who suffers from hypertension. He is a regional salesman for a fast-food chain. His physician has told him to stop adding salt to any food he cooks and to cut his table salt consumption in half. Jerry has been following this advice, but his blood pressure is still 160/98. After further discussion, the physician learns that Jerry seldom cooks and he eats at least five of seven lunches per week at fast-food restaurants. He eats frozen dinners at least three nights a week and cheese and crackers with milk at bedtime.

ASSESSMENT

1. What data has the physician collected so far?
2. What needs to change in Jerry's diet?
3. What information does Jerry need?

DIAGNOSIS

4. What behaviors are keeping Jerry's blood pressure so high?
5. What further education does Jerry need?

PLAN/GOAL

6. If you were the dietitian, what two goals would you set for Jerry?

IMPLEMENTATION

7. What are the main topics that you would teach Jerry about a low-fat, low-sodium diet?
8. Give three or four examples of foods that Jerry could eat in a fast-food restaurant and adhere to his new diet.
9. List three or four examples of low-sodium instant meals Jerry could make at home for dinner.
10. What could he substitute for his current bedtime snack?

EVALUATION/OUTCOME CRITERIA

11. How will the doctor know if Jerry is successful?

C A S E   S T U D Y

At 29, Jennifer was finally pregnant. She and her husband, Adam, had been planning for a family for over 3 years. She had been eating with pregnancy in mind. She had been watching her weight and running or bicycling to keep fit. Once she had verified she was pregnant, she even started taking daily vitamins on her own. By the time she was 3 months pregnant, she was doing well. She had very little morning sickness, but she did have frequent periods of dizziness and shortness of breath with exercise. She thought that was not unusual in pregnancy.

She looked forward to the arrival of the baby. She hoped to teach the child to respect other people and animals. Her child would also be a vegetarian, as she had been since her freshman year at college. For the duration of the pregnancy, she did add chicken and fish to her diet.

At her next prenatal appointment, she was crushed when the nurse practitioner (NP) told her she was anemic. The NP was concerned about her diet and suggested she take prenatal vitamins with iron.

ASSESSMENT

1. What information do you have about Jennifer and her prenatal problem?
2. How much iron does Jennifer need during her pregnancy?
3. How are her symptoms related to the anemia?

DIAGNOSIS

4. What was the cause of Jennifer's anemia?

PLAN/GOAL

5. Write a measurable specific goal for Jennifer's anemia.

IMPLEMENTATION

6. Respecting Jennifer's desire to be a vegetarian, suggest some foods she could eat that are high in iron.
7. What could she eat to enhance the absorption of the iron she eats?

EVALUATION/OUTCOME CRITERIA

8. How could Jennifer know if the plan is successful?
9. What would the NP check to see if the plan is successful?
10. What are the consequences if the plan fails?

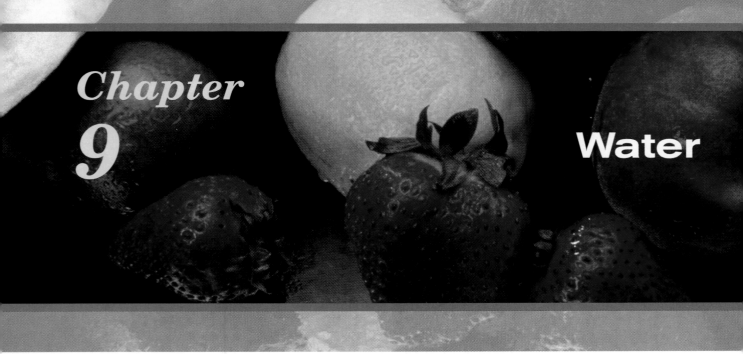

Chapter 9

Water

Key Terms

acid-base balance

acidosis

alkalosis

buffer systems

cellular edema

dehydration

extracellular fluid

homeostasis

hypothalamus

interstitial fluid

intracellular fluid

milliequivalent

osmolality

osmosis

pH

solute

solvent

vascular osmotic pressure

intracellular fluid
water within cells; approximately
65% of total body fluid

Objectives

After studying this chapter, you should be able to:

● Describe the functions of water in the body

● Explain fluid balance and its maintenance

● Name causes and consequences of water depletion

● Give causes and consequences of positive fluid balance

● Describe the acid-base balance of the human body

FUNCTIONS OF BODY WATER

Although humans can live about 8 weeks without food, it is possible to live only a few days without water. Water is a component of all body cells and constitutes from 50 to 60% of the body weight of normal adults. The percentage is higher in males than females because men usually have more muscle tissue than women. The water content of muscle tissue is higher than that of fat tissue. The percentage of water content is highest in newborns (75%) and decreases with age.

Body water is divided into two basic compartments: intracellular and extracellular. **Intracellular fluid** (ICF) is water within the cells and accounts for about 65% of

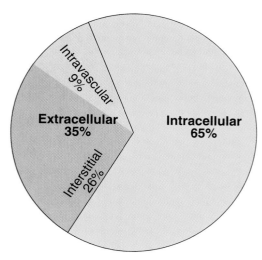

FIGURE 9-1 Body fluid compartments as percentage of total body fluid. All fluid in the body can be classified as either intracellular or extracellular.

total body fluid (Figure 9-1). **Extracellular fluid** (ECF) is water outside the cells and accounts for about 35% of total body fluid. Extracellular fluid is found in the intravascular fluid (water in the blood stream), **interstitial fluid**, and glandular secretions.

Although it is a component of all body tissues, water is the major component of blood plasma. It is a **solvent** for nutrients and waste products and helps transport both to and from body cells by way of the blood. It is necessary for the hydrolysis of nutrients in the cells, making it essential for metabolism. It functions as a lubricant in joints and in digestion. In addition, it cools the body through perspiration and may, depending on its source, provide some mineral elements (Table 9-1).

The best source of water is drinking water. Beverages of all types are the second-best source. A considerable amount is also found in foods, especially fruits, vegetables, soups, milk, and gelatin desserts. In addition, energy metabolism produces water. When carbohydrates, fats, and proteins are metabolized, their end products include carbon dioxide and water (Table 9-2).

extracellular fluid
water outside the cells; approximately 35% of total body fluid

interstitial fluid
fluid between cells

solvent
liquid part of a solution

TABLE 9-1 Functions of Water

Component of all body tissues
Solvent for nutrients and body wastes
Provides transport for nutrients and wastes
Essential for hydrolysis and thus metabolism
Lubricant of joints and in digestion
Helps regulate body temperature

TABLE 9-2 Estimated Daily Fluid Intake for an Adult

Ingested liquids	1,500 ml
Water in foods	700 ml
Water from oxidation	200 ml
Total	2,400 ml

FLUID AND ELECTROLYTE BALANCE

homeostasis
state of physical balance;
stable condition

milliequivalent
the concentration of electrolytes
in a solution

osmosis
movement of a substance
through a semipermeable
membrane

solute
the substance dissolved in
a solution

For optimum health there must be **homeostasis**. For this to exist, the body must be in *fluid and electrolyte balance*. This means the water lost by healthy individuals through urination, feces, perspiration, and the respiratory tract must be replaced both in terms of volume and electrolyte content. Electrolytes are measured in **milliequivalents** (mEq/L). An illness causing vomiting and diarrhea can result in large losses of water and electrolytes and must be addressed quickly. Water lost through urine is known as sensible (noticeable) water loss. Insensible (unnoticed) water loss is in feces, perspiration, and respiration. The body must excrete 500 ml of water as urine each day in order to get rid of the waste products of metabolism (Table 9-3).

Water moves through cell walls by **osmosis** (Figure 9-2). Water flows from the side with the lesser amount of **solute** to the side with the greater solute concentration. The electrolytes sodium, chloride, and potassium are the solutes that maintain the balance between intracellular and extracellular fluids. Potassium is the principal electrolyte in

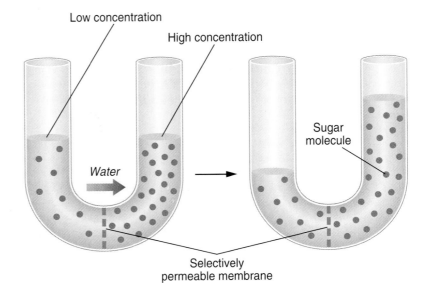

Low concentration

High concentration

Water

Sugar
molecule

Selectively
permeable membrane

Before Osmosis   **After Osmosis**

FIGURE 9-2 In osmosis, water passes through the selectively permeable cell membrane from an area of low solute concentration to an area of high solute concentration.

intracellular fluid. Sodium is the principal electrolyte in extracellular fluid. **Osmolality** is the measure of particles in a solution.

When the electrolytes in the extracellular fluid are *increased*, ICF moves to the ECF in an attempt to equalize the concentration of electrolytes on both sides of the membrane. This movement reduces the amount of water in the cells. The cells of the **hypothalamus** (regulates appetite and thirst) then become dehydrated, as do those in the mouth and tongue, and the body experiences thirst. The hypothalamus stimulates the pituitary gland to excrete ADH (antidiuretic hormone) whenever the electrolytes become too concentrated in the blood or whenever blood volume or blood pressure is too low. (This measurement is called **vascular osmotic pressure**.). The ADH causes the kidneys to reabsorb water rather than excrete it. At such times, thirst causes the healthy person to drink fluids, which provide the water and electrolytes needed by the cells.

When the sodium in the ECF is reduced, water flows from the ECF into the cells, causing **cellular edema**. When this occurs, the adrenal glands secrete aldosterone, which triggers the kidneys to increase the amount of sodium reabsorbed. When the missing sodium is replaced in the ECF, the excess water that has been drawn from the ECF into the cells moves back to the ECF, and the edema is relieved.

The amount of water used and thus needed each day varies, depending on age, size, activity, environmental temperature, and physical condition. The average adult water requirement is 1 ml (milliliter) for every kcal in food consumed. For example, for every 1,800 kcal in food consumed, one needs to drink 7.5 glasses of fluid. For optimal health, it is recommended that adults drink eight 8-ounce glasses of fluid a day, preferably eight glasses of water but at least four of water and four of other fluids. Youth, fever, diarrhea, unusual perspiration, and hyperthyroidism increase the requirement.

Dehydration

When the amount of water in the body is inadequate, **dehydration** can occur. It can be caused by inadequate intake or abnormal loss. Such loss can occur from severe diarrhea, vomiting, hemorrhage, burns, diabetes mellitus, excessive perspiration, excessive urination, or the use of certain medications such as diuretics. Symptoms of dehydration include low blood pressure, thirst, dry skin, fever, and mental disorientation.

As water is lost, electrolytes are also lost. Thus, treatment includes replacement of electrolytes and fluids. Electrolyte content must be checked and corrections made if necessary. A loss of 10% of body water can cause serious problems. Blood volume and nutrient absorption are reduced, and kidney function is upset. A loss of 20% of body water can cause circulatory failure and death. Infants, for example, are at high risk of dehydration when fever, vomiting, and diarrhea occur. Intravenous fluids are often necessary if sufficient fluids cannot be consumed by mouth.

The thirst sensation often lags behind the body's need for water, especially in the elderly, children, athletes, and the ill. Feeling thirsty is not a reliable indicator of when the body needs water. Fluids should be drunk throughout the day to prevent dehydration (Figure 9-3 and Table 9-4).

osmolality
number of particles per kilogram of solution; solutions with high osmolality exert more pressure than do those with fewer particles

hypothalamus
area at base of brain that regulates appetite and thirst

vascular osmotic pressure
high concentration of electrolytes in the blood; low blood volume or blood pressure

cellular edema
swelling of body cells caused by inadequate amount of sodium in extracellular fluid

dehydration
loss of water

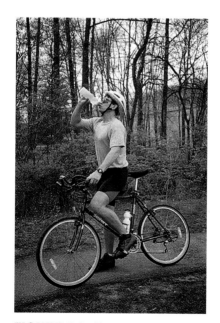

FIGURE 9-3 Preventing dehydration is an important element of proper nutrition.

Dehydration can occur in hot weather when one perspires excessively but fails to drink sufficient water to replace the amount lost through perspiration. Failure to replace water lost through perspiration could lead to one of the four stages of heat illness or could progress through all four. The four stages of heat illness are: (1) *Heat fatigue*, which causes thirst, feelings of weakness, or fatigue. To combat this, one should go to a cool place, rest, and drink fluids. (2) *Heat cramp*, due to the loss of sodium and potassium, which causes leg cramps and thirst. One should go to a cool place, rest, and drink fluids. (3) *Heat exhaustion*, which causes thirst, dizziness, nausea, headache, and profuse sweating. Treatment includes sponge baths with cool water, a 2- to 3-day rest, and the ingestion of a great deal of water. (4) *Heat stroke*, which involves fever and could produce brain and kidney damage.

TABLE 9-3 Factors That Lead to Fluid Imbalances

	FLUID DEFICIT	FLUID EXCESS
Enviromental factors	Exposure to sun or high atmospheric temperatures	
Personal behaviors	Fasting Fad diets Exercise without adequate fluid replacement	Excessive sodium or water intake Venous compression due to pregnancy
Psychological influences	Decreased motivation to drink due to Fatigue Depression Excessive use of Laxatives Enemas Alcohol Caffeine	Low protein intake due to anorexia
Consequences of diseases	Fluid losses due to Fever Wound drainage Vomiting Diarrhea Heavy menstrual flow Burns Difficulty swallowing due to Oral pain Fatigue Neuromuscular weakness Excessive urinary output due to uncontrolled Diabetes mellitus Diabetes insipidus	Fluid retention due to Renal failure Cardiac conditions Congestive heart failure Valvular diseases Left ventricular failure Cirrhosis Cancer Impaired venous return

TABLE 9-4 Signs of Dehydration

Health history reveals inadequate intake of fluids.

Decrease in urine output.

Weight loss (% body weight): 3–5% for mild, 6–9% for moderate, and 10–15% for severe dehydration.

Eyes appear sunken; tongue has increased furrows and fissures.

Oral mucous membranes are dry.

Decreased skin turgor (normal skin resiliency).

Changes in neurological status may occur with moderate to severe dehydration.

Emergency medical service (911) should be called and the patient should be put in chilled water and transported to the hospital. People can die from heat stroke. People who are unable to perspire are at high risk for any of the stages of heat illness.

Excess Water Accumulation

Some conditions cause an excessive accumulation of fluid in the body. This condition is called positive water balance. It occurs when more water is taken in than is used and excreted, and edema results. Hypothyroidism, congestive heart failure, hypoproteinemia (low amounts of protein), some infections, some cancers, and some renal conditions can cause such water retention because sodium is not being excreted normally. Fluids and sodium may then be restricted.

ACID-BASE BALANCE

In addition to maintaining fluid and electrolyte balance, the body must also maintain acid-base balance. This is the regulation of hydrogen ions in body fluids (pH balance).

In a water solution, an acid gives off hydrogen ions and a base picks them up. Hydrochloric acid is an example of an acid found in the body. It is secreted by the stomach and is necessary for the digestion of proteins. Ammonia is a base produced in the kidneys from amino acids.

Acidic substances run from pH 1 to 7, with the lowest numbers representing the most acidic (which contain the most hydrogen ions). Alkaline substances run from pH 7 to 14, with the alkalinity increasing with the number (as the number of hydrogen ions decreases). A pH 7 is considered neutral. Blood plasma runs from pH 7.35 to 7.45. Intracellular fluid has a pH of 6.8. The kidneys play the primary role in maintaining the acid-base balance by selecting which ions to retain and which to excrete. For the most part, what a person eats affects the acidity not of the body but of the urine.

acid-base balance
the regulation of hydrogen ions in body fluids

pH
symbol for the degree of acidity or alkalinity of a solution

Buffer Systems

The body has **buffer systems** that regulate hydrogen ion content in body fluids. Such a system is a mixture of a weak acid and a strong base that reacts to protect the nature of the solution in which it exists. In a normal buffer system, the ratio of base to acid is 20:1. For example, when a strong acid is added to a buffered solution, the base takes up the hydrogen ions of the strong acid, thereby weakening it. When a strong base is added to a solution, the acid of the buffer system combines with this base and weakens it.

A mixture of carbonic acid and sodium bicarbonate forms the body's main buffer system. Carbonic acid moves easily to buffer a strong alkali and sodium bicarbonate moves easily to buffer a strong acid. Amounts are easily adjusted by the lungs and kidneys to suit needs. For example, the end products of metabolism are carbon dioxide and water, and together they can form carbonic acid. The hemoglobin in the blood carries carbon dioxide to the lungs, where the excess is excreted. If the amount of carbon dioxide is more concentrated than it should be, the medulla oblongata in the brain causes the breathing rate to increase. This increase, in turn, increases the rate at which the body rids itself of carbon dioxide. Excess sodium bicarbonate is excreted via the kidneys. The kidneys can excrete urine from pH 4.5 to pH 8. The pH of average urine is 6.

Acidosis and Alkalosis

The healthy person eating a balanced diet does not normally have to think about acid-base balance. Upsets can occur in some disease conditions, however. Renal failure, uncontrolled diabetes mellitus, starvation, or severe diarrhea can cause **acidosis**. This is a condition in which the body is unable to balance the need for bases with the amount of acids it is retaining. **Alkalosis** can occur when the body has suffered a loss of hydrochloric acid from severe vomiting or has ingested too much alkali, such as too many antacid tablets.

CONSIDERATIONS FOR THE HEALTH CARE PROFESSIONAL

Patients who are required to limit both their salt and liquid intake will probably be unhappy with their diets. In such cases, it is helpful when the dietitian can discuss realistic ways of planning menus for them and *with* them. These menus should be based, of course, on good nutrition, but they also must be based on the patient's normal habits and desires as much as is possible. The patient's former diet should be reviewed with the patient. The high-salt and high-liquid foods should be pointed out and alternative foods presented in a positive manner.

● SUMMARY

Water is a component of all tissues. It is a solvent for nutrients and body wastes and provides transport for both. It is essential for hydrolysis, lubrication, and maintenance of normal temperature. Its best sources are water, beverages, fruits, vegetables, soups, and water-based desserts.

Fluid balance and electrolyte balance are dependent upon one another. An upset in one can cause an upset in the other. An inadequate supply of water can result in dehydration, which can be caused by severe diarrhea, vomiting, hemorrhage, burns, or excessive perspiration or urination. Symptoms include thirst, dry skin, fever, lowered blood pressure, and mental disorientation. Dehydration can result in death. Positive water balance is an excess accumulation of water in the body. It causes edema.

Acid-base balance is the regulation of hydrogen ions in the body. Excessive acids or inadequate amounts of base can cause acidosis. Excessive base or inadequate amounts of acids can cause alkalosis.

Healthy people eating a balanced diet need not be concerned about fluid, electrolyte, or acid-base balance, as the body has intricate maintenance systems for all.

● DISCUSSION TOPICS

1. Why can people live longer without food than without water?

2. Why does water constitute a larger proportion of a man's body weight than of a woman's?

3. Describe homeostasis.

4. How do the lungs help to prevent excess acid from developing in the body?

5. What happens to the skin when it touches a red-hot pan? How might such developments on a large scale upset the body's fluid and electrolyte balance?

6. What is alkalosis? What causes it?

7. Explain how dehydration is dangerous in adults and in infants and children.

8. What does pH mean? How is it related to the homeostasis of the body?

● SUGGESTED ACTIVITIES

1. Ask a nurse to describe what happens to body tissue when it is badly burned. Also ask about the treatment of burn patients, including diet.

2. Ask a nurse to describe a diabetic coma, explaining what causes it, why it can be life-threatening, and how it can be treated.

● REVIEW

Multiple choice. Select the *letter* that precedes the best answer.

1. Fluid within the cells is called
   a. interstitial fluid
   b. extracellular fluid
   c. intracellular fluid
   d. none of the above

2. Intravascular fluid contains
   a. interstitial fluid
   b. extracellular fluid
   c. intracellular fluid
   d. none of the above

3. In a mixture of sugar and water, water is the
   a. solvent
   b. solute
   c. solution
   d. none of the above

4. Water
   a. is essential for hydrolysis
   b. causes hydrogenation
   c. reduces hypoproteinemia
   d. is produced by hypothyroidism

5. Good sources of water include
   a. oranges and melon
   b. seafood and meats
   c. baked desserts and rice
   d. all of the above

6. The solute in the extracellular fluid principally responsible for maintaining fluid balance is
   a. potassium
   b. phosphorus
   c. calcium
   d. sodium

7. The solute in the intracellular fluid principally responsible for maintaining fluid balance is
   a. potassium
   b. phosphorus
   c. calcium
   d. sodium

8. ADH causes the kidneys to
   a. conserve fluid
   b. reabsorb additional sodium
   c. release additional sodium
   d. excrete increased amounts of urine

9. The amount of water needed by individuals
   a. varies from day to day
   b. is not affected by one's activities
   c. decreases with fever
   d. all of the above

10. Positive water balance
    a. means one's intake is equal to output
    b. can cause hydrogenation
    c. may cause edema
    d. is a good thing

C A S E   S T U D Y

The Remerons were spending the day at the beach. The three children were impatient during the hour drive. As they drove, Mrs. Remeron was double-checking that she had packed everything she wanted to bring. She asked her husband if he had taken his diuretic for his hypertension before he left the house. He had not, and she was glad she always had some with her. He took the pill with his cup of coffee. The second they arrived, the children catapulted out of the van and raced down to the beach.

It was a perfect June day. While the children built sand castles, swam, and played games, Mr. and Mrs. Remeron sunbathed, read, and relaxed. The children devoured their lunch and juice at noon. Mr. Remeron slept through lunch. Late in the afternoon, when it was time for one last dip, Mr. Remeron stood up quickly to chase the children. He was suddenly dizzy and almost fainted. He couldn't focus his eyes and felt nauseated and sweaty. His wife made him get in the shade, checked his pulse, and handed him a box of juice to drink.

ASSESSMENT

1. What data do you have about Mr. Remeron's problem?

2. What questions would you ask Mr. Remeron?

3. What did Mrs. Remeron suspect?

DIAGNOSIS

4. Complete the nursing diagnosis statement. Mr. Remeron's fluid volume deficit is related to _____ as evidenced by his behavior of _____.

PLAN/GOAL

5. What is your immediate concern or goal for Mr. Remeron?

6. What is your next concern for the next 24 hours?

IMPLEMENTATION

7. What fluid is most helpful to Mr. Remeron? Why?

8. How much fluid does he need to drink?

9. What else should be done to treat Mr. Remeron?

EVALUATION/OUTCOME CRITERIA

10. What should Mrs. Remeron be looking for, when the plan is effective?

C A S E   S T U D Y

Jack was a 72-year-old male with a recent diagnosis of congestive heart failure (CHF) and hypertension. Jack didn't understand what all the fuss was about. The only thing he had a problem with was the swelling around his ankles. He didn't notice any heart problem. His problem was in his feet! Jack was being discharged from the hospital after a 2-day stay. He was to start on new diuretics and a potassium supplement. The doctor had written a referral for a home health nurse and a dietitian to work with Jack. Jack was expected to eat a low-sodium diet and to observe a fluid restriction in addition to taking his prescribed medication.

ASSESSMENT

1. What do you know about Jack?
2. What is the significance of water to Jack's health problem?

DIAGNOSIS

3. Why was Jack placed on a fluid restriction?
4. What diet education would be appropriate and why?

PLAN/GOAL

5. List the changes Jack needs to make to maintain his health.

IMPLEMENTATION

6. List several strategies for teaching Jack about his diet changes.

7. List several reasons why Jack should listen to your teaching.
8. Create some visual aids for Jack to help him adhere to his new diet. Where would you place them in his house?
9. What does Jack need to know about cooking methods for this diet?
10. What other resources, agencies, or persons could help Jack stick to his diet?

EVALUATION/OUTCOME CRITERIA

11. What could be measured by the home health nurse to see if the plan is effective?

Section 2

MAINTENANCE OF HEALTH THROUGH GOOD NUTRITION

Chapter
10

Food-Related Illnesses and Allergies

Key Terms

abstinence
allergens
allergic reaction
allergy
botulism
carrier
dermatitis
desensitize
dysentery
elimination diet
enterotoxins

food poisoning
hypersensitivity
insecticide
mold
neurotoxins
pathogens
salmonella
skin tests
staph
trichinosis
urticaria

pathogens
disease-causing agents

Objectives

After studying this chapter, you should be able to:

- Identify diseases caused by contaminated food, their signs, and the means by which they are spread

- List signs of food contamination

- State precautions for protecting food from contamination

- Describe allergies and elimination diets and their uses

ILLNESSES CAUSED BY PATHOGENS

The most nutritious food can cause illness if it is contaminated with **pathogens** (disease-causing agents) or certain chemicals. Some of the pathogens that can cause foodborne illness include certain bacteria, viruses, molds, worms, and protozoa. The chemicals may be a natural component of specific foods, intentionally added during production or processing, or accidentally added through carelessness or pollution.

There are always microorganisms in the environment. Some are useful, such as the bacteria used to make yogurt and certain cheeses. Others are pathogens.

food poisoning
foodborne illness

enterotoxins
toxins affecting mucous
membranes

neurotoxins
toxins affecting the nervous
system

botulism
deadliest of food poisonings;
caused by the bacteria
Clostridium botulinum

Pathogens may be in the air, on equipment, in food, on the skin, or in mucus and feces. Food is a particularly good breeding place for them because it provides nutrients, moisture, and often, warmth. Although pathogens can be found in all food groups, they are most commonly found in foods from animal sources. Contaminated food seldom smells, looks, or tastes different from noncontaminated food.

Food poisoning is a general term for foodborne illness. When food poisoning develops as a result of a pathogen's infecting someone, it is a *foodborne infection*. When it is caused by toxins produced by the pathogen, it is called *food intoxication* and, in the case of botulism, can kill. Toxins can be produced by bacteria during food preparation or storage, or in one's digestive tract. **Enterotoxins** affect mucous membranes in the digestive tract and **neurotoxins** affect the nervous system.

It is thought that as many as one-third of the population of the United States may experience food poisoning each year. Its typical symptoms include vomiting, diarrhea, headache, and abdominal cramps. Many never know they are suffering from food poisoning and assume they have the flu. Others, especially young children, the elderly, or those with compromised immune systems (such as people who are HIV-positive) may become very ill and some may die.

Bacteria That Cause Foodborne Illness

Campylobacter jejuni, Clostridium botulinum, Clostridium perfringens, Cyclospora Cayentanensis, Escherichia coli 0157:H7, Listeria monocytogenes, Salmonella, Shigella, and *Staphylococcus aureas* are examples of bacteria that can cause foodborne illness.

Campylobacter Jejuni. *Campylobacter jejuni* is believed to be one of the most prevalent causes of diarrhea. It is commonly found in the intestinal tracts of cattle, pigs, sheep, chickens, turkeys, dogs, and cats, and can contaminate meat during slaughter. It is caused by the ingestion of live bacteria.

It can take from two to five (or more) days to develop after infection, and may last up to ten days. Symptoms include diarrhea (sometimes bloody), fever, headache, muscle and abdominal pain, and nausea. It can be transmitted to humans via unpasteurized milk, contaminated water, and raw or undercooked meats, poultry, and shellfish.

Clostridium Botulinum. *Clostridium botulinum* is found in soil and water, on plants, and in the intestinal tracts of animals and fish. The spores of this bacteria can divide and produce toxin in the absence of oxygen. (Spores are single cells that are produced asexually, each of which is able to develop into a new organism. They have thick, protective walls that allow them to survive unfavorable conditions.) This means that toxin can be produced in sealed containers such as cans, jars, and vacuum-packaged foods.

The spores are extremely heat resistant and must be boiled for six hours before they will be destroyed. Such a lengthy time will, of course, destroy the food they have infected. The toxin, however, can be destroyed by boiling for twenty minutes. This toxin causes **botulism**, which is perhaps the rarest but most deadly of all food poisonings. Symptoms usually appear within 4 to 36 hours after eating and include double vision, speech difficulties, inability to swallow, and respiratory paralysis. If botulism is not properly treated, death will result in 3 to 10 days. The fatality rate in the United States is about 65%.

Great care must be taken to prevent botulism when canning foods at home. The FDA and USDA reported five deaths from botulism traced to commercially canned foods in the United States between 1925 and 1974, but 700 deaths from home-canned foods during that same time period. If a can bulges, *Clostridium botulinum* may be present and can be fatal. A good rule of thumb is: "If in doubt, throw it out" where children and animals cannot reach it.

Clostridium Perfringens. *Clostridium perfringens* is often called the "cafeteria" or "buffet germ" because it tends to infect those who eat food that has been standing on buffets or steam tables for long periods. *Clostridium perfringens* is found in soil dust, sewage, and the intestinal tracts of animals. It is a spore-forming pathogen that needs little oxygen. The bacteria are destroyed by cooking, but the spores can survive it.

Clostridium perfringens is transmitted by eating heavily contaminated food. Symptoms include nausea, diarrhea, and inflammation of the stomach and intestine. Symptoms may appear within 6 to 24 hours of ingestion and last approximately 24 hours.

To best prevent it, hot foods should be kept at or above 140°F and cold foods below 40°F. Leftovers should be heated to 165°F before serving. Foods should be stored at temperatures of 40°F or lower. People with compromised immune systems should be very cautious concerning *Clostridium perfringens*.

Cyclospora Cayentanensis. *Cyclospora cayentanensis* is a parasite that causes gastroenteritis. Until 1996 most cases were experienced by overseas travelers, but several domestic outbreaks have been reported in recent years. This bacteria is commonly found in the feces of an infected person and can be transmitted by poor hygiene. It has been found in unclean water.

Symptoms are watery diarrhea, abdominal cramps, decreased appetite, and a low-grade fever. These symptoms could last off and on for several weeks. Those with compromised immune systems, children, and the elderly are at greatest risk of complications.

Cyclospora has an incubation period of one week, is associated with invasion of the small intestine, and is manifested by the preceding symptoms. The parasite's natural ecology, infective dose, and host range are unknown. It is known that *Cyclospora* does not multiply outside the host.

It is strongly recommended that clean water be used for drinking and the irrigation of produce. Thorough washing of fruits and vegetables and the practice of good hygiene by food handlers help to prevent the spread of this bacteria.

Escherichia Coli (E. coli 0157:H7). *Escherichia coli,* commonly called "E. coli," is a group of bacteria that can cause illness in humans. E. coli 0157:H7 is a very infectious strain of this group. These bacteria can be found in the intestines of some mammals (including humans and animals used for food), in raw milk, and in water contaminated by animal or human feces.

E. coli are transmitted to humans through contaminated water, unpasteurized milk or apple juice, raw or rare ground beef products, unwashed fruits or vegetables, and directly from person to person. Plant foods can be contaminated by fertilization with raw manure or irrigation with contaminated water.

Symptoms include severe abdominal cramps, diarrhea that may be watery or bloody, and nausea. Sometimes, however, E. coli 0157:H7 can cause hemorrhagic colitis (inflammation of the colon). This in turn can result in *hemolytic uremic syndrome* (HUS) in children, which can damage the kidneys.

E. coli can be controlled by careful choice and cooking of foods. All meats and poultry should be cooked thoroughly. Ground beef, veal, and lamb should be cooked to 160°F, and ground poultry to at least 165°F. Fruits and vegetables should be carefully washed, and unpasteurized milk and other dairy products and vegetable and fruit juices should be avoided. People with compromised immune systems should be especially vigilant.

Listeria Monocytogenes. *Listeria monocytogenes* is a bacteria often found in human and animal intestines, and in milk, leafy vegetables, and soil. It can grow in the refrigerator and can be transmitted to humans by unpasteurized dairy foods such as milk, soft cheeses, and ice creams, and via leafy, raw vegetables and processed meats.

Listeria monocytogenes can affect a person from 12 hours to 3 weeks after ingestion. Symptoms include fatigue, fever, chills, headache, backache, abdominal pain, and diarrhea. It can develop into more serious conditions and cause respiratory distress, spontaneous abortion, or meningitis.

To prevent infection by *Listeria monocytogenes,* meats and poultry should be thoroughly cooked and salad greens carefully washed. Attention must be paid to all dairy products—especially the unfamiliar from new sources—to be certain they have been pasteurized.

Salmonellosis. Salmonellosis (commonly called *salmonella*) is an infection caused by the *Salmonella* bacteria (see Table 10-1). **Salmonella** can be found in raw meats, poultry, fish, milk, and eggs. It is transmitted by eating contaminated food or by contact with a carrier. Salmonellosis is characterized by headache, vomiting, diarrhea, abdominal cramps, and fever. Symptoms generally begin from 6 to 48 hours after eating. In severe cases, it can result in death. One species of *Salmonella* causes typhoid fever. Those who suffer the most severe cases are typically the very young, the elderly, and the weak or incapacitated.

Refrigeration (40°F or lower) inhibits the growth of these bacteria, but they can remain alive in the freezer and in dried foods. *Salmonella* bacteria are destroyed by heating to at least 140°F for a minimum of 10 minutes.

To prevent contamination, thaw poultry and meats in the refrigerator or microwave and cook immediately. Avoid cross-contamination of raw and cooked foods by carefully cleaning utensils and counter surfaces that were in contact with raw food. Raw or undercooked eggs, or

salmonella

an infection caused by the Salmonella bacteria

TABLE 10-1 Foodborne Illnesses

BACTERIA	TRANSMISSION	SYMPTOMS	PREVENTION
Campylobacter jejuni	Unpasteurized milk, contaminated water, raw and undercooked meat and shellfish.	Diarrhea, fever, headache, abdominal pain, and nausea.	Avoid unpasteurized milk and questionable water. Cook meat and fish thoroughly.
Clostridium botulinum	Home-canned and, rarely, improperly prepared commercially canned food.	Double vision, speech difficulties, inability to swallow, respiratory paralysis.	Avoid bulging cans. Boil home-canned green beans for 10 min.
Clostridium perfringens	Sometimes referred to as the "cafeteria germ." Outbreaks occur when large quantities of food are served at room temperature or from a steam table. Meat, poultry, cooked dried beans, and gravies are the most common carriers.	Diarrhea and gas pains beginning between 6 and 24 hours after ingestion and lasting approximately 24 hours.	Keep hot food hot (at or above 140°F) and cold food cold (at or below 40°F). Leftovers should be heated to at least 165°F before serving. Wash all soil from vegetables.
Cyclospora cayentanensis	Feces-contaminated food or water.	Watery diarrhea, abdominal cramps, decreased appetite, and low-grade fever. Could last off and on for several weeks.	Thorough hand washing, washing fruit before eating, using and drinking only clean water.
Escherichia coli (E. coli 0157:H7)	Eating contaminated foods such as undercooked hamburger, ground poultry, and unpasteurized milk and apple juice.	Abdominal cramps, watery diarrhea, nausea, and vomiting. Serious complications: bloody diarrhea and severe abdominal cramps. Onset within 3–9 days. Duration 2–9 days, if no complications.	Cook ground meat to 160°F. Eat no raw ground meat. Wash all fruits and vegetables before eating.
Listeria monocytogenes	Unpasteurized milk, raw and cooked poultry, and meat, raw, and leafy vegetables	Sudden onset of fever, chills, headache, backache, and occasional abdominal pain and diarrhea.	Avoid unpasteurized milk and dairy products. Cook ground meats to 160°F, ground poultry to 165°F. Hot foods should be kept hot and cold foods cold. Wash produce thoroughly.
Salmonella	Raw or undercooked food such as eggs, poultry, unpasteurized milk, or other dairy products and meats. Cross-contamination by uncooked foods.	Headache, abdominal pain, diarrhea, fever, and nausea. Onset: 6–48 hours. Duration: 1–8 days.	Avoid cross-contamination of raw and cooked foods. Do not eat raw eggs. Cook ground beef to 160°F. Keep hot foods hot and cold foods cold. Do not eat any unpasteurized raw or undercooked food of animal origin.
Shigella	Contamination of food by infected food handlers. Primarily transmitted in cold salads such as tuna, chicken, and potato.	Severe diarrhea, nausea, headaches, chills, and dehydration. Onset 1 day to a week.	Good hygiene of food handlers and sanitary food preparation. Keep hot foods hot and cold foods cold. Always wash hands in hot soapy water after going to the bathroom and before preparing or eating food.
Staphylococcus aureas	Transmitted by infected food handlers.	Vomiting, diarrhea, abdominal cramps. Onset: ½–8 hours. Duration: 1–2 days.	Good hygiene of food handlers. Always wash hands thoroughly in hot soapy water before preparing food. Keep hot food hot and cold food cold.

Adapted from *Safe Food Backgrounder,* National Live Stock and Meat Board, 1994.

foods that contain them, should not be eaten. Even a taste of raw cookie dough or Caesar salad dressing made with raw egg yolk can cause contamination. People with compromised immune systems should be especially careful.

Shigella. *Shigella* bacteria are found in the intestinal tract and thus the feces of infected individuals. The disease they cause is called *shigellosis*. These bacteria are typically passed on by an infected food handler who did not wash his or her hands properly after using the toilet. They are also found on plants that were fertilized with untreated animal feces or given contaminated water. *Shigella* are destroyed by heat, but infected cold foods such as tuna, chicken, or egg salads are common carriers.

Shigellosis can occur from one day to a week following infection. Symptoms include diarrhea (sometimes with blood and mucus), fever, chills, headache, nausea, and abdominal cramps, and can lead to dehydration. Some people, however, experience no symptoms.

Staphylococcus Aureus. *Staphylococcus aureas* bacteria are found on human skin, in infected cuts and pimples, and in noses and throats. Staphylococcal poisoning is commonly called "**staph**." These bacteria grow in meats; poultry; fish; egg dishes; salads such as potato, egg, macaroni, and tuna; and in cream-filled pastries. This poisoning is transmitted by carriers and by eating foods that contain the toxin these bacteria create.

Symptoms, which include vomiting, diarrhea, and abdominal cramps, begin within one-half to 8 hours after ingestion of the toxin, and last from 24 to 48 hours. "Staph" is considered a mild illness.

The growth of these bacteria is inhibited if foods are kept at temperatures above 140°F or below 40°F. Their toxin can be destroyed by boiling the food for several hours or by heating it in a pressure cooker at 240°F for 30 minutes. Both of these methods would destroy both the appeal and nutrient content of the infected foods. It is more practical to safely discard foods suspected of being contaminated.

Other Substances That Cause Food Poisoning

Mold is a type of fungus. Its roots go down, into the food, and it grows a stalk upward on which spores form. The green, "fuzzy" part that can be seen by the naked eye is where the spores are found. Some spores cause respiratory problems and/or allergic reactions for some people. For this reason, moldy food should never be smelled.

Some molds produce a dangerous mycotoxin called aflatoxin that can cause cancer. It can develop in spoiled peanuts and peanut butter, soybeans, grains, nuts, and spices. Symptoms of such an infection include abdominal pain, vomiting, and diarrhea, and may occur from 1 day to several months after ingestion. It can cause liver and skin damage and, ultimately, cancer.

The Food and Drug Administration observes the aflatoxin content of foods closely and, although this toxin cannot as yet be totally eradicated, foods containing more than a very minute amount of it cannot be sold by one state to another.

staph
staphylococcal poisoning

mold
is a type of fungus

Neither cooking nor refrigeration destroys this toxin. Cheese may develop mold and that part should be cut away to a depth of at least an inch. (Cheeses such as bleu or Roquefort that were intentionally ripened by harmless molds are safe to eat.) Fruits and vegetables showing signs of mold should not be purchased.

Trichinella spiralis is a parasitic worm that causes trichinosis. This disease is transmitted by eating inadequately cooked pork from pigs that are infected with the *Trichinella spiralis* parasite. Symptoms include abdominal pain, vomiting, fever, chills, and muscle pain. Symptoms occur about 24 hours after ingesting infected pork. Cooking all pork to an internal temperature of at least 170°F kills the organism and prevents this disease. It can also be destroyed by freezing.

Dysentery is a disease caused by protozoa (tiny, one-celled animal). The protozoa are introduced to food by carriers or contaminated water. They cause severe diarrhea that can occur intermittently until the patient is treated appropriately.

trichinosis
disease caused by the parasitic roundworm *Trichinella spiralis*; can be transmitted through undercooked pork

dysentery
disease caused by microorganism; characterized by diarrhea

Prevention of Foodborne Illnesses

Strict federal, state, and local laws regulate the commercial production of food in the United States, and dairies, canneries, bakeries, and meat-packing plants are all subject to government inspection. Nevertheless, errors and accidents can and do occur, and illness can result. *Most foodborne illnesses occur because of the ignorance or carelessness of people who handle food.* People can introduce pathogens to food, prevent them from reaching it, or kill them with appropriate cooking temperatures.

Cleanliness is especially important in preventing foodborne illness. When kitchen equipment such as a cutting board, meat grinder, or countertop is used for preparing pathogen-infected foods and not cleaned properly afterward, noninfected food that is subsequently prepared with this equipment can become infected by the same pathogen(s). This is called cross-contamination. Dishes used to hold uncooked meat, poultry, fish, or eggs must always be washed before cooked foods are placed on them.

When food workers fail to wash their hands after blowing their noses or using the toilet, they can "share" their germs very easily. Mucus and feces are favorite breeding areas of pathogens.

Food workers who have even small cuts on their hands must wear gloves because a wound could carry a pathogen. Foods must be covered and stored properly to keep dust, insects, and animals from reaching and possibly contaminating them. Water from unknown sources should not be used for cooking because it, too, can carry pathogens.

Temperatures during preparation and storage of food must be carefully observed. When infected foods are undercooked, the pathogen is not destroyed and can be passed to consumers (see Table 10-2). Foods allowed to stand at temperatures between 40 and 140°F provide an ideal breeding place for pathogens.

Leftover food should always be refrigerated as soon as the meal is finished, and covered when it is cold. It should not be allowed to cool to room temperature before it is refrigerated. Frozen food should either be cooked from the frozen state or thawed in the refrigerator. (When cooked from the frozen state, cooking time will generally increase by at

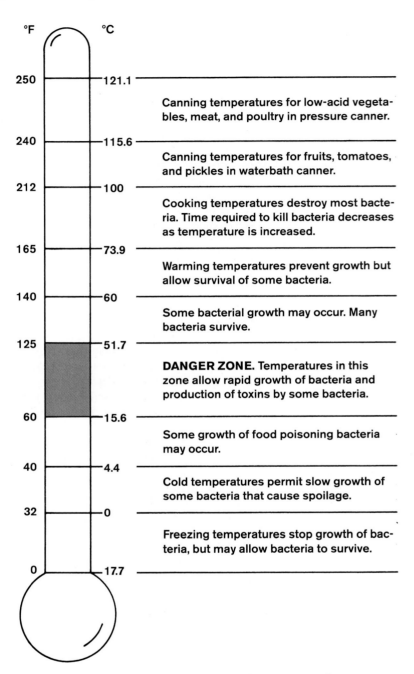

FIGURE 10-1 Temperatures of food for control of bacteria. (Adapted from USDA Home and Garden Bulletin No. 247, 1990.)

least 50 percent.) Frozen food should not be thawed at room temperature. Food must always be protected from dust, insects, and animals.

Carriers are people (or animals) capable of transmitting infectious (disease-causing) organisms. Often the carrier suffers no effects from the organism and therefore is unaware of the danger she or he

carrier

one who is capable of transmitting an infectious organism

TABLE 10-2 Cooking Temperatures

PRODUCT	FAHRENHEIT
Eggs & Egg Dishes	
Eggs	Cook until yolk & white are firm
Egg dishes	160
Fresh Beef, Veal, Lamb	
Ground products like hamburger	
(Prepared as patties, meat loaf,	
meatballs, etc.)	160
Roasts, steaks, and chops	
Medium Rare	145
Medium	160
Well done	170
Fresh Pork	
All cuts including ground product	
Medium	160
Well done	170
Poultry	
Ground chicken, turkey	165
Whole chicken, turkey	
Medium, unstuffed	170
Well done	180
Whole bird with stuffing	
(Stuffing must reach 165°)	180
Poultry breasts, roasts	170
Thighs, wings	Cook until juices run clear
Ham	
Fresh (raw)	160
Fully cooked, to reheat	140

Source: U.S. Department of Agriculture Food Safety and Inspection Service, Home and Garden Bulletin No. 254, May 1994. Washington, D.C.

represents. Food workers should be tested regularly to confirm that they are not carriers of communicable diseases.

Selection of food should be made with great care. Packages and jars should be properly sealed. Cans should not bulge. Foods that look or smell at all unusual and foods showing signs of mold should be left in the store. Only pasteurized milk and dairy products should be used (see Table 10-3).

TABLE 10-3 To Prevent Food Poisoning

- Keep kitchen and equipment thoroughly clean.
- Wash hands after blowing nose or using bathroom.
- Wear gloves if cooking with any hand wound.
- Cover and store foods to prevent microbes or animals from reaching it.
- Cook foods to appropriate temperatures.
- Limit standing time at temperatures between 40°F and 140°F.
- Prevent known carriers from preparing foods.
- Select only packages and jars that were sealed by the manufacturer.
- Avoid bulging cans, foods that look or smell odd, and foods showing signs of mold.

MISCELLANEOUS FOOD POISIONINGS

Occasionally, food poisoning is caused by ingesting certain plants or animals that contain poison. Examples are plants such as poisonous mushrooms, rhubarb leaves, and fish from polluted water.

Poisoning also can result from ingesting cleaning agents, **insecticides**, or excessive amounts of a drug. Children may swallow cleaning agents or medicines. The cook may mistakenly use a poison instead of a cooking ingredient. Sometimes insecticides cling to fresh fruits and vegetables. It is essential that all potential poisons be kept out of the reach of young children and kept separate from all food supplies. Fresh fruits and vegetables should be thoroughly washed before being eaten.

FOOD ALLERGIES

An **allergy** is an altered reaction of the tissues of some individuals to substances that, in similar amounts, are harmless to other people. The substances causing **hypersensitivity** are called **allergens**. Some common allergens are pollen, dust, animal dander (bits of dried skin), drugs, cosmetics, and certain foods. This discussion will be limited to allergic reactions to foods. A food allergy occurs when the immune system reacts to a food substance, usually a protein. When such a reaction occurs, antibodies form and cause allergic symptoms. An altered reaction to a specific food that does not involve the immune system is called (the specific food) *intolerance*.

Types of Allergic Reactions

Sometimes allergic reactions are immediate, and sometimes several hours elapse before signs occur. Allergic individuals seem most prone to allergic reactions during periods of stress. Typical signs of food allergies include hay fever, **urticaria**, edema, headache, **dermatitis**, nausea, dizziness, and asthma (which causes breathing difficulties).

insecticide
agent that destroys insects

allergy
sensitivity to specific substance(s)

hypersensitivity
abnormally strong sensitivity to certain substance(s)

allergens
substance-causing allergy

urticaria
hives; common allergic reaction

dermatitis
inflammation of the skin

Allergic reactions are uncomfortable and can be detrimental to health. When breathing difficulties are severe, they are life-threatening.

Allergic reactions to the same food can differ in two individuals. For example, the fact that someone gets hives from eating strawberries does not mean that an allergic reaction to strawberries will appear as hives in another member of the same family. Allergic reactions can even differ from time to time with the same individual.

Treatment of Allergies

The simplest treatment for allergies is to remove the item that causes the allergic reaction. However, because of the variety of allergic reactions, finding the allergen can be difficult.

When food allergies are suspected, it is wise for the patient to keep a food diary for several days and to record all food and drink ingested as well as allergic reactions and the time of their onset. Such records can help pinpoint specific allergens. Some common food allergens are listed in Table 10-4. It is common for other foods in the same class as the allergens to cause allergic reactions as well. Cooking sometimes alters the foods and can eliminate allergic reactions in some people.

Laboratory tests may be used to find the allergen or allergens. The RAST (radio allergosorbent test), for example, may be used to determine which compounds are causing allergic reactions. **Skin tests** are sometimes used to detect allergies. However, food allergies can be difficult to determine from skin tests.

After completion of the allergy testing, the patient is usually placed on an **elimination diet**. For one or two weeks the patient does not eat any of the tested compounds that gave a positive reaction. The patient includes in the diet the foods that almost no one reacts to, such as rice, fresh meats, and poultry, noncitrus fruits, and vegetables. Sometimes, these diets allow only a limited number of foods and can be nutritionally inadequate. If that is the case, vitamin and mineral supplements may be prescribed.

When relief is found from the allergic symptoms, the patient is continued on the diet, and, gradually, other foods are added to the diet at a rate of only one every 4 to 7 days. Those foods most likely to produce allergic reactions are added last until an allergic reaction occurs. The allergy can then be pinpointed, and the offending foods eliminated from the diet. Knowing the cause of the allergy enables the patient to lead a healthy, normal life, provided that eliminating these foods does not affect her or his nutrition.

allergic reaction
adverse physical reaction to specific substance(s)

skin tests
allergy tests using potential allergens on scratches on the skin

elimination diet
limited diet in which only certain foods are allowed; intended to find the food allergen causing reaction

TABLE 10-4 Common Food Allergens

Milk	Strawberries	Soybeans
Wheat	Tomatoes	Pork
Corn	Legumes	Fish
Eggs	Nuts	
Citrus fruit	Chocolate	

If the elimination of the allergen results in a diet deficient in certain nutrients, suitable substitutes for those nutrients must be found. For example, if a patient is allergic to citrus fruits, other foods rich in vitamin C to which the patient is not allergic must be found. If the allergy is to milk, soybean milk may be substituted.

The patient must be taught the food sources of the nutrient or nutrients lacking so that other foods can be substituted that are nutritionally equal to those causing the allergy. It is essential that the patient be taught to read the labels on commercially prepared foods and to check the ingredients of restaurant foods carefully. Baked products, mixes, meatloaf, or pancakes may contain egg, milk, or wheat that may be responsible for the allergic reaction.

Sometimes, however, the allergies require such a restriction of foods that the diet does become nutritionally inadequate. As in all cases of allergy, and particularly in such cases, it is hoped that the patient can become **desensitized** to the allergens so that a nutritionally balanced diet can be restored. The patient is desensitized by eating a minute amount of food allergen after a period of complete **abstinence** from it. The amount of the allergen is gradually increased until the patient can tolerate it.

desensitize

to gradually reduce the body's sensitivity (allergic reaction) to specific items

abstinence

avoidance

CONSIDERATIONS FOR THE HEALTH CARE PROFESSIONAL

Some patients will need simple instructions from the health care professional about avoiding microbial contamination of food supplies at home. Many, if not most, should be warned not to thaw food at room temperature. Others should be reminded that leftover foods should *not* be cooled at room temperature before being refrigerated.

Patients with food allergies will require careful training to avoid their specific allergens. They must be taught to read food labels carefully and to ask the ingredients of foods in restaurants and at friends' homes. Role-playing is an effective way to help such patients.

● SUMMARY

Infection or poisoning traced to food is usually caused by human ignorance or carelessness. The serving of safe meals is essentially the responsibility of the cook. Food should not be prepared by anyone who has or carries a contagious disease. All fresh fruits and vegetables should be washed before being eaten. Meats, poultry, fish, eggs, and dairy products should be refrigerated. Pork should always be cooked to the well-done stage. Food should be covered to prevent contamination by dust, insects, or animals. Garbage should also be covered so that it does not attract insects. Hands that prepare foods should be clean and free of cuts or wounds. Kitchen equipment should be spotless. Finally, the food itself should be safe. People should avoid foods containing natural poisons.

Food allergies can cause many different and unpleasant symptoms. Elimination diets are used to determine their causes. Some of the most common food allergens have been found to be milk, chocolate, eggs, tomatoes, fish, citrus fruit, legumes, strawberries, and wheat.

● DISCUSSION TOPICS

1. Name four types of foodborne illness. If any class member has suffered from one, ask the person to describe the symptoms.
2. How does food become contaminated?
3. Why should foods be refrigerated?
4. What are allergies? What can cause them?
5. What are some common allergic reactions to food? How can they be avoided?
6. Do people inherit allergies? Explain.
7. Of what use is a food diary in relation to allergies? What are elimination diets, and when are they used?
8. What is the most difficult part of treating food allergies?
9. How can an allergic patient be desensitized?
10. Is an elimination diet always nutritious? Explain.
11. Explain how eggs, wheat, or milk may be hidden in each of the following foods: mayonnaise, bread, rye crackers, potato salad, gravy, meatloaf, breaded veal cutlet, bologna, malted milk.

● SUGGESTED ACTIVITIES

1. Ask a doctor or registered nurse to explain skin tests to the class. Discuss these tests after the lecture.
2. Ask someone with food allergies to speak to the class. Follow this talk with questions from the audience.
3. Visit a restaurant kitchen. Look for practices that may lead to potential food poisoning. Note the practices and uses of equipment designed to prevent food poisoning.

● REVIEW

Multiple choice. Select the *letter* that precedes the best answer.

1. A microorganism is a(n)
   a. unit of measurement
   b. tiny animal or plant
   c. component of a microscope
   d. individual human cell
2. Salmonella bacteria are destroyed by heating foods to 140°F for a minimum of
   a. 2 minutes
   b. 10 minutes
   c. 30 minutes
   d. 2 hours

3. Someone who is capable of spreading an infectious organism but is not sick is called a
   a. food handler
   b. carrier
   c. transport
   d. fomite

4. When an organism is infectious, it is
   a. disease-causing
   b. prone to infections
   c. not contagious
   d. always fatal

5. Most cases of food poisoning in the United States are caused by
   a. careless processing in commercial factories
   b. lack of government inspection
   c. careless handling of food in the kitchen
   d. house pets

6. Food poisoning symptoms generally include
   a. joint pain
   b. constipation
   c. abdominal upset and headache
   d. swelling of the feet

7. Salmonella infections and staphylococcal poisoning are caused by
   a. a virus
   b. bacteria
   c. protozoa
   d. worms

8. The deadliest of the bacterial food poisonings is
   a. staphylococcal poisoning
   b. salmonellosis
   c. botulism
   d. perfringens poisoning

9. The disease caused by a parasite sometimes found in pork is
   a. tularemia
   b. dysentery
   c. avitaminosis
   d. trichinosis

10. The disease caused by a protozoan and characterized by severe diarrhea is
   a. salmonellosis
   b. botulism
   c. dysentery
   d. infectious hepatitis

11. Foods may be contaminated by
   a. people
   b. overcooking them
   c. refrigeration
   d. all of the above

12. The temperatures in the danger zone that encourage bacterial growth are from
   a. 0 to 32°F
   b. 32 to 60°F
   c. 60 to 125°F
   d. 125 to 212°F

13. Leftover foods should be
   a. put in the refrigerator immediately after meals
   b. cooled to room temperature before refrigerating
   c. cooled in the refrigerator for at least an hour before freezing
   d. stored unwrapped in the refrigerator

14. Frozen foods should be
   a. thawed at room temperature
   b. refrozen if not used immediately after thawing
   c. thawed in the refrigerator
   d. any of the above

15. An adverse physical reaction to a food is called a food
    a. refusal   c. symptom
    b. allergy   d. allergen

16. Substances that cause altered physical reactions are called
    a. symptoms   c. allergens
    b. allergies   d. abstinence

17. One of the typical symptoms of food allergies is
    a. diabetes mellitus   c. hives
    b. colitis   d. atherosclerosis

18. The simplest treatment for a food allergy is
    a. a skin test
    b. avoiding all fruit
    c. elimination of the allergen
    d. the use of penicillin

19. In cases of food allergy, an elimination diet may be prescribed to
    a. desensitize the patient   c. avoid surgery
    b. avoid medication   d. find the allergen

20. Some foods that frequently cause an allergic reaction are
    a. milk, eggs, and wheat   c. canned pears and tapioca
    b. lamb, rice, and sugar   d. rice and pears

C A S E   S T U D Y

Mrs. J. has known that Krista was allergic to milk, since Krista was two months old. She had to put her on soy milk as an infant. Now that Krista is 5 years old and will be going to school in the fall, Mrs. J. wonders whether she has "outgrown" her milk allergy. Krista and Mrs. J. have an appointment with the pediatrician to discuss the possibility.

The Saturday before the doctor's appointment, the entire family attended a wedding. It was a beautiful ceremony, and the dinner at the reception was delicious. It was the first time the children had ever had Caesar salad and cocktail meatballs. As always, Mrs. J. reminded the family about Krista's milk allergy. Later at the reception, when the adults were visiting and dancing, the children helped distribute the vanilla and chocolate wedding cake. Krista ate one piece with her mother and part of her brother's. He had the rich dark chocolate part of the cake with milk chocolate frosting.

On Sunday morning, Krista woke up crying, complaining of severe stomach pain and diarrhea. Mrs. J. noticed a red rash on her neck and chest.

ASSESSMENT

1. What did Mrs. J. observe on Sunday morning?
2. What other data do you have about Krista's health?
3. What do you suspect is the problem?
4. Which foods are most likely the cause?

DIAGNOSIS

5. Krista's abdominal pain and diarrhea could have been caused by _____.
6. Mrs. J needs more education about_____ ?

PLAN/GOAL

7. What is the immediate goal for Krista?
8. What is the long-range goal?

IMPLEMENTATION

9. At the doctor's appointment, what should Mrs. J. discuss?
10. What is the doctor likely to do to verify Krista's food allergies?
11. What is the doctor likely to recommend in regard to Krista's drinking milk at school? What else could Krista drink at school?
12. What does Mrs. J. need to learn?

EVALUATION/OUTCOME CRITERIA

13. When the intervention is completed, how will Mrs. J. know if it has been effective?

CASE STUDY

Ito and Maia were very excited about babysitting their 6-year-old grandson, Chang, for the day. They had discussed the day's activities in advance with Chang and his parents. The plan was finalized: a trip to the zoo in the morning, lunch at McDonalds, and the afternoon in the park. Chang rarely went to fast-food restaurants. His parents didn't frequent them because they didn't think it was a healthy diet.

Chang loved the elephants, and the monkeys made him laugh. By lunchtime, Chang was ready to eat even though Grandpa Ito had let him have some chocolate milk at the zoo. He couldn't wait to bite into his cheeseburger and fries. Grandpa brought his own lunch because he was on a special diet.

The afternoon was great fun at the park. The slides, hide and seek, and chasing the pigeons all kept Chang busy. Chang couldn't wait to tell Mom and Dad about his great day. As Chang was showing his mother his imitation of a monkey, his stomach started to hurt and he had to run to the bathroom. Suddenly he didn't feel so good; he had diarrhea and his head hurt.

ASSESSMENT

1. What data do you have about Chang?
2. What do you suspect caused Chang's sudden change in health?
3. What foods are most likely the cause?

DIAGNOSIS

4. What was the likely cause of Chang's abdominal pain?
5. Why did Chang have diarrhea?

PLAN/GOAL

6. What is the goal for Chang?

IMPLEMENTATION

7. What other symptoms might Chang experience?
8. What should his mother tell him about his illness?
9. What is Chang at high risk for as a young child?
10. What should Chang's mother be encouraging him to drink while he has diarrhea?
11. Would an antidiarrheal medication be helpful? Appropriate?

EVALUATION/OUTCOME CRITERIA

12. How will Chang's mother know if her treatment is effective?

Diet During Pregnancy and Lactation

Key Terms

adolescent

amniotic fluid

anemia

eclamptic stage

fetal alcohol
  syndrome (FAS)

fetal malformations

fetus

gestational diabetes

hyperemesis
  gravidarum

hyperglycemia

hypoglycemia

lactation

macrosomia

morning sickness

obstetrician

parenteral nutrition

pica

placenta

pregnancy-induced
  hypertension (PIH)

proteinuria

retardation

spontaneous
  abortion

trimester

fetus
infant in utero

amniotic fluid
surrounds fetus in the uterus

placenta
organ in the uterus that links blood
supplies of mother and infant

Objectives

After studying this chapter, you should be able to:

● Identify nutritional needs during pregnancy and lactation

● Describe nutritional needs of pregnant adolescents

● Modify the normal diet to meet the needs of pregnant and lactating women

THE IMPORTANCE OF GOOD NUTRITION DURING PREGNANCY

Good nutrition during the 38–40 weeks of a normal pregnancy is essential for both mother and child. In addition to her normal nutritional requirements, the pregnant woman must provide nutrients and kcal for the fetus, amniotic fluid, the placenta, and for the increased blood volume and breast, uterine, and fat tissue.

The pregnant woman who follows a nutritionally adequate diet is more apt to feel better, retain her health, and bear a healthy infant than one who chooses her foods thoughtlessly.

Studies have shown a relationship between the mother's diet and the health of the baby at birth. It is also thought that the woman who consumed a nutritious diet before pregnancy is more apt to bear a healthy infant than one who did not. Malnutrition of the mother is believed to cause growth and mental retardation in the fetus. Low-birthweight infants (less than 5.5 pounds) have a higher mortality (death) rate than those of normal birthweight.

WEIGHT GAIN DURING PREGNANCY

Weight gain during pregnancy is natural and necessary for the infant to develop normally and the mother to retain her health. in addition to the developing infant, the mother's uterus, breasts, placenta, blood volume, body fluids, and fat must all increase to accommodate the infant's needs (Table 11-1).

The average weight gain during pregnancy is 25 to 35 pounds. During the first trimester of pregnancy, there is an average weight gain of only 2 to 4 pounds. Most of the weight gain occurs during the second and third trimesters of pregnancy, when it averages about 1 pound a week. This is because there is a substantial increase in maternal tissue during the second trimester, and the fetus grows a great deal during the third trimester.

Weight gain varies, of course. A pregnant adolescent who is still growing will gain more weight than a mature woman of the same size. Underweight women should gain 28 to 40 pounds. Women of average weight should avoid excessive weight gain and try to stay within the 25 to 35 pound average gain. If the woman is pregnant with twins, then the recommended weight gain is 35 to 45 pounds. Obese women can afford to gain less than the average woman, but not less than 15 pounds.

No one should lose weight during pregnancy, because it could cause nutrient deficiencies for both mother and infant. On average, a pregnant adult requires no additional kcal during the first trimester of pregnancy and only an additional 300 kcal a day during the second and third trimesters.

retardation
slowing

trimester
3-month period; commonly used to denote periods of pregnancy

adolescent
person between the ages of 13 and 20

TABLE 11-1 Components of Weight Gain During Pregnancy, with Approximate Amounts of Gain

COMPONENT	AMOUNT OF GAIN
Fetus	7.5 pounds
Placenta	1 pound
Amniotic fluid	2 pounds
Uterus	2 pounds
Breasts	1-3 pounds
Blood volume	4 pounds
Maternal fat	4+ pounds

PREPREGNANCY NUTRITIONAL NEEDS

Research has shown that adequate prepregnancy nutrition is critical for the prevention of neural tube defects such as spina bifida. During the first trimester, many women do not realize that they are pregnant. If they did not have an adequate intake of folate before becoming pregnant, the baby may be damaged. Lifestyle and habits also need to be taken into consideration before becoming pregnant. Certain medications, smoking, illegal drugs, and alcohol can all be detrimental to the embryo. Good nutrition is essential before becoming pregnant and during pregnancy.

NUTRITIONAL NEEDS DURING PREGNANCY

Some specific nutrient requirements are increased dramatically during pregnancy, as can be seen in Table 11-2. These figures are recommended for the general U.S. population; the physician may suggest alternative figures based on the patient's nutritional status, age, and activities.

The protein requirement is increased by 20% for the pregnant woman over 25 and by 25% for the pregnant adolescent. Proteins are essential for tissue building, and protein-rich foods are excellent sources of many other essential nutrients, especially iron, copper, zinc, and the B vitamins.

TABLE 11-2 Recommended Dietary Allowances During Pregnancy and Lactation

	Weight		Height		Protein	FAT-SOLUBLE VITAMINS			WATER-SOLUBLE VITAMINS			
Age	(kg)	(lb)	(cm)	(in)	(g)	Vitamin A (μg RE)	Vitamin D (μg)	Vitamin E (μg α-TE)	Vitamin K (μg)	Vitamin C (mg)	Thiamin (mg)	Riboflavin (mg)
11−14 years												
Not pregnant	46	101	157	62	46	800	5	8	45	50	1.1	1.3
Pregnant					60	800	5	10	65	70	1.5	1.6
Lactating												
1st 6 months					65	1,300	5	12	65	95	1.6	1.8
2nd 6 months					62	1,200	5	11	65	90	1.6	1.7
15−18 years												
Not pregnant	55	120	163	64	44	800	5	8	55	60	1.1	1.3
Pregnant					60	800	5	10	65	70	1.5	1.6
Lactating												
1st 6 months					65	1,300	5	12	65	95	1.6	1.8
2nd 6 months					62	1,200	5	11	65	90	1.6	1.7
19−24 years												
Not pregnant	58	128	164	65	46	800	5	8	60	60	1.1	1.3
Pregnant					60	800	5	10	65	70	1.5	1.6
Lactating												
1st 6 months					65	1,300	5	12	65	95	1.6	1.8
2nd 6 months					62	1,200	5	11	65	90	1.6	1.7
25 years +												
Not pregnant	63	138	163	64	50	800	5	8	60	60	1.1	1.3
Pregnant					60	800	5	10	65	70	1.5	1.6
Lactating												
1st 6 months					65	1,300	5	12	65	95	1.6	1.8
2nd 6 months					62	1,200	5	11	65	90	1.6	1.7

Reprinted with permission from **Recommended Dietary Allowances: 10th Edition.** Copyright © 1989 by the National Academy of Sciences. Courtesy of the National Academy Press, Washington, D.C., 1989 for all but vitamin D, calcium, phosphorus, and magnesium. These last four recommendations are from Dietary Reference Intakes, National Academy of Sciences, 1997.

Current research indicates there is no need for increased vitamin A during pregnancy. Excessive intake of vitamin A can cause birth defects. The vitamin D requirement during pregnancy remains the normal 10 μg for women 24 years and younger, but doubles from the normal 5 μg to 10 μg for women 25 years and older. The requirement for vitamin E is increased from 8 to 10 mg for all pregnant women. The vitamin K requirement is 65 μg for pregnant women of all ages. This represents *no* increase for pregnant women 25 and older, but it is a very large increase for pregnant girls between 11 and 14, whose normal vitamin K requirement is 45 μg. It is also a large increase for pregnant girls between 15 and 18, whose normal requirement is 55 μg, and it is a considerable increase for pregnant women between 19 and 24, whose normal vitamin K requirement is 60 <μg.

WATER-SOLUBLE VITAMINS				MINERALS								
Niacin (mg NE)	Vitamin B₆	Folate (μg)	Vitamin B₁₂ (μg)	Calcium (mg)	Phosphorus (mg)	Magnesium (mg)	Fluoride (mg)	Iron (mg)	Zinc (mg)	Iodine (μg)	Selenium (μg)
15	1.4	150	2.0	1,300	1,055	200	2.0	15	12	150	45
17	2.2	400	2.2	1,300	1,055	200	2.0	30	15	175	65
20	2.1	280	2.6	1,300	1,055	200	2.0	15	19	200	75
20	2.1	260	2.6	1,300	1,055	200	2.0	15	16	200	75
15	1.5	180	2.0	1,300	1,055	300	2.9	15	12	150	50
17	2.2	400	2.2	1,300	1,055	335	2.9	30	15	175	65
20	2.1	280	2.6	1,300	1,055	300	2.9	15	19	200	75
20	2.1	260	2.6	1,300	1,055	300	2.9	15	16	200	75
15	1.6	180	2.0	1,000	580	255	3.1	15	12	150	55
17	2.2	400	2.2	1,000	580	290	3.1	30	15	175	65
20	2.1	280	2.6	1,000	580	255	3.1	15	19	200	75
20	2.1	260	2.6	1,000	580	255	3.1	15	16	200	75
15	1.6	180	2.0	1,000	580	265	3.1	15	12	150	55
17	2.2	400	2.2	1,000	580	300	3.1	30	15	175	65
20	2.1	280	2.6	1,000	580	265	3.1	15	19	200	75
20	2.1	260	2.6	1,000	580	265	3.1	15	16	200	75

The requirements for all the water-soluble vitamins are increased during pregnancy. Additional vitamin C is needed for collagen development and to increase the absorption of iron. The B vitamins are needed in greater amounts because of their roles in metabolism and the development of red blood cells.

The requirements for the minerals calcium, iron, zinc, iodine, and selenium are all increased during pregnancy. Calcium is, of course, essential for the development of the infant's bones and teeth as well as for blood clotting and muscle action.

The need for iron increases because of the increased blood volume during pregnancy. In addition, the fetus increases its hemoglobin level to 20 to 22g per 100 ml of blood. This is nearly twice the normal human hemoglobin level of 13 to 14 mg per 100 ml of blood.

The infant's hemoglobin level is reduced to normal shortly after birth as the extra hemoglobin breaks down. The resulting iron is stored in the liver and is available when needed during the infant's first few months of life, when the diet is essentially breast milk or formula. Therefore, an iron supplement is commonly prescribed during pregnancy. However, if the pregnant woman's hemoglobin remains at an acceptable level without a supplement, the physician will not prescribe one.

FULFILLMENT OF NUTRITIONAL NEEDS DURING PREGNANCY

To meet the nutritional requirements of pregnancy, the woman should base her diet on the Food Guide Pyramid. Special care should be taken in the selection of food so that the necessary kcal are provided by nutrient-dense foods.

One of the best ways of providing these nutrients is by drinking additional milk each day or using appropriate substitutes. The extra milk will provide protein, calcium, phosphorus, thiamin, riboflavin, and niacin. If whole milk is used, it will also contribute saturated fat and cholesterol and provide 150 kcal per 8 ounces of milk. Fat-free milk contributes no fat or cholesterol, provides 90 kcal per 8 ounce serving, and is the better choice.

obstetrician

doctor who cares for the mother during pregnancy and delivery

To be sure that the vitamin requirements of pregnancy are met, obstetricians, nurse midwives, and physician's assistants (PAs) may prescribe a vitamin supplement in addition to an iron supplement. However, it is *not* advisable for the mother to take any unprescribed nutrient supplement, as an excess of vitamins or minerals can be toxic to mother and infant. Excessive vitamin A, for example, can cause birth defects.

The unusual cravings for certain foods during pregnancy do no harm unless eating them interferes with the normal balanced diet or causes excessive weight gain.

CONCERNS DURING PREGNANCY
Nausea

Sometimes nausea (the feeling of a need to vomit) occurs during the first trimester of pregnancy. This type of nausea is commonly known as morning sickness, but it can occur at any time. It typically passes as the pregnancy proceeds to the second trimester. The following suggestions can help relieve morning sickness:

- Eat dry crackers or dry toast before rising.
- Eat small, frequent meals.
- Avoid foods with offensive odors.
- Avoid liquids at mealtime.

In rare cases, the nausea persists and becomes so severe that it is life-threatening. This condition is called hyperemesis gravidarum. The mother may be hospitalized and given parenteral nutrition. This means the patient is given nutrients via a vein. This is discussed more fully in Chapter 22. Such cases are difficult, and the patients need support and optimism from those who help them.

Constipation

Constipation and hemorrhoids can be relieved by eating high-fiber foods, getting daily exercise, drinking eight glasses of liquid each day, and responding immediately to the urge to defecate.

Heartburn

Heartburn is a common complaint during pregnancy. As the fetus grows, it pushes on the mother's stomach, which may cause stomach acid to move into the lower esophagus and create a burning sensation there. Heartburn may be relieved by eating small, frequent meals, avoiding spicy or greasy foods, avoiding liquids with meals, waiting at least an hour after eating before lying down, and waiting at least 2 hours before exercising.

Excessive Weight Gain

If weight gain becomes excessive, the pregnant woman should reevaluate her diet and eliminate foods (except for the extra pint of milk) that do not fit within the Food Guide Pyramid. Examples include candy, cookies, rich desserts, potato chips, salad dressings, and sweet beverages. In addition, she might drink fat-free milk, if not doing so, which would reduce her kcal, but not her intake of proteins, vitamins, and minerals. Except in cases in which the woman cannot tolerate lactose (the sugar in milk), it is not advisable to substitute calcium pills for milk because the substitution reduces the protein, vitamin, and mineral content of the diet.

A bowl of clean, crisp, raw vegetables such as broccoli or cauliflower tips, carrots, celery, cucumber, zucchini sticks, or radishes can provide interesting snacks that are nutritious, filling, satisfying, and low in kcal. Fruits and custards made with fat-free milk make nutritious, satisfying desserts that are not high in kcal. Broiling, baking, or boiling foods instead of frying can further reduce the caloric content of the diet.

morning sickness
early morning nausea common to some pregnancies

hyperemesis gravidarum
nausea so severe as to be life-threatening

parenteral nutrition
nutrition provided via a vein

Pregnancy-Induced Hypertension

Pregnancy-induced hypertension (PIH) was formerly called *toxemia* or *preeclampsia*. It is a condition that sometimes occurs during the third trimester of pregnancy. It is characterized by high blood pressure, the presence of albumin in the urine (**proteinuria**), and edema. The edema causes a somewhat sudden increase in weight. If the condition persists and reaches the **eclamptic** (convulsive) **stage**, convulsions, coma, and death of mother and child may occur. The cause of this condition is not known, but it occurs more frequently among pregnant women on inadequate diets (particularly when the diets are inadequate in protein) than among pregnant women on nutritionally adequate good diets. There is also a higher rate of PIH among pregnant adolescents than among pregnant adults.

Pica

Pica is the craving for nonfood substances such as starch, clay (soil), or ice. The reasons people get such a craving are not clear. Although both men and women are affected, pica is most common among pregnant women. Some believe it relieves nausea. Others think the practice is based on cultural heritage. It should be discouraged because it can cause blockage of the colon and create nutritional deficiencies. If the soil binds with minerals, the body cannot absorb them. If these substances take the place of nutrient-rich foods in the diet, there can be multiple nutritional deficiencies. Eating laundry starch in addition to a regular diet will add unwanted calories.

Anemia

Anemia is a condition caused by an insufficiency of red blood cells, hemoglobin, or blood volume. The patient suffering from it does not receive sufficient oxygen from the blood and consequently feels weak and tired, has a poor appetite, and appears pale. *Iron deficiency* is its most common form. During pregnancy, the increased volume of blood creates the need for additional iron for the hemoglobin of this blood. When this need is not met by the diet or by the iron stores in the mother's body, iron deficiency anemia develops. This may be treated with a daily iron supplement.

Folate deficiency can result in a form of megaloblastic anemia that can occur during pregnancy. It is characterized by too few red blood cells and by large immature red blood cells. The body's requirement for folic acid increases dramatically when new red blood cells are being formed. Consequently, the obstetrician might prescribe a folate supplement of 400 μg a day during pregnancy.

Alcohol, Caffeine, Drugs, and Tobacco

Alcohol consumption is associated with subnormal physical and mental development of the fetus. This is called **fetal alcohol syndrome (FAS)**. Many infants with FAS are premature and have a low birthweight. Physical characteristics may include a small head, short eye slits that make eyes appear to be set far apart, a flat midface, and a

---

pregnancy-induced hypertension (PIH)
typically occurs during late pregnancy; characterized by high blood pressure, albumin in the urine, and edema

proteinuria
protein in the urine

eclamptic stage
convulsive stage of toxemia

pica
abnormal craving for nonfood substance

anemia
condition caused by insufficient number of red blood cells, hemoglobin, or blood volume

fetal alcohol syndrome (FAS)
subnormal physical and mental development caused by mother's excessive use of alcohol during pregnancy

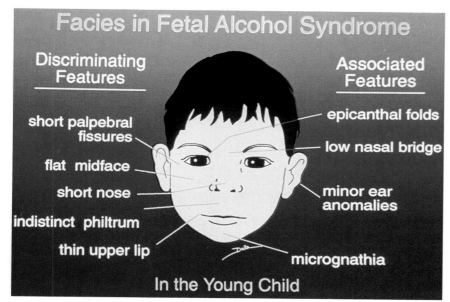

FIGURE 11-1 Discriminating and Associated Features in FAS
From "Unit 5: Alcohol, Pregnancy, and the Fetal Alcohol Syndrome: Second Edition" of the Project Cork Institute Medical School Curriculum (slide lecture series) on *Biomedical Education: Alcohol Use and Its Medical Consequences,* by A. P. Streissguth and R. E. Little, 1994, Dartmouth, NH: Dartmouth Medical School.

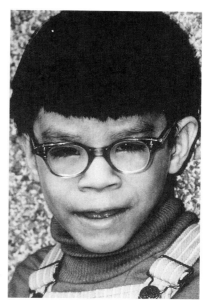

FIGURE 11-2 The growth and development of a patient with FAS from 8–18 years of age. From "Natural History of the fetal alcohol syndrome: A 10-year follow-up of eleven patients," by A. P. Streissguth, A. K. Clarren, and K. L. Jones, 1985, *The Lancet, 2,* pp. 85–91.

thin upper lip. There is usually a growth deficiency (height, weight), placing the child in the lowest tenth of age norms. There is also evidence of central nervous system dysfunction, including hyperactivity, seizures, attention deficits, and microcephaly (small head). See Figure 11-1 and 11-2. When the mother drinks alcohol, it enters the fetal bloodstream in the same concentration as it does the mother's. Unfortunately, the fetus does not have the capacity to metabolize it as quickly as the mother, so it stays longer in the fetal blood than it does in the maternal blood. Abstinence is recommended.

Caffeine is known to cross the placenta, and it enters the fetal bloodstream. Birth defects in newborn rats whose mothers were fed very high doses of caffeine during pregnancy have been observed, but there are no data on humans showing that moderate amounts of caffeine are harmful. As a safety measure, however, it is suggested that pregnant women limit their caffeine intake to two cups of caffeine-containing beverages each day.

Drugs vary in their effects, but self-prescribed drugs, including vitamins and mineral supplements and dangerous illegal drugs, can all damage the fetus. Drugs derived from vitamin A can cause **fetal malformations** and **spontaneous abortions**. Illegal drugs can cause the infant to be born addicted to whatever substance the mother used and, possibly, to be born with the human immunodeficiency virus (HIV). If a pregnant woman is known to be infected with HIV, her physician may prescribe AZT in an attempt to prevent the spread of the disease to the developing fetus.

Tobacco smoking by pregnant women has for some time been associated with babies of reduced birthweight. The more the mother

fetal malformations
physical abnormalities of the fetus

spontaneous abortion
occurring naturally; miscarriage

smokes, the smaller her baby will be because smoking reduces the oxygen and nutrients carried by the blood. Other risks associated with smoking include SIDS (sudden infant death syndrome), fetal death, spontaneous abortion, and complications at birth. Smoking during pregnancy may also affect the intellectual and behavioral development of the baby as it grows up.

Because the substances discussed in this section may cause fetal problems, it is advisable that pregnant women avoid them.

DIET FOR THE PREGNANT WOMAN WITH DIABETES

Diabetes mellitus is a group of diseases in which one cannot use or store glucose normally because of inadequate production or use of insulin. This impaired metabolism causes glucose to accumulate in the blood, where it causes numerous problems if not controlled. (See Chapter 17 for additional information on diabetes mellitus.)

gestational diabetes
diabetes occurring during pregnancy; usually disappears after delivery of the infant

Some women have diabetes mellitus when they become pregnant. Others may develop **gestational diabetes** during pregnancy. In most cases, this latter type disappears after the infant is born. Either type increases the risks of physical or mental defects in the infant, stillbirth, and **macrosomia** (birthweight over 9 pounds) unless blood glucose levels are carefully monitored and maintained within normal limits.

macrosomia
birthweight over 9 pounds

Every pregnant woman should be tested for diabetes between 16 and 28 weeks of gestation. Those found to have the disease must learn to monitor their diets to maintain normal blood glucose levels and to avoid both **hypoglycemia** and **hyperglycemia**.

hypoglycemia
subnormal levels of blood sugar

In general, the nutrient requirements of the pregnant woman with diabetes are the same as for the normal pregnant woman. The diet should be planned with a registered dietitian or a certified diabetes educator, because it will depend on the type of insulin and the time and number of injections. Patients with gestational diabetes and diabetic patients who do not normally require insulin to control their diabetes may require insulin during pregnancy to control blood glucose levels. Oral hypoglycemic agents should not be used as they may harm the baby. Between-meal feedings help maintain blood glucose at a steady level. Artificial sweeteners have been researched extensively and found to be safe for use during pregnancy.

hyperglycemia
excessive amounts of sugar in the blood

PREGNANCY DURING ADOLESCENCE

Teenage pregnancy is an increasing concern. The nutritional, physical, psychological, social, and economic demands on a pregnant adolescent are tremendous. With the birth of the infant, they increase. Young women who are themselves still in need of nurturing and financial support are suddenly responsible for helpless newborns. If the mother does not have sufficient help, the total effect on her, the child, and society can be devastating.

Prenatal health care; infant care; and psychological, nutritional, and economic counseling, as well as help in locating appropriate housing may all be needed. And at this time, the young woman's family may or may not be supportive.

At such a time, nutritional habits can seem to some as being of slight importance. They are, however, of primary importance. An adolescent's eating habits may not be adequate to fulfill the nutritional needs of her own growing body. When she adds the nutritional burden of a developing fetus, both are put at risk. Adolescents are particularly vulnerable to pregnancy-induced hypertension (PIH) and premature delivery. PIH can cause cardiovascular and kidney problems later. Premature delivery is a leading cause of death among newborns. Inadequate nutrition of the mother is related to both mental and physical birth defects.

These young women will need to know their own nutritional needs and the additional nutritional requirements of pregnancy (see Table 11-2). WIC (Women, Infants, and Children) can help with all prenatal care, nutrition education, and adequate food for the best outcome possible. Pregnant teenagers will need much counseling and emotional support from caring, experienced people before nutritional improvements can be suggested.

LACTATION

A woman needs to decide whether to breastfeed before her infant is born. Almost all women can breastfeed; breast size is no barrier. **Lactation**, the production and secretion of breast milk for the purpose of nourishing an infant, is facilitated by an interplay of various hormones after delivery of the infant. Oxytocin and prolactin instigate the lactation process. Prolactin is responsible for milk production, and oxytocin is involved in milk ejection from the breast. The infant's sucking initiates the release of oxytocin, which causes the ejection of milk into the infant's mouth. This is called the let-down reflex. It is a supply-and-demand mechanism. The more an infant nurses, the more milk the mother produces.

lactation
the period during which the mother is nursing the baby

It will take 2 to 3 weeks to fully establish a feeding routine; therefore, it is recommended that no supplemental feedings be given during this time. Human milk is formulated to meet the nutrient needs of infants for the first 6 months of life with the exceptions of iron, vitamin D, and flouride. To be able to produce the needed milk to feed her infant, the mother must pay special attention to her nutritional needs during lactation.

kcal Requirements during Lactation

The mother's kcal requirement increases during lactation. The kcal requirement depends on the amount of milk produced. Approximately 85 kcal are required to produce 100 ml (3⅓ oz) of milk. During the first 6 months, average daily milk production is 750 ml (25 oz) and for this the mother requires approximately an extra 640 kcal a day. During the second 6 months, when the baby begins to eat food in addition to breast milk, average daily milk production slows to 600 ml (20 oz) and the kcal requirement is reduced to approximately 510 extra kcal a day.

The Food and Nutrition Board suggests an increase of 500 kcal a day during lactation. This is less than the actual need because it is assumed that some fat has been stored during pregnancy, which can be used for milk production. The precise number of kcal the mother needs depends on the size of the infant and its appetite and on the size and activities of the mother. Each ounce of human milk contains 20 kcal.

If the kcal content of the mother's diet is insufficient, the quantity of milk will be reduced. Thus, lactation is not a good time to go on a strict weight-loss diet. There will be some natural weight loss caused by the burning of the stored fat for milk production.

Nutrient Requirements during Lactation

In general, most nutrient requirements are increased during lactation. The amounts depend on the age of the mother (see Table 11-2). Protein is of particular importance because it is estimated that 10g of protein are secreted in the milk each day.

The Food Guide Pyramid will be helpful in meal planning for the lactating mother. She should be sure to include sufficient fruits and vegetables, especially those rich in vitamin C. Extra fat-free milk will provide many of the additional nutrients and kcal required during lactation. Potato chips, sodas, candies, and desserts provide little more than kcal.

Vegetarians will need to be especially careful to be sure they have sufficient kcal, iron, zinc, copper, protein, calcium, and vitamin D. A vitamin B_{12} supplement can be prescribed for them.

It is important that the nursing mother have sufficient fluids to replace those lost in the infant's milk. Water and real fruit juice are the best choices.

The mother should be made aware that she must reduce her caloric intake at the end of the nursing period to avoid adding unwanted weight.

Medicines, Caffeine, Alcohol, and Tobacco

Most chemicals enter the mother's milk, so it is essential that the mother check with her obstetrician before using any medicines or nutritional supplements. Caffeine can cause the infant to be irritable. Alcohol in excess, tobacco, and illegal drugs can be very harmful.

CONSIDERATIONS FOR THE HEALTH CARE PROFESSIONAL

Good nutrition during pregnancy can make the difference between a healthy, productive life and one shattered by health and economic problems—for both mother and child.

Most pregnant women will want the best nutrition for themselves and their children. They also will be concerned about their weight during and after pregnancy. It is essential that they receive advice from a properly trained health care professional. Articles in newspapers and magazines or in pamphlets from health food stores may or may not be correct and should not be taken at face value unless approved by a professional in the dietetic field.

Nutrition is currently a popular topic, and people are inclined to believe what is printed. It can be difficult to persuade people that the information they read is incorrect. As always, the health care professional must use great patience in reeducating those patients who may require it.

The pregnant teenager can present the greatest challenge. Her needs are vast but her experience, and thus her perspective, is limited. Teaching pregnant adolescents about good nutrition may be difficult but, if successful, can help not only that particular patient but her child and her friends.

● SUMMARY

A pregnant woman is most likely to remain healthy and bear a healthy infant if she follows a well-balanced diet. Research has shown that maternal nutrition can affect the subsequent mental and physical health of the child. Anemia and PIH are two conditions that can be caused by inadequate nutrition. Caloric and most nutrient requirements increase for pregnant women (especially adolescents) and women who are breastfeeding. The average weight gain during pregnancy is 25 to 35 pounds.

● DISCUSSION TOPICS

1. Discuss the statement "A pregnant woman must eat for two."

2. Why is it especially important for a pregnant woman to have a highly nutritious diet?

3. Discuss weight gain during pregnancy from the first month through the ninth. Why is an excessive weight gain during pregnancy undesirable? Is pregnancy a good time to reduce? Explain.

4. Of what value are protein-rich foods during pregnancy?

5. It is common for an iron supplement to be prescribed during pregnancy. Why? What may happen if the mother-to-be does not receive an adequate supply of iron? How might such a condition affect her baby? Discuss the advisability of the pregnant woman's taking a self-prescribed iron or vitamin supplement in addition to that prescribed by the obstetrician.

6. Discuss why the obstetrician regularly checks the pregnant woman's blood pressure, urine, and weight during pregnancy.

7. Discuss the effects of lactation on the mother's diet.

8. What is morning sickness, and how can it be alleviated? If any class member has been pregnant, ask her questions regarding morning sickness. Can this be a truly serious problem? Explain.

9. Why is it a good idea for a pregnant woman to include a citrus fruit or melon with every meal?

10. Why is the average weight gain 25 to 35 pounds during pregnancy when the infant weights approximately 7½ pounds?

11. Why does the need for protein increase so dramatically during pregnancy?

12. Describe pica. Why is it undesirable?

13. Discuss the dangers to the fetus if the mother uses drugs.

14. How can the mother's diabetes affect the fetus?

● SUGGESTED ACTIVITIES

1. Ask a dietitian to speak to the class on the importance of adequate nutrition before and during pregnancy. Ask the speaker questions regarding the effects of good and poor nutrition on the health of the mother, prenatal development, infant mortality, and the growth and development of the child. Ask the speaker's opinion regarding the use of alcohol, caffeine, and tobacco during pregnancy. During lactation.

2. Invite a nurse practitioner to speak to the class on the symptoms and dangers of PIH.

3. Invite a certified diabetes educator to speak to the class on the problems that can occur during the pregnancy of a diabetic mother.

● REVIEW

Multiple choice. Select the *letter* that precedes the best answer.

1. The infant developing in the mother's uterus is called the
a. sperm   c. placenta
b. fetus   d. ovary

2. A common form of anemia is caused by
a. pica   c. a lack of iron
b. an excess in vitamin A   d. improper cooking of meat

3. High blood pressure, edema, and albumin in the urine are symptoms of
a. nausea   c. pica
b. anemia   d. pregnancy-induced hypertension

4. A common name given nausea in early pregnancy is
a. morning sickness
b. pica
c. pregnancy-induced hypertension
d. mortality

5. Folate and vitamin B_{12} requirements increase during pregnancy because of their roles in
a. building strong bones and teeth
b. fighting infections in the placenta
c. building blood
d. enzyme action

6. The average additional daily energy requirement for the pregnant woman during the last two trimesters is
   a. 100 calories
   b. 300 calories
   c. 500 calories
   d. 1,000 calories

7. The additional nutrients required during pregnancy can be met by
   a. eating steak each day
   b. drinking a malted milk each day
   c. using an additional pint of fat-free milk each day
   d. using an iron supplement

8. Craving nonfood substances during pregnancy is known as
   a. anemia
   b. megaloblastic anemia
   c. nausea
   d. pica

9. During pregnancy, the average weight gain is
   a. 15 to 24 pounds
   b. 25 to 35 pounds
   c. 11 to 24 kilograms
   d. 15 to 24 kilograms

10. The period during which a mother nurses her baby is known as
    a. pregnancy
    b. trimester
    c. lactation
    d. obstetrics

11. Some appropriate substitutes for milk include
    a. orange juice and tomato juice
    b. cheese and custard
    c. breads and cereals
    d. vegetables and fruit juices

12. The RDA for additional kcal for a nursing mother is
    a. 100
    b. 300
    c. 500
    d. 1,000

13. The daily diet during pregnancy and lactation should
    a. be based on the Food Guide Pyramid
    b. include at least two quarts of milk
    c. be limited to 1,900 kcal
    d. all of the above

14. Appropriate snacks for pregnant and lactating women include
    a. fruits and raw vegetables
    b. potato chips and pretzels
    c. sodas
    d. hard candies

15. the duration of a normal pregnancy is
    a. 34–36 weeks
    b. 36–38 weeks
    c. 38–40 weeks
    d. 40–42 weeks

16. The fluid surrounding the fetus in the uterus is the
    a. parenteral fluid
    b. intracellular fluid
    c. amniotic fluid
    d. synovial fluid

17. During pregnancy, parenteral nutrition may be necessary for patients
    a. with excessive weight gain
    b. suffering from hyperemesis gravidarum
    c. who cannot tolerate milk
    d. who do not eat meat

18. Heartburn may be prevented by
a. eating small, frequent meals
b. lying down immediately after eating
c. taking an aspirin
d. increasing liquid at meals

19. Pregnancy-induced hypertension
a. is relieved with salty food
b. may occur when diets contain insufficient protein
c. tends to be a precursor of iron deficiency
d. causes megaloblastic anemia

20. Gestational diabetes
a. tends to cause low-birthweight babies
b. always develops into Type I insulin-dependent diabetes mellitus
c. usually disappears after the baby is born
d. presents no danger to mother or child

21. Maternal malnutrition
a. has little effect on the fetus
b. may cause an increase in the fetal hemoglobin level
c. often causes macrosomia
d. can lead to developmental or mental retardation

22. The need for iron increases during pregnancy because
a. it prevents maternal goiter
b. it is essential to bone development
c. it is necessary to fetal metabolism
d. of the increased blood volume

23. Nutrient-dense foods provide substantial amounts of
a. vitamins, minerals, and proteins
b. kcal per gram of food
c. carbohydrates, fats, and water
d. sodium, chloride, and water

24. Excessive vitamin A should be avoided during pregnancy because it may
a. cause birth defects
b. cause gestational diabetes
c. contribute to gallstones in the fetus
d. reduce the mother's appetite

C A S E   S T U D Y

When 28-year-old Carolyn learned she was pregnant, she decided this would be a good time to lose that extra 15 pounds and save money on food at the same time. The doctor told her that most women gain about 25 to 35 pounds during pregnancy. She reasoned that if she didn't gain any weight, she should be about 10 to 15 pounds lighter after the baby was born.

Sticking to her "diet" was easy at first; she felt nauseated about food anyway. When she was about 4 months pregnant, though, the nausea passed and her appetite increased. She fought the desire to eat and ate very little. In the morning, she had juice, coffee, toast, and jelly. At lunch, she had coffee, yogurt, and fruit. At dinner, she ate vegetables, usually as soup, toast, and lots of salted popcorn.

She started feeling tired nearly all the time but passed it off to the pregnancy. She often felt bloated. She skipped several doctors' appointments to save money. By her twentieth week her face and hands were puffy, her shoes were tight even in the morning, and she got scared. At the doctor's office, her blood pressure was 150/98 (normal blood pressure is 120/80). She had gained 8 pounds. He took a urine sample looking for proteinuria. He checked her reflexes and asked her about headaches and blurred vision. The doctor explained what was happening. He reviewed her eating habits with her and explained the possible consequences to herself and to the baby. She vowed to put the baby's interests first and to lose weight after the baby was born. She was instructed to take a blood-pressure-lowering medication and stay on bed rest until her next appointment.

ASSESSMENT

1. What information do you have about Carolyn?
2. What may be causing Carolyn's symptoms?
3. What is the problem with the timing of Carolyn's weight-loss program?

DIAGNOSIS

4. Carolyn's knowledge deficit of ___ is related to ___ as shown by her choice to _____.
5. Carolyn's poor nutrition, less than requirements during pregnancy, is related to ____.
6. Carolyn's decreased cardiac output as evidenced by an elevated blood pressure is related to _____.

PLAN/GOAL

7. What is your immediate goal for Carolyn?

8. What is your long-term goal for Carolyn?
9. What are your education goals for Carolyn?

IMPLEMENTATION

10. What major topics need to be discussed with Carolyn regarding a healthy pregnancy?
11. What topics need to be taught in regard to her elevated blood pressure?
12. What signs and symptoms does Carolyn need to be taught concerning her hypertension?
13. How can breastfeeding help Carolyn lose weight?

EVALUATION/OUTCOME CRITERIA

14. At her next doctor's appointment, what will the doctor be checking to determine whether the treatment was successful?

C A S E   S T U D Y

Carleta was a beautiful black-haired 16-year-old sophomore at Central High. She was smart, had A's and B's in all her classes, and had career ambitions for after graduation. Her boyfriend, Enrico, was 18 years old and a senior. He had a black Camaro and didn't care much for school—just cars and Carleta. He was handsome and seemed too mature for high school. He worked part time in his uncle's auto body shop. He couldn't wait to get out of high school.

Carleta always met Enrico before and after school. When semester exams came, Carleta studied, was stressed, and missed her period. She didn't think much about it. She enjoyed all the extra hours of sleep over Christmas break but still felt tired when it was time to go back to school.

When she couldn't eat breakfast and felt nauseated all morning, she thought she might be pregnant. She bought a home pregnancy kit at the drug store and used it one day after school. It was positive. She was scared to tell her mother, who had "warned" her repeatedly about Enrico.

By the time she decided to go to the free clinic to see the nurse practitioner (NP) she was 3 months pregnant. The NP advised her to stop smoking and to increase her calories and protein. She gave her a prescription for prenatal vitamins. She asked Carleta to see her on a regular basis for the rest of her pregnancy. Carleta wanted to have a healthy baby, but she didn't want to be fat. She gained only 10 pounds during the rest of her pregnancy. She smoked only when she was with Enrico.

At 37 weeks, Juanita Maria was born. She weighed 5 pounds 1 ounce and was 18 inches long. She had periods of apnea in which she temporarily stopped breathing so she had to wear an apnea monitor when she went home. The neonatologist discussed how to treat the apnea at home and made sure Carleta and Enrico knew CPR.

ASSESSMENT

1. What objective data do you have about Carleta?

2. What information are you guessing about in regard to Carleta's nutrition?

3. What information do you have about Juanita?

4. What factors most likely caused Juanita's health problems?

DIAGNOSIS

5. What caused Carleta to eat the way she did?

6. What was the cause of Carleta's noncompliance?

7. Complete the diagnosis statement. Juanita's rate of growth was related to _____.

8. Complete the following statement. Juanita was at high risk for _____ secondary to _____.

PLAN/GOAL

9. What is your goal for Carleta's health after the birth?

10. What is your goal for Juanita's health?

IMPLEMENTATION

11. What topics do you need to teach Carleta about Juanita?

12. Who else needs to be present for the teaching?

13. As a teenage mother with a low-birthweight baby, Carleta needs what type of medical and nursing follow-up? Would home health care nursing visits help?

14. What is your primary concern for Juanita?

EVALUATION/OUTCOME CRITERIA

15. At the next visit, what criteria will the NP be using to see if Carleta and Juanita are healthy?

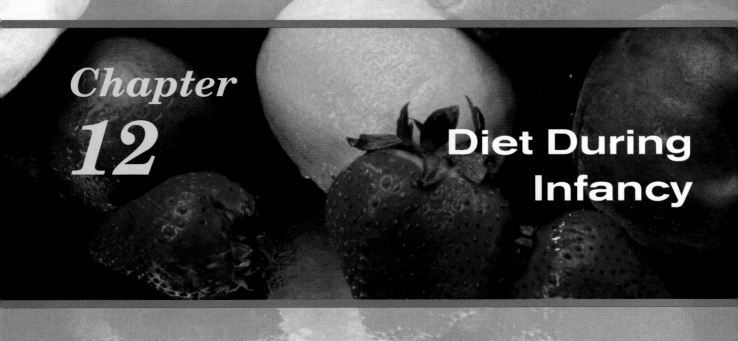

Chapter
12

Diet During Infancy

Key Terms

amniocentesis
bonding
galactosemia
galactosuria
immunity
inborn errors of
  metabolism
isoleucine
leucine
Lofenalac
maple syrup urine
  disease (MSUD)
mutations

on demand
phenylalanine
phenylalanine
  hydroxylase
phenylketonuria
psychosocial
  development
regurgitation
sterile
transferase
valine
weaning

**psychosocial
development**
relating to both psychological
and social development

Objectives

After studying this chapter, you should be able to:

● State the effect inadequate nutrition has on an infant

● Identify the ingredients used in infant formulas

● Describe when and how foods are introduced into the baby's diet

● Describe inborn errors of metabolism and their dietary treatment

Food and its presentation are extremely important during the baby's first year. Physical and mental development are dependent on the food itself, and **psychosocial development** is affected by the time and manner in which the food is offered.

Infants react to their parents' emotions. If food is forced on a child, or withheld until the child is uncomfortable, or if the food is presented in a tense manner, the child reacts with tension and unhappiness. If the parent is relaxed, an infant's mealtime can be a pleasure for both parent and child (Figure 12-1).

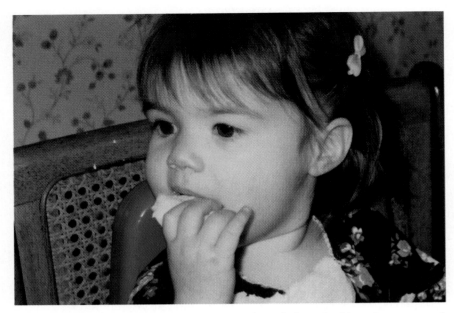

FIGURE 12-1 Food is better accepted and digested in a happy and relaxed atmosphere.

on demand

feeding infants as they desire

Although babies have been fed according to prescribed time schedules in the past, it is preferable to feed infants **on demand**. Feeding on demand prevents the frustrations that hunger can bring and helps the child develop trust in people. The newborn may require more frequent feedings, but normally the demand schedule averages approximately every 4 hours by the time the baby is 2 or 3 months old.

NUTRITIONAL REQUIREMENTS OF THE INFANT

The first year of life is a period of the most rapid growth in one's life. A baby doubles its birth weight by 6 months of age and triples it within the first year. This explains why the infant's energy, vitamin, mineral, and protein requirements are higher per unit of body weight than those of older children or adults. It is important to remember, however, that growth rates vary from child to child. Nutritional needs will depend largely on a child's growth rate.

During the first year, the normal child needs about 100 kcal per kilogram of body weight each day. This is approximately two to three times the adult requirement. Low-birthweight infants and infants who have suffered from malnutrition or illness require more than the normal number of kcal per kilogram of body weight. The nutritional status of infants is reflected by many of the same characteristics as those of adults (see Table 1-2).

The basis of the infant's diet is breast milk or formula. Either one is a highly nutritious, digestible food containing proteins, fats, carbohydrates, vitamins, minerals, and water.

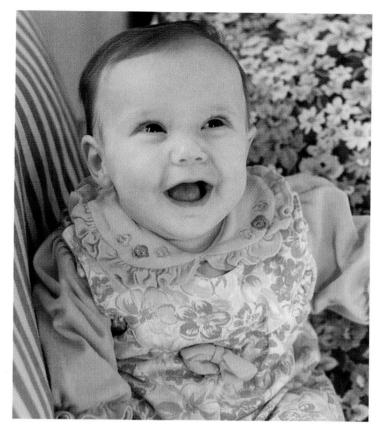

FIGURE 12-2 A happy, healthy, well-fed 6-month-old child.

It is recommended that infants up to 6 months of age have 2.2g of protein per kilogram of weight each day, and from 6 to 12 months, 1.56g of protein per kilogram of weight each day. This is satisfactorily supplied by human milk or by infant formulas (Figure 12-2).

Infants have more water per pound of body weight than do adults. Thus, they usually need 1.5 ml of water per kcal. This is the same ratio of water to kcal as is found in human milk and in most infant formulas.

Essential vitamins and minerals can be supplied in breast milk, formula, and food. Except for vitamin D, breast milk provides all the nutrients an infant needs for the first 4 to 6 months of life. An infant is born with a 3- to 6-month supply of iron. When the infant reaches 6 months of age, the pediatrician usually starts the infant on iron-fortified cereal.

Human milk usually supplies the infant with sufficient vitamin C. Iron-fortified formula is available, and its use is recommended by the American Academy of Pediatricians. The pediatrician can prescribe a vitamin D supplement for infants who are nursed and who are not exposed to sunlight on a regular basis. Newborns lack intestinal bacteria to synthesize vitamin K, so they are routinely given a vitamin K supplement shortly after birth. In addition, some pediatricians prescribe fluoride for breastfed babies or for formula-fed babies living in areas where the water contains little fluoride.

Care must be taken that infants do not receive excessive amounts of either vitamin A or D because both can be toxic in excessive amounts. Vitamin A can damage the liver and cause bone abnormalities, and vitamin D can damage the cardiovascular system and kidneys.

BREASTFEEDING

Although babies will thrive whether nursed or formula fed, there is little doubt that breastfeeding provides advantages that formulas cannot match. Breastfeeding is nature's way of providing a good diet for the baby. It is, in fact, used as the guide by which nutritional requirements of infants are measured.

immunity
ability to resist certain diseases

sterile
free of infectious organisms

bonding
emotional attachment

Mother's milk provides the infant with temporary immunity to many infectious diseases. It is economical, nutritionally adequate, and sanitary, and it saves time otherwise spent in shopping for or preparing formula. It is sterile, easy to digest, and usually does not cause gastrointestinal disturbances or allergic reactions. Breastfed infants grow more rapidly during the first few months of life than formula-fed babies, and they have fewer infections (especially ear infections). And, because breast milk contains less protein and minerals than infant formula, it reduces the load on the infant's kidneys. Breastfeeding also promotes oral motor development in infants.

The breast should be offered about every 2 hours in the first several weeks. As the infant grows and develops, a stronger sucking ability will allow more milk to be extracted at each feeding, and the frequency of nursing sessions will decrease. It is recommended that an infant nurse at each breast for approximately 10 to 15 minutes each session. Growth spurts occur at about 10 days, 2 weeks, 6 weeks, and 3 months. During this time, the infant will nurse more frequently to increase the supply of nutrients needed to support growth. As mentioned previously, the amount of milk needed is the amount the mother produces.

One can be quite confident the infant is getting sufficient nutrients and kcal from breastfeeding if (1) there are six or more wet diapers a day; (2) there is normal growth; (3) there are one or two mustard-colored bowel movements a day; and (4) the breast becomes soft during nursing.

From the mother's perspective at least, the bonding that occurs during breastfeeding is unmatched. In addition, breastfeeding helps the mother's uterus return to normal size after delivery and controls postpartum bleeding. Research has shown a correlation between breastfeeding and a decreased risk of breast cancer in premenopausal women.

Breastfeeding had been on the decline for many years, but a growing number of mothers are now nursing their babies. If the mother works and cannot be available for every feeding, breast milk can be expressed earlier, refrigerated or frozen, and used at the appropriate time, or a bottle of formula can be substituted. Never warm the breast milk in a microwave oven because the antibodies will be destroyed.

BOTTLE FEEDING

Despite the foregoing, some mothers choose to bottle feed their babies. Certain women are unable to produce enough breast milk. Some lack emotional support from their families, and some simply find it foreign to their culture. Others who are employed or involved in many activities outside the home find bottle feeding more convenient. Either way is acceptable provided the infant is given love and attention during the feeding.

The infant should be cuddled and held in an upright position during the feeding (Figure 12-3). It appears that babies fed this way are less inclined to develop middle ear infections than those fed lying down. It is believed that the upright position prevents fluid from pooling at the back of the throat and entering tubes from the middle ear. During and after the feeding, the infant should be burped to release gas in the stomach, just as the breastfed infant should be burped (Figure 12-4). Burping helps prevent **regurgitation**.

If the baby is to be bottle fed, the pediatrician will provide information on commercial formulas and feeding instructions. Formulas are usually based on cow's milk because it is abundant and easily modified to resemble human milk. It must be modified because it has more protein and mineral salts and less milk sugar (lactose) than human milk. Formulas are developed so that they are similar to human milk in nutrient and kcal values.

When an infant is extremely sensitive or allergic to infant formulas, a synthetic formula may be given. Synthetic milk is commonly made from soybeans. Formulas with predigested proteins are used for infants unable to tolerate all other types of formulas.

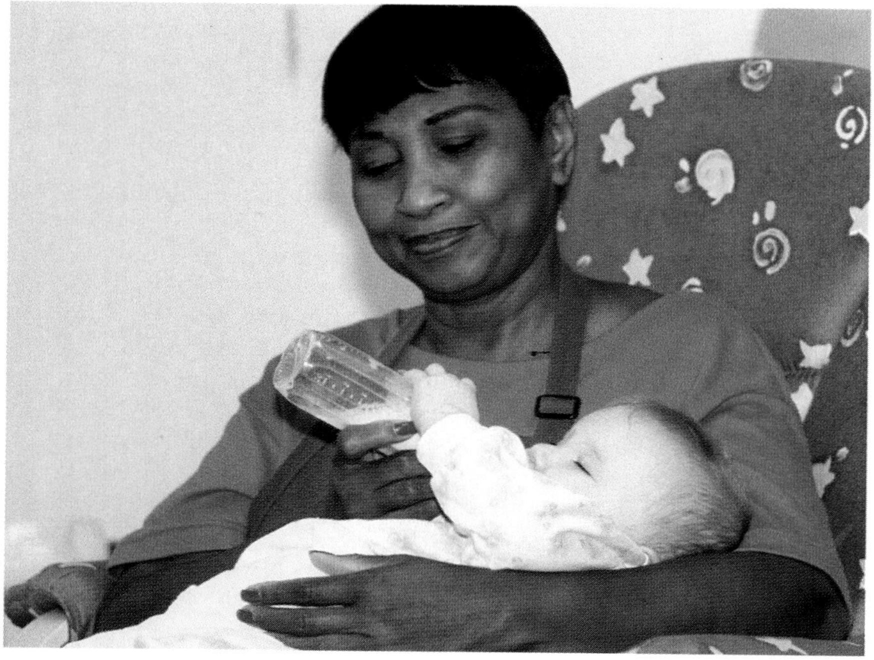

regurgitation
vomiting

FIGURE 12-3 Feeding is a good time to provide the infant with love and attention.

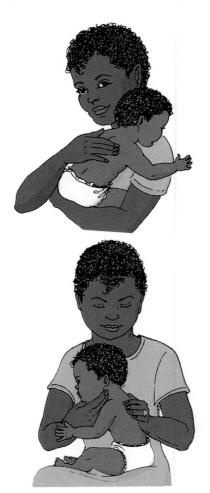

FIGURE 12-4 To burp a baby, hold him or her in one of the two positions shown and gently stroke his or her back.

Formulas can be purchased in ready-to-feed, concentrated, or powdered forms. Sterile water must be mixed with the concentrated and powdered forms. The most convenient type is also the most expensive.

If the type purchased requires the addition of water, it is essential that the amount of water added be correctly measured. Too little water will create too heavy a protein and mineral load for the infant's kidneys. Too much water will dilute the nutrient and kcal value so that the infant will not thrive.

Infants under the age of 1 year should not be given regular cow's milk. Because its protein is more difficult and slower to digest than that of human milk, it can cause gastrointestinal blood loss. The kidneys are challenged by its high protein and mineral content, and dehydration and even damage to the central nervous system can result. In addition, the fat is less bioavailable, meaning it is not absorbed as efficiently as that in human milk.

Formula may be given cold, at room temperature, or warmed, but it should be given at the same temperature consistently. To warm the formula for feeding, place the bottle in a saucepan of warm water or a bottle warmer. The bottles should be shaken occasionally to warm contents evenly. Warming the bottle in the microwave is not advisable because milk can heat unevenly and burn the infant's mouth. The temperature of the milk can be tested by shaking a few drops on one's wrist. The milk should feel lukewarm.

Infants should not be put to bed with a bottle. Saliva, which normally cleanses the teeth, diminishes as the infant falls asleep. The milk then bathes the upper front teeth, causing tooth decay. Also, the bottle can cause the upper jaw to protrude and the lower to recede. The result is known as the baby bottle mouth or nursing bottle syndrome. It is preferable to feed the infant the bedtime bottle, cleanse the teeth and gums with some water from another bottle or cup, and then put the infant to bed.

SUPPLEMENTARY FOODS

The age at which infants are introduced to solid and semisolid food has varied considerably over the years. At the beginning of this century, doctors advocated that children be fed only breast milk during their first 12 months. By the 1950s, in response to parental demand, some pediatricians advised the introduction of solid food before the age of 1 month. Now, the general recommendation is that the infant's diet be limited to breast milk or formula until the age of 4 to 6 months and that breast milk or formula remain the major food source until the child is 1 year old. With the appropriate supplements of iron and vitamin D, and possibly vitamin C and fluoride, breast milk or formula fulfills the nutritional requirements of most children until they reach the age of 6 months.

The introduction of solid foods before the age of 4 to 6 months is not recommended. The child's gastrointestinal tract and kidneys are not sufficiently developed to handle solid food before that age. Further, it is thought that the early introduction of solid foods may increase the likelihood of overfeeding and the possibility of the development of food allergies, particularly in children whose parents suffer from allergies.

An infant's readiness for solid foods will be demonstrated by (1) the physical ability to pull food into the mouth rather than always pushing the tongue and food out of the mouth, (2) a willingness to participate in the process, (3) the ability to sit up with support, (4) having head and neck control, and (5) the need for additional nutrients. If the infant is drinking more than 32 ounces of formula or nursing 8 to 10 times in 24 hours, then solid food should be started.

Solid foods must be introduced gradually and individually. One food is introduced and then no other new food for 4 or 5 days. If there is no allergic reaction, another food can be introduced, a waiting period allowed, then another, and so on. The typical order of introduction begins with cereal, usually iron-fortified rice, then oat, wheat, and mixed cereals. Cooked and pureed vegetables follow, then cooked and pureed fruits, egg yolk, and finally, finely ground meats. Between 6 and 12 months, toast, zwieback, teething biscuits, custards, puddings, and ice cream can be added. Honey should never be given to an infant because it could be contaminated with *Clostridium botulinum* bacteria. When the infant learns to drink from a cup, juice can be introduced. Juice should never be given from a bottle because babies will fill up on it and not get enough calories from other sources. Pasteurized apple juice is usually given first. It is recommended that only 100% juice products be given because they are nutrient-dense.

By the age of 1 year, most babies are eating foods from all of the Food Guide Pyramid's groups and may have most any food that is easily chewed and digested (Figures 12-5 and 12-6). However, precautions must be taken to avoid offering foods on which the child can choke. Examples include hot dogs, nuts, whole peas, grapes, popcorn, small candies, and small pieces of tough meat or raw vegetables. Foods should be selected according to the advice of the pediatrician. It is not necessary to use the commercially prepared "junior" foods. Table foods generally can be used.

The Food Guide Pyramid provides excellent help in determining the baby's menu. Its use will help supply the appropriate nutrients and

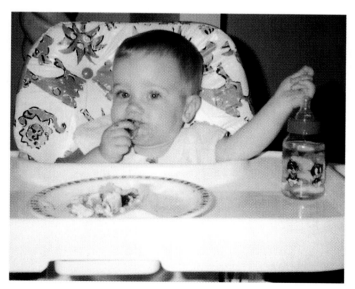

FIGURE 12-5 Finger foods encourage self-feeding.

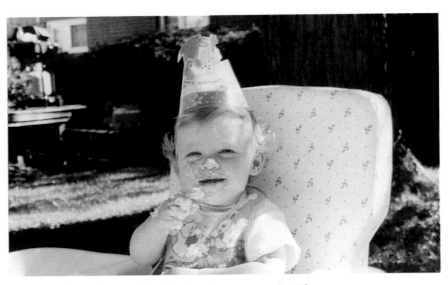

FIGURE 12-6 Finger foods can be messy but fun.

develop good eating habits. It is particularly important at this time to avoid excess sugar and salt in the infant's diet so that the child does not develop a taste for them and, consequently, overuse them throughout life.

weaning

training an infant to drink from the cup instead of the nipple

Weaning actually begins when the infant is first given food from a spoon (Figure 12-7). It progresses as the child shows an interest in, and an ability to drink from, a cup. The child will ultimately discard the bottle or refuse the breast. If the child shows great reluctance to discard the bottle or still seeks the breast, the pediatrician's advice should be sought.

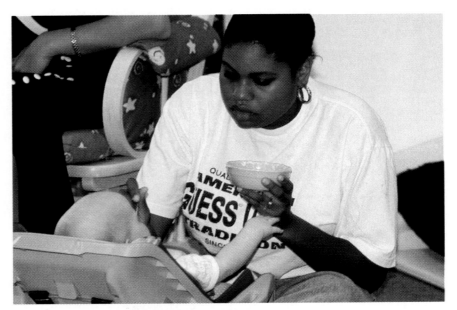

FIGURE 12-7 Weaning an infant from the bottle actually begins when food is given with a spoon.

SPECIAL NUTRITIONAL NEEDS

Premature Infants

An infant born before 37 weeks gestation is considered to be premature. These babies have special needs. The sucking reflex is not developed until 34 weeks gestation, and infants born earlier must be fed by total parenteral nutrition, tube feedings, or bolus feedings. The best food for a premature infant is its mother's breast milk which contains more protein, sodium, and some other minerals than does the milk produced by mothers of full-term infants. Other concerns in preterm infants are low birthweight, underdeveloped lungs, immature GI tract, inadequate bone mineralization, and lack of fat reserves. Many specialized formulas are available for premature infants.

Cystic Fibrosis

Cystic fibrosis (CF) is an inherited disease affecting the exocrine glands (their secretions flow through a duct). The exocrine glands produce thick, sticky secretions (mucus) in CF patients. This thick mucus affects the lungs and intestines. The CF infant has fat-soluble vitamin deficiencies because much of the fat eaten is not absorbed by the body. These infants produce excess mucus, which can block release of enzymes from the pancreas. Replacement enzymes are taken orally with meals. Malnutrition is due to malabsorption and problems with the digestion of needed nutrients.

Failure to Thrive

Failure to thrive (FTT) can be determined by plotting the infant on the growth chart (Figures 12-8 and 12-9). If the weight for length is less than the fifth percentile, then a diagnosis is made of FTT. Also, if an infant goes down a percentile in weight then FTT is suspected. This rule applies only to full-term infants. Failure to thrive can have many causes, such as watering down formula (poverty), congenital abnormalities, AIDS, lack of bonding, child abuse, or neglect.

METABOLIC DISORDERS

Some infants are born with metabolic disabilities. These congenital disabilities prevent the normal metabolism of specific nutrients. They are called **inborn errors of metabolism**. They are caused by **mutations** in the genes. There is great variation in the seriousness of the conditions caused by these defects. Some cause death at an early age, and some can be minimized so that life can be supported by adjustments in the normal diet. Among children born with these defects, there is, however, the common danger of damage to the central nervous system because of their abnormal body chemistry. This results in mental retardation and sometimes retarded growth. Early diagnosis of these inborn errors combined with diet therapy increases the chances of preventing retardation. Hospitals test newborns for some of these disorders as a matter of course. If there is a family history of a certain

inborn errors of metabolism
congenital disabilities preventing normal metabolism

mutations
changes in the genes

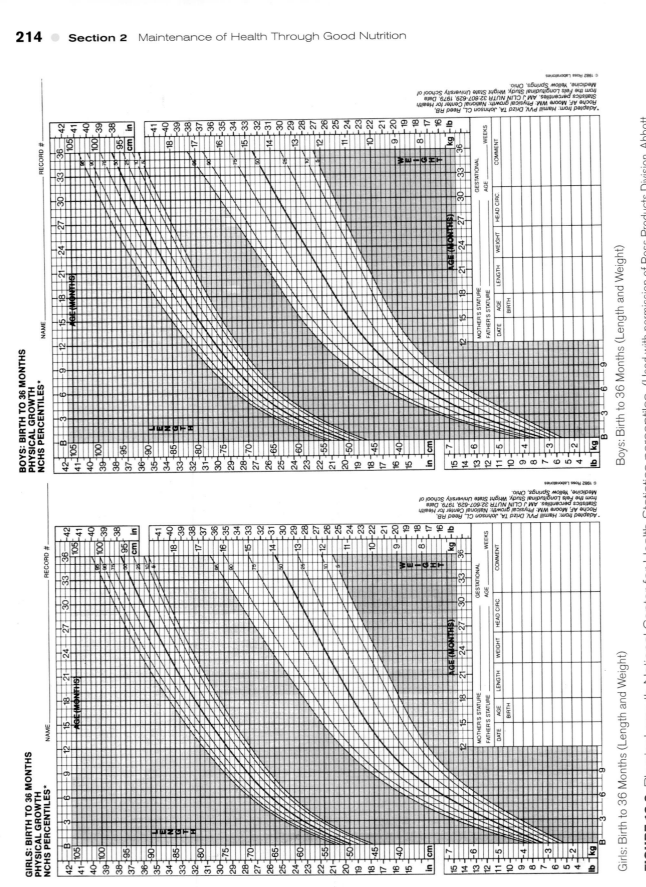

FIGURE 12-8 Physical growth National Center for Health Statistics percentiles. (Used with permission of Ross Products Division, Abbott Laboratories, Columbus, OH 43216. From Ross Laboratories. © 1982 Ross Products Division, Abbott Laboratories.)

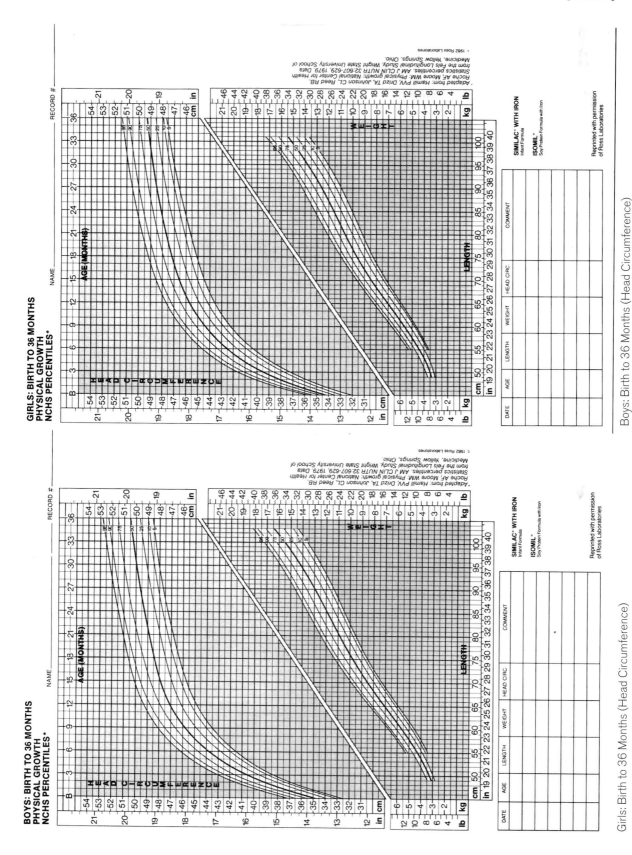

Boys: Birth to 36 Months (Head Circumference)

Girls: Birth to 36 Months (Head Circumference)

FIGURE 12-8 *continued*

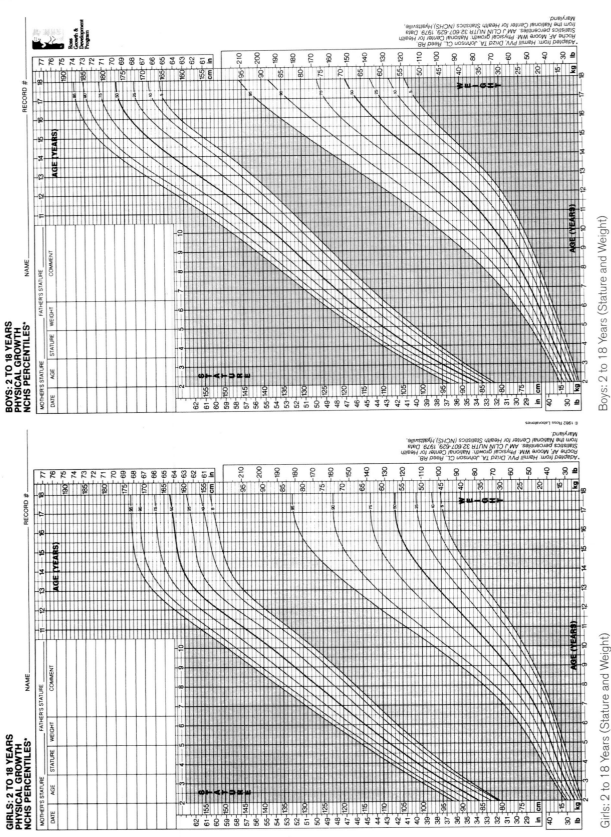

FIGURE 12-9 Physical growth National Center for Health Statistics percentiles. (Used with permission of Ross Products Division, Abbott Laboratories, Columbus, OH 43216. From Ross Laboratories. © 1982 Ross Products Division, Abbott Laboratories.)

Girls: 2 to 18 Years (Stature and Weight)

Boys: 2 to 18 Years (Stature and Weight)

genetic disorder, genetic screening can be done. In addition, some of these abnormalities can be discovered by **amniocentesis**.

Galactosemia

Galasctosemia is a condition in which there is a lack of the liver enzyme **transferase**. Transferase normally converts galactose to glucose. Galactose is the simple sugar resulting from the digestion of lactose, the sugar found in milk (see Chapter 4). When transferase is missing, and the infant ingests anything containing galactose, the amount of galactose in the blood becomes so excessive that it is toxic. The newborn suffers diarrhea, vomiting, edema, and the child's liver does not function normally. Cataracts may develop, **galactosuria** occurs, and mental retardation ensues.

Diet Therapy.   Diet therapy for galactosemia is the exclusion of anything containing milk from any mammal. During infancy, the treatment is relatively simple because parents can feed the baby lactose-free, commercially prepared formula and can provide supplemental minerals and vitamins. As the child grows and moves on to adult foods, parents must be extremely careful to avoid any food, beverage, or medicine that contains lactose. Nutritional supplements of calcium, vitamin D, and riboflavin must be given so that the diet is nutritionally adequate. This restricted diet may be necessary throughout life, but some physicians allow a somewhat liberalized diet as the child reaches school age. This may mean only small amounts of baked or processed foods that contain small amounts of milk. Even this restricted diet must be accompanied by careful and regular monitoring for galactosuria.

Phenylketonuria (PKU)

In **phenylketonuria**, infants lack the liver enzyme **phenylalanine hydroxylase**, which is necessary for the metabolism of the amino acid **phenylalanine**. Infants seem to be normal at birth, but if the disease is not treated, most of them become hyperactive, suffer seizures between 6 and 18 months, and become mentally retarded. Most hospitals today screen newborns for phenylketonuria. PKU babies typically have light-colored skin and hair.

Diet Therapy.   There is a special, nutritionally adequate, commercial infant formula available for PKU babies. It is called **Lofenalac**. It has had 95% of phenylalanine removed from its protein source. It provides just enough phenylalanine for basic needs but no excess. The specific amount depends on the infant's size and growth rate. Regular blood tests determine the adequacy of the amounts. Diets are carefully monitored for kcal and nutrient content and are adjusted frequently as needs change. Except for fats and sugars, there is some protein in all foods. Some of that protein is phenylalanine, so diets for the growing child eating normal food must be carefully planned. There are two varieties of synthetic milk available for older children. They are *Phenyl-free* and *PKU-1, -2,* or *-3*. None of these contains any phenylalanine. They can be used as beverages or in puddings and baked products. Diets

amniocentesis
a test to determine the status of the fetus in utero

galactosemia
inherited error in metabolism that prevents normal metabolism of galactose

transferase
liver enzyme that converts galactose to glucose

galactosuria
galactose in the urine

phenylketonuria (PKU)
condition caused by an inborn error of metabolism in which the infant lacks an enzyme necessary to metabolize the amino acid phenylalanine

phenylalanine hydroxylase
liver enzyme necessary to metabolize the amino acid phenylalanine

phenylalanine
amino acid

Lofenalac
commercial infant formula with 95% of phenylalanine removed

TABLE 12-1

FOODS ALLOWED PEOPLE WITH PKU	FOODS NOT ALLOWED PEOPLE WITH PKU
Special low-phenylalanine formulas	Meats
The following which contain no phenylalanine:	Fish
Fats	Poultry
Sugars	Eggs
Jellies	Milk
Some candies	Cheese
The following which contain some phylalanine:	Nuts
Fruits	Dried beans/peas
Vegetables	Commercially prepared products made from regular flour
Cereals	

should be monitored throughout life to avoid mental retardation and to control hyperactivity and aggressive behavior (Table 12-1).

Maple Syrup Urine Disease (MSUD)

maple syrup urine disease (MSUD)
disease caused by an inborn error of metabolism in which the body cannot metabolize certain amino acids

leucine
an amino acid

isoleucine
an amino acid

valine
an amino acid

Maple Syrup Urine Disease (MSUD) is a congenital defect resulting in the inability to metabolize three amino acids: leucine, isoleucine, and valine. It is named for the odor of the urine of these patients. When the infant ingests food protein, there are increased blood levels of these amino acids. Hypoglycemia, apathy, and convulsions occur very early. If the disease is not treated promptly, the child will die.

Diet Therapy. The diet must provide sufficient kcal and nutrients, but with extremely restricted amounts of leucine, isoleucine, and valine. A special formula and low-protein foods are used. Diet therapy appears to be necessary throughout life.

WOMEN, INFANTS AND CHILDREN (WIC)

The Women, Infants and Children (WIC) program is federally funded and provides monthly food packages of infant formula or milk, cereal, eggs, cheese, peanut butter, and juice for a mother who is breastfeeding. Infants and children who qualify are given monthly food vouchers until the age of 5. Eligibility depends on nutritional risk, history of miscarriage or premature birth, abnormal growth, anemia, and low income. Nutrition education is a component of the services provided.

CONSIDERATIONS FOR THE HEALTH CARE PROFESSIONAL

Although the physical and mental development of infants depend on the nutrients and kcal they receive, their psychosocial development depends on *how and when* these nutrients and kcal are provided. Some new parents will have a solid knowledge of the nutrition information needed but lack a real understanding of the importance of how and when food should be presented to infants. They may hold the infant during feedings but focus instead on the television or newspaper.

Other parents may know instinctively how important cuddling and attention are to an infant, but they lack accurate knowledge of infant nutrition.

Parents from both groups are apt to have opinions based on their parents' knowledge that may or may not be correct. The health care professional will help these parents most if she or he listens carefully to them. Then, if a *two-way discussion* follows, the parents are more inclined to listen to the advice and suggestions of the health care professional.

● SUMMARY

It is particularly important that babies have adequate diets so that their physical and mental development are not impaired. Breastfeeding is nature's way of feeding an infant, although formula feeding is quite acceptable. Cow's milk is usually used in formulas because it is most available and is easily modified to resemble human milk. Milk typically is modified by adding sugar and water to evaporated milk. The young child's diet is supplemented on the advice of the pediatrician. Added foods should be based on the Food Guide Pyramid.

Inborn errors of metabolism cause various problems, ranging from mental retardation to death, if not properly treated. In these conditions, diet therapy is the primary tool in maintaining the patient's health.

Premature, CF, and FTT infants have special nutritional needs.

● DISCUSSION TOPICS

1. Do any of the students know a woman who has breastfed her baby? What were her reactions to the experience?

2. Why is breastfeeding not always possible?

3. Discuss the possible effects of regularly propping the baby's bottle instead of holding the baby during feeding.

4. Why is a rigid time schedule for feeding a baby not advisable? Explain why feeding infants on demand the first few months can lead to a regular feeding schedule.

5. How may weaning be accomplished?

6. What is meant by inborn errors of metabolism? What causes them? How might they affect people?

7. Discuss PKU. Include its cause, symptoms, effects, and treatment.

● SUGGESTED ACTIVITIES

1. Have a panel discussion on the advantages and disadvantages of breastfeeding. Invite lactation specialists, doctors, and parents as panelists.

2. Observe a demonstration of the actual feeding and burping of a baby.

3. Visit a store that carries prepared infant formulas and compare their prices.

4. Invite a physician to give a talk on inborn errors of metabolism.

● REVIEW

A. Multiple choice. Select the *letter* that precedes the best answer.

1. The most rapid growth in a child's life occurs during
   a. its first month
   b. the month following weaning
   c. its first year
   d. its sixth year

2. The amount of protein needed by a child during its first year
   a. is greater during the first 6 months than during the second
   b. is greater during the second 6 months than during the first
   c. does not change from the first month to the twelfth
   d. increases on a weekly basis

3. After the initial supplement of vitamin K following birth, breast milk provides all the nutrients an infant needs during the first 4 to 6 months except for
   a. vitamin A   c. vitamin C
   b. vitamin B   d. vitamin D

4. The vitamin in question 3 might be provided
   a. by injection
   b. in diluted orange juice
   c. by regular walks in the sunshine
   d. in pasteurized apple juice

5. Breastfed babies are more resistant to infection than are bottle-fed babies because mother's milk provides
   a. a sterile environment   c. leucine
   b. synthetic antibiotics   d. immunity

6. The development of emotional attachment to a child is called
   a. transferase
   b. bonding
   c. psychosocial development
   d. immunity

7. It is recommended that, at each feeding, an infant nurse at each breast for approximately
   a. 3–5 minutes   c. 10–15 minutes
   b. 5–10 minutes   d. 20 minutes

8. It can be said that infant formulas
   a. are usually based on cow's milk
   b. have the same protein content as cow's milk
   c. contain fewer minerals than cow's milk
   d. contain no sugar

9. Infants with sensitivities or allergies to cow's milk may be given
   a. goat's milk
   b. synthetic milk, often made from soybeans
   c. formula with predigested carbohydrates
   d. any of the above

10. By the age of 6 months, a child
   a. may be introduced to a new formula
   b. is usually completely weaned
   c. is usually introduced to solid foods
   d. is no longer given milk

B. Briefly answer the following questions.

   1. Why should the mother give her baby special attention during feedings?

   2. How is a bottle warmed? Is it always necessary to warm the bottle? Explain. Why is a microwave oven not recommended?

   3. Why is it not advisable to give an 8-month-old child peanuts?

CASE STUDY

Ingrid was a 32-year-old Amish woman who was having her fourth child. Jacob was 7 pounds, 9 ounces and 20 inches long at birth. Ingrid left the hospital with Jacob within 24 hours after his birth. She was anxious to go home. Her mother, Elsa, had the house prepared so that Ingrid could concentrate on the new baby. A week after Jacob was born, Levi, Ingrid's husband, was killed in an auto-buggy accident. Ingrid's life was suddenly in turmoil. What was she going to do with four children and a farm and no husband?

Ingrid sobbed for weeks over Levi. Elsa could hardly get her to eat, let alone take care of Jacob. Ingrid would sit and rock in isolation for hours. Jacob was cranky and didn't feed well. At times, Elsa would bottle feed Jacob just so she knew he was fed.

When Jacob was 3 months old Ingrid and Elsa took him to see the nurse practitioner (NP) at the family clinic. Elsa said something to the NP about Levi and about how Jacob was being fed. The NP talked to Ingrid about Jacob's slow growth and development. He wasn't smiling or tracking objects. The NP asked Ingrid to return monthly and to monitor Jacob closely.

At the 5-month appointment, the NP plotted Jacob's growth. He weighed 10 pounds and measured 22 inches long. The NP told Ingrid that Jacob was in trouble. He had failure to thrive. Ingrid was devastated.

ASSESSMENT

1. What data do you have about Ingrid?
2. What data do you have about Jacob?
3. What factors contributed to Jacob's problem?
4. Using the growth charts in Figure 12-8, determine normal weight and height at 5 months. What should Jacob weigh and how long should he be?
5. What should Jacob be doing at 5 months?
6. How severe is Jacob's failure to thrive?

DIAGNOSIS

7. Complete the following. Jacob's failure to thrive is related to_____.
8. Complete the following. Jacob's poor nutrition, less than body requirements, is secondary to _____.
9. Complete the following. Ingrid's ineffective breastfeeding is a result of _____.
10. Complete the following. Ingrid's strain as caregiver is a result of_____.

PLAN/GOAL

11. What is your immediate goal for Jacob?
12. What is your longer term goal for Jacob?
13. What is your goal for Ingrid?

IMPLEMENTATION

14. What needs to be changed for Jacob to thrive?
15. What does the NP need to teach Ingrid?
16. How else can the NP help Ingrid?
17. How can Elsa help Ingrid?
18. How can the Amish community help Ingrid?

EVALUATION/OUTCOME CRITERIA

19. After the plan has been in place for 6 weeks, what changes should Ingrid see in Jacob?
20. What will the NP measure and observe in Jacob and Ingrid if the plan is successful?

C A S E   S T U D Y

Paula M. was a 37-year-old married television journalist. She and her husband, Aaron, were eagerly awaiting the birth of their first child. Paula knew it was going to be rough to juggle her career and take care of the baby. Her career was just taking off. Her boss was very flexible and supportive. He suggested that she work on background research while she was on maternity leave. He was willing to let her bring the baby to the office when she returned to work.

Paula had been interviewing nannies for her return to work. Cody was a good baby, but Paula had had no idea that breastfeeding was so time-consuming. She nursed Cody

successfully for 6 weeks while she tried to maintain her career.

In consultation with her doctor, she made the transition to bottle feeding and a nanny at 8 weeks instead of the twelfth week as originally planned. Cody cried more with the bottle feeding, but he drank the formula. The nanny took care of Cody 5 hours a day when she started. When Paula returned to full-time work at 12 weeks the nanny took care of Cody while Paula and Aaron were working. Paula had imagined a different maternity leave. She enjoyed the time at home with Cody after she returned each day, and was pleased that she had nursed him for 6 weeks.

ASSESSMENT

1. What data do you have about the problem?
2. What factor contributed the most of the change in Paula's breastfeeding plans?
3. What benefit did Cody get from 6 weeks of breastfeeding?
4. What can you guess is the status of bonding between Paula and Cody?
5. What do you suspect will be the relationship between Cody and the nanny?

DIAGNOSIS

6. Why did Paula switch to bottle feeding earlier than she had planned?
7. Does the change from breastfeeding to bottle feeding remain nutritionally adequate?
8. Could Cody's problems with crying be emotionally related?

PLAN/GOAL

9. What is your primary goal for Cody?
10. What needs have to be met for Cody to develop?

IMPLEMENTATION

11. What are the advantages of breast milk over formula?
12. What else happens other than nutritional intake when a mother is breastfeeding that is important to a child's development?
13. What else could Paula have done if she didn't have time to breastfeed but wanted Cody to get her breast milk?
14. What needs to be done after bottle feeding?
15. What criteria can Paula use to evaluate whether Cody is getting enough kcal and nutrients?

EVALUATION/OUTCOME CRITERIA

16. After Paula had been back at work about 1 month, what criteria could she use to assure that Cody was happy and developing on time?

Chapter 13

Diet During Childhood and Adolescence

Key Terms

acne

adolescence

alcoholism

amenorrhea

anorexia nervosa

anxiety

bulimia

cirrhosis

dental caries

depression

fast foods

fermentation

glycogen loading (carboloading)

peer group

self-esteem

Objectives

After studying this chapter, you should be able to:

● Identify nutritional needs of children aged 1 to 12 and of adolescents

● State the effects of inadequate nutrition during the growing years

● Describe eating disorders that can occur during adolescence

● Evaluate the nutritive value of the fast-food products available in the United States today

CHILDREN AGED ONE TO TWELVE

Although specific nutritional requirements change as children grow, nutrition always affects physical, mental, and emotional growth and development. Studies indicate that the mental ability and size of an individual are directly influenced by nutrition during the early years. Children who have an inadequate supply of nutrients—especially of protein—and kcal during their early years may be shorter and less intellectually able than children who receive an adequate diet.

Eating habits develop during childhood. Once developed, poor eating habits will be difficult to change. They can exacerbate emotional and physical problems such as irritability, depression, anxiety, fatigue, and illness.

Because children learn partly by imitation, learning good eating habits is easier if the parents have good habits and are calm and relaxed about the child's. Nutritious foods should be available at snack time as well as at mealtime (Figure 13-1), and meals should include a wide variety of foods to ensure good nutrient intake.

Parents should be aware that it is not uncommon for children's appetites to vary. The rate of growth is not constant. As the child ages, the rate of growth actually slows. The approximate weight gain of a child during the second year of life is only 5 pounds. In addition, children's attention is increasingly focused on their environment rather than their stomachs. Consequently, their appetites and interest in food commonly decrease during the early years. Children between the ages of 1 and 3 undergo vast changes. Their legs grow longer; they develop muscles; they lose their baby shape; they begin to walk and talk; and they learn to feed and generally assert themselves (Figure 13-2). A 2-year-old child's statement "No!" is his or her way of saying "Let me decide!"

As children continue to grow and develop, they will increasingly and healthfully assert themselves. They want and need to show their growing independence. Parents should respect this need as much as possible. Children's likes and dislikes may change. New foods should be introduced gradually, in small amounts, and as attractively as possible. Allowing the child to assist in purchasing and preparing a new food is often a good way of arousing interest in the food and a desire to eat it.

Children should be offered nutrient-dense foods because the amount eaten will be small. Fats should not be limited before the age of 2 years, but meals and snacks should not be fat-laden either. Whole

depression
an indentation; or feelings of extreme sadness

anxiety
apprehension

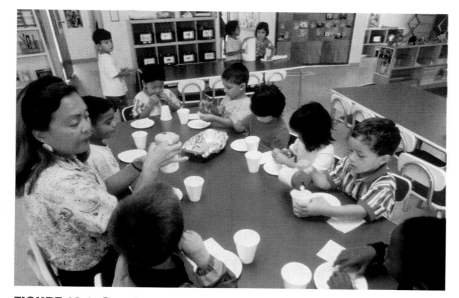

FIGURE 13-1 Snacks are enjoyed with friends in the playroom.

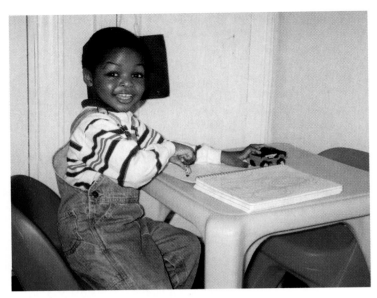

FIGURE 13-2 A healthy three-year-old at play

milk is recommended until the age of 2, but lowfat or fat-free should be served from 2 on. The guideline for fat intake after the age of 2 is 30% or less of total kcal per day with no more than 10% from saturated fats. It is recommended that children not salt their food at the table or have foods prepared with a lot of salt.

Children are especially sensitive to and reject hot (temperature) foods, but they like crisp textures, mild flavors, and familiar foods. They are wary of foods covered by sauce or gravy. Parents should set realistic goals and expectations as to the amount of food a child needs. A good rule of thumb for preschool children is one tablespoon for each year of age. Table 13-1 details serving sizes according to age. Calorie needs will depend on rate of growth, activity level, body size, metabolism, and health.

TABLE 13-1 Food plan for preschool and school-age children based on the Food Guide Pyramid

FOOD GROUP	NO. OF SERVINGS	AGE 1–2	APPROXIMATE SERVING SIZE* AGE 3–4	AGE 5–6	AGE 7–12
Milk, yogurt, and cheese:	3	½–¾ cup or 1 oz	¾ cup or 1½ oz	1 cup or 2 oz	1 cup or 2 oz
Meat, poultry, fish, dry beans, eggs, and nuts:	2 or more	1 oz or 1–2 tbsp	1½ oz or 3–4 tbsp	1½ oz or ½ cup	2 oz or ½ cup
Vegetables:	3 or more	1–2 tbsp	3–4 tbsp	½ cup	½ cup
Fruits:	2 or more	1–2 tbsp or ½ cup juice	3–4 tbsp or ½ cup juice	½ cup or ½ cup juice	½ cup or ½ cup juice
Bread, cereal, rice, and pasta:	6 or more	½ slice or ½ cup	1 slice or ½ cup	1 slice or ¾ cup	1 cup or ¾ cup

Adapted from Food and Nutrition Service, US Department of Agriculture: *Meal pattern requirements and offer versus serve manual,* FNS-265, 1990.

*Use as a starting point. Increase serving size as energy yields dictate, but maintain variety in the diet by making sure all food groups are still appropriately represented.

Children can have food jags, such as eating only one or two foods, or rituals, such as not letting foods touch on the plate, or using a different spoon for each food eaten. Choking is prevalent in young children. To prevent choking, do not give children under 4 years of age peanuts, grapes, hot dogs, raw carrots, hard candy, or thick peanut butter.

A child needs a snack every 3 to 4 hours for continued energy. Children often prefer finger foods for snacks. Snacks should be nutrient-dense and as nutritious as food served at mealtime. Cheese, saltines, fruit, milk, and unsweetened cereals make good snacks.

Mealtime should be pleasant, and food should not be forced on the child. *The parent's primary responsibility is to provide nutritious food in a pleasant setting, and the child's responsibility is to decide how much food to eat and whether to eat,* according to child expert Ellyn Satter. See Table 13-2 for a list of parental behaviors that will help to enhance children's eating. When a child is hungry, he or she will eat. Forcing a child to eat can cause disordered eating and, ultimately, chronic overeating, anorexia nervosa, or bulima (discussed later in this chapter).

anorexia nervosa
psychologically induced lack of appetite

bulimia
condition in which patient alternately binges and purges

TABLE 13-2 Feeding Children

WHAT PARENTS SHOULD DO:

- Choose and buy food
- Make and offer meals
- Have meals and snacks at regular times
- Don't give children food handouts
- Include children in family meals
- Make food easy to eat
- Make food safe
- Let children eat like children
- Let them eat as much as they want
- Make mealtimes pleasant
- Talk and smile, but don't be distracting
- Keep mealtimes calm
- Teach children to behave at meals

WHAT CHILDREN SHOULD DO:

- Decide whether or not to eat
- Decide how much to eat
- Grow the way nature intended

From *Ellyn Satter's Feeding with Love and Good Sense: Video and Teacher's Guide* by Ellyn Satter. Copyright © 1995 by Ellyn Satter. Reprinted with permission.

kcal and Nutrient Needs of Young Children

The *rate* of growth diminishes from the age of 1 until about 10, thus the kcal requirement per pound of body weight also diminishes during this period. For example, at 6 months, a girl needs about 54 kcal per pound of body weight, but by the age of 10, she will require only 35 kcal per pound of body weight.

Nutrient needs, however, do not diminish. From the age of 6 months to 10 years, nutrient needs actually *increase* because of the increase in body size. Therefore, it is especially important that young children are given nutritious foods *that they will eat.*

The Food Guide Pyramid is a good foundation for developing meal plans that, with adjustments, will suit all family members. A variety of foods should be offered, and, when possible, the child should be offered some choices of foods. Such a choice at the table helps the child's psychosocial development.

In general, the young child will need 2 to 3 cups of milk each day, or the equivalent in terms of calcium. However, excessive use of milk should be avoided because it can crowd out other, iron-rich foods and possibly cause iron-deficiency. The number of servings of the other food groups is the same for adults, but the sizes will be smaller. The use of sweets should be minimized because the child is apt to prefer them to nutrient-rich foods. Sweetened fruit juices, especially, should be avoided. Children also need water and fiber in their diets. They need to drink 1 ml of water for each kcal. If food valued at 1,200 kcal is eaten then five 8-ounce glasses of water are needed. Fiber needs are calculated according to age. After age 3, a child's fiber needs are "age + 5g" and no more than "age + 10g." A child who eats more fiber than that might be too full to eat enough other foods to provide all the kcal needed for growth and development. Fiber should be added slowly, if not already in the diet, and fluids must also be increased. Childhood is a good time to develop the lifelong good habit of getting enough dietary fiber to prevent constipation and diseases such as colon cancer and diverticulitis.

ADOLESCENCE

adolescent

person between the ages of 13 and 20

acne

pimples

Adolescence is a period of rapid growth that causes major changes. It tends to begin between the ages of 10 and 13 in girls and between 13 and 16 in boys. The growth rate may be 3 inches a year for girls and 4 inches for boys. Bones grow and gain density, muscle and fat tissue develop, and blood volume increases. Sexual maturity occurs. Boys' voices change; girls experience the onset of menses; and both may experience **acne**. Acne is not caused by specific foods but by overactivity of the sebaceous glands of the skin.

These changes are obvious and have a tremendous effect on an adolescent's psychosocial development. No two individuals will develop in the same way. One girl may become heavier than she might like; another may be thin; a boy may not develop the muscle or the height he desires; some may develop serious complexion problems. It can be a time of great joy, but it also can be a time when counseling is needed.

Adolescent Food Habits

Adolescents typically have enormous appetites. When good eating habits have been established during childhood and there is nutritious food available, the teenager's food habits should present no serious problem.

Adolescents are imitators, like children, but instead of imitating adults, adolescents prefer to imitate their peers and do what is popular. Unfortunately, the foods that are popular often have low nutrient density such as potato chips, sodas, and candy. These foods provide mainly carbohydrates and fats and very little protein, vitamins, and minerals, except for salt, which is usually provided in excess. Adolescents' eating habits can be seriously affected by busy schedules, part-time jobs, athletics, social activities, and the lack of an available adult to prepare nutritious food when adolescents are hungry or have time to eat (Figure 13-3).

When the adolescent's food habits need improvement, it is wise for the adult to tactfully inform her or him of nutritional needs and of the poor nutrition quality of the foods she or he is eating. The adolescent has a natural desire for independence and may resent being told what to do.

Before attempting to change an adolescent's food habits, carefully check her or his food choices for nutrient content. It is too easily assumed that because the adolescent chooses the food, the food is automatically a poor choice in regard to nutrient content. It might be a good choice. An adolescent who has a problem maintaining an appropriate weight may need some advice regarding diet.

peer group
group of people approximately one's own age

kcal and Nutrient Needs of Adolescents

Because of adolescents' rapid growth, kcal requirements naturally increase. Boys' kcal requirements tend to be greater than girls' because boys are generally bigger, tend to be more physically active, and have more lean muscle mass than do girls.

Except for vitamin D, nutrient needs increase dramatically at the onset of adolescence. Because of menstruation, girls have a greater need for iron than do boys. The RDA's for vitamin D, vitamin C, vitamin B$_{12}$, calcium, phosphorus, and iodine are the same for both sexes. the RDAs for the remaining nutrients are higher for boys than they are for girls.

ADOLESCENT PROBLEMS RELATED TO NUTRITION

Adolescence is a stressful time for most young people. They are unexpectedly faced with numerous physical changes; an innate need for independence; increased work and extra curricular demands at school; in many cases, jobs; and social and sexual pressures from their peers. For many teens, such stress can cause one or more of the following problems.

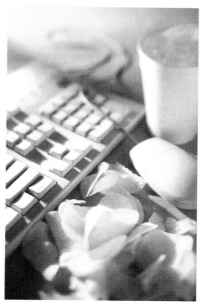

FIGURE 13-3 Due to their busy schedules and independence, adolescents may not always choose nutritious foods for snacks or meals.

Anorexia Nervosa

In general, adolescent boys in the United States are considered well nourished. Studies show, however, that girls sometimes have diets deficient in kcal and protein, iron, calcium, vitamin A, or some of the B vitamins.

These deficiencies can be due to poor eating habits caused by concern about weight. A moderate concern about weight is understandable, and possibly even beneficial, provided it does not cause diets to be deficient in essential nutrients or lead to a potentially fatal condition called anorexia nervosa.

Anorexia nervosa, commonly called *anorexia,* is a psychological disorder more common to women than men. It can begin as early as late childhood, but usually begins during the teen years or the early twenties. It causes the patient to so drastically reduce kcal that the reduction disrupts metabolism and causes hair loss, low blood pressure, weakness, **amenorrhea**, brain damage, and even death.

amenorrhea

the stoppage of the monthly menstrual flow

The causes of anorexia are unclear. Someone with this disorder (an anorexic) has an inordinate fear of being fat. Some anorexics have been overweight and have irrational fears of regaining lost weight. Some young women with demanding parents perceive this as their only means of control. Some may want to resemble slim fashion models. Some fear growing up. Many are perfectionistic overachievers who want to control their body. It pleases them to deny themselves food when they are hungry.

These young women usually set a maximum weight for themselves and become expert at "counting calories" to maintain their chosen weight. If the weight declines too far, the anorexic will ultimately die.

Treatment requires:

1. Development of a strong and trusting relationship between the patient and the health care professional involved in the case;
2. That the patient learn and accept that weight gain and a change in body contours are normal during adolescence;
3. Diet therapy so the patient will understand the need for both nutrients and kcal and how best to obtain them;
4. Individual and family counseling so the problem is understood by everyone;
5. Close supervision by the health care professional; and
6. Time and patience from all involved.

Bulimia

Bulimia is a syndrome in which the patient alternately binges and purges by inducing vomiting and using laxatives and diuretics to get rid of ingested food. Bulimics are said to fear that they cannot stop eating. They tend to be high achievers who are perfectionistic, obsessive, and depressed. They generally lack a strong sense of self and have a need to seem special. They know their binge-purge syndrome is abnormal but also fear being overweight. This condition is more common among women than men and can begin any time from the late teens into the thirties.

A bulimic usually binges on high-kcal foods such as cookies, ice cream, pastries, and other "forbidden" foods. The binge can take only a few moments or can run several hours—until there is no space for more food. It occurs when the person is alone. Bulimia can follow a period of excessive dieting, and stress usually increases the frequency of binges.

Bulimia is not usually life-threatening, but it can irritate the esophagus and cause electrolyte imbalances, malnutrition, dehydration, and dental caries.

Treatment usually includes limiting eating to mealtimes and close supervision after meals to prevent self-induced vomiting. Diet therapy helps teach the patient basic nutritional facts so that he or she will be more inclined to treat the body with respect. Psychological counseling will help the patient to understand his or her fears about food. Group therapy also can be helpful.

Both bulimia and anorexia can be problems that will have to be confronted throughout the patient's life.

Overweight

Overweight during adolescence is particularly unfortunate because it is apt to diminish the individual's self-esteem and, consequently, can exclude her or him from the normal social life of the teen years, further diminishing self-esteem. Also, it tends to make the individual prone to overweight as an adult.

self-esteem
feelings of self-worth

Although numerous studies have been done, the cause of overweight is difficult to determine. Heredity is believed to play a role. Just as one inherits height, color of hair, or artistic talents, it appears that one may inherit the tendency (or lack of it) to overweight. Overfeeding during infancy and childhood also can be a contributing factor. Then, once a person is overweight, the overweight itself contributes further to the problem.

For example, if a teenager becomes the center of his classmates' jokes, he or she may prefer to spend time alone, perhaps watching television, and finding comfort in food. This behavior adds more kcal, reduces activity, and, thus, worsens the condition.

The problem of overweight during adolescence is especially difficult to solve until the individual involved makes the independent decision to lose weight. After making such a decision, the teenager should see a physician to ensure that his or her health is good, to work out the amount of weight that should be lost, the time required for such a loss, and daily kcal requirements.

After a physician's examination, the individual will be helped by discussing the plan with a registered dietitian. Meals should be planned carefully to include the necessary nutrients, but avoid exceeding the kcal allotment. In general, a plan developed using the Food Guide Pyramid is the easiest for the dieting teen to understand and follow. It is essential that the nutrient and kcal content of fast foods be understood by the teen and these foods plus other snacks can be built into the weight-loss plan. Exercise should also be included in any overweight adolescent's weight-loss plan. This helps burn calories and may also inspire the young person to meet new people and to try new activities, such as dancing, baseball, or aerobics.

TABLE 13-3 Nutrient and kcal Contents of Some Fast Foods Compared with RDAs for 16-Year-Old Female

	WEIGHT (oz)	KCAL	PROTEIN (g)	FAT (g)	CALCIUM (mg)	IRON (mg)	SODIUM (mg)	VITAMIN A (RE)	THIAMIN (mg)	RIBOFLAVIN (mg)	NIACIN (mg)	VITAMIN C (mg)
Hamburger	3½	250	12	11	56	2.2	463	14	0.23	0.24	3.8	1
French fries	2	160	2	8	10	0.4	108	0	0.09	0.01	1.6	5
Chocolate milk shake	10	335	9	8	374	0.9	314	59	0.13	0.63	0.4	0
Pizza	4	300	15	9	220	1.6	700	106	0.34	0.29	4.2	2
Soda	12	160	0	0	11	0.2	18	0	0	0	0	0
Doughnut	2	210	3	12	22	1.0	192	5	0.12	0.12	1.1	0
Potato chips	2	315	3	21	15	0.6	300	0	0.09	0	2.4	24
Chocolate bar with peanuts	1½	225	6	16	75	0.6	30	12	1.0	1.0	2.1	0
RDAs for 16-year-old girl		2,200	44	73	1,200	15	500	800	1.1	1.3	15	60

Fast Foods

Many Americans have become extremely fond of "**fast foods**." Many others are highly critical of their nutrient content. Examples of these foods—most of which are favorites of teenagers—include hamburgers, cheeseburgers, milkshakes, pizza, sodas, hot chocolate, tacos, chili, fried chicken, and onion rings. Because of the criticism they have received, some fast-food companies have run tests to determine the nutrient content of their products. These results are usually available in the fast-food restaurant.

Generally speaking, fast foods are excessively high in fat and sodium, as well as kcal, and contain only limited amounts of vitamins and minerals (other than sodium) and little fiber. In Table 13-3, the nutrient content of some varieties of fast foods are shown compared with the RDA for a 16-year-old girl. This shows the potential for problems with a diet that regularly consists of these foods to the exclusion of others.

Nevertheless, these foods are more nutritious than sodas, cakes, and candy. When used with discretion in a balanced diet, they are not harmful.

Alcohol and the Adolescent

In a process called fermentation, sugars and starches can be changed to alcohol. Enzyme action causes this change. Alcohol is typically made from fruit, corn, rye, barley, rice, or potatoes. It provides 7 kcal per gram but almost no nutrients.

Alcohol is a drug that can have serious side effects. Initially, it causes the drinker to feel "happy" because it lowers inhibitions. This feeling affects the drinker's judgment and can lead to accidents and crime. Ultimately, alcohol is a depressant; continued drinking leads to sleepiness, loss of consciousness, and, when too much is consumed in a short period, death.

Abuse (overuse) of alcohol is called alcoholism. Alcoholism can destroy lives and families and devastate the drinker's nutritional status and thus health. It affects absorption and normal metabolism of glucose, fats, proteins, and vitamins. When thiamin and niacin cannot be absorbed, the cells cannot use glucose for energy. Blood cells, which depend on glucose for energy, are particularly affected. Accumulation of fat in the liver can lead to cirrhosis of the liver if the alcohol abuse continues. Alcohol causes kidneys to excrete larger than normal amounts of water, resulting in an increased loss of minerals. In a poor nutritional state, the body is less able to fight off disease.

In addition, excessive, long-term drinking can cause high blood pressure and can damage the heart muscle. It is associated with cancer of the throat and the esophagus and can damage the reproductive system.

The risks to the drinker are obvious. When a pregnant or lactating woman drinks, however, she puts the fetus or the nursing infant at risk as well. Alcohol can lower birthweight and cause fetal alcohol syndrome (see Chapter 11).

Unfortunately, many teenagers ignore the dangers of alcohol and use it in an effort to appear adult. In addition to the damage to their own health and the accidents and the random acts of violence caused

fast foods
restaurant food that is ready to serve before orders are taken

fermentation
changing of sugars and starches to alcohol

alcoholism
chronic and excessive use of alcohol

cirrhosis
generic term for liver disease characterized by cell loss

by their drinking, their behavior inspires younger children to emulate them. The health professional is in a good position to spread the message that alcohol is a drug and can cause severe economic and family problems, as well as addiction, disease, and death.

Marijuana

Marijuana use continues to increase among teenagers. Marijuana makes one hungry, especially for sweets. One marijuana cigarette is as harmful as four or five tobacco cigarettes because the marijuana smoke is held in the lungs for a longer period of time. As marijuana is smoked, the lungs absorb the primary active ingredient, delta-9-tetrahydro-cannabinol (THC), and this fat-soluble substance is transported via lipoproteins to various body tissues for storage (Indiana Prevention Resource Center, 1992). Experts believe that the use of marijuana can lead to the use of other drugs such as cocaine. Common street names for marijuana include grass, weed, pot, and dope.

Cocaine

Cocaine is highly addictive and extremely harmful. It causes restlessness, heightened self-confidence, euphoria, irritability, insomnia, depression, confusion, hallucinations, loss of appetite, and a tendency to withdraw from normal activities. Cocaine can cause cardiac irregularities, heart attacks, and cardiac arrests resulting in death. Weight loss is very common; addicts would give up food for the drug. The smokable form of cocaine is *crack,* which is more addictive than any other drug. It is estimated that half of all crimes against property committed in major cities are related to the use of crack cocaine and the addict's need for money to buy the drug.

Tobacco

Cigarette smoking is addictive. Cigarette smoking by teenagers is very prevalent. Teenagers smoke to "be cool," to look older, or because of peer pressure. Smoking can influence appetite, nutrition status, and weight. Smokers need two times the RDA for vitamin C because smoking alters the metabolism. Low intakes of vitamin C, vitamin A, beta-carotene, folate, and fiber are common in smokers. Smoking increases the risk of lung cancer and heart disease.

Other Addictive Drugs

Methamphetamine is the most potent form of amphetamine. Amphetamines cause heart, breathing, and blood pressure rates to increase. The mouth is usually dry, and swallowing is difficult. Urination is also difficult. Appetite is depressed. The users' pupils are dilated, and reflexes speed up. As the drug wears off, feelings of fatigue or depression are experienced. Street names include crank, speed, crystal, meth, zip, and ice.

Inhalants are chemicals whose fumes are inhaled into the body and produce mind-altering effects. Some inhalants are gasoline, lighter fluid, tool-cleaning solvents, model airplane glue, typewriter correction fluid, and permanent ink in felt-tip pens. Inhalants are both physically and psychologically addictive. Individuals who inhale may risk depression and apathy, nosebleeds, headaches, eye pain, chronic fatigue, heart failure, loss of muscle control, and death.

Dental Caries

Dental Caries are promoted by the use of sugar in the diet. Sugar aids the development of certain harmful bacteria in the mouth that produce acids that can erode tooth enamel.

Dental caries can be prevented by avoiding sticky sugar foods unless the teeth can be brushed or the mouth can be rinsed immediately after eating them.

When fluoride is added to the drinking water, the number of dental caries is reduced. Fluoride toothpaste also is believed to be helpful. Fluoride is a normal component of bones and teeth but must not be used in excessive amounts, because it can be toxic and can affect bone and soft tissues.

dental caries
decayed areas on teeth; cavities

Nutrition for the Athlete

Good nutrition during the period of life when one is involved in athletics can prevent unnecessary wear and tear on the body as well as maintain the athlete in top physical form. The specific nutritional needs of the athlete are not numerous, but they are important. The athlete needs additional water, kcal, thiamin, riboflavin, niacin, sodium, potassium, iron, and protein.

The body uses water to rid itself of excess heat through perspiration. This lost water must be regularly replaced during the activity to prevent dehydration (Figure 13-4). Plain water is the recommended liquid because it rehydrates the body more quickly than sweetened liquids or the drinks that contain electrolytes. The "electrolyte" drinks are useful to replenish fluids after an athletic event but not during one. Salt tablets are not recommended because, despite the loss of salt and potassium through perspiration, the loss is not equal to the amount contained in the tablets. If there is an insufficient water intake, these salt tablets can increase the risk of dehydration.

The increase in kcal depends on the activity and the length of time it is performed. The requirement could be double the normal, up to 6,000 kcal per day. Because glucose and fatty acids, not protein, are used for energy, the normal diet proportions of 50 to 55% carbohydrate, 30% fat, and 10 to 15% protein are advised.

There is an increased need for B vitamins because they are necessary for energy metabolism. They are provided in the breads, cereals, fruits, and vegetables needed to bring the kcal count to the total required. Some extra protein is used during training, when muscle mass and blood volume are increasing. This amount is included in the RDA for age and is provided in the normal diet. Protein needs are not increased by physical activity. In fact, excess protein can cause increased urine production, which can lead to dehydration.

The minerals sodium and potassium are needed in larger amounts because of loss through perspiration. This amount of sodium can usually be replaced just by salting food to taste, and orange juice or bananas can provide the extra potassium.

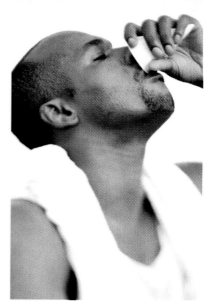

FIGURE 13-4 All athletes must take time out to rest and replace lost fluids.

A sufficient supply of iron is important to the athlete, particularly to the female athlete. Iron-rich foods eaten with vitamin C–rich foods should provide sufficient iron. The onset of menstruation can be delayed by the heavy physical activity of the young female athlete, and amenorrhea may occur in those already menstruating.

When weight is a concern of the athlete, such as with wrestlers, care should be taken that the individual does not become dehydrated by refusing liquids in an effort to "make weight" for the class.

When weight must be added, the athlete will need an additional 2,500 kcal to develop 1 pound of muscle mass. The additional foods eaten to reach this amount of kcal should contain the normal proportion of nutrients. A high-fat diet should be avoided because it increases the potential for heart disease. Athletes should reduce kcal when training ends. Unused muscle will be converted to fat.

In general, the athlete should select foods using the Food Guide Pyramid. The pregame meal should be eaten 3 hours before the event and should consist primarily of carbohydrates and small amounts of protein and fat. Concentrated sugar foods are not advisable because they may cause extra water to collect in the intestines, creating gas and possibly diarrhea.

Glycogen loading (carboloading) is sometimes used for long activities. To increase muscle stores of glycogen, the athlete begins 6 days before the events. For 3 days, the athlete eats a diet consisting of only 10% carbohydrate and mostly protein and fat as she or he performs heavy exercise. This depletes the current store of glycogen. The next 3 days, the diet is 70% carbohydrate, and the exercise is very light so that the muscles become loaded with glycogen. This practice may cause an abnormal heartbeat and some weight gain.

Currently, it is recommended that the athlete exercise heavily and eat carbohydrates as desired. Then, during the week before the competition, exercise should be reduced. On the day before competition, the athlete should eat a high-carbohydrate diet and rest.

After the event, the athlete may prefer to drink fruit juices until relaxed and then satisfy the appetite with sandwiches or a full meal.

There are no magic potions or diet supplements that will increase an athlete's prowess, as may be touted by health food faddists. *Steroid* drugs should not be used to build muscles (Figure 13-5). They can affect the fat content of the blood, damage the liver, change the reproductive system, and even the facial appearance. Good diet, good health habits, and practice combined with innate talent remain the essentials for athletic success.

glycogen loading

process in which the muscle store of glycogen is maximized; also called carboloading

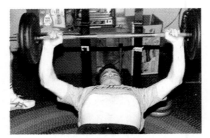

FIGURE 13-5 Building muscles requires using *them*—NOT steroid drugs. (Courtesy of Delmar Publishers, Albany, NY)

CONSIDERATIONS FOR THE HEALTH CARE PROFESSIONAL

The health care professional who works with young children will be challenged by the poor appetites of her or his patients. Compounding this problem will be the anxiety of the patients' parents. They will understandably be concerned about their children's appetites and physical conditions. The health care professional can be most helpful to all concerned by exhibiting patience and understanding and by listening to parents and patient.

The problems of adolescent patients, perhaps particularly those with disordered eating, can be especially vexing. For example, telling an anorexic patient to eat could be counterproductive. Health care professionals working with such patients should consult with the patient's psychological counselor. Parents of patients with disordered eating must be included in both nutritional and family counseling.

● SUMMARY

Children's nutritional needs vary as they grow and develop. The rate of growth slows between the ages of 1 and 10, and the child's kcal requirement per pound of body weight slows accordingly. However, nutrient needs gradually increase during these years. During adolescence, growth is rapid, and nutritional and kcal requirements increase substantially. Anorexia nervosa, bulimia, and obesity are problems of weight control that can occur during adolescence. Fast foods are acceptable when used with discretion in a balanced diet. Alcohol can be a serious problem for adolescents, and it is essential that adolescents understand its potential dangers. The nutritional needs of athletes are similar to those of nonathletes except for increased needs for kcal, B vitamins, sodium, potassium, and iron.

● DISCUSSION TOPICS

1. Discuss how parents' anxieties about children's food habits may affect those habits.
2. In what ways does overweight affect an adolescent's self-esteem?
3. Why can it be especially difficult for a parent to influence her or his adolescent's attitudes about food?
4. Discuss the nutrient content of some fast foods. Explain why they can be useful additions to the diet and also why they should not be used exclusively.
5. What could result if a 30-year-old lawyer continued to eat as he did as a 17-year-old football player?
6. Describe anorexia nervosa. Ask if anyone in the class has suffered from it or knows of anyone who has. Ask that individual for descriptions of the patient's attitude, physical condition, possible causes, and case results.
7. Discuss how snack foods can affect one's overall nutrition. Why should they be included in an adolescent's weight-loss plan?
8. Describe a "typical" bulimic patient. What role does stress often play in bulimia? Why do bulimics often binge on cakes, cookies, and ice cream? How does bulimia upset one's electrolyte balance? How does it irritate the esophagus? How can it cause dental carries? What could happen in uncontrolled bulimia?

● SUGGESTED ACTIVITIES

1. List your favorite snack foods. List nutritious snack foods. Check kcal values of these foods (see Table A-4 in the appendix) and compare lists for nutrition and taste. Discuss possible improvements in your list of favorite snacks.

2. Plan a talk for fourth-grade students on the importance of good food habits. Begin with an outline, and develop it into a narrative that 9-year-old children will understand. If possible, ask permission of a fourth-grade teacher to deliver this talk to the class.

3. Role-play a situation in which your younger sister, who is considerably overweight, has just asked you how she can lose weight. Ask her why she wants to lose weight; how much weight she wants to lose; if she is willing to change her eating habits for the rest of her life; what her favorite foods are; when she eats; the amounts she eats; where she eats; and with whom she eats.

4. Invite a registered dietitian to talk to the class on any or all of the following: glycogen loading; fast foods; anorexia nervosa; bulimia; overweight in adolescence.

5. Invite a psychiatrist who specializes in adolescent eating disorders to speak to the class.

6. Hold a panel discussion on alcohol and drugs. Assign the following topics to individual class members. They should prepare themselves by doing outside research before the panel discussion.

   What is alcohol?
   What are some commonly abused drugs?
   Why do people use alcohol or drugs?
   How do alcohol and drugs affect the human body?
   How can alcohol and drug abuse affect one's nutritional status?
   What are the dangers of drinking or using drugs during pregnancy?

● REVIEW

Multiple choice. Select the *letter* that precedes the best answer.

1. Anorexia nervosa
   a. is characterized by binges and purges
   b. causes severe acne
   c. is a psychological disorder
   d. typically causes overweight

2. A child's eating habits
   a. can reflect his or her desire to assert self
   b. seldom change after the child reaches the age of 1 year
   c. usually improve when parents force the child to try new foods
   d. have no relation to the child's growth rate

3. Children's appetites
   a. vary
   b. are static
   c. are irrelevant to their nutritional status
   d. are entirely dependent on the size of the child

4. Of the following foods, children are most apt to prefer
   a. carrot-zucchini casserole
   b. creamed carrots with peas
   c. raw carrot sticks
   d. carrot and pineapple gelatin salad

5. A psychological disorder that causes people to drastically and chronically reduce kcal content of their food is called
   a. bulimia   c. anorexia nervosa
   b. amenorrhea   d. metabolic psychosis

6. Children's iron requirement is high because it is needed for
   a. healthy bones and teeth   c. prevention of night blindness
   b. fighting infections   d. blood building

7. As a child grows, his or her kcal requirement per pound of body weight
   a. remains unchanged   c. becomes less
   b. increases   d. doubles each year

8. Meatloaf is a good source of
   a. protein   c. calcium
   b. vitamin C   d. all of the above and more

9. Low nutrient dense foods provide
   a. carbohydrate and fat
   b. proteins, minerals, and vitamins
   c. no calories
   d. fiber

10. Although adolescent boys usually need more kcal than adolescent girls, the girls usually need more
   a. protein   c. iron
   b. vitamin C   d. vitamin D

C A S E   S T U D Y

Tanya L. was a dark-haired, exotic-looking, 19-year-old champion ice skater. She dreamed of going to the next Olympics. Tanya had been skating since she was 6 years old. She spent 4 or 5 hours a day practicing, perfecting her technique. She watched videos of herself doing spins and jumps to perfect her required elements. Tanya had always been slim as a child and teenager. Recently, between weight lifting and late-adolescent changes, Tanya had become obsessed about her weight. She thought she was getting fat. She reasoned that if she lost some weight her jumps would be easier.

At first, she cut out snacks and sodas after practice. Then she started counting the calories of everything she ate. That led to cutting her total by 25%. She lost 5 pounds, but that wasn't enough. She noticed cellulite on her upper thighs, so she added leg lifts to her practice sessions and further reduced her intake.

Tanya's mother noticed some changes in Tanya. She began having difficulty getting up in the morning. Her hair looked dull, and there were clumps of it in the bathroom sink. One day, Tanya's mother noticed her reading food labels and muttering about calories.

Two weeks later, Tanya's skating coach called her mother from the ice rink. Tanya had taken a bad fall, and they thought she should go to the hospital. In the emergency room, they checked Tanya's blood pressure and found it very low. Tanya said she couldn't understand why she got so dizzy and felt so weak. When they weighed her, she had lost 15 pounds. The doctor talked to Tanya about being an athlete and dieting. He also talked to Tanya's mother about anorexia and recommended a treatment plan.

ASSESSMENT

1. What data do you have about Tanya?
2. Why was Tanya at risk for anorexia?
3. Why did the doctor suspect anorexia?
4. How significant is this problem?

DIAGNOSIS

5. What are the detrimental effects of decreasing kcal below needs?
6. What signs of anorexia does Tanya exhibit?

PLAN/GOAL

7. What is Tanya's desired goal?
8. What will the doctor's goal be for Tanya?

IMPLEMENTATION

The doctor recommended a visit to his office once a week after practice so that Tanya could weigh in and visit with the psychiatric nurse practitioner.

9. What could Tanya be taught regarding her diet plan?
10. What could her family be taught to help her?
11. How might the weekly visits to her doctor's office help?
12. How can the NP help?
13. How long should Tanya be monitored?

EVALUATION/OUTCOME CRITERIA

14. What criteria will have been met when the NP recommends stopping the weekly visits?
15. Can anorexia be cured?
16. Could Tanya relapse?

C A S E   S T U D Y

Daneta was an attractive 17-year-old black girl with beautiful, shiny hair. She was 5 feet 7 inches tall and weighed 135 pounds. She was a very good student but didn't have a lot of friends, except for her boyfriend, Jamall. She was really upset when her boyfriend broke up with her. She thought it was because she was too fat. One day on a city bus, she overheard a tall, slim, pretty young woman tell her friend that she regularly forced herself to vomit after eating a large dinner. She said it helped her control her weight.

Daneta decided this would be her secret to getting slim and getting her boyfriend back. She began her new "routine" that evening.

Soon, she was using laxatives and borrowing her grandmother's diuretics. When she was really hungry, she'd buy two boxes of her favorite cookies and a pint of ice cream and eat them all in an hour. Then she'd force herself to vomit.

Within 2 months, her weight dropped to 115 pounds. She had thought she would be happy, but she was too tired to care. She thought her boyfriend would come running back to her, but he hadn't even noticed. Her girlfriend noticed that her hair was limp and dull. Her mother noticed her weight loss and caught her gagging herself one night.

ASSESSMENT

1. What information do you have about Daneta?

2. Calculate Daneta's ideal weight according to Table 16-2.

3. What did Daneta's mother suspect when she observed Daneta gagging herself?

4. What are the psychological needs of a teen who suffers from bulimia?

DIAGNOSIS

5. Complete this statement: Daneta's decreased intake of kcal less than requirements is secondary to _____.

6. What signs of bulimia does Daneta exhibit?

PLAN/GOAL

7. What is the major nutrition goal for Daneta?

8. What is the priority for Daneta's coping skills?

IMPLEMENTATION

9. What should Daneta and her mother be taught about good nutrition?

10. What needs to be taught about bulimia? Who else needs this information besides her mother?

11. How can a counselor help Daneta? How long does she require counseling?

12. How can her teachers help Daneta?

13. What can be done to prevent or decrease the recurrence of bulimia?

EVALUATION/OUTCOME CRITERIA

14. What criteria would her mother use to demonstrate that her bulimia was under control?

15. Can bulimia be cured?

Chapter
14

Diet During Young and Middle Adulthood

Key Terms

energy imbalance
hypertension
kcal value
kcal requirement
lean muscle mass
nutrient requirement
obesity

Objectives

After studying this chapter, you should be able to:

● Identify the nutritional needs of young adults and the middle-aged

● Explain sensible, long-range weight control for these people

● Adapt menus to meet their nutritional and kcal requirements

Adulthood can be broadly divided into three periods: young, middle, and late adulthood. The first two periods will be discussed in this chapter. Late adulthood is discussed in Chapter 15.

Young adulthood is a time of excitement and exploration. The age range runs from about 18 to 40 years of age. Individuals are alive with plans, desires, and energy as they begin searching for and finding their places in the mainstream of adult life. They appear to have boundless energy for both social and professional activities. They are usually interested in exercise for its own sake and often participate in athletic events as well.

The middle period ranges from about 40 to 65 years of age. This is a time when the physical activities of young adulthood typically begin to decrease, resulting in lowered kcal requirement for most individuals. During these years, people seldom have young children to supervise, and the strenuous physical labor of some occupations may be delegated to younger people. Middle-aged people may tire more easily than they did when they were younger. Therefore, they may not get as much exercise as they did in earlier years. Because appetite and food intake may not decrease, there is a common tendency toward weight gain during this period.

NUTRIENT REQUIREMENTS

Growth is usually complete by the age of 25. Consequently, except during pregnancy and lactation, the essential nutrients are needed only to maintain and repair body tissue and to produce energy. During these years, the **nutrient requirements** of healthy adults change very little. (See the Recommended Dietary Allowances on the inside front cover.)

Despite men's generally larger size, only 11 of the given RDAs are greater for men than for women. Six of the RDAs are the same for both sexes. The iron requirement for women throughout the childbearing years remains higher than that for men. Extra iron is needed to replace blood loss during menstruation and to help build both the infant's and the extra maternal blood needed during pregnancy. After menopause, this requirement for women matches that of men.

Protein needs for adults are thought to be 0.8g per kilogram of body weight. To determine the specific amount, one must divide the weight in pounds by 2.2 to obtain the weight in kilograms and then multiply the weight in kilograms by 0.8.

The current requirement for calcium for adults from 19 to 50 is 1,000 mg, and for vitamin D, 5 mg. Both calcium and vitamin D are essential for strong bones, and both are found in milk. Bone loss begins slowly, at about the age of 35 to 40, and can lead to osteoporosis later. Therefore, it is wise for young people, especially women, who are more prone to osteoporosis than men, to consume foods that provide more than the requirements for these two nutrients. Three glasses of milk a day fulfill the requirement for each of these nutrients. Increasing this amount could prevent osteoporosis. Fat-free milk or foods made from fat-free milk should be used to limit the amount of fat consumed.

nutrient requirement
amount of specific nutrient needed by the body

KCAL REQUIREMENTS

The **kcal requirement** begins to diminish after the age of 25, as basal metabolism rates (REE) are reduced by approximately 2 to 3% a decade (Table 14-1). This is a small amount each year, but, after 25 years, a person will gain weight if the total **kcal value** of the food eaten is not reduced accordingly. An individual's actual need, of course, will be determined primarily by activity and amount of **lean muscle mass**. Those who are more active will require more kcal than those with a high proportion of fat tissue.

kcal requirement
number of kcal required daily to meet energy needs

kcal value
number of kcal in a specific amount of specific food or beverage

lean muscle mass
percentage of muscle tissue

TABLE 14-1 Median Weights and Heights and Recommended Daily Energy Intake for Adults

CATEGORY	AGE (years) OR CONDITION	WEIGHT (kg)	WEIGHT (lb)	HEIGHT (cm)	HEIGHT (in)	REE (kcal/day)	AVERAGE ENERGY ALLOWANCE (KCAL) Multiples of REE	AVERAGE ENERGY ALLOWANCE (KCAL) per kg	AVERAGE ENERGY ALLOWANCE (KCAL) per day
Males	19–24	72	160	177	70	1,780	1.67	40	2,900
	25–50	79	174	176	70	1,800	1.60	37	2,900
	51+	77	170	173	68	1,530	1.50	30	2,300
Females	19–24	58	128	164	65	1,350	1.60	38	2,200
	25–50	63	138	163	64	1,380	1.55	36	2,200
	51+	65	143	160	63	1,280	1.50	30	1,900

Reprinted with permission from Recommended Dietary Allowances: 10th Edition. Copyright © 1989 by the National Academy of Sciences. Courtesy of the National Academy Press, Washington, D.C.

NUTRITION-RELATED CONCERNS

Eating Habits

It is especially important to maintain good eating habits during young and middle adulthood. Women, who may be concerned about weight, cost of food, or time, can easily develop nutrient deficiencies. For example, a woman who settles for a piece of pie at lunchtime while her husband eats a hamburger and salad is being very foolish. If she continues to eat like this, she will jeopardize her health.

A hamburger can have 250 to 400 kcal. The salad will contain less than 50 kcal without dressing, and the dressing could be limited to one tablespoon, or approximately 100 kcal, for a total intake of about 400 to 550 kcal. Pies average 100 kcal per one-inch slice. Most slices are about 3½ inches. A scoop of ice cream on the pie would bring the total to at least another 100 kcal.

Although the kcal intakes of the husband and wife would be comparable, the nutrient intakes would differ. The wife's would be inadequate. If the woman is of childbearing age and plans to have children, she or her children could suffer from such habits.

In general, people today are concerned about nutrition and want to limit fats, cholesterol, sugar, salt, and kcal and increase fiber. Many know the sources of these items; others do not. Unfortunately, both groups tend to select their food because of convenience and flavor rather than nutritional content. It is easier to drive through a fast-food restaurant or heat a prepared frozen dinner in the microwave and complete the meal with ice cream than it is to shop for individual food items, cook them, and wash up after the meal. Consequently, many people ingest more fats, sugar, salt, and high-calorie foods and less fiber and other nutrients than they should.

WEIGHT CONTROL

Weight control is one of the top concerns of U.S. adults. Whether for reasons of vanity, health, or both, most people are interested in controlling their weight. It is advisable, because overweight can introduce health problems. Cases of diabetes mellitus and **hypertension** are more numerous among the overweight than among those of normal weight. Overweight individuals are poor risks for surgery, and their lives are generally shorter than are those of people who are not overweight. They are prone to social and emotional problems because **obesity** can reduce self-esteem.

The causes of overweight are not always known, but the most common cause appears to be **energy imbalance**. In other words, if one is overweight, chances are that more kcal have been taken in than were needed for energy.

An intake of 3,500 kcal more than the body needs for maintenance and activities will result in one extra pound. An individual who overeats by only 200 kcal a day can gain 20 pounds in one year. Obviously, when nutrient requirements remain static but kcal requirements decrease, people must select their foods carefully to fulfill their nutrient requirements. (See Table 14-2.) Genetics and a hypothyroid condition can also contribute to overweight.

hypertension

higher than normal blood pressure

obesity

excessive body fat, 20% above average

energy imbalance

eating either too much or too little for the amount of energy expended

TABLE 14-2 2,000-kcal Daily Menus

Breakfast		
½ cup orange juice	50 kcal	
1 cup dry cereal	100	
½ cup fat-free milk	43	
2 teaspoons sugar	35	
2 slices toast	150	
½ tablespoon margarine	50	
1 cup black coffee	0	428 kcal
	428	
Lunch		
Roast beef sandwich:		
3 oz roast beef	200	
2 slices toast	150	
1 tablespoon mayonnaise	100	
lettuce	10	
1 cup fat-free milk	85	
1 orange	75	620 kcal
	620	
Dinner		
2 oz broiled fish	150	
1 baked potato	100	
1½ tablespoon margarine	150	
½ cup green peas	50	
tossed salad with 1 Tbsp. dressing	150	
1 cup fat-free milk	86	
¾ cup ice cream	200	
1 oatmeal cookie	100	986 kcal
	986	2,034

Individuals who are overweight simply because of energy imbalance can solve the problem by eating less, and increasing physical exercise. Exercise will increase the number of kcal burned. However, unless the exercise is sufficient to burn more kcal than the ingested food contains, exercise alone will not solve the problem. By far the most effective method of weight loss is increased exercise combined with reduced kcal. This will help tone the muscles as the excess adipose tissue is lost.

When weight reduction is to be undertaken, the patient should confirm with his or her physician that he or she is in good health. Then, with the help of a registered dietitian, a healthy eating plan should be developed that will fit the dieter's lifestyle. A diet is easiest to follow when it is based on the Food Guide Pyramid. This plan will aid the dieter in obtaining needed nutrients, will help change previously unsatisfactory eating habits, and will allow him or her to adapt, and thus enjoy home, party, or restaurant meals. For additional information about weight-loss diets, see Chapter 16.

CONSIDERATIONS FOR THE HEALTH CARE PROFESSIONAL

The young and middle years of life are busy. Most people feel they have too many things to do and too little time to accomplish them. Most have families, jobs, and social obligations and, thus, more responsibilities.

When health problems occur during these years, people can be psychologically devastated. They worry about their children, bills, and jobs. Some patients this age will require psychological counseling; others will need the assistance of a social service agency; some will need both. Others will simply need reassurance that they will recover and that their lives will continue much as before their accident or illness.

The health care professional can do patients a great service by alerting her or his superiors to serious problems when they exist and, in simpler cases, by helping the patient see that there is a light at the end of the tunnel.

● SUMMARY

Although kcal requirements diminish after the age of 25, most nutrient requirements do not. Consequently, food must be selected with increasing care as one ages to ensure that nutrient requirements are met without exceeding the kcal requirement.

Overweight can cause health problems. If it is caused by energy imbalance, a program of weight loss should be undertaken. A sensible weight-loss program includes exercise. The diet should be based on the Food Guide Pyramid, and eating habits should be improved during the diet so that the lost weight will not be regained later.

● DISCUSSION TOPICS

1. Why do kcal requirements tend to diminish after the age of 25? Why do nutrient requirements not diminish at the same time?

2. How can only an extra 200 kcal a day result in overweight?

3. Why does a 40-year-old carpenter require more kcal than a 40-year-old architect?

4. How would you advise your 30-year-old sister, who boasts about eating only an English muffin and coffee at lunch?

5. Why is overweight inadvisable?

6. Why are middle-aged adults more inclined to overweight than young adults?

7. Why is 35-year-old Vera putting on weight even though she doesn't eat any more than she did as a 17-year-old cheerleader?

● SUGGESTED ACTIVITIES

1. Keep a food diary for a day and check off each food under the Food Guide Pyramid headings, as shown in the form below.

	FAT/ SWEET	DAIRY	MEATS	VEG.	FRUIT	BREAD/ CEREAL
Recommended no. of servings/day	Use sparingly	2–3	2–3	3–5	2–4	6–11
Breakfast						
Lunch						
Dinner						
Total						

    a. Total the entries in the vertical columns. Which columns have the highest totals?

    b. Discuss the shortages or excesses and the possible dangers of each

    c. Discuss realistic ways of improving your diet

    d. Repeat this exercise in a week. Evaluate for improvements.

● REVIEW

Multiple choice. Select the *letter* that precedes the best answer.

1. The number of kcal one needs each day is called one's
   a. nutrient requirement
   b. kcal intake
   c. kcal requirement
   d. nutritional requirement

2. Overweight during middle age is often due to
   a. obesity
   b. hypertension
   c. adipose tissue
   d. energy imbalance

3. The measure of energy in foods eaten is one's
   a. kcal requirement
   b. kcal intake
   c. nutrient requirement
   d. energy imbalance

4. Because of menstruation and pregnancy during the young and middle years, women have a greater need than men for
   a. proteins
   b. B vitamins
   c. iodine
   d. iron

5. kcal requirements
   a. increase with age
   b. decrease with age
   c. remain unchanged throughout adult life
   d. none of the above

6. To lose one pound of weight, one must reduce kcal intake by
   a. 1,000 kcal
   b. 800 kcal
   c. 3,500 kcal
   d. none of the above

7. Daily protein needs of adults are thought to be
   a. .5g per kilogram of body weight
   b. .8g per kilogram of body weight
   c. 10g per kilogram of body weight
   d. 8mg per day regardless of body weight

8. Exercise
   a. is more important to men than to women
   b. has no effect on muscles after the age of 40
   c. eliminates the need for postmenopausal women to drink milk
   d. helps to burn kcal as it tones the muscles

9. Nutrient requirements during adult life generally
   a. increase with age
   b. decrease with age
   c. remain unchanged
   d. none of the above

10. Women's kcal requirements as compared with men's are generally
    a. higher
    b. lower
    c. the same as
    d. none of the above

C A S E   S T U D Y

Ravi was a 40-year-old man from India who felt that he had finally succeeded in business. He had been working 10–12 hour days, 6 days a week for the past 12 years. His chain of dry-cleaning stores was finally profitable. Now that he had five stores and a manager in each one, he felt he could finally relax a little and take a vacation.

Ravi had planned for years to return to India to visit his family. He wanted to lose about 20–25 pounds before he went home. He had developed some bad eating habits and had not been exercising. He had about 5 months before the date of his departure. He also hoped to return to a more native Indian diet in the process. He knew his parents would have been very disappointed if they knew he had become so westernized.

ASSESSMENT

1. What do you know about Ravi?

2. What values has he acted on for 12 years? What values does he want to act on in the future?

3. What do you suspect Ravi has been eating?

4. How much weight could Ravi safely lose in 5 months?

DIAGNOSIS

5. What are possible causes of Ravi's weight problem?

6. What education is needed to help Ravi lose weight?

PLAN/GOAL

7. What are the two major goals for Ravi's health?

IMPLEMENTATION

8. What are the most important diet changes that Ravi needs to make to lose weight?

9. What foods does he need to include to return to a more native diet?

10. What does he need to do about exercise?

11. How can his family help?

12. Would he be more successful losing weight alone or in a group?

EVALUATION/OUTCOME CRITERIA

13. One month after starting the above plan, what changes will be in place?

14. If the above plan is successful, what will Ravi report in 5 months?

C A S E   S T U D Y

Jill was a 35-year-old mother of four boys. The last boy was in school, and she was looking forward to a little time to herself. She was used to running all day, doing laundry, running errands, making meals, and chauffeuring the boys to their after-school sports. She would miss her afternoons with the youngest, Jason. They played one-on-one basketball, kickball, and soccer until the older boys were out of school. Meals were always light and simple at Jill's house. Lots of salads, vegetables, and cold baked chicken were the order of the day, so that all the boys could eat with their different schedules.

Within a month, Jill had settled into a new routine of crafts and cooking a hot meal. She finally had the opportunity to do some "girl" things, as she called them, and she loved it. She also took great pride in having a hot meal on the table and even served dessert. She had lunch out with the girls and invited neighbors and friends over for casual dinners. She was thoroughly enjoying herself, except for one thing. Within 3 months, she had gained 8 pounds. She let it slide. When that figure was up to 15 pounds, Jill decided she had better do something about it.

ASSESSMENT

1. What objective information do you have about Jill?

2. What is the most significant change in her life?

3. How has that change affected her?

4. How long should Jill expect to take to lose the 15 pounds she gained?

DIAGNOSIS

5. What caused Jill to change her eating habits?

6. What were the consequences of the change in Jill's activity level?

PLAN/GOAL

7. What changes does Jill need to make in her diet and activities?

IMPLEMENTATION

8. List some strategies that match Jill's new priorities.

9. What can she do with the boys that would help?

10. What can the boys do to help her lose weight?

EVALUATION/OUTCOME CRITERIA

11. What criteria would Jill use to determine the success of the plan?

Diet During Late Adulthood

Key Terms

arthritis
atherosclerosis
dentition
estrogen
food faddists
geriatrics
gerontology
hypertension
occlusions
osteoporosis
periodontal disease
physiological
plaque
skeletal system

gerontology
the study of aging

physiological
relating to bodily functions

Objectives

After studying this chapter, you should be able to

- Explain the nutritional and kcal needs of people 65 and over

- Explain the development of given chronic diseases

- Identify physiological, economic, and psychosocial problems that can affect a senior citizen's nutrition

Currently, the fastest-growing age group in the United States is that of people age 85 and older. The average life expectancy in this country is now 79 years for women and 72 years for men. It is expected that by the year 2000 there will be 26 million people in the United States 80 years and older. Consequently, gerontology, the study of aging, is of increasing importance.

The rate of aging varies. Each person is affected by heredity, emotional and physical stress, and nutrition. Experiments continue to teach more about the causes of aging and the role of nutrition in the aging process.

THE EFFECTS OF AGING

As people age, physiological, psychosocial, and economic changes occur that affect nutrition.

dentition

arrangement, type, and number of teeth

Physiological Changes

The body's functions slow with age, and its ability to replace worn cells is reduced. The metabolic rate slows; bones become less dense; lean muscle mass is reduced; eyes do not focus on nearby objects as they once did and some grow cloudy from cataracts; poor dentition is common; the heart and kidneys become less efficient; and hearing, taste, and smell are less acute. If poor nutrition has been chronic, the immune system may be compromised.

Digestion is affected because the secretion of hydrochloric acid and enzymes is diminished. This in turn decreases the intrinsic factor synthesis, which leads to a deficiency of vitamin B_{12}. The tone of the intestines is reduced and the result may be constipation or, in some cases, diarrhea.

Psychosocial Changes

Feelings do not decrease with age. In fact, psychosocial problems can increase as one grows older. Age does not diminish the desire to feel useful and appreciated and loved by family and friends. Retirement years may not be "golden" if one suffers a loss of self-esteem from feelings of uselessness. Grief over the loss of a spouse or close friend, combined with the resulting loneliness can be devastating. Physical disabilities that develop in the senior years and prevent one from going out independently can destroy a social life. Becoming a fifth wheel in a grown child's home or a resident of a nursing home can lead to severe depression. Problems such as these can diminish a person's appetite and ability to shop and cook.

Economic Changes

Retirement typically results in decreased income. Unless one has carefully prepared for it, this can affect one's quality of life by reducing social activities, adding worry about meeting bills, and causing one to select a less than healthy diet by choosing foods on the basis of cost rather than nutrient content.

Sidestepping Potential Problems

Healthy eating habits throughout life, an exercise program suited to one's age, and social activities that please can prevent or delay physical deterioration and psychological depression during the senior years. Their benefits can be said to be circular. The first two contribute largely to one's physical condition, and social activities can prevent or diminish depression, which, if unchecked, can also depress appetite. They give purpose to the day, joy to the heart, and zest to the appetite. Whenever an elderly person is depressed, the patient's nutrition and lifestyle should be carefully reviewed.

Food-drug interactions must be monitored closely in the elderly. Frequently, specific foods will prevent, decrease, or enhance the absorption of a particular drug. Dairy products should not be consumed within 2 hours of taking the antibiotic tetracycline or it will not be absorbed. A person taking a blood clot–reducing drug such as coumadin or warfarin (often called blood thinners) needs to consume vitamin

K–rich food in moderation as they counteract blood thinners. Even vitamin supplements can cause interactions. The antioxidant vitamins are not to be taken with blood clot–reducing medications because they also have a tendency to thin the blood.

Drug-drug interactions as well as food-drug interactions can contribute to decreased nutritional status. These interactions could affect appetite as well as absorption of nutrients from the food eaten. Careful monitoring is recommended. (See Table A-2 in the appendix.)

NUTRITIONAL REQUIREMENTS OF SENIOR CITIZENS

Although the nutritional needs of growth disappear with age, the normal nutritional needs for maintaining a constant state of good health remain throughout life. Good nutrition can speed recovery from illness, surgery, or broken bones and generally can improve the spirits and the quality, and even the length, of life.

Despite the physical changes the body undergoes after the age of 51 or so, only a few of the RDAs for people in that age category are less than those for younger people.

The protein requirement remains at the average 50g per day for women and 63g for men. This is based on the estimated need of 0.8g per kilogram of body weight. After age 65, it may be advisable to increase one's daily protein intake to 1.0g per kilogram of body weight. In general, vitamin requirements do not change after the age of 51, except for a slight decrease in the RDAs for thiamin, riboflavin, and niacin. The need for these three vitamins depends largely on the kcal intake, and kcal requirement is reduced after the age of 51. The need for iron is decreased after age 51 in women because of menopause. (See the Recommended Dietary Allowances on the inside front cover.)

The kcal requirement decreases approximately 2 to 3% a decade because metabolism slows and activity is reduced (see Table 15-1). If the kcal intake is not reduced, weight will increase. This additional weight would increase the work of the heart and put increased stress on the **skeletal system**. It is important that the kcal requirement not be exceeded and just as important that the nutrient requirements be

skeletal system
body's bone structure

TABLE 15-1 Median Weights and Heights and Recommended Daily Energy Intake for Adults

CATEGORY	AGE (years) OR CONDITION	WEIGHT (kg)	(lb)	HEIGHT (cm)	(in)	REE (kcal/day)	AVERAGE ENERGY ALLOWANCE (kcal) Multiples of REE	per kg	per day
Males	25–50	79	174	176	70	1,800	1.60	37	2,900
	51+	77	170	173	68	1,530	1.50	30	2,300
Females	25–50	63	138	163	64	1,380	1.55	36	2,200
	51+	65	143	160	63	1,280	1.50	30	1,900

Source: **Recommended Dietary Allowances: 10th Edition. Copyright © 1989 by the National Academy of Sciences. Courtesy of the National Academy Press, Washington, D.C.**

fulfilled to maintain good nutritional status. An exercise plan appropriate for one's age and health can be helpful in burning excess kcal and toning and strengthening the muscles.

FOOD HABITS OF SENIOR CITIZENS

If the established food habits of the older person are poor, such habits will undoubtedly have been a long time in the making. These habits will not be easy to change. Poor food habits that begin during old age can also present problems. Decreased income during retirement, physical disability, and inadequate cooking facilities may cause difficulties in food selection and preparation. Anorexia caused by grief, loneliness, boredom, or difficulty in chewing can decrease food consumption. Dementia and/or Alzheimers may cause the elderly to think they have eaten when they may not have.

Studies indicate that many senior citizens consume diets deficient in protein; vitamins C, D, B_6, B_{12}, and folate; and the minerals calcium, zinc, iron, and sometimes kcal.

An elderly patient's diet plan should be based on the Food Guide Pyramid and the nutrients contained compared with the RDA. Older persons' needs can vary considerably, depending on their conditions, so each person should be examined by a physician to determine specific requirements. If the patient consumes less that 1,500 kcal a day a multivitamin-mineral supplement is recommended.

Variety and nutrient-dense foods should be encouraged, as should the use of water. Water is important to help prevent constipation, to maintain urinary volume, and to prevent dehydration. When there is serious protein and kcal malnutrition (PEM), the reason may be economic or psychosocial. Elderly people who have long hospital stays can develop PEM in the hospital. They may dislike the food; drugs may dull the appetite; and they may be lonely and depressed. Sometimes poor or missing teeth can make eating protein foods difficult (Figure 15-1). In such cases, protein-rich soups can be used.

If overweight is a problem, it may be caused by overeating, lack of exercise, drugs, or alcohol.

Any adjustment in food habits will require great tact, and plans for changes must be based on the individual's total situation.

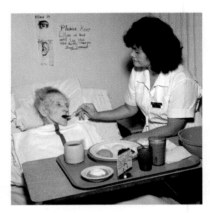

FIGURE 15-1 Older adults may have health problems that affect their ability to self-feed. (Courtesy of Delmar Publishers, Albany, NY)

FOOD FADS AND THE ELDERLY

Some older people are consciously or unconsciously searching for eternal life, if not youth. Consequently, they are frequently susceptible to the claims of **food faddists** who seek to profit from their ignorance. Senior citizens spend money on unnecessary vitamins, minerals, and special honey, molasses, bread, milk, and other foods that may be guaranteed by the salesperson to prevent or cure various diseases. This money could be much more effectively used on ordinary foods from the Food Guide Pyramid that would cost considerably less.

food faddists
people who have certain beliefs about particular foods or diets

NUTRITION AND CHRONIC DISEASES COMMON TO SENIOR CITIZENS

It is estimated that 85% of people over 65 have one or more chronic diseases or physical problems. Examples include osteoporosis, arthritis, cataracts, cancer, diabetes mellitus, hypertension, heart disease, and periodontal disease. The branch of medicine that is involved with diseases of older people is called geriatrics.

Osteoporosis

Osteoporosis is a condition in which the amount of calcium in bones is reduced, making them porous. It is estimated that up to 50% of elderly people have osteoporosis, and the majority of these are women. A bone density scan can be done with a special X-ray to determine if one has osteoporosis. It is typically unnoticed at its onset, which occurs at approximately age 45, and it may not be noticed at all until a fracture occurs. One of its symptoms is a gradual reduction in height.

Doctors are not certain of its cause. It is thought that years of a sedentary life coupled with a diet deficient in calcium, vitamin D, and fluoride contribute to it, as does estrogen loss, which occurs after menopause. Physicians are recommending estrogen replacement therapy (ERT) to help prevent osteoporosis and heart disease. Some doctors are also advising patients to consume 1,500 mg of calcium, which would require the daily consumption of over one quart of milk or its equivalent. Calcium tablets, preferably calcium carbonate, could be used instead, but the patient would also require supplementary vitamin D if sunshine were unavailable or if the patient were home-bound. A diet with sufficient calcium and vitamin D plus an appropriate exercise program begun early in the adult years are thought to help prevent this disease.

Another possible cause of osteoporosis may be a diet containing excessive amounts of phosphorus, which can speed bone loss. It is known that Americans are ingesting increasing amounts of phosphorus. Sodas and processed foods contain phosphorus, and their consumption is increasing as milk consumption is decreasing in the United States. Some believe that periodontal disease may be a harbinger of osteoporosis. Periodontal disease is characterized by bone loss in the jaw, which can lead to loosened teeth and infection in the gums.

Arthritis

Arthritis is a disease that causes the joints to become painful and stiff. It results in structural changes in the cartilage of the joints. A patient with arthritis should be especially careful to avoid overweight because the extra weight adds stress to joints that are already painful. If the patient is overweight, a weight reduction program should be instituted.

The regular use of aspirin by these patients may cause slight bleeding in the stomach lining and subsequent anemia, so their diets may require additional iron. Arthritis can greatly complicate a patient's

geriatrics
the branch of medicine involved with diseases of the elderly

osteoporosis
condition in which bones become brittle because there have been insufficient mineral deposits, especially calcium

estrogen
hormone secreted by the ovaries

periodontal disease
disease of the mouth and gums

arthritis
chronic disease involving the joints

life because it may partially or completely immobilize the patient so much that shopping, moving around, and cooking become difficult.

Aspirin and other anti-inflammatory drugs do help relieve the pain of arthritis, but there is as yet no cure. Patients should be well informed of this to prevent them from wasting their money on so-called miracle cures recommended by health food faddists or quacks.

Cancer

Research about the role of nutrition in cancer development continues. The American Cancer Society has indicated that diets consistently high in fat or low in fiber and vitamin A may contribute to cancer (see Chapter 21).

Diabetes Mellitus

Diabetes mellitus is a chronic disease. It develops when the body does not produce sufficient amounts of insulin or does not use it effectively for normal carbohydrate metabolism. Diet is very important in the treatment of diabetes. Chapter 17 discusses this treatment in detail.

Hypertension

hypertension
higher than normal blood pressure

occlusions
blockages

plaque
fatty deposit on interior of artery walls

atherosclerosis
a form of arteriosclerosis affecting the intima (inner lining) of the artery walls

Hypertension, or high blood pressure, can lead to strokes. It is associated with diets high in salt or possibly low in calcium. Most Americans ingest from two to six times the amount of salt needed each day. It is thought that the earlier a person reduces salt intake, the better that person's chances of avoiding hypertension, particularly if there is a family history of it. Hypertension is discussed in detail in Chapter 18.

Heart Disease

Heart attack and stroke are the major causes of death in the United States. They occur when arteries become blocked (occluded), preventing the normal passage of blood. These occlusions (blockages) are caused by blood clots that form and are unable to pass through an unnaturally narrowed artery. Arteries are narrowed by plaque, a fatty substance containing cholesterol that accumulates in the walls of the artery. This condition is called atherosclerosis. It is believed that excessive cholesterol and saturated fats in the diet over many years contribute to this condition. The therapeutic diet appropriate for atherosclerosis is discussed in Chapter 18.

Effects of Nutrition

Current research about the role of nutrition in preventing or relieving these chronic diseases continues. The effects of nutrition are cumulative over many years. The effects of a lifetime of poor eating habits cannot be cured overnight. When diets have been poor for a long time, prevention of these chronic diseases may not be possible. It may be possible, however, to use nutrition to help stabilize the condition of a patient who has one of these diseases. The prevention of many of the diseases of the elderly should begin in one's youth (Figure 15-2).

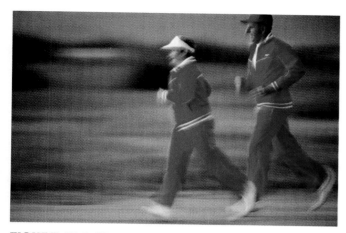

FIGURE 15-2 Exercising for good health is not limited to the young. (Courtesy of Delmar Publishers, Albany, NY)

APPROPRIATE DIETS FOR SENIOR CITIZENS

The diets of senior citizens should be planned around the Food Guide Pyramid (Figure 2-1). When special health problems exist, the normal diet should be adapted to meet individual needs (see Section 3, Diet Therapy).

The federal government provides the states with funds to serve senior citizens hot meals at noon in senior centers across the country. These senior centers become social clubs and are immensely beneficial to the elderly. They provide companionship in addition to nutritious food. Frequently the noon meal at "the center" becomes the focal point of an older person's day.

The federal government also provides transportation for those who are otherwise unable to reach the senior center for the meal. When individuals are completely homebound, arrangements can be made for the meals to be delivered to their homes. Some communities have Meals-on-Wheels projects. Participating people pay according to ability. In addition, food stamps are available and can sometimes be used for the Meals-on-Wheels programs.

CONSIDERATIONS FOR THE HEALTH CARE PROFESSIONAL

It is essential that the health care professional remember that each patient is an individual with individual needs. It is easy for someone working exclusively with geriatric patients to group them together, but doing so diminishes the quality of the care they receive and adds to their unhappiness. The 80-year-old patient is just as pleased to see a smile on the face of a nurse as is an 18-year-old patient. The 70-year-old overweight arthritic patient deserves as much help with a weight-loss program as the 45-year-old patient. The 85-year-old patient

TABLE 15-2 2,200-kcal Daily Menus

Breakfast

½ cup orange juice	50 kcal	
1 cup dry cereal	100	
½ cup fat-free milk	43	
2 teaspoons sugar	35	
2 slices whole grain bread, toasted	150	
½ tablespoon margarine	50	
1 tablespoon jelly	50	
1 cup black coffee	0	478 kcal
	478	

Lunch

¾ cup macaroni and cheese	300	
1 tomato, sliced	25	
½ cup green beans	25	
1 cup fat-free milk	85	
⅔ cup custard	200	635 kcal
	635	

Dinner

½ cup pineapple juice	75	
3 oz broiled hamburger	240	
½ cup rice	100	
½ cup shredded lettuce	10	
1 tablespoon salad dressing	75	
1 cup fat-free milk	85	
Fresh fruit	100	685 kcal
	685	

Snacks

1 banana	100	
5 dried prunes	100	
2 oatmeal cookies	200	400 kcal
	400	2,198

suffering from senility still enjoys a bright hello and a gentle pat on the back. People's feelings must never be forgotten. The incapacitation that can accompany old age is a terrible indignity, and these patients deserve special care.

● SUMMARY

The elderly are becoming an increasingly large segment of the U.S. population, and their nutritional needs are of growing concern. It is becoming apparent that many of the chronic diseases of the elderly could be delayed or avoided by maintaining good nutrition throughout life. Most nutrient requirements do not decrease with age, but kcal

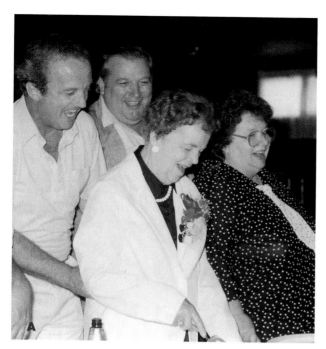 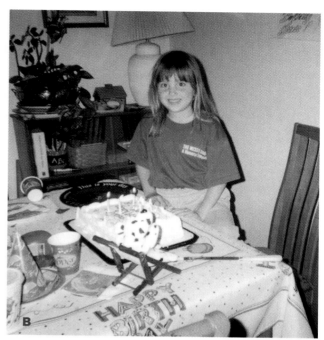

FIGURE 15-3 Celebrating one's eightieth birthday (A) is as much fun as celebrating one's eighth (B) when health is good.

requirements do. When food habits of senior citizens must be changed, adjustments require great tact and patience on the part of the dietitian. Older people are easily attracted to food fads that promise good health and prolonged life.

● DISCUSSION TOPICS

1. Why are the normal nutrient requirements of people in their seventies the same as those of people in their fifties?

2. Why does the iron requirement usually diminish for women after the age of 50?

3. Why might elderly people suffer from anorexia?

4. How might arthritis affect one's eating habits?

5. In what ways can emotional stress affect eating habits? What kinds of emotional stress do the elderly sometimes suffer?

6. Why are older people inclined to believe food faddists' stories?

7. What is the difference between geriatrics and gerontology?

8. What is periodontal disease, and what is its possible significance?

9. What is osteoporosis?

10. Why do kcal requirements diminish as people age?

● SUGGESTED ACTIVITIES

1. Arrange a talk on nutrition for senior citizens at a congregate meal site.

2. If possible, visit a nursing home at mealtime. Write your evaluation of the food and a description of patient reactions to it and to you, the visitor.

3. Describe an appropriate response to your 65-year-old aunt, who has just become captivated by a salesperson in a local health food store and has announced that she is buying a 6-month supply of vinegar-honey tablets that are guaranteed to prevent arthritis.

4. Plan a talk on nutrition for the Parents' Association of a local high school. The talk is entitled "Invest Now for Future Dividends—Eat Well."

● REVIEW

Multiple choice. Select the *letter* that precedes the best answer.

1. Gerontology is of increasing interest because it is
   a. the branch of medicine involved with diseases of older people
   b. the study of nutrition
   c. hoped that experimentation in this field will explain the causes of aging
   d. the study of heart disease

2. After the age of 51, nutrient requirements generally
   a. increase
   b. decrease
   c. remain unchanged
   d. none of the above

3. After the age of 51, kcal requirements generally
   a. increase
   b. decrease
   c. remain unchanged
   d. none of the above

4. The iron requirement for women after the age of approximately 51 generally
   a. increases
   b. decreases
   c. remains unchanged
   d. none of the above

5. As the metabolic rate slows with age,
   a. the kcal requirement is increased
   b. the kcal requirement is decreased
   c. there is a decreased need for vitamin A, D, and K
   d. cataracts can develop

6. Osteoporosis is a disease that causes
   a. poor appetite
   b. a reduction in the number of red blood cells
   c. joints to become painful and stiff
   d. bones to become porous

7. Arthritis is a disease that causes
   a. poor appetite
   b. a reduction in the number of red blood cells
   c. joints to become painful and stiff
   d. bones to become porous

8. Hypertension is related to diets high in
    a. cholesterol   c. calcium
    b. vitamin D   d. salt

9. Diets high in cholesterol content are thought to contribute to
    a. diabetes mellitus   c. heart disease
    b. hypertension   d. cataracts

CASE STUDY

Chester and Mildred have been married for 54 years. They have enjoyed 12 years of retirement in their Florida home. Since their forties, they have tried to eat right, exercise, and be proactive about their health. Since Mildred had her hysterectomy, Chester has made sure she takes her estrogen. Mildred has been concerned about Chester recently because he cracked a molar and had to have a replacement. When the dentist saw the X-rays, he commented that Chester had lost some bone density in his jaw. The dentist also noticed that two of Chesters' teeth were loose. Chester told Mildred that the dentist gave him a questionnaire to fill out with questions like "Have you suffered any broken bones recently?" and "Have you noticed a loss of height?"

ASSESSMENT

1. What do you know about Chester's health?
2. What did the dentist suspect about Chester?
3. How significant is this problem?
4. How common is this problem in elders?

DIAGNOSIS

5. What could be the cause of Chester's loss of bone density?
6. What education does Chester need regarding his condition?

PLAN/GOAL

7. What needs to change in Chester's diet?

IMPLEMENTATION

8. What additions or alterations in Chester's diet would prevent further osteoporosis? What are the best sources of calcium?
9. What information does Chester need to make this change?
10. Who can help him learn?
11. Why doesn't Mildred show any of these signs?
12. Can osteoporosis be cured?

EVALUATION/OUTCOME CRITERIA

13. In 6 months, when the dentist examines Chester again, what will Chester report?
14. How long will it take before the dentist can measure an improvement on an X-ray?

C A S E   S T U D Y

Harold was an 82-year-old long-time widower who lived alone in his own home. He was a big rough-looking man who had spent most of his life doing hard physical labor. In his forties, he weighed over 230 pounds. He proudly reported he was 6 feet 3 inches tall. His modest home was paid off. He lived off his pension and social security and had little else left at the end of the month. His passion was woodworking, which he did in the garage. The lights used to be on late into the evening in the garage, but not in the last 6 months.

Harold had so many physical complaints that few of his neighbors really listened to him. Harold shaved about every 3 or 4 days now and wore an unbuttoned plaid flannel shirt over his long underwear. He seemed to wear the same shirt for days at a time. After several weeks of no lights in the garage in the evening and no sightings of Harold outside, the neighbors elected Gertrude to check on him. Gertrude brought Harold's mail to the front door. When she inquired about his health and whereabouts, she did listen to his complaints. Up close he looked thinner than the last time she had seen him, and she noticed he had some red sores on and around his mouth. He complained about being tired and said his arthritis was really bad right now.

Gertrude asked Harold if he had been eating. Harold could remember eating cold cereal and coffee. At lunch he had a bowl of soup. For dinner he had a cooked potato and a can of tuna. Gertrude asked Harold about eating any vegetables or fruits. Harold just snapped at her and became impatient with her "butting in" and muttered something about how much all that stuff costs and walked back into the house. Gertrude was still worried about Harold, so, after conferring with the other neighbors, she called his son, Phil. Phil persuaded Harold to go to the doctor. The doctor referred Harold to a gerontology nurse practitioner.

ASSESSMENT

1. What do you know about Harold and his health?

2. What do you know is a barrier in Harold's life to maintaining health?

3. What nutrients are missing from Harold's diet? Why are they missing?

4. How significant is the problem? What are the long-term consequences of the problem?

DIAGNOSIS

5. What are some reasons for Harold's nutrition problem?

6. What nutrition education does Harold need?

PLAN/GOAL

7. What are your goals for Harold's health problems?

IMPLEMENTATION

8. Identify how each of the following resources can help Harold solve this problem and prevent further problems.

   a. Gertrude and the other neighbors
   b. his son, Phil
   c. his church
   d. local agencies such as Meals on Wheels and the free food pantry

9. What are the least expensive sources of vitamins C, D, B_6, B_{12}, and folate?

10. How can the nurse practitioner help?

EVALUATION/OUTCOME CRITERIA

11. At Harold's next NP appointment, what changes would the NP expect to note? What would the NP expect Phil to report?

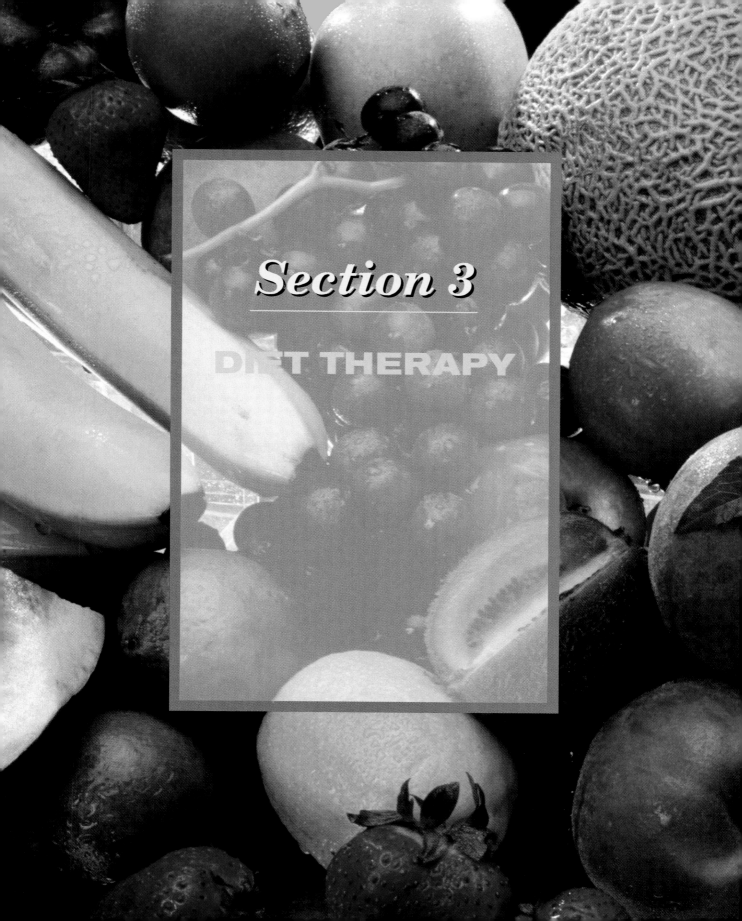

Section 3

DIET THERAPY

Chapter 16

Diet and Weight Control

Key Terms

amphetamines
appetite
caliper
crash diets
diabetes mellitus
diuretics
energy imbalance
fad diets
fat cell theory
gastric bypass
hunger
hypertension
hyperthyroidism

hypothyroidism
jejunum
morbid
normal weight
obesity
overweight
phenylpropanol-
    amine
plateau period
set point theory
stomach banding
underweight
yo-yo effect

normal weight
average weight for size and age

Objectives

After studying this chapter, you should be able to:

● Discuss the causes and dangers of overweight

● Discuss the causes and dangers of underweight

● Identify foods suitable for high-kcal diets and those suitable for low-kcal diets

One needs to understand some commonly used terms before discussing weight control. The term *normal weight* can mean average, desired, or standard. **Normal weight** is that which is appropriate for the maintenance of good health for a particular individual at a particular time. The following is a simple method of determining one's ideal body weight. It is known as the "rule of thumb" method.

1. Males assume 106 pounds for the first 5 feet (60 inches) and add 6 pounds for each inch over 60.

2. Females assume 100 pounds for the first 5 feet (60 inches) and add 5 pounds for each inch over 60.

3. Large-boned individuals of both sexes *increase* the first sum by 10%.

4. Small-boned individuals of both sexes *decrease* the first sum by 10%.

This method is quick, but one must remember that it is only an estimate.

overweight

weight 10–20% above average

obesity

excessive body fat, 20% above average

underweight

weight that is 10–15% below average

Overweight can be defined as weight 10 to 20% above average. **Obesity** can be defined as excessive body fat, with weight 20% above average. **Underweight** is weight 10 to 15% below average.

The medical standard used to define obesity is the body mass index (BMI). It is used to determine whether a person is at health risk from excess weight. The BMI is obtained by dividing weight in kilograms by height in meters squared. Fewer health risks are associated with a BMI range of 19 to 25 than with BMI above or below that range. A BMI greater than 25 indicates obesity and health risks. Table 16-1 presents a range of BMIs using English units, so one needn't do the metric conversion.

The *distribution* of fat is another indicator of possible health problems. Fat in the abdominal cavity *(visceral fat)* has been shown to be associated with a greater risk for hypertension, diabetes, coronary heart disease, Type 2 diabetes, and certain types of cancer than has fat in the thigh, buttocks, and hip area. A pear-shaped body has a lower risk for disease than does the apple-shaped body. A waist-to-hip ratio also can give an indication of risk. This is determined by dividing the waist measurement by the hip measurement. A ratio greater than 1.0 in men and 0.8 in women indicates risk for the same diseases as given above.

TABLE 16-1 Body Mass Index (BMI)

HEIGHT (in feet and inches)	WEIGHT (in pounds)													
4′10″	91	96	100	105	110	115	119	124	129	134	138	143	167	191
4′11″	94	99	104	109	114	119	124	128	133	138	143	148	173	198
5′	97	102	107	112	118	123	128	133	138	143	148	153	179	204
5′1″	100	106	111	116	122	127	132	137	143	148	153	158	185	211
5′2″	104	109	115	120	126	131	136	142	147	153	158	164	191	218
5′3″	107	113	118	124	130	135	141	146	152	158	163	169	197	225
5′4″	110	116	122	128	134	140	145	151	157	163	169	174	204	232
5′5″	114	120	126	132	138	144	150	156	162	168	174	180	210	240
5′6″	118	124	130	136	142	148	155	161	167	173	179	186	216	247
5′7″	121	127	134	140	146	153	159	166	172	178	185	191	223	255
5′8″	125	131	138	144	151	158	164	171	177	184	190	197	230	262
5′9″	128	135	142	149	155	162	169	176	182	189	196	203	236	270
5′10″	132	139	146	153	160	167	174	181	188	195	202	207	243	278
5′11″	136	143	150	157	165	172	179	186	193	200	208	215	250	286
6′	140	147	154	162	169	177	184	191	199	206	213	221	258	294
6′1″	144	151	159	166	174	182	189	197	204	212	219	227	265	302
6′2″	148	155	163	171	179	186	194	202	210	218	225	233	272	311
6′3″	152	160	168	176	184	192	200	208	216	224	232	240	279	319
6′4″	156	164	172	180	189	197	205	213	221	230	238	246	287	328
BMI	19	20	21	22	23	24	25	26	27	28	29	30	35	40

TABLE 16-2 USDA Acceptance Weights for Adults

HEIGHT WITHOUT SHOES (in feet and inches)	WEIGHT WITHOUT CLOTHES (in pounds), BY AGE*	
	19 to 34 Years	35 Years or Older
5′0″	97–128	108–138
5′1″	101–132	111–143
5′2″	104–137	115–148
5′3″	107–141	119–152
5′4″	111–146	122–157
5′5″	114–150	126–162
5′6″	118–155	130–167
5′7″	121–160	134–172
5′8″	125–164	138–178
5′9″	129–169	142–183
5′10″	132–174	146–188
5′11″	136–179	151–194
6′0″	140–184	155–199
6′1″	144–189	159–205
6′2″	148–195	164–210
6′3″	152–200	168–216
6′4″	156–205	173–222
6′5″	160–211	177–228
6′6″	164–216	182–234

Source: From The Human Nutrition Information Service. USDA. Report of the Dietary Guidelines Advisory Committee on the Dietary Guidelines for Americans—1990. Hyattsville, MD: U.S. Government Printing Office, June 1990, p. 8.
*The higher weights in the ranges generally apply to men, who tend to have more muscle and bone than women; the lower weights more often apply to women.

Body weight is composed of fluids, organs, fat, muscle, and bones, so large variation exists among people. In addition to height, age, physical condition, heredity, gender, and general frame size (small, medium, or large) are all critical factors in determining desired weight. For example, a 6′2″ man with a 44″ chest, 36″ long arms, and 8½″ wrists will weigh more than a 6′2″man with a 40″ chest, 35″ long arms, and 7½″ wrists because he has more body tissue. Table 16-2 gives lists of acceptable weights according to age, sex, and height for adults that reflect realistic weight goals. The Metropolitan Height and Weight tables (Appendix A-1), which are categorized by height, sex, and frame size, can also be used.

Some people can weigh more than is indicated on Table 16-2 and still be in good physical condition. Professional football players, because of the amount of lean muscle mass they develop, are examples. However, when they retire and reduce their physical activity, that same muscle can change to fat. If their weights remain the same, they then will be considered overfat because the proportion of fat will have

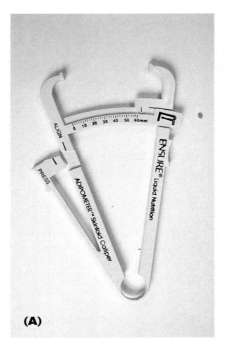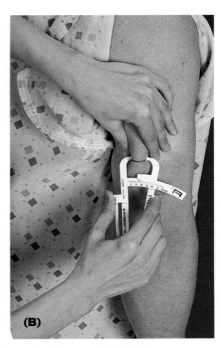

(A)   **(B)**

FIGURE 16-1 (A) A skinfold caliper. (B) Measuring triceps skinfold thickness.

caliper

mechanical device used to measure percentage of body fat by skinfold measurement

diabetes mellitus

chronic disease in which the body lacks the normal ability to metabolize glucose

hypertension

higher than normal blood pressure

energy imbalance

eating either too much or too little for the amount of energy expended

become too high. Some can weigh what Table 16-2 indicates they should weigh and yet be overfat because too great a percentage of the weight is made up of fat.

Body fat is measured with a **caliper**. Using a caliper correctly requires practice and skill. Because the fat under the skin on the stomach and on the upper arm is representative of the percentage of overall body fat, it is usually measured when knowledge of the percentage of body fat is required. If it is more than 1½ inches, one is considered overweight. If it is under ½ inch, one is considered underweight (Figure 16-1).

A moderate amount of fat is a necessary component of the body. It protects organs from injury, and acts as insulation. The final determination of desirable weight depends on common sense. One can usually see when one is overweight.

OVERWEIGHT AND OBESITY

Overweight is a serious health hazard. It puts extra strain on the heart, lungs, muscles, bones, and joints, and it increases the susceptibility to **diabetes mellitus** and **hypertension**. It increases surgical risks, shortens the lifespan, causes psychosocial problems, and is associated with heart disease and some forms of cancer.

Causes

There is no one cause for obesity. Genetic, physiological, metabolic, biochemical, and psychological factors can all contribute to it. **Energy imbalance** is a significant cause of overweight. People eat more than they need. Excess weight can accumulate during and after middle age because people reduce their level of activity and metabolism slows with age. Consequently, weight accumulates unless kcal intake is reduced. **Hypothyroidism** is a possible, but rare, cause of obesity. In this condition, the basal metabolic rate (BMR) is low, thereby reducing the number of kcal needed for energy. Unless corrected this condition can result in excess weight.

There are two popular theories about weight loss: the fat cell theory and the set point theory. According to the **fat cell theory**, obesity develops when the size of fat cells increases. When their size decreases, as during a reducing diet, the individual is driven to eat in order for the fat cells to regain their former size. Therefore, it is difficult to lose weight and keep it off.

According to the **set point theory**, everyone has a set point or natural weight at which the body is so comfortable that it does not allow for deviation. This is said to be the reason why some people cannot lose weight below a "set point" or why, if they do, they quickly regain to that "set point." The only way to lower a "set point" is through exercising three to five times a week.

Healthy Weight

Not everyone fits the USDA weight table shown in Table 16-2 or the "healthy weight target," which is a BMI of 19 to 25. For anyone with a BMI of 25 or higher, a more realistic approach would be a reduction of one or two BMI points to reduce health problems and disease risks. After this loss have been maintained for 6 months, further lowering of the BMI needs to be attempted. A "healthy weight" may be the weight at which one is eating nutritiously, exercising, has no health problems, and is free from disease.

DIETARY TREATMENT OF OVERWEIGHT AND OBESITY

Obviously, if a significant cause of overweight is overeating, the solution is to reduce one's food intake. This is seldom easy. To accomplish it, one must undertake a weight-reduction (low-kcal) diet. For the diet to be effective, one must have a genuine desire to lose weight.

The simplest and, therefore, perhaps the best weight-reduction diet is the normal diet based on the Food Guide Pyramid but with the kcal content controlled. If necessary, its consistency can also be adapted to meet individual needs by using a food processor or a blender.

Exchange lists provide another excellent method frequently used to healthfully control the kcal value of the diet. These lists were originally developed by the American Diabetes Association and the American Dietetic Association for the use of diabetic patients. They are organized to provide specific numbers of kcal and nutrients according to six lists and are discussed in detail in Chapter 17.

Counting fat grams is another way sometimes used to lower kcal intake. Each gram of fat contains 9 kcal, so the reduction of only a few grams of fat per day will result in weight loss. However, for optimal

hypothyroidism
condition in which the thyroid gland secretes too little thyroxine and T_3; body metabolism is slower than normal

fat cell theory
belief that fat cells have a natural drive to regain any weight lost

set point theory
belief that everyone has a natural weight ("set point") at which the body is most comfortable

TABLE 16-3 Figuring Your Fat-Gram Allowance*

Step 1: Determine how many calories you need to maintain your ideal weight. Start by finding your ideal weight in Table 16-2.

Step 2: a. To find your kcal needs, multiply your ideal weight by 15 if you are moderately active or by 20 if you are very active.

b. From that total, subtract the following according to your age:

Age 25–34, subtract 0

Age 35–44, subtract 100

Age 45–54, subtract 200

Age 55–64, subtract 300

Age 65+, subtract 400

Step 3: To find your fat-gram allowance, multiply your daily kcal by the percentage of fat desired (10%, 20%, or 30%), then divide by 9 kcal/g.

SUGGESTED DAILY FAT INTAKE TABLE			
KCAL	30%	20%	10%
1,200	40g	26g	13g
1,400	47g	31g	16g
1,600	53g	36g	18g
1,800	60g	40g	20g
2,000	67g	44g	22g
2,200	73g	49g	24g
2,400	80g	53g	27g

*The maximum amount of fat you can eat every day and still keep your blood cholesterol at a safe level.

absorption of fat-soluble vitamins, one requires that at least 10% of daily kcal intake come from fats, and 30% is the recommended amount. Therefore, in diets limiting fats to 30% of total kcal, one must consume 3g of fat per 100 kcal; in those limiting fats to 20% of total kcal, one must consume 2g fat per 100 kcal; and in those limiting fats to 10% of total kcal, one needs 1g fat per 100 kcal. See Table 16-3 to calculate individual fat-gram allowances.

A reduction of 3,500 kcal will result in a weight loss of one pound. Physicians frequently recommend that no more than one or two pounds of weight be lost in one week. To accomplish this, one must reduce one's weekly kcal by 3,500–7,000, or daily intake by 500–1,000. Diets should not be reduced below 1,200 kcal a day or the dieter will not receive the necessary nutrients. The diet should consist of 15 to 20% protein, 45 to 55% carbohydrate, and 30% or less of fat: in other words, normal proportions of nutrients but in reduced amounts. The number of meals and snacks each day should be determined by the dieter's needs and desires, but the total number of kcal must not be exceeded.

There is no magic way of losing weight and maintaining the reduced weight, but there is a key to it. That *key is changing eating habits.* In fact, unless eating habits are truly changed, it is likely that the lost weight will be regained once the weight reduction has been accomplished because at that point the dieter may be euphoric about the weight loss and forget its cost. The cost of slimness is eating less than one might prefer and exercising at least three to five times a week for 30 minutes.

Food Selection

The dieter must learn to "eat smart." Daily kcal counting is not necessary if one learns the kcal and fat-gram values of favorite foods and considers them before indulging. Some foods are good choices on weight-loss diets because of their low kcal/low fat-gram values and some foods should be used in moderation because of their high kcal and high fat-gram values (see Table 16-4). The low kcal, low fat-gram foods should be used during weight loss and thereafter.

Substitutions of foods with very low kcal contents should be made for those with high kcal contents whenever possible. The following are examples:

- Fat-free milk for whole milk
- Evaporated fat-free milk for evaporated milk
- Yogurt or low-fat sour cream for regular sour cream
- Lemon juice and herbs for heavy salad dressings
- Fat-free salad dressings for regular salad dressings
- Fruit for rich appetizers or desserts
- Consommé or bouillon instead of cream soups
- Water-packed canned foods rather than those packed in oil or syrup

TABLE 16-4 Foods to Allow or to Use in Moderation on a Low-kcal Diet

FOODS TO ALLOW	FOODS TO USE IN MODERATION	
Fat-free milk, low-fat buttermilk, low-fat yogurt	Cream soups	Jellies and jams
Low-fat cottage cheese and other fat-free-milk cheeses	Cream sauces	Processed meats
Eggs, except prepared with fat	Cream in any form	Salad dressing
Lean beef, lamb, veal, pork, chicken, turkey, fish	Gravies	Cakes
Clear soup	Rich desserts	Cookies
Whole grain or enriched bread	Sweet drinks and sodas	Pastries
Vegetables low in carbohydrates	Alcoholic beverages	Oily fish
Fresh fruits and those canned in their own juice or in water	Candy	Whole milk
Coffee or tea, without milk and sugar	Fried foods	Butter
Salt, pepper, herbs, garlic, and onions	Cheese	Sugar
	Nuts	

There are many low-kcal, fat-free, low-fat, sugar-free, and dietetic foods on the market. A food that is said to be fat-free or sugar-free is not kcal-free. The food label must be read to determine if the product can fit into a healthy eating plan for weight reduction. Dietetic foods are usually reserved for diabetics. Diet soda can act as a diuretic and can make one hungry, and it should be used in moderation. Ice water with lemon or lime slices makes a pleasant kcal-free drink and helps prevent dehydration.

Some foods that can be eaten with relative disregard for kcal content (provided they are served without additional kcal-rich ingredients) are listed in Table 16-5.

TABLE 16-5 Low-kcal Foods That May Be Used Freely on a Weight-Loss Diet

Black coffee	Cauliflower
Plain tea or tea with lemon	Broccoli
Cantaloupe	Celery
Strawberries	Cucumbers
Lettuce	Red and green peppers
Cabbage	Bean sprouts
Asparagus	Mushrooms
Tomatoes	Spinach
Zucchini	

Cooking Methods

Cooking methods should be considered. Broiling, grilling, baking, roasting, poaching, or boiling are the preferred methods because they do not require the addition of fat, as frying does. Skimming of fat from the tops of soups and meat dishes, reduces their fat content, as does trimming fat from meats before cooking. The addition of extra butter or margarine to foods should be avoided.

Exercise

Exercise, particularly aerobic exercise, is an excellent adjunct to any weight-loss program. Aerobic exercise uses energy from the body's fat reserves as it increases the amount of oxygen the body takes in. Examples are dancing, jogging, bicycling, skiing, rowing, and power walking. Such exercise helps tone the muscles, burns kcal, increases the BMR so food is burned faster, and is fun for the participant. Any exercise program must begin slowly and increase over time so that no physical damage occurs.

Exercise alone can only rarely replace the actual diet, however. The dieter should be made aware of the number of kcal burned by specific exercises so as to avoid overeating after the workout.

Behavior Modification for Weight Loss

Behavior modification means change in habits. The fundamental behavior modifications for a weight-loss program are the development of a new and healthy eating plan and the development of an exercise program that can be used over the long term. These are both major lifestyle changes, and one may need to participate in a support group or undergo psychological counseling in order to successfully adapt to these changes.

It is important that one learn the difference between hunger and appetite. **Hunger** is the physiological need for food that is felt 4 to 6 hours after eating a full meal. **Appetite** is a learned psychological reaction to food caused by pleasant memories of eating it. For example, after eating a full meal one is unlikely to be hungry. Yet, when dessert is served, appetite causes one to want to eat it. One must learn to listen to one's body and recognize the difference between hunger and appetite. Additional behavior modifications are given below.

hunger
physiological need for food

appetite
learned psychological reaction to food caused by pleasant memories of eating

1. Weigh regularly (for example, once a week), but do not weigh yourself daily.
2. Don't wait too long between meals.
3. Join a support group and go to meetings during and after the weight loss.
4. Eat slowly.
5. Use a small plate.
6. Use low-kcal garnishes.
7. Eat whole, fresh foods. Avoid processed foods.
8. Treat yourself with something other than food.
9. Anticipate problems (e.g., banquets and holidays). "Undereat" slightly before and after.
10. "Save" some kcal for snacks and treats.
11. If something goes wrong, don't punish yourself by eating.
12. If there is no weight loss for one week, realize that lean muscle mass is being produced from exercising or there may be retention of water.
13. If a binge does occur, don't punish yourself by continuing to binge. Stop it! Go for a walk, to a movie, to a museum. Call a friend.
14. Adapt family meals to suit your needs. Don't make a production of your diet. Avoid the heavy-kcal items. Limit yourself to a spoonful of something too rich for a weight-loss diet. Substitute something you like that is low in kcal.
15. Take small portions.
16. Eat vegetables and bread without butter or margarine.
17. Include daily exercise. Park further from work and walk.

Patience and encouragement are needed throughout the adoption of a healthful diet and exercise regime. Temptation is everywhere, and the dieter should be forewarned. Just one piece of chocolate cake could set the diet back for half a day (400 to 500 kcal) and lower resistance to

TABLE 16-6 Sample Menus for a Low-kcal Diet—1,200 kcal

BREAKFAST	LUNCH	DINNER
Orange juice (½ cup = 50 kcal)	Sliced chicken	Half grapefruit (80 kcal)
Poached egg (80 kcal)	(½ breast = 3 oz at 140 kcal)	Lean roast beef (3 oz = 200 kcal)
Whole wheat toast (1 slice = 75 kcal)	Asparagus on lettuce	Baked potato (100 kcal)
Margarine (1 tsp = 33 kcal)	(4 spears = 10 kcal + lettuce leaves	Cooked carrots (½ cup = 35 kcal)
Fat-free milk (½ cup = 45 kcal)	at 5 kcal) with cottage cheese	Lettuce and tomato salad
Black coffee	(2 oz = 50 kcal)	(⅛ head lettuce = 8 kcal;
	Bread (1 slice = 75 kcal)	½ tomato = 15 kcal)
	Margarine (1 tsp. = 33 kcal)	Bread (½ slice = 35 kcal)
	Cantaloupe (½ melon = 50 kcal)	Margarine (1 tsp = 33 kcal)
	Black coffee or tea	Strawberries (1 cup fresh = 55 kcal)
		Fat-free milk (½ cup = 45 kcal)
		Black coffee or tea

future temptation. Breaking the diet one day will make it seem easy to break it a second day, and so on. Fresh vegetables and drinks of water may be used to harmlessly prevent or soothe the hunger pains that are bound to appear. The human body needs 8 glasses of water each day, and water can give one a feeling of being full. A short walk or a few minutes of exercise may help to turn the dieter's thoughts from food. Sample menus for a low-kcal diet are shown in Table 16-6.

Fad Diets

Many of the countless fad diets regularly published in magazines and books are **crash diets**. This means they are intended to cause a very rapid rate of weight reduction. Often **fad diets** require the purchase of expensive foods. Others are part of a weight-loss plan including exercise with special equipment. Expensive food items and equipment can add to the burden of dieting.

A crash diet usually does result in an initial rapid weight loss. However, the weight loss is thought to be caused by a loss of body water and lean muscle mass rather than body fat. Sudden weight loss of this type is followed by a **plateau period**: that is, a period in which weight does not decrease. Disillusionment is apt to occur during this period and may cause the dieter to go on an "eating binge." This can result in regaining the weight that was lost and sometimes more. This weight gain in turn causes the dieter to try another weight-loss diet, creating a **yo-yo effect**.

Some popular reducing diets severely limit the foods allowed, providing a real danger of nutrient deficiencies over time, and their restricted nature makes them boring. Some provide too much cholesterol and fat, contributing to atherosclerosis. Some contain an excess of protein, which puts too great a demand on the kidneys. The powdered varieties of weight-loss diets available are not only expensive and

crash diets

fad-type diets intended to reduce weight very quickly; in fact they reduce water, not fat tissue

fad diets

currently popular weight-reducing diets; usually nutritionally inadequate and not useful or permanent methods of weight reduction

plateau period

period in which there is no change

yo-yo effect

refers to crash diets; the dieter's weight goes up and down over short periods because these diets do not change eating habits

inconvenient (if one is not at home to prepare them), they can be life-threatening if they fail to supply sufficient potassium for the heart.

These diets ultimately fail because they defeat the dual purpose of the dieter, which is to lose weight and prevent its returning. Both can be accomplished only if eating habits are changed, and crash diets do not do this.

Surgical Treatment of Obesity

When obesity becomes morbid (damaging to health) and dieting and exercising are not working, surgery could be indicated. Two of the surgical procedures used are the gastric bypass and stomach banding. Both procedures reduce the size of the stomach.

In gastric bypass, most of the stomach is stapled off, creating a pouch in the upper part. The pouch is attached directly to the jejunum so that the food eaten bypasses most of the stomach (Figure 16-2). In stomach banding, the stomach is also stapled but to a slightly lesser degree than in gastric bypass. The food moves to the duodenum, but the outlet from the upper stomach is somewhat restricted (Figure 16-2). In both procedures the reduced stomach capacity limits the amount of food that can be eaten, and fewer nutrients are absorbed. Consequently weight is lost.

morbid
damaging to health

gastric bypass
surgical reduction of the stomach

stomach banding
surgical reduction of stomach, but to lesser degree than bypass

jejunum
the middle section comprising about two-fifths of the small intestine

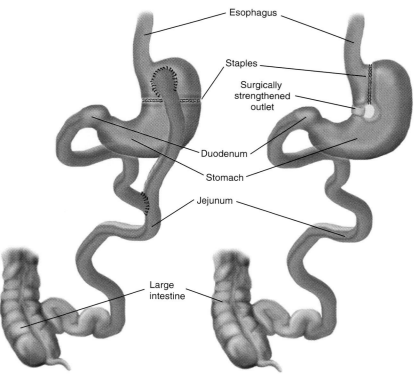

GASTRIC BYPASS   STOMACH BANDING

FIGURE 16-2 Gastric bypass and stomach banding.

These procedures are done only on morbidly obese patients who have been very carefully screened. Patients undergoing either procedure need follow-up with a dietitian in order to develop nutritionally sound diets and appropriate behavior modification.

Some obese people think that such a procedure would be their salvation, believing that, after it, they could eat as much as they wanted and still lose weight. It may not be salvation. Common complications of this type of surgery include diarrhea and consequent electrolyte and fluid imbalances, liver problems, kidney stones, and bone disease—the last probably caused by reduced absorption of minerals and vitamins.

Pharmaceutical Treatment of Obesity

The use of any weight-loss medication, whether by prescription or over the counter, should be considered very carefully. Miracles are still in short supply.

amphetamines
drugs intended to inhibit appetite

Amphetamines (pep pills) have been prescribed for the treatment of obesity because they depress the appetite. However, it has been learned that their effectiveness is reduced within a relatively short time. The dosage must be regularly increased; they cause nervousness and insomnia; and they can become habit-forming. Consequently, they are rarely prescribed now. Over-the-counter diet pills are available. They are intended to reduce appetite but are not thought to be effective. In addition to caffeine and artificial sweeteners, they contain **phenylpropanolamine**, which can damage blood vessels and should be avoided.

phenylpropanolamine
constituent of diet pills; can damage blood vessels

diuretics
substances used to increase the amount of urine excreted

Some people believe that **diuretics** and laxatives promote weight loss. They do, but only of water. They do not cause a reduction of body fat, which is what the dieter is seeking. An excess of either could be dangerous because of possible upsets in fluid and electrolyte balance. In addition, laxatives can become habit-forming. They should not be used on any frequent or regular basis without the supervision of a physician.

Although there is no magic pill to help those with excess weight reduce, the wish for one remains, and pharmaceutical companies continue the search. Some of the products developed in recent years were approved by the Food and Drug Administration (FDA) but subsequently were recalled when it was learned that they appeared to cause heart valve damage in 30% of patients using them. Two of these, fenfluramine (Pondimin®) and dexfenfluramine (Redux™), depress appetite. When either of these drugs is combined with phentermine, an amphetamine-like drug, the combination is called "fen-phen." Phentermine increases the rate at which kcal are used by the body.

UNDERWEIGHT
Dangers

Underweight can cause complications of pregnancy and various nutritional deficiencies. It may lower one's resistance to infections and, if carried to the extreme, can cause death.

Causes

Underweight can be caused by inadequate consumption of nutritious food because of depression, disease, anorexia nervosa, bulimia, or poverty, or it can be genetically determined. It also can be caused by excessive activity, the tissue wasting of certain diseases, poor absorption of nutrients, infection, or **hyperthyroidism**. For further discussion of anorexia nervosa and bulimia, see Chapter 13.

Treatment

Underweight is treated by a high-kcal diet or by a high-kcal diet combined with psychological counseling if the condition is psychological in origin as, for example, in depression or anorexia nervosa. In many cases, a high-kcal diet will be met with resistance. It can be as difficult for an underweight person to gain weight as it is for an overweight person to lose it.

The diet should be based on the Food Guide Pyramid so that it can be easily adapted from the regular, family menus or to a soft-textured diet. The total number of kcal prescribed per day will vary from person to person, depending on the person's activity, age, size, gender, and physical condition.

If the individual is to gain one pound a week, 3,500 kcal in addition to the individual's basic normal weekly kcal requirement are prescribed. This means an extra 500 kcal must be taken in each day. If a weight gain of two pounds per week is required, an additional 7,000 kcal each week, or an additional 1,000 kcal per day, are necessary. This diet cannot be immediately accepted at full kcal value. Time will be needed to gradually increase the daily kcal value. In this diet, there is an increased intake of foods rich in carbohydrates, some fats, and protein. Vitamins and minerals are supplied in adequate amounts. If there are deficiencies of some vitamins and minerals, supplements are prescribed.

Nearly all nutritious foods are allowed in the high-kcal diet, but easily digested food (carbohydrates) are recommended. Because an excess of fat can be distasteful and spoil the appetite, fatty foods must be used with discretion. Fried foods are not recommended. Bulky foods should be used sparingly. Bulk takes up stomach space that could be better used for more concentrated, high kcal foods. See Table 16-7 for high-kcal and high-protein shakes and spread that could be used to increase kcal intake.

Persons requiring this diet frequently have poor appetites, so meals should be made especially appetizing. Favorite foods should be served, and portions of all foods should be small to avoid discouraging the patients. Many of the extra kcal needed may be gotten as snacks between meals, unless these snacks reduce the patient's appetite for meals and consequently reduce daily kcal total. Some patients do better if the number of meals is reduced, thereby increasing the appetite for each meal served. When the causes of underweight are psychological, therapy is required before the diet is begun, and the diet counselor and therapist may well need to consult one another before and during treatment. Foods to be avoided in a high-kcal diet are foods the patient dislikes, fatty foods, and bulky, low-kcal foods.

hyperthyroidism
condition in which the thyroid gland secretes too much thyroxine and T_3; the body's rate of metabolism is unusually high

TABLE 16-7 High-kcal and High-Protein Shakes and Spread

HIGH-KCAL SHAKE: 6 OZ SERVING

½ cup vanilla ice cream	1 Tbsp. vegetable oil
½ cup corn syrup	1 tsp. chocolate syrup
2 Tbsp. whole milk	

Place ingredients in blender and blend at high speed until smooth. Drink immediately.

kcal, 530; protein, 4g; sodium, 165 mg; potassium, 180 mg; phosphorus, 135 mg

HIGH-KCAL, HIGH-PROTEIN SHAKE: 8 OZ SERVING

¼ cup Egg Beaters	2 Tbsp. corn syrup, honey, or sugar
½ cup whipping cream	½ tsp. vanilla, if desired**
½ cup vanilla ice cream*	

Beat Egg Beaters until frothy. Add other ingredients and beat until well blended. Refrigerate. This recipe may be made by the quart and stored for 2–3 days. *Strawberry ice cream may be substituted. **Substitute ½ tsp. maple, black walnut, rum, or chocolate flavoring for vanilla.

kcal, 685; protein, 14g; sodium, 155 mg; potassium, 325 mg; phosphorus, 225 mg

PEANUT BUTTER SNACK SPREAD: ⅛ CUP SERVING

1 Tbsp. instant dry milk	1 Tbsp. honey
1 tsp. water	3 heaping Tbsp. peanut butter
1 tsp. vanilla	

Combine dry milk, water, and vanilla, stirring to moisten. Add honey and peanut butter, stirring slowly until liquid blends with peanut butter. Spread between graham crackers or soda crackers. The spread can also be formed into balls, chilled, and eaten as candy. Keeps well in refrigerator, but is difficult to spread when cold.

kcal, 440; protein, 17g

CONSIDERATIONS FOR THE HEALTH CARE PROFESSIONAL

Even for the most determined patients, a successful weight-loss program will be charged with anxiety. There will be days of disappointment. It will take a long time to reach the ultimate goal. The health care professional will need to supply psychological support and nutritional advice when disappointing results create the need for emotional support. It is essential that the health care professional see the problems, support the patient, and then effectively lead her or him back to the diet. The key words for the health care professional are *support* and *encouragement*.

● SUMMARY

Excessive weight endangers health and should be lost by the use of a restricted-kcal diet based on the Food Guide Pyramid. Such a diet helps the dieter change eating habits and avoid regaining the lost weight. Excess weight is usually caused by energy imbalance. Exercise is beneficial to weight-loss regimens but rarely can replace the restricted-kcal diet. Fad diets are expensive, boring, and may lead to nutritional deficiencies. They ultimately fail because they do not change eating habits. Underweight is also dangerous to health, and psychological counseling as well as a high-kcal diet may be required for proper treatment. Behavior modification must be an essential component of any weight-loss or weight-gain regimen.

● DISCUSSION TOPICS

1. Discuss *overweight, obesity,* and *underweight.* Tell how someone may be overweight according to the weight charts and still be considered to be in good physical condition. What factors contribute to the determination of one's correct weight?

2. What are some causes of overweight? Discuss why some people eat more than they need. Discuss how overeating can be prevented or changed.

3. Explain why changing eating habits is essential to an effective weight-loss program.

4. Name 10 foods that may be used without concern as to kcal during a weight-loss program. Explain why.

5. Describe the use of exercise during a weight-loss program. Could it be used in lieu of the diet? Why?

6. Describe one or two popular reducing diets. Could such a diet have any effect on the nutrition of those people who subscribe to it? If so, what? Ask if anyone in the class has used such a diet. If anyone has, ask that person to describe the diet, the physical effects felt during the diet, and the ultimate result.

7. Explain why a high-kcal diet could be unpleasant for a patient.

8. Discuss the causes and dangers of underweight.

● SUGGESTED ACTIVITIES

1. Using Table A-4 in the Appendix, look for kcal values of ten favorite foods. Make two lists. On the left, list which of the ten foods would be suitable for a high-kcal diet. On the right side, list those foods suitable for a low-kcal diet.

2. Make a list of foods eaten yesterday. Circle those foods that would not be suitable for a low-kcal diet. Explain why.

3. Find recipes that are suitable for the high-kcal diet and others that are suitable for the low-kcal diet. Compare and discuss.

● REVIEW

Multiple choice. Select the *letter* that precedes the best answer.

1. The general type of foods that should be avoided in the low-kcal diet are
   a. fatty foods
   b. foods the patient likes
   c. breads and cereals
   d. coffee and tea

2. In the high-kcal diet, the energy value
   a. is increased
   b. is decreased
   c. is reduced to minimal levels
   d. remains the same as on the regular diet

3. The low-kcal diet may be prescribed for
   a. obesity
   b. anorexia nervosa
   c. hyperthyroidism
   d. severe allergies

4. In the low-kcal diet, the energy value
   a. remains the same as for the regular diet
   b. is decreased
   c. is increased
   d. should equal that of the clear liquid diet

5. A proper weight reduction plan allows for loss of
   a. 1 to 2 pounds per day
   b. 1 to 2 pounds per week
   c. 3 to 5 pounds per week
   d. 15 to 20 pounds per month

6. Popular crash diets
   a. are always effective and totally harmless
   b. are useful for teenagers
   c. result in a slow, even loss of weight
   d. are potentially hazardous

7. Normal weight
   a. is always the same for two people of the same sex and height
   b. does not change during one's lifetime
   c. may be greater than the amounts indicated on the weight charts
   d. all of the above

8. A caliper is used
   a. to measure the amount of weight to be lost
   b. to determine the percentage of body fat
   c. to determine the percentage of bone tissue
   d. only in cases of gross obesity

9. The most common cause of overweight is
   a. hypothyroidism
   b. hyperthyroidism
   c. energy imbalance
   d. all of the above

10. The dysfunction of the thyroid gland in which the basal metabolic rate is lowered and the need for kcal is reduced is called
    a. hypothyroidism
    b. hyperthyroidism
    c. energy imbalance
    d. all of the above

11. The dysfunction of the thyroid gland in which the basal metabolic rate is raised and the need for kcal is increased is called
    a. hypothyroidism
    b. hyperthyroidism
    c. energy imbalance
    d. goiter

12. To lose 2 pounds per week, one must reduce weekly kcal by
    a. 500
    b. 1,000
    c. 3,500
    d. 7,000

13. To lose 1 pound per week, one must reduce weekly kcal by
    a. 500
    b. 1,000
    c. 3,500
    d. 7,000

14. The key to losing weight and maintaining the reduced weight is
    a. skipping lunch
    b. fasting one day each week
    c. changing eating habits
    d. assiduously counting kcal each meal

15. Strawberries, yogurt, poached egg, and whole wheat toast would
    a. be allowed on a kcal-restricted diet
    b. not be allowed on a low-kcal diet
    c. constitute a poor breakfast for someone on a high-kcal diet
    d. not be a nutritious breakfast for someone on a weight-control diet

16. Baking, roasting, broiling, boiling, and poaching are recommended for
    a. low-kcal diets only
    b. high-kcal diets only
    c. both high- and low-kcal diets
    d. none of the above

17. Large green salads with creamy dressings are recommended for
    a. low-kcal diets
    b. high-kcal diets
    c. both low- and high-kcal diets
    d. neither low- nor high-kcal diets

18. Fad diets are not recommended as reducing diets because they
    a. usually cause illness
    b. alter eating habits excessively
    c. do not alter eating habits
    d. require an excessive amount of time before weight loss occurs

19. Someone on a weight-reduction diet with the goal of losing 80 pounds
   a. will undoubtedly have a BMI of 20 or less
   b. can eat fat-free foods with abandon
   c. should avoid all carbohydrates
   d. should not weigh himself daily

20. Amphetamines are
   a. an excellent method of maintaining a depressed appetite
   b. interchangeable with diuretics
   c. frequently used today
   d. dangerously habit-forming

C A S E   S T U D Y

Ken was a 35-year-old father of two who had been divorced for four years. Ken wanted to start dating again. He missed having an adult to talk to as a friend. But he was embarrassed by the extra weight he had gained. He was about 5 feet 10 inches tall and currently weighed 220 pounds. He knew he was overweight, and he had not been faithful about exercising. Ken was a fair cook and could make basic meals. A typical dinner was some meat, vegetables, cut-up fresh fruit, and milk. He let the kids have candy or sweets only on special occasions. He made sure they ate breakfast together before school. In warm weather, breakfast was cold cereal and juice. Even the little kids could handle that themselves. In the winter, breakfast was oatmeal and hot chocolate. Ken was proud of the fact that neither of the kids was in trouble or had poor grades at school. He made sure they were both busy in after-school sports programs until he came home from work.

He passed his physical with his doctor and told the doctor of his plan to get back in shape and lose weight. The doctor advised him to avoid the fad weight-loss pills and advertised quick-weight-loss plans. The doctor gave Ken a couple of pamphlets on safe weight-loss programs that he wanted Ken to consider. The doctor asked Ken to check back in 3 months so that he could monitor his progress.

ASSESSMENT

1. What do you know about Ken and his current priorities? What is a new priority he wants to add to his life?

2. Use the rule of thumb to determine Ken's ideal weight.

3. How long will it take him to reach his ideal weight if he loses 1 or 2 pounds a week?

4. What major changes does Ken need to make to lose weight?

5. Use the BMI to determine whether he is at risk for health problems at his current weight.

DIAGNOSIS

6. What would be the best method for Ken to lose weight?

7. Was Ken eating nutritiously?

8. What changes do you think Ken needs to make in his diet?

PLAN/GOAL

9. What are some reasonable measurable goals for Ken?

IMPLEMENTATION

10. What are the advantages and disadvantages of each of the following methods of weight loss for Ken?
    a. Weight Watchers
    b. Jenny Craig
    c. Slimfast and low-fat diet

11. What are the advantages of each of the following exercise plans for Ken?
    a. Self-guided plan
    b. Health club near home
    c. Hospital-based facility

12. Looking at the options in questions 10 and 11 above and taking into consideration Ken's priorities, what type of program would you recommend for Ken?

(continued)

C A S E S T U D Y
(continued)

13. How can the children help?

14. What low-kcal foods can Ken keep at work and at home that he can eat when he is hungry between meals?

15. What does Ken need to learn to drink to help with his weight loss?

EVALUATION/OUTCOME CRITERIA

16. In 3 months when Ken returns to the doctor, what changes will Ken be able to report, and what will the doctor be able to measure?

17. If Ken follows your program, how long will it take before he will have lost enough weight to consider dating?

C A S E S T U D Y

Margaret was a 55-year-old German-born woman who was 5 feet 3 inches tall and weighed 250 pounds. She had been heavy all of her life but ballooned to over 200 pounds in the last 5 years. Margaret loved buttered French bread toasted in the oven. For variety, she would melt different cheeses on the bread. She loved peanut butter and jelly sandwiches, cream cheese on bagels, and every kind of dessert. She ate fruit and vegetables, but they weren't her favorite foods. She had tried fad diets. She would lose 10–15 pounds, but, as she tired of the diet, she would gain it all back and more. Food had always been her friend and source of comfort.

She was recently put on hypertension medication. It seemed as if she was always tired. In the past 3 months she had been unable to even walk from her car to the office without getting short of breath and having to stop several times. She was experiencing sleep apnea at night. She was getting pretty upset with the situation and concerned about her health. She asked her doctor about gastric bypass surgery. He reluctantly agreed to have her screened. He discussed at length the necessary lifestyle and dietary and exercise changes she would have to make for the surgery to be successful.

She was scheduled for the surgery after 2 months of research on her part and assessment by physicians to ensure it was safe. After the surgery, she was placed on a rigorous, closely supervised recovery program. Her sister had to agree to move in with her for this period to be her recovery coach. Margaret attended classes about the meaning of food, how to eat, weight loss, exercise, and behavior modification.

ASSESSMENT

1. What do you know about Margaret? What was her new priority?

2. What is her ideal weight?
   a. How many pounds does she need to lose?
   b. How long should it take to be done safely?

3. What is her current risk for health problems on the basis of her BMI?

4. What are her known health problems?

5. At what weight will her health risk be reasonable?

(continued)

C A S E S T U D Y
(continued)

6. How long will it take to reach that reasonable health risk weight?

DIAGNOSIS

7. What are Margaret's nutritional problems?

8. What nutrition education is needed? Is there any other education needed?

9. What other diagnoses apply to Margaret?

PLAN/GOAL

10. Write at least three goals for Margaret that are reasonable and measurable.

11. What are some low-kcal vegetables that Margaret could eat freely?

12. What are some food substitutions that Margaret needs to learn?

13. What does she need to learn about reading food labels? What is the difference between fat-free, sugar-free, and dietetic?

14. What seasonings would help give Margaret some variety?

15. What is essential for Margaret to learn about controlling the size of portions of foods she wants to eat?

16. What are some behavior modification hints or tips related to where and when she eats that would help her?

17. Before she was accepted for surgery, Margaret had to join a hospital-based health club or purchase a home treadmill. Given her level of activity intolerance, what is reasonable to expect of Margaret in the first month? In 3 months? In 6 months?

18. Margaret was instructed to turn in her home scale to the doctor's office and to see him every Friday morning to weigh in and have her blood pressure checked. What is the rationale for these directions?

19. What is the rationale for having her sister move in with her?

20. What does Margaret need to learn in behavior modification class in order to lose weight and keep it off?

EVALUATION/OUTCOME CRITERIA

21. What changes should the doctor see, hear, and be able to measure that are indicative of success?

Chapter 17

Diet and Diabetes Mellitus

Key Terms

acidosis
aspartame
coma
diabetes mellitus
diabetic coma
endogenous insulin
etiology
exchange lists
exogenous insulin
gestational diabetes
glucagon
glycosuria
hyperglycemia
hypoglycemia
insulin
insulin-dependent
  diabetes mellitus
  (type 1 or IDDM)

insulin reaction
ketonemia
ketones
ketonuria
neuropathy
non-insulin-
  dependent
  diabetes mellitus
  (type 2 or NIDDM)
oral diabetes
  medications
pancreas
polydipsia
polyphagia
polyuria
renal threshold
retinopathy
vascular system

Objectives

After studying this chapter, you should be able to:

● Describe diabetes mellitus and identify the types

● Describe the symptoms of diabetes mellitus

● Explain the relationship of insulin to diabetes mellitus

● Discuss appropriate nutritional management of diabetes mellitus

Diabetes mellitus is the name for a group of serious and chronic (long-standing) disorders affecting the metabolism of carbohydrates. These disorders are characterized by **hyperglycemia** (abnormally large amounts of glucose in the blood). Diabetes mellitus afflicts between 10 and 12 million people in the United States. It is a major cause of death; blindness; heart and kidney disease; amputations of toes, feet, and legs; and infections.

Hundreds of years ago, a Greek physician named it *diabetes*, which means "to flow through," because of the large amounts of urine generated by victims. Later, the Latin word *mellitus*, which means "honeyed," was added because of the amount of glucose in the urine.

Diabetes insipidus is a different disorder. It also generates large amounts of urine, but it is "insipid," not sweet. This is a rare condition, caused by a damaged pituitary gland. It is not discussed in this chapter.

The body needs a constant supply of energy, and glucose is its primary source. Carbohydrates provide most of the glucose, but about 10% of fats and up to nearly 60% of proteins can be converted to glucose if necessary.

The distribution of glucose must be carefully managed for the maintenance of good health. Glucose is transported by the blood, and its entry into the cells is controlled by hormones. The primary hormone in this work is insulin.

Insulin is secreted by the beta cells of the islets of Langerhans in the pancreas gland. When there is inadequate production of insulin or the body is unable to use the insulin it produces, glucose cannot enter the cells and it accumulates in the blood, creating hyperglycemia. This condition can cause serious complications.

Another hormone, glucagon, which is secreted by the alpha cells of the islets of Langerhans, helps release energy when needed by converting glycogen to glucose. Somatostatin is a hormone produced by the delta cells of the islets of Langerhans and the hypothalamus. It is thought to participate in the regulation of insulin secretion.

The amount of glucose in the blood normally rises after a meal. The pancreas reacts by providing insulin. As the insulin circulates in the blood, it binds to special insulin receptors on cell surfaces. This binding causes the cells to accept the glucose. The resulting reduced amount of glucose in the blood in turn signals the pancreas to stop sending insulin.

SYMPTOMS OF DIABETES MELLITUS

The abnormal concentration of glucose in the blood of diabetic patients draws water from the cells to the blood. When hyperglycemia exceeds the renal threshold, the glucose is excreted in the urine (glycosuria). With the loss of the cellular fluid, the patient experiences polyuria (excessive urination) and polydipsia (excessive thirst) typically results.

The inability to metabolize glucose causes the body to break down its own tissue for protein and fat. This response causes polyphagia (excessive appetite), but at the same time a loss of weight, weakness, and fatigue occur. The body's use of protein from its own tissue causes it to excrete nitrogen.

Because the untreated diabetic patient cannot use carbohydrates for energy, excessive amounts of fats are broken down, and consequently the liver produces ketones from the fatty acids. In healthy people, ketones are subsequently broken down to carbon dioxide and water, yielding energy. In diabetic patients, fats break down faster than the body can handle them. Ketones collect in the blood (ketonemia) and must be excreted in the urine (ketonuria). Ketones are acids that lower blood pH, causing acidosis. Acidosis can lead to diabetic coma, which can result in death if the patient is not treated quickly with fluids and insulin.

In addition to the symptoms previously mentioned, diabetic patients suffer from diseases of the vascular system. Atherosclerosis (a condition in which there is a heavy buildup of fatty substances inside artery walls, reducing blood flow) is a major cause of death among diabetic

---

diabetes mellitus
chronic disease in which the body lacks the normal ability to metabolize glucose

hyperglycemia
excessive amounts of sugar in the blood

insulin
secretion of the islets of Langerhans in the pancreas gland; essential for the proper metabolism of glucose

glucagon
hormone from alpha cells of pancreas; helps cells release energy

pancreas
gland that secretes enzymes essential for digestion and insulin, which is essential for glucose metabolism

renal threshold
kidneys' capacity

glycosuria
excess sugar in the urine

polyuria
excessive urination

polydipsia
abnormal thirst

polyphagia
excess hunger

ketones
substances to which fatty acids are broken down in the liver

ketonemia
ketones collected in the blood

ketonuria
ketone bodies in the urine

acidosis
condition in which excess acids accumulate or there is a loss of base in the body

diabetic coma
unconsciousness caused by a state of acidosis due to too much sugar or too little insulin

vascular system
circulatory system

retinopathy
damage to small blood vessels in the eyes

neuropathy
nerve damage

etiology
cause

insulin-dependent diabetes mellitus (type 1 or IDDM)
diabetes occurring suddenly between the ages of 1 and 40; patients secrete little, if any, insulin and require insulin injections and a carefully controlled diet

non-insulin-dependent diabetes mellitus (type 2 or NIDDM)
diabetes occurring after age 40; onset is gradual and production of insulin gradually diminishes; can usually be controlled by diet and exercise

patients. Damage to the small blood vessels can cause retinal degeneration. Retinopathy is the leading cause of blindness in the United States. Nerve damage (neuropathy) is not uncommon, and infections, particularly of the urinary tract, are frequent problems.

ETIOLOGY

The etiology (cause) of diabetes mellitus is not confirmed. Although it appears that diabetes mellitus may be hereditary, environmental factors also may contribute to its occurrence. For example, viruses or obesity may precipitate the disease in people who have a genetic predisposition.

The World Health Organization indicates that the prevalence of the disease is increasing worldwide, especially in areas showing improvement in living standards.

CLASSIFICATION

The two major types of diabetes mellitus are IDDM or type 1, which is also known as insulin-dependent diabetes mellitus, and NIDDM or type 2, also known as non-insulin-dependent diabetes mellitus.

Type 1 was formerly classified as juvenile-onset diabetes mellitus. It occurs between the ages of 1 and 40 and includes from 10 to 20% of all diabetes cases. These patients secrete little, if any, insulin and thus become insulin-dependent, requiring both insulin injections and a carefully controlled diet. This type of diabetes occurs suddenly, exhibiting many of the symptoms described in the preceding section. It can be difficult to control.

Type 2 was previously called adult-onset diabetes. It is less severe than type 1. It usually occurs after the age of 40. Its onset is gradual as the amount of insulin produced each day gradually diminishes. It is not uncommon for the patient to have no symptoms and to be totally ignorant of her or his condition until it is discovered accidentally during a routine urine or blood test or after a heart attack or stroke.

This type of diabetes can usually be controlled by diet and exercise, or by diet, exercise, and an oral glucose-lowering medication. Table 17-1 shows four types of oral glucose-lowering medications in order from newest and most frequently used to oldest and least frequently used. The goals of medical nutrition therapy for patients with type 2 include maintaining healthy glucose, blood pressure, and lipid levels. Also, because approximately 80% of type 2 patients are overweight, these patients may be placed on weight-reduction diets after their blood glucose levels are within acceptable range. Thus, monitoring their weight loss also becomes part of their therapy.

gestational diabetes
diabetes occurring during pregnancy; usually disappears after delivery of the infant

Gestational diabetes can occur between the sixteenth and twenty-eighth week of pregnancy. If it is not responsive to diet and exercise, insulin injection therapy will be used. It is recommended that a dietitian and or a diabetic educator be consulted to plan an adequate diet that will control blood sugar for mother and baby.

TABLE 17-1 Four Types of Oral Diabetes (Glucose-Lowering) Medications

NON-SULFONYLUREA	
Glucophage (Metformin)	
ALPHA-GLUCOSIDASE INHIBITOR	
Precose (Acarbose)	
SECOND-GENERATION SULFONYLUREAS	
Diabeta	Glucotrol (Glipizide)
Micronase (Glyburide)	Gluctrol XL
Glynase prestabs	Amaryl (Glimepiride)
FIRST-GENERATION SULFONYLUREAS	
Diabinese (Chlorpropimide)	Tolinase (Tolazamide)
Orinase (Tolbutamide)	Dymelor (Acetoheximide)

oral diabetes medications
oral hypoglycemic agents, medications that may be given to type 2 diabetes mellitus patients to lower blood glucose

Concentrated sugars should be avoided. Weight gain should continue, but not in excessive amounts. Usually, gestational diabetes disappears after the infant is born. However, diabetes mellitus can develop 5 to 10 years after the pregnancy (see Chapter 11).

Secondary diabetes mellitus occurs infrequently and is caused by certain drugs or by a disease of the pancreas.

TREATMENT OF DIABETES MELLITUS

The treatment of diabetes mellitus is intended to:

1. Control blood glucose levels
2. Provide optimal nourishment for the patient
3. Prevent symptoms and thus delay the complications of the disease

Treatment is typically begun when blood tests indicate hyperglycemia or when other previously discussed symptoms occur. Normal blood glucose levels (called fasting blood sugar, FBS) are from about 70 to 110 mg/dl.

Treatment can be by diet alone or by a diet combined with insulin or a glucose-lowering medication plus regulated exercise and the regular monitoring of the patient's blood glucose levels.

The physician and dietitian can provide essential testing, information, and counseling and can help the patient delay potential damage. The ultimate responsibility, however, rests with the patient. When a person with diabetes mellitus uses nicotine, eats carelessly, forgets insulin, ignores symptoms, and neglects appropriate blood tests, she or he increases the risk of developing permanent tissue damage.

NUTRITIONAL MANAGEMENT OF DIABETES MELLITUS

The dietitian will need to know the patient's diet history, food likes and dislikes, and lifestyle at the onset. The patient's kcal needs will depend on age, activities, lean muscle mass, size and REE.

It is recommended that carbohydrates provide 50 to 60% of the kcal. Approximately 40 to 50% should be from complex carbohydrates (starches). The remaining 10 to 20 percent of carbohydrates could be from simple sugar.

Research provides no evidence that carbohydrates from simple sugars are digested and absorbed more rapidly than are complex carbohydrates, and they do not appear to affect blood sugar control. It is the *total amount of carbohydrates eaten* that affects blood sugar levels rather than the type. Being able to substitute foods containing sucrose for other carbohydrates increases flexibility in meal planning for the diabetic.

Fats should be limited to 30% of total kcal, and proteins should provide from 15 to 20% of total kcal. Lean proteins are advisable because they contain limited amounts of fats.

Regardless of the percentages of energy nutrients prescribed, the foods ultimately eaten should provide sufficient vitamins and minerals as well as energy nutrients.

The patient with type 1 diabetes needs a nutritional plan that balances kcal and nutrient needs with insulin therapy and exercise. It is important that meals and snacks be composed of similar nutrients and kcal, and eaten at regular times each day. Small meals plus two or three snacks may be more helpful in maintaining steady blood glucose levels for these patients than three large meals each day.

The patient with type 1 diabetes should anticipate the possibility of missing meals occasionally and carry a few crackers and some cheese or peanut butter to prevent **hypoglycemia**, which can occur in such a circumstance.

hypoglycemia
subnormal levels of blood sugar

The patient with type 2 diabetes may be overweight. The nutritional goal for this patient is not only to keep blood glucose levels in the normal range but to lose weight as well. Exercise can help attain both goals.

Carbohydrate Counting

Carbohydrate counting is the newest method for teaching a diabetic how to control blood sugar with food. The starch/breads, milk, and fruits have all been put under the heading of "carbohydrates." This means that these three food groups can be interchanged within one meal. One would still have the same number of servings of carbohydrates, but it would not be the typical number of starches, or fruits and milk that one usually eats. For example, one is to have four carbohydrates for breakfast (2 breads, 1 fruit, and 1 milk). If there is no milk available, a bread or fruit must be eaten in place of the milk. The exchange lists are utilized in carbohydrate counting as well as in traditional meal planning. Protein, approximately 3–4 oz., is eaten for lunch and dinner. One or two fat exchanges are recommended for each meal. Two carbohydrates should be eaten for an evening snack. These are only beginning guidelines. A dietitian or diabetic educator can help tailor this to the individual patient.

Diets Based on Exchange Lists

The method of diet therapy most commonly used for diabetic patients is that based on **exchange lists**. These lists were developed by the American Diabetes Association in conjunction with the American Dietetic Association and are summarized in Table 17-2 and included completely in Table 17-3.

exchange lists

lists of foods with interchangeable nutrient and kcal contents; used in specific forms of diet therapy

TABLE 17-2 Summary of Exchange Lists

GROUP/LIST	CARBOHYDRATE (grams)	PROTEIN (grams)	FAT (grams)	KCAL
Carbohydrate Group				
Starch	15	3	1 or less	80
Fruit	15	–	–	60
Milk				
Fat-free	12	8	0–3	90
Reduced-fat (2%)	12	8	5	120
Whole	12	8	8	150
Other carbohydrates	15	varies	varies	varies
Vegetables	5	2	–	25
Meat and Meat Substitute Group				
Very lean	–	7	0–1	35
Lean	–	7	3	55
Medium-fat	–	7	5	75
High-fat	–	7	8	100
Fat Group	–	–	5	45

Source: Exchange List for Meal Planning. The American Diabetes Association and The American Dietetic Association, 1995.

TABLE 17-3 Exchange Lists for Meal Planning

STARCH EXCHANGE LIST	
One starch exchange equals 15g carbohydrate, 3g protein, 0–1g fat, and 80 kcal	
Bread/Starches	
Bagel	½ (1 oz)
Bread, reduced-calorie	2 slices (1½ oz)
Bread, white, whole-wheat, pumpernickel, rye	1 slice (1 oz)
Bread sticks, crisp, 4 in. long × ½ in.	2 (⅔ oz)
English muffin	½
Hot dog or hamburger bun	½ (1 oz)
Pita, 6 in. across	½
Raisin bread, unfrosted	1 slice (1 oz)
Roll, plain, small	1 (1 oz)

(continued)

TABLE 17-3 *continued*

Bread (*continued*)

Tortilla, corn, 6 in. across	1
Tortilla, flour, 7–8 in. across	1
Waffle, 4½ in. square, reduced-fat	1

Beans, Peas, and Lentils (*Count as 1 starch exchange, plus 1 very lean meat exchange.*)

Beans and peas (garbanzo, pinto, kidney, white, split, black-eyed)	½ cup
Lima beans	⅔ cup
Lentils	½ cup
Miso*	3 Tbsp.

* = 400 mg or more sodium per exchange.

Cereals and Grains

Bran cereals	½ cup
Bulgur	½ cup
Cereals	½ cup
Cereals, unsweetened, ready-to-eat	¾ cup
Cornmeal (dry)	3 Tbsp.
Couscous	⅓ cup
Flour (dry)	3 Tbsp.
Granola, low-fat	¼ cup
Grape-Nuts®	¼ cup
Grits	½ cup
Kasha	½ cup
Millet	¼ cup
Muesli	¼ cup
Oats	½ cup
Pasta	½ cup
Puffed cereal	1½ cups
Rice milk	½ cup
Rice, white or brown	⅓ cup
Shredded Wheat®	½ cup
Sugar-frosted cereal	½ cup
Wheat germ	3 Tbsp.

Crackers and Snacks

Animal crackers	8
Graham crackers, 2½ in. square	3
Matzoh	¾ oz
Melba toast	4 slices
Oyster crackers	24
Popcorn (popped, no fat added or low-fat microwave)	3 cups

(*continued*)

TABLE 17-3 *continued*

Crackers and Snacks (*continued*)

Pretzels	¾ oz
Rice cakes, 4 in. across	2
Saltine-type crackers	6
Snack chips, fat-free (tortilla, potato)	15–20 (¾ oz)
Whole-wheat crackers, no fat added	2–5 (¾ oz)

Starchy Vegetables

Baked beans	⅓ cup
Corn	½ cup
Corn on cob, medium	1 (5 oz)
Mixed vegetables with corn, peas, or pasta	1 cup
Peas, green	½ cup
Plantain	½ cup
Potato, baked or boiled	1 small (3 oz)
Potato, mashed	½ cup
Squash, winter (acorn, butternut)	1 cup
Yam, sweet potato, plain	½ cup

Starchy Foods Prepared with Fat (*Count as 1 starch exchange, plus 1 fat exchange.*)

Biscuit, 2½ in. across	1
Chow mein noodles	½ cup
Corn bread, 2 in. cube	1 (2 oz)
Crackers, round butter type	6
Croutons	1 cup
French-fried potatoes	16–25 (3 oz)
Granola	¼ cup
Muffin, small	1 (1½ oz)
Pancake, 4 in. across	2
Popcorn, microwave	3 cups
Sandwich crackers, cheese or peanut butter filling	3
Stuffing, bread (prepared)	⅓ cup
Taco shell, 6 in. across	2
Waffle, 4½ in. square	1
Whole-wheat crackers, fat added	4–6 (1 oz)

MEAT AND SUBSTITUTES LIST

Very Lean Meat and Substitutes List *One exchange equals 0g carbohydrate, 7g protein, 0–1g fat, and 35 kcal*

- One very lean meat exchange is equal to any one of the following items.

Poultry: Chicken or turkey (white meat, no skin),
Cornish hen (no skin)   1 oz

(continued)

TABLE 17-3 *continued*

Very Lean Meat and Substitutes List (*continued*)

Fish: Fresh or frozen cod, flounder, haddock, halibut, trout; tuna fresh or canned in water	1 oz
Shellfish: Clams, crab, lobster, scallops, shrimp, imitation shellfish	1 oz
Game: Duck or pheasant (no skin), venison, buffalo, ostrich	1 oz
Cheese with 1 gram or less fat per ounce:	
Nonfat or low-fat cottage cheese	¼ cup
Fat-free cheese	1 oz
Other: Processed sandwich meat with 1 gram or less fat per ounce, such as deli thin, shaved meats, chipped beef*, turkey ham	1 oz
Egg whites	2
Egg substitutes, plain	¼ cup
Hot dogs with 1 gram or less fat per ounce*	1 oz
Kidney (high in cholesterol)	1 oz
Sausage with 1 gram or less fat per ounce	1 oz

• Count as one very lean meat and one starch exchange.

Beans, peas, lentils (cooked)	½ cup

* = 400 mg or more sodium per exchange.

Lean Meat and Substitutes List *One exchange equals 0g carbohydrate, 7g protein, 3g fat, and 55 kcal*

• One lean meat exchange is equal to any one of the following items.

Beef: USDA Select or Choice grades of lean beef trimmed of fat, such as round, sirloin, and flank steak; tenderloin; roast (rib, chuck, rump); steak (T-bone, porterhouse, cubed), ground round	1 oz
Pork: Lean pork, such as fresh ham; canned, cured, or boiled ham; Canadian bacon *; tenderloin, center loin chop	1 oz
Lamb: Roast, chop, leg	1 oz
Veal: Lean chop, roast	1 oz
Poultry: Chicken, turkey (dark meat, no skin), chicken (white meat, with skin), domestic duck or goose (well-drained of fat, no skin)	1 oz
Fish:	
Herring (uncreamed or smoked)	1 oz
Oysters	6 medium
Salmon (fresh or canned), catfish	1 oz
Sardines (canned)	2 medium
Tuna (canned in oil, drained)	1 oz

(*continued*)

TABLE 17-3 *continued*

Lean Meat and Substitutes List (*continued*)

Game: Goose (no skin), rabbit	1 oz
Cheese:	
4.5%-fat cottage cheese	¼ cup
Grated Parmesan	2 Tbsp.
Cheeses with 3 grams or less fat per ounce	1 oz
Other:	
Hot dogs with 3 grams or less fat per ounce *	1½ oz
Processed sandwich meat with 3 grams or less fat per ounce, such as turkey pastrami or kielbasa	1 oz
Liver, heart (high in cholesterol)	1 oz

Medium-Fat Meat and Substitutes List *One exchange equals 0g carbohydrate, 7g protein, 5g fat, and 75 kcal*

• One medium-fat meat exchange is equal to any one of the following items.

Beef: Most beef products fall into this category (ground beef, meatloaf, corned beef, short ribs, Prime grades of meat trimmed of fat, such as prime rib)	1 oz
Pork: Top loin, chop, Boston butt, cutlet	1 oz
Lamb: Rib roast, ground	1 oz
Veal: Cutlet (ground or cubed, unbreaded)	1 oz
Poultry: Chicken (dark meat, with skin), ground turkey or ground chicken, fried chicken (with skin)	1 oz
Fish: Any fried fish product	1 oz
Cheese: With 5 grams or less fat per ounce	
Feta	1 oz
Mozzarella	1 oz
Ricotta	¼ cup (2 oz)
Other:	
Eggs (high in cholesterol, limit to 3 per week)	1
Sausage with 5 grams or less fat per ounce	1 oz
Soy milk	1 cup
Tempeh	¼ cup
Tofu	4 oz or ½ cup

High-Fat Meat and Substitutes List *One exchange equals 0g carbohydrate, 7g protein, 8g fat, and 100 kcal*

Remember these items are high in saturated fat, cholesterol, and calories and may raise blood cholesterol levels if eaten on a regular basis.

• One high-fat meat exchange is equal to any one of the following items.

Pork: Spareribs, ground pork, pork sausage	1 oz	
Cheese: All regular cheeses, such as American*, cheddar, Monterey Jack, Swiss	1 oz	(*continued*)

TABLE 17-3 *continued*

High-Fat Meat and Substitutes List (*continued*)

Other: Processed sandwich meats with 8 grams
or less fat per ounce, such as bologna, pimento
loaf, salami | 1 oz
  Sausage, such as bratwurst, Italian, knockwurst,
    Polish, smoked | 1 oz
  Hot dog (turkey or chicken)* | 1 (10/lb)
  Bacon | 3 slices (20 slices/lb)

• Count as one high-fat meat plus one fat exchange.

Hot dog (beef, pork, or combination)* | 1 (10/lb)
Peanut butter (contains unsaturated fat) | 2 Tbsp.

* = 400 mg or more sodium per exchange.

FRUIT EXCHANGE LIST

Fruit *One Fruit exchange equals 15g carbohydrate and 60 kcal*
The weight includes skin, core, seeds, and rind.

Apple, unpeeled, small	1 (4 oz)
Applesauce, unsweetened	½ cup
Apples, dried	4 rings
Apricots, fresh	4 whole (5½ oz)
Apricots, dried	8 halves
Apricots, canned	½ cup
Banana, small	1 (4 oz)
Blackberries	¾ cup
Blueberries	¾ cup
Cantaloupe, small	⅓ melon (11 oz) or 1 cup cubes
Cherries, sweet, fresh	12 (3 oz)
Cherries, sweet, canned	½ cup
Dates	3
Fruit cocktail	½ cup
Grapefruit, large	½ (11 oz)
Grapefruit sections, canned	¾ cup
Grapes, small	17 (3 oz)
Honeydew melon	1 slice (10 oz) or 1 cup cubes
Kiwi	1 (3½ oz)
Mandarin oranges, canned	¾ cup
Mango, small	½ cup
Nectarine, small	1 (5 oz)
Orange, small	1 (6½ oz)
Papaya	½ fruit (8 oz) or 1 cup cubes
Peach, medium, fresh	1 (6 oz)
Peaches, canned	½ cup *(continued)*

TABLE 17-3 *continued*

Fruit (*continued*)

Pear, large, fresh	½ (4 oz)
Pears, canned	½ cup
Pineapple, fresh	¾ cup
Pineapple, canned	½ cup
Plums, small	2 (5 oz)
Prunes, dried	3
Raisins	2 Tbsp.
Raspberries	1 cup
Strawberries	1¼ cup whole berries
Tangerines, small	2 (8 oz)
Watermelon	1¼ cup cubes

Fruit Juice

Apple juice/cider	½ cup
Cranberry juice cocktail	⅓ cup
Cranberry juice cocktail, reduced-calorie	1 cup
Fruit juice blends, 100% juice	⅓ cup
Grape juice	⅓ cup
Grapefruit juice	½ cup
Orange juice	½ cup
Pineapple juice	½ cup
Prune juice	⅓ cup

MILK EXCHANGE LIST

Fat-free and Very Low-fat Milk:

Each item on this list contains 12g of carbohydrate, 8g of protein, a trace of fat, and 90 kcal. One exchange is equal to any one of the following items:

Fat-free	1 cup
½% milk	1 cup
Low-fat milk (1%)	1 cup
Low-fat buttermilk	1 cup
Evaporated fat-free milk	½ cup
Dry nonfat milk	⅓ cup
Plain nonfat yogurt	¾ cup
Nonfat or Low-fat fruit flavored yogurt sweetened with aspartame	1 cup

Low-fat Milk:

Each item on this list contains 12g of carbohydrate, 8g of protein, 5g of fat, and 120 kcal. One exchange is equal to any one of the following items:

Reduced-fat milk (2%)	1 cup
Plain low-fat yogurt (with added nonfat milk solids)	¾ cup

(continued)

TABLE 17-3 *continued*

Whole Milk:

Each item on this list contains 12g of carbohydrate, 8g of protein, 8g of fat, and 150 kcal. One exchange is equal to any one of the following items:

Whole milk	1 cup
Evaporated whole milk	½ cup
Whole plain yogurt	8 oz

FAT EXCHANGE LIST

Each item on this list contains 5g of fat, and 45 kcal.
One exchange is equal to any one of the following items:

Unsaturated

Avocado	⅛ medium or 1 oz.
Margarine	1 tsp.
Margarine, diet	1 Tbsp.
Mayonnaise	1 tsp.
Mayonnaise, reduced-calorie	1 Tbsp.
Nuts and Seeds:	
Almonds, dry roasted	6 whole
Cashews, dry roasted	6 whole
Pecans	2 whole
Peanuts	10 nuts
Peanut butter	2 tsp.
Seeds, pine nuts, sunflower, (without seeds)	1 Tbsp.
Oil (canola, corn, cottonseed, safflower, soybean, sunflower, olive, peanut)	1 tsp.
Olives, ripe; black	8 large
Olives, green, stuffed	10 large
Salad dressing, mayonnaise-type	2 tsp.
Salad dressing, mayonnaise type, reduced-calorie	1 Tbsp.
Salad dressing (all varieties)	1 Tbsp.
Salad dressing, reduced-calorie	2 Tbsp.

Saturated

Butter	1 tsp.
Bacon	1 slice
Chitterlings, boiled	½ oz
Coconut, shredded	2 Tbsp.
Cream (light, coffee, table)	2 Tbsp.
Cream, sour	2 Tbsp.
Cream (half and half)	2 Tbsp.
Cream cheese	1 Tbsp.
Salt Pork	1″ × 1″ × ¼″ if eaten

Source: The American Diabetes Association and the American Diabetic Association.

TABLE 17-3 *continued*

OTHER CARBOHYDRATES EXCHANGE LIST

One exchange equals 15g carbohydrate, or 1 starch, or 1 fruit, or 1 milk.

FOOD	SERVING SIZE	EXCHANGES PER SERVING
Angel food cake, unfrosted	1/12 cake	2 carbohydrates
Brownie, small, unfrosted	2 in. square	1 carbohydrate, 1 fat
Cake, unfrosted	2 in. square	1 carbohydrate, 1 fat
Cake, frosted	2 in. square	2 carbohydrates, 1 fat
Cookie, fat-free	2 small	1 carbohydrate
Cookie or sandwich cookie with creme filling	2 small	1 carbohydrate, 1 fat
Cranberry sauce, jellied	¼ cup	1½ carbohydrates
Cupcake, frosted	1 small	2 carbohydrates, 1 fat
Doughnut, plain cake	1 medium (1½ oz)	1½ carbohydrates, 2 fats
Doughnut, glazed	3¾ in. across (2 oz)	2 carbohydrates, 2 fats
Fruit juice bars, frozen, 100% juice	1 bar (3 oz)	1 carbohydrate
Fruit snacks, chewy (pureed fruit concentrate)	1 roll (¾ oz)	1 carbohydrate
Fruit spreads, 100% fruit	1 Tbsp.	1 carbohydrate
Gelatin, regular	½ cup	1 carbohydrate
Gingersnaps	3	1 carbohydrate
Granola bar	1 bar	1 carbohydrate, 1 fat
Granola bar, fat-fee	1 bar	2 carbohydrates
Honey	1 Tbsp.	1 carbohydrate
Hummus	⅓ cup	1 carbohydrate, 1 fat
Ice cream	½ cup	1 carbohydrate, 2 fats
Ice cream, light	½ cup	1 carbohydrate, 1 fat
Ice cream, fat-free, no sugar added	½ cup	1 carbohydrate
Jam or jelly, regular	1 Tbsp.	1 carbohydrate
Milk, chocolate, whole	1 cup	2 carbohydrates, 1 fat
Pie, fruit, 2 crusts	⅙ pie	3 carbohydrates, 2 fats
Pie, pumpkin or custard	⅛ pie	1 carbohydrate, 2 fats
Potato chips	12–18 (1 oz)	1 carbohydrate, 2 fats
Pudding, regular (made with low-fat milk)	½ cup	2 carbohydrates
Pudding, sugar-free (made with low-fat milk)	½ cup	1 carbohydrate
Salad dressing, fat-free*	¼ cup	1 carbohydrate
Sherbet, sorbet	½ cup	2 carbohydrates
Spaghetti or pasta sauce, canned*	½ cup	1 carbohydrate, 1 fat
Sugar	1 Tbsp.	½ carbohydrate
Sweet roll or Danish	1 (2½ oz)	2½ carbohydrates, 2 fats
Syrup, light	2 Tbsp.	1 carbohydrate
Syrup, regular	1 Tbsp.	1 carbohydrate
Syrup, regular	¼ cup	4 carbohydrates
Tortilla chips	6–12 (1 oz)	1 carbohydrate, 2 fats
Vanilla wafers	5	1 carbohydrate, 1 fat
Yogurt, frozen, low-fat, fat-free	⅓ cup	1 carbohydrate, 0–1 fat
Yogurt, frozen, fat-free, no sugar added	½ cup	1 carbohydrate
Yogurt, low-fat with fruit	1 cup	3 carbohydrates, 0–1 fat

* = 400 mg or more sodium per exchange.

Under this plan, foods are categorized by type and included in the lists in Table 17-3.

The foods within each list contain approximately equal amounts of kcal, carbohydrates, protein, and fats. This means that any one food on a particular list can be substituted for any other food on that *particular list* and still provide the patient with the prescribed types and amounts of nutrients and kcal.

The amounts of nutrients and kcal on one list are not the same as those on any other list. Each list includes serving size by volume or weight and the kcal value of each food item, in addition to the grams of carbohydrates, and, when appropriate, proteins and fats. The number of kcal needed will determine the number of items prescribed from any particular list. These lists also can be used to control kcal content of diets and are thus appropriate for low-kcal diets.

The total energy requirements for adult diabetic patients who are not overweight will be the same as for nondiabetic individuals. When patients are overweight, a reduction in kcal will be built into the diet plans, typically allowing for a weight loss of one pound a week.

The diet is given in terms of exchanges rather than as particular foods. For example, the menu pattern for breakfast may include 1 fruit exchange, 1 meat exchange, 2 bread exchanges, and 2 fat exchanges. The patient may choose the desired foods from the exchange lists for each meal but must adhere to the specific exchange lists named and the specific number of exchanges on each list. Vegetables (nonstarchy) are relatively free and can be eaten in amounts up to 1½ cups cooked or 3 cups raw. If more than this amount is eaten at one meal, count the additional amount as one more carbohydrate. Snacks are built into the plan. In this way, the patient has variety in a simple yet controlled way.

When there are changes in one's physical condition, such as pregnancy or lactation, or in one's lifestyle, the diet will need to be modified. A change in job or in working hours can affect nutrient and kcal requirements. When such changes occur, the patient should be advised to consult her or his physician or dietitian so that kcal and insulin needs can be promptly adjusted.

MISCELLANEOUS CONCERNS OF THE DIABETIC PATIENT

Fiber

The therapeutic value of fiber in the diabetic diet has become increasingly evident. High fiber intake appears to reduce the amount of insulin needed because it lowers blood glucose. It also appears to lower the blood cholesterol and triglyceride levels. High fiber may mean 25 or 35g of dietary fiber a day. Such high amounts can be difficult to include. High-fiber foods should be increased very gradually, as an abrupt increase can create intestinal gas and discomfort. When increasing fiber in the diet one must also increase intake of water. An increased fiber intake can affect mineral absorption.

Alternative Sweeteners

Saccharin has been shown to produce bladder cancer in rats when used in large quantities. Aspartame is the generic name for an additional sweetener composed of two amino acids, phenylalanine and aspartic acid. It does not require insulin for metabolism. Both have been approved by the FDA, and the American Diabetes Association has given its approval for their use. Sucralose, a sweetener made from a sugar molecule that has been altered in such a way that the body will not absorb it, was also recently approved by the FDA.

aspartame
artificial sweetener made from amino acids; does not require insulin for metabolism

Dietetic Foods

The use of diabetic or dietetic foods is generally a waste of money and can be misleading to the patient. Often the containers of foods will contain the same ingredients as containers of foods prepared for the general public, but the cost is typically higher for the dietetic foods. There is potential danger for diabetic patients who use these foods if they do not read the labels on the food containers and assume that because they are labeled "dietetic," they can be used with abandon. In reality, their use should be in specified amounts only, because these foods will contain carbohydrates, fats, and proteins that must be calculated in the total day's diet.

It is advisable for the diabetic patient to use foods prepared for the general public but to avoid those packed in syrup or oil. The important thing is for the diabetic patient to *read the label* on all food containers purchased.

Alcohol

Although alcohol is not recommended for diabetic patients, its limited use is sometimes allowed if approved by the physician. However, some diabetic patients who use hypoglycemic agents cannot tolerate alcohol. When used, it must be included in the diet plan.

Exercise

Exercise helps the body use glucose by increasing insulin receptor sites and stimulating the creation of glucagon. It lowers cholesterol and blood pressure and reduces stress and body fat as it tones the muscles. For patients with type 2 diabetes, exercise helps improve weight control, glucose levels, and the cardiovascular system.

However, for patients with type 1 diabetes, exercise can complicate glucose control. As it lowers glucose levels, hypoglycemia can develop. Exercise must be carefully discussed with the patient's physician. If done, it should be on a regular basis, and it must be considered carefully as the meal plans are developed so that sufficient kcal and insulin are prescribed.

Insulin Therapy

Patients with type 1 diabetes must have injections of insulin every day to control their blood glucose levels (Figure 17-1). This insulin is called

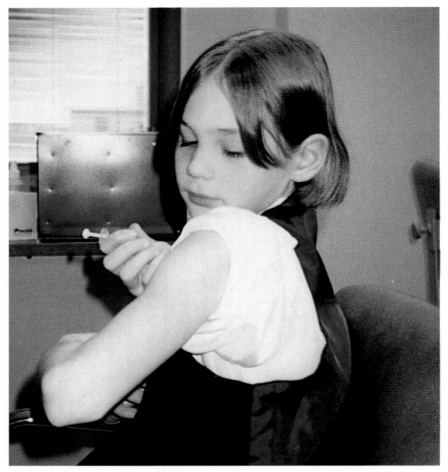

FIGURE 17-1 This young diabetic is self-injecting insulin into the upper arm. (Courtesy of the Diabetes Center of Albany Memorial Hospital, Albany, NY)

exogenous insulin
is produced outside the body

endogenous insulin
insulin produced within the body

exogenous insulin because it is produced outside the body. **Endogenous insulin** is produced by the body.

Exogenous insulin must be injected because it is a protein and, if swallowed, it would be digested and would not reach the bloodstream as the complete hormone. After insulin treatment is begun, it is usually necessary for the patient to continue it throughout life.

Human insulin is the most common insulin given to patients. This insulin does not come from humans but is made synthetically by a chemical process in a laboratory. Human insulin is preferred because it is very similar to insulin made by the pancreas. Animal insulin comes from cows or pigs and is called beef or pork insulin. These insulins are not used as often as human insulin because they contain antibodies that make them less pure than human insulin.

There are various types of insulin available. They differ in the length of time required before they are effective and in the length of time they continue to act. This latter category is called insulin action. Consequently, they are classified as very rapid-, rapid-, intermediate-, and long-acting. Those most commonly used are intermediate-acting types that work within 2 to 8 hours and are effective for 24 to 28 hours. For type 1 diabetes, insulin is often given in two or more injections daily and may contain more than one type of insulin. Injections are given at prescribed times.

Insulin Reactions

When patients do not eat the prescribed diet but continue to take the prescribed insulin, hypoglycemia can result. This is called an **insulin reaction**, or *hypoglycemic episode,* and may lead to **coma**. Symptoms include headache, blurred vision, tremors, confusion, poor coordination, and eventual unconsciousness. Insulin reaction is dangerous because if frequent or prolonged, brain damage can occur. (The brain must have sufficient amounts of glucose in order to function.) The physician should be consulted if an insulin reaction occurs or seems imminent.

Conscious patients may be treated by giving them a glucose tablet, a sugar cube, or a beverage containing sugar followed by a complex carbohydrate. If the patient is unconscious, intravenous treatment of dextrose and water is given. It is advisable for the diabetic patient to carry identification explaining the condition so that people do not think he or she is drunk when, in reality, the person is experiencing an insulin reaction.

insulin reaction
hypoglycemia leading to insulin coma caused by too much insulin or too little food

coma
state of unconsciousness

CONSIDERATIONS FOR THE HEALTH CARE PROFESSIONAL

It is important to point out to the diabetic patient that one can live a near-normal life if the diet is followed, medication is taken as prescribed, and time is allowed for sufficient exercise and rest. The importance of eating all of the prescribed food must be emphasized. It is important for meals to be eaten at regular times so that the insulin-glucose balance can be maintained. It is imperative that the patient learn to read carefully all labels on commercially prepared foods.

Adjustments must be made in shopping, cooking, and eating habits so that the diet plan can be followed. Family meals can be simply adapted for the diabetic diet. The diabetic patient soon learns which exchange lists are to be included at each meal and at snack times and the foods within each exchange list. (See Table 17-3 for the exchange lists, Table 17-4 for free foods, and Table 17-5 for seasonings that can be used.)

● SUMMARY

The diabetic diet is used in treating diabetes mellitus, a metabolic disease caused by the improper functioning of the pancreas that results in inadequate production or utilization of insulin. If the condition is left untreated, the body cannot use glucose properly, and then serious complications, even death, can occur. Treatment includes diet, medication, and exercise. Diabetic diets are prescribed by the physician or dietitian in consultation with the patient.

TABLE 17-4 Free Foods Allowed on the Exchange List

FREE FOOD LIST

A *free food* is any food or drink that contains less than 20 kcal or less than 5g of carbohydrate per serving. Foods with a serving size listed should be limited to three servings per day. Be sure to spread them out throughout the day. Eating all three servings at one time could affect your blood glucose level. Foods listed without a serving size can be eaten as often as you like.

Fat-Free or Reduced-Fat Foods

Cream cheese, fat-free	1 Tbsp.
Creamers, nondairy, liquid	1 Tbsp.
Creamers, nondairy, powdered	2 tsp.
Mayonnaise, fat-free	1 Tbsp.
Mayonnaise, reduced-fat	1 tsp.
Margarine, fat-free	4 Tbsp.
Margarine, reduced-fat	1 tsp.
Miracle Whip®, nonfat	1 Tbsp.
Miracle Whip®, reduced-fat	1 tsp.
Nonstick cooking spray	
Salad dressing, fat-free	1 Tbsp.
Salad dressing, fat-free, Italian	2 Tbsp.
Salsa	¼ cup
Sour cream, fat-free, reduced-fat	1 Tbsp.
Whipped topping, regular light	2 Tbsp.

Drinks

Bouillon, broth, consommé*	
Bouillon or broth, low-sodium	
Carbonated or mineral water	
Club soda	
Cocoa powder, unsweetened	1 Tbsp.
Coffee	
Diet soft drinks, sugar-free	
Drink mixes, sugar-free	
Tea	
Tonic water, sugar-free	

Sugar-Free or Low-Sugar Foods

Candy, hard, sugar-free	1 candy
Gelatin dessert, sugar-free	
Gelatin, unflavored	
Gum, sugar-free	
Jam or jelly, low-sugar or light	2 tsp.
Syrup, sugar-free	2 Tbsp.

Sugar substitutes, alternatives, or replacements that are approved by the Food and Drug Administration (FDA) are safe to use. Common brand names include:

- Equal® (aspartame)
- Sprinkle Sweet® (saccharin)
- Sweet One® (acesulfame K)
- Sweet-10® (saccharin)
- Sugar Twin® (saccharin)
- Sweet 'n Low® (saccharin)

Condiments

Catsup	1 Tbsp.
Horseradish	
Lemon juice	
Lime juice	
Mustard	
Pickles, dill*	1½ large
Soy sauce, regular or light*	
Taco sauce	1 Tbsp.
Vinegar	

Source: The American Diabetes Association and the American Dietetic Association.

* = 400 mg or more of sodium per exchange.

TABLE 17-5 Useful Seasonings

Read the label, and choose those seasonings that do not contain sodium or salt.

Basil (fresh)	Garlic	Oregano
Celery seeds	Garlic powder	Paprika
Cinnamon	Herbs	Pepper
Chili powder	Hot pepper sauce	Pimento
Chives	Lemon	Spices
Curry	Lemon juice	Soy sauce
Dill	Lemon pepper	Soy sauce, low-sodium ("lite")
Flavoring extracts	Lime	Wine, used in cooking (¼ cup)
(vanilla, almond,	Lime juice	Worcestershire sauce
walnut, peppermint,	Mint	
lemon, butter, etc.)	Onion powder	

Source: The American Diabetes Association and the American Dietetic Association.

● DISCUSSION TOPICS

1. Describe diabetes mellitus. Explain why it is a serious disease.

2. What is insulin? What is its use? Why can it not be taken orally?

3. What is the function of oral diabetes medication? For which type of diabetes is it usually prescribed?

4. Explain the differences between type 1 and type 2 diabetes.

5. Describe the symptoms of type 1 diabetes. Include the following terms: hyperglycemia, renal threshold, glycosuria, polydipsia, polyuria, polyphagia, ketones, ketonuria, and acidosis.

6. Explain why it is essential that diabetic patients read labels on food.

7. Why are "dietetic" foods not recommended for diabetic patients?

8. Discuss how an insulin reaction might occur.

9. Why must a diabetic patient's tray be checked carefully after meals?

10. Why is the use of exchange lists the most commonly used method of dietary treatment of type 1 diabetes mellitus?

11. How would pregnancy affect the diet of a patient with type 1 diabetes? How would lactation affect the diet of a patient with type 1 diabetes?

12. Discuss the effects of exercise on glucose utilization.

● SUGGESTED ACTIVITIES

1. Ask a physician or dietitian or diabetic educator to speak to the class on diabetes mellitus and its treatment.

2. Ask a diabetic educator to explain and demonstrate carbohydrate counting.

3. Visit a local supermarket and compare regular and "dietetic" containers of food in terms of cost, kcal, and nutrient content.

4. Invite someone with type 1 diabetes to talk to the class about his or her condition.

5. Invite someone with type 2 diabetes to talk to the class about his or her condition.

● REVIEW

Multiple choice. Select the *letter* that precedes the best answer.

1. Diabetes mellitus is a metabolic disorder
   a. caused by malfunction of the thyroid gland
   b. for which a low-fiber diet may be ordered
   c. in which glucose accumulates in the blood
   d. that is contagious

2. The metabolism of glucose
   a. depends on insulin secreted by the islets of Langerhans
   b. depends on enzymes present in pancreatic juice
   c. is totally dependent on the acid content of the stomach
   d. is directly related to secretions from the thyroid gland

3. Type 1 diabetes mellitus is treated by the
   1. administration of insulin
   2. exclusion of foods that contain glucose
   3. administration of thyroxine
   4. use of a low-fat diet

4. The physician may recommend as part of the nutritional management of diabetes mellitus that the diet
   a. consist of 40 to 50% proteins
   b. consist of no more than 30% carbohydrates
   c. contain 15 to 20% proteins
   d. exclude all simple sugars

5. Diets based on the exchange lists
   a. are appropriate for patients with type 1 diabetes mellitus
   b. are not appropriate for patients with type 2 diabetes mellitus
   c. eliminate all carbohydrates
   d. should not be used by nondiabetic persons who want to control their kcal

6. When an excessive amount of glucose accumulates in the blood, the condition
   a. is called hypoglycemia
   b. leads to glycosuria
   c. is known as acidosis
   d. always leads to coma

7. Diabetic coma
   a. is called alkalosis
   b. is caused by inadequate insulin
   c. is caused by an excessive amount of insulin
   d. causes polyuria

8. Type 2 diabetes mellitus
   a. usually occurs before the age of 40
   b. usually occurs after the age of 40
   c. usually requires insulin
   d. cannot be controlled by diet and a glucose-lowering medication

9. Glucose-lowering medications
   a. have exactly the same effect as insulin
   b. cannot be used for patients over 40
   c. stimulate the pancreas to produce insulin
   d. are only used for patients with type 1 diabetes mellitus

10. Diabetic diets based on the exchange lists regulate amounts of
    a. carbohydrate
    b. kcal
    c. protein and fat
    d. all of the above

C A S E   S T U D Y

Penny was a 45-year-old female who was admitted to the hospital for rotator cuff surgery. The preoperative lab work revealed a fasting blood sugar (FBS) of 320 mg/dl, which surprised Penny and her doctor. After the doctor ran more tests, it was determined that Penny had NIDDM (type 2 diabetes). She currently weighed 145 pounds and stood 5 feet 7 inches.

The doctor decided to delay the surgery until Penny could get stabilized on a diabetic diet.

The doctor referred Penny to a diabetic education program to work with the diabetic nurse specialist and the registered dietitian. Penny thought that she wouldn't have to make many changes because she ate a balanced diet already. At her first class, the dietitian asked her to write down everything she had eaten yesterday. The following list is what Penny recorded.

Breakfast
8-oz glass of orange juice
2 fried eggs
1 slice of whole wheat toast
    with 2 pats of margarine
    and 2 Tbsp. grape jelly
coffee with milk

Lunch
1 cup of cream of chicken
    soup
1 grilled cheese sandwich
    with lettuce and tomatoes
1 apple
8-oz glass of milk
½ cup of rice pudding

Dinner
2 slices of meatloaf
1 medium baked potato with
    3 pats of margarine
½ cup of broccoli
1 cup of gelatin dessert with fruit
8-oz glass of milk

For an afternoon snack, she had a cup of yogurt and canned fruit.

ASSESSMENT

1. What do you know about Penny so far?
2. Using the rule of thumb in chapter 16, what is Penny's ideal weight? Does she need to lose weight?
3. What do you know about her food choices from the one-day list?
   a. Is her diet as well balanced as she thinks it is?

DIAGNOSIS

4. What diagnoses has the doctor given Penny? What changes are needed in her current diet?

PLAN/GOAL

5. What are reasonable, measurable goals for Penny?

IMPLEMENTATION

The dietitian suggested an 1,800-kcal diet for Penny with the following distribution of categories: milk, 4; bread, 9; meat, 6; fat, 7.

6. Looking at Penny's list of foods, identify which category each food is in.
   a. Label the food so you can total each category.
   b. Add up the totals in each category.
   c. Compare the totals in each category.
   d. What are the differences?
7. Modify her food list to reflect the dietitian's recommended number of exchanges. Which foods need to be eliminated?
8. After Penny learns the exchange system, what else does she need to do to manage her diabetes?

EVALUATION/OUTCOME CRITERIA

9. At her 2-month follow-up with the diabetic team, what should Penny's FBS be?
   a. What should she be able to write out or describe?
   b. What should her weight be?

C A S E   S T U D Y

Alonzo was a 19-year-old college student who, early in his fall term, developed an insatiable appetite, yet he didn't gain any weight. His roommate, Ricardo, was irritated by the fact that Alonzo was in the bathroom so often. Alonzo complained of being thirsty all the time. He resorted to carrying his water bottle with him around campus. When Ricardo and his buddies wanted to go out Friday evening, Alonzo was too tired. Alonzo used to love to party and dance until the early hours of the morning. Alonzo thought he was tired from studying too much and shrugged off his fatigue.

When Alonzo's parents came to visit on parent's weekend in late October, they were shocked to see how thin he had become. Alonzo agreed to see a doctor on Monday. The doctor took his history and tested his urine and blood and then admitted Alonzo to the hospital.

ASSESSMENT

1. What data do you have about Alonzo?
2. What do you suspect is wrong with Alonzo?
3. What tests are necessary for confirmation of your suspicion?

DIAGNOSIS

4. What is the probable diagnosis that the doctor will give Alonzo?
5. What education will be needed for Alonzo's probable diagnosis?
6. What other diagnoses, either actual or potential, apply to Alonzo?

PLAN/GOAL

7. What goals are appropriate and measurable for Alonzo?

IMPLEMENTATION

The doctor has prescribed a mixed insulin injection for Alonzo twice a day and a diabetic diet.

8. What topics are essential for Alonzo to learn?
9. What skills does Alonzo need to master before he goes home?
10. Who else needs to be in class with Alonzo?
11. What general information about Alonzo's condition does Ricardo need to know? What does he need to know about an emergency?
12. How can Alonzo handle the Friday evening beer-drinking parties?

EVALUATION/OUTCOME CRITERIA

13. At Alonzo's 2-week follow-up appointment with the diabetic educators, what should his fasting blood sugar be?
14. What should he be able to verbalize and demonstrate?
15. What should happen to his symptoms?

Chapter 18

Diet and Cardiovascular Disease

Key Terms

angina pectoris
arteriosclerosis
atherosclerosis
cardiovascular
  disease (CVD)
cerebral vascular
  accident (CVA)
cholesterol
compensated heart
  disease
congestive heart
  failure (CHF)
decompensated
  heart disease
diuretics
edema
endocardium
essential hypertension
hyperlipidemia
hypertension

hypokalemia
infarct
ischemia
lumen
monosodium
  glutamate (MSG)
myocardial
  infarction (MI)
myocardium
pericardium
peripheral vascular
  disease (PVD)
plaque
primary hyper-
  tension
secondary hyper-
  tension
serum cholesterol
thrombus
vascular disease

Objectives

After studying this chapter, you should be able to:

● Identify factors that contribute to heart disease

● Explain why cholesterol and saturated fats are
  limited in some cardiovascular conditions

● Identify foods to avoid or limit in a cholesterol-
  controlled diet

● Explain why sodium is limited in some cardiovascular conditions

● Identify foods that are limited or prohibited in
  sodium-controlled diets

Cardiovascular disease (CVD) affects the heart and
blood vessels. It is the leading cause of death and permanent disability in the United States today. The grief and
economic distress it causes are staggering. Organiza-
tions, especially the American Heart Association, are
promoting programs designed to alert people to the risk
factors for cardiovascular disease and thereby reduce its
frequency.

Cardiovascular disease can be acute (sudden) or
chronic. **Myocardial infarction**, or **MI**, is an example
of the acute form. Chronic heart disease develops over
time and causes the loss of heart function. If the heart
can maintain blood circulation, the disease is classified

as **compensated heart disease**. Compensation usually requires that the heart beat unusually fast. Consequently, the heart enlarges. If the heart cannot maintain circulation, the condition is classified as **decompensated heart disease**, and congestive heart failure (CHF) occurs. The heart muscle (**myocardium**), the valves, the lining (**endocardium**), the outer covering (**pericardium**), or the blood vessels may be affected by heart disease.

ATHEROSCLEROSIS

Arteriosclerosis is the general term for **vascular disease** in which arteries harden (become thickened), making the passage of blood difficult and sometimes impossible. **Atherosclerosis** is the form of arteriosclerosis that most frequently occurs in developed countries. It is believed to begin in childhood and is considered one of the major causes of heart attack.

Atherosclerosis affects the inner lining of arteries (the intima), where deposits of **cholesterol**, fats, and other substances accumulate over time, thickening and weakening artery walls. These deposits are called **plaque**. (Figure 18-1). Plaque deposits gradually reduce the size of the **lumen** of the artery and, consequently, the amount of blood flow. The reduced blood flow causes an inadequate supply of nutrients and oxygen delivery to and waste removal from the tissues. This condition is called **ischemia**.

The reduced oxygen supply causes pain. When the pain occurs in the chest and radiates down the left arm, it is called **angina pectoris** and should be considered a warning. When the lumen narrows so that a blood clot (**thrombus**) occurs in a coronary artery and blood flow is cut off, a heart attack occurs. The dead tissue that results is called an **infarct**. The heart muscle that should have received the blood is the myocardium. Thus, such an attack is commonly called an acute myocardial infarction (MI). Some patients who experience an MI will require surgery to bypass the clogged artery. The procedure is a coronary artery bypass graft (CABG), which is commonly referred to as bypass surgery.

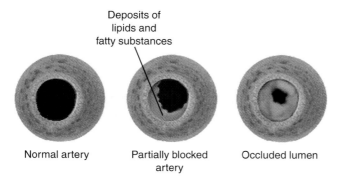

Deposits of
lipids and
fatty substances

Normal artery   Partially blocked   Occluded lumen
artery

FIGURE 18-1 Progression of atherosclerosis. (Courtesy of Delmar Publishers, Albany, NY)

---

cardiovascular disease (CVD)
disease affecting heart and blood vessels

myocardial infarction (MI)
heart attack; caused by the blockage of an artery leading to the heart

compensated heart disease
heart disease in which the heart is able to maintain circulation to all body parts

decompensated heart disease
heart disease in which the heart cannot maintain circulation to all body parts

myocardium
heart muscle

endocardium
lining of the heart

pericardium
outer covering of the heart

vascular disease
disease of the blood vessels

atherosclerosis
a form of arteriosclerosis affecting the intima (inner lining) of the artery walls

cholesterol
fatlike substance that is a constituent of body cells; is synthesized in the liver; also found in animal foods

plaque
fatty deposit on interior of artery walls

lumen
the hollow area in a tube

ischemia
reduced blood flow causing inadequate supply of nutrients and oxygen to, and wastes from, tissues

angina pectoris

pain in the heart muscle due to inadequate blood supply

thrombus

blood clot

infarct

dead tissue resulting from blocked artery

cerebrovascular accident (CVA)

either a blockage or bursting of blood vessel leading to the brain

peripheral vascular disease (PVD)

narrowed arteries some distance from the heart

hyperlipidemia

excessive amounts of fats in the blood

serum cholesterol

cholesterol in the blood

When blood flow to the brain is blocked in this way or blood vessels burst and blood flows into the brain, a stroke, or **cerebrovascular accident (CVA)**, results. When it occurs in tissue some distance from the heart, it is called **peripheral vascular disease (PVD)**.

Risk Factors

Hyperlipidemia, hypertension (high blood pressure), and smoking are major risk factors for the development of atherosclerosis. Other contributory factors are believed to include obesity, diabetes mellitus, male sex, heredity, personality type (ability to handle stress), age (risk increases with years), and sedentary lifestyle. Although some of these factors are beyond one's control, some factors are not.

It is known that dietary cholesterol and triglycerides (fats in foods and in adipose tissue) contribute to hyperlipidemia. Foods containing saturated fats increase **serum cholesterol**, whereas mono- and unsaturated fats tend to reduce it.

Lipoproteins carry cholesterol and fats in the blood to body tissues. Low-density lipoprotein (LDL) carry most of the cholesterol to the cells, and elevated blood levels of LDL are believed to contribute to atherosclerosis. High-density lipoprotein (HDL) carry cholesterol from the tissues to the liver for eventual excretion. It is believed that low serum levels of HDL can contribute to atherosclerosis.

Diet can alleviate hypertension (discussed later in this chapter), reduce obesity, and help control diabetes mellitus. A sedentary lifestyle can be changed. Exercise can help the patient lose weight, lower blood pressure, and increase the HDL ("good") cholesterol level. It must be done in consultation with the physician and be increased gradually. Also, one can stop smoking. In sum, a person can considerably reduce the risk of atherosclerosis and thus an MI, CVA, and PVD.

MEDICAL NUTRITIONAL THERAPY FOR HYPERLIPIDEMIA

Medical nutritional therapy is the primary treatment for hyperlipidemia. It involves reducing the quantity and types of fats and often kcal in the diet. When the amount of dietary fat is reduced, there is typically a corresponding reduction in the amount of cholesterol and saturated fat ingested and a loss of weight. In overweight persons, weight loss alone will help reduce serum cholesterol levels.

The American Heart Association categorizes blood cholesterol levels of 200 mg/dl or less to be desirable, 200–239 mg/dl to be borderline high, and 240 mg/dl and greater to be high.

In an effort to prevent heart disease, the American Heart Association has developed guidelines in which it is recommended that adult diets contain less than 300 mg of cholesterol per day and that fats provide no more than 30% of kcal, with a maximum of 10% from saturated fats, a maximum of 10% from polyunsaturated fats, and a maximum of 10% of monounsaturated fats. Carbohydrates should make up 50 to 55% of the kcal, and proteins from 12 to 20% of them. Currently, it is believed that nearly 40% of the kcal in the average U.S. diet come from fats.

A fat-restricted diet can be difficult for the patient to accept. A diet very low in fat will seem unusual and highly unpalatable (unpleasant-tasting) to most patients. It takes approximately 2 or 3 months to adjust to a low-fat diet. If the physician will allow it, the change in the nutrient makeup of the diet should be made gradually (Table 18-1).

Information about the fat content of foods and methods of preparation that minimize the amount of fat in the diet are essential to the patient. The patient must be taught to select whole, fresh foods and to prepare them without the addition of any fat. Only lean meat should be selected, and all visible fat must be removed. Fat-free milk and fat-free

TABLE 18-1 Foods to Include and Foods to Avoid on Fat-Restricted Diets

FOODS TO INCLUDE	FOODS TO AVOID
Breads and Cereals	
Whole grain breads and rolls	Breads made with egg or cheese, croissants
Plain buns, bagels, pita bread	Bakery products
Cereals without coconut	Butter crackers
Saltines, matzos, rusks	
Rice, pasta	
Vegetables and Fruits	
Any fresh fruit or vegetable, except	Coconut, palm oil
those on the "Avoid" list	Avocados, olives
Meats, Poultry, and Fish	
After trimming fat and removing skin before eating:	Fatty or prime-grade meats; pastrami; spareribs;
Fish, but limited shrimp or lobster	sausage; bacon; luncheon meats; domestic ducks
Lean beef, pork, lamb, veal	and geese; organ meats
Egg whites, yolks	
Dairy	
Fat-free milk or low-fat milk	Milk with more than 1% fat, cream, nondairy creamers
Dry curd or low-fat cottage cheese	Most cheese, especially process or blue
Buttermilk	
Puddings made with fat-free milk	
Other Foods	
Oils (canola, olive, peanut)	Butter
Syrup	Lard
Gelatin	Bakery desserts
Jelly	Ice creams
Honey	Fried foods
Fat-free broths	Commercially prepared meals; salad dressings
Margarine made from liquid corn, sesame, olive,	Cream soups
or sunflower oil (in limited amounts)	Cream sauces; gravies
Limited nuts	
Limited home-made salad dressings	
Sherbet	
Hard candy	

milk cheeses should be used instead of whole milk and natural cheeses. Desserts containing whole milk, eggs, and cream are to be avoided.

In a fat-controlled diet, one must be particularly careful when using animal foods. Cholesterol is found only in animal tissue. Organ meats, egg yolks, and some shellfish are especially rich in cholesterol and should be used in limited quantities, if at all. Saturated fats are found in all animal foods and in coconut, chocolate, and palm oil. They tend to be solid at room temperature. Polyunsaturated fats are derived from plants and some fish and are usually soft or liquid at room temperature. Soft margarine containing mostly liquid vegetable oil is substituted for butter, and liquid vegetable oils are used in cooking.

Studies indicate that water-soluble fiber, such as that found in oat bran, legumes, and fruits, bind with cholesterol-containing substances and prevent their reabsorption by the blood. Twenty-five to 35g of soluble fiber a day is thought to effectively reduce serum cholesterol by as much as 15%. This is a large amount of fiber and must be introduced gradually to the diet along with increased fluids or the patient will suffer from flatulence. Table 18-2 lists foods to limit on a low-cholesterol diet.

Some patients will find the use of the diabetic exchange lists useful for controlling the fat content of their diets. When fat-controlled diets are severely restricted, limiting kcal intake to 1,200, they may be deficient in fat-soluble vitamins. Consequently, a vitamin supplement may be prescribed.

If appropriate blood lipid levels cannot be attained within 3 to 6 months by the use of fat-restricted diet alone (see Table 18-3 for menus), the physician can prescribe a cholesterol-lowering drug such as lovastatin (Mevacor) or simvastatin (Zocor).

TABLE 18-2 Foods to Limit on a Low-Cholesterol Diet

Fats on meats and fish	Natural cheeses
Lard	Commercially fried foods
Organ meats	Commercially prepared baked goods
Bacon	Commercially prepared meat loaf
Luncheon meats	Commercially prepared mayonnaise
Prime-grade meats marbled with fat	Quiche Lorraine
Duck	Chicken à la king
Skin on chicken and turkey	Cheeseburgers
Crab meat	Chicken livers
Shrimp	Custard
Lobster	Soufflé
Egg yolks	Lemon meringue pie
Butter	Cheesecake
Cream	Ice cream
Whole milk	Eggnog

TABLE 18-3 Sample Menus for a Fat-Controlled Diet

BREAKFAST	LUNCH	DINNER
Orange juice	Tomato juice	3 oz chicken
Cream of wheat with	Uncreamed cottage	Baked potato
1 Tbsp. sugar and	cheese on fruit salad	Baked acorn squash
1 cup fat-free milk	(no avocado)	with 1 Tbsp. honey
1 slice toast	2 slices toast with	Lettuce salad
1 Tbsp. jelly	2 Tbsp. honey	1 slice bread
Coffee	Angelfood cake	1 Tbsp. jelly
	1 cup fat-free milk	Canned peaches
	Tea	1 cup fat-free milk
		Tea

MYOCARDIAL INFARCTION

Myocardial infarction (MI) is caused by the blockage of a coronary artery supplying blood to the heart. The heart tissue denied blood because of this blockage dies. Atherosclerosis is a primary cause, but hypertension, abnormal blood clotting, and infection such as that caused by rheumatic fever (which damages heart valves) are also contributory factors.

After the attack, the patient is in shock. This causes a fluid shift, and the patient may feel thirsty. The patient should be given nothing by mouth (NPO), however, until the physician evaluates the condition. If the patient remains nauseated after the period of shock, IV infusions are given to prevent dehydration.

After several hours, the patient may begin to eat. A liquid diet may be recommended for the first 24 hours. Following that, a low-cholesterol–low-sodium diet is usually given, with the patient regulating the amount eaten.

Foods should not be extremely hot or extremely cold. They should be easy to chew and digest and contain little roughage so that the work of the heart will be minimal. Both chewing and the increased activity of the gastrointestinal tract that follow ingestion of high-fiber foods cause extra work for the heart. The percentage of energy nutrients will be based on the particular needs of the patient, but, in most cases, the types and amounts of fats will be limited. Sodium is usually limited to prevent fluid accumulation. Some physicians will order a restriction on the amount of caffeine for the first few days after an MI. The dual goal is to allow the heart to rest and its tissue to heal.

CONGESTIVE HEART FAILURE

Congestive heart failure (CHF) is an example of decompensation, or severe heart disease. It can result from injury to the heart muscle due to atherosclerosis, hypertension, or rheumatic fever. In this situation, when damage is extreme and the heart cannot provide adequate

congestive heart failure (CHF)
a form of decompensated heart disease

edema

the abnormal retention of fluid
by the body

diuretics

substances used to increase
the amount of urine excreted

hypokalemia

low level of potassium in the
blood

circulation, the amount of oxygen taken in is insufficient for body needs. Shortness of breath is common, and chest pain can occur on exertion.

Because of the reduced circulation, tissues retain fluid that would normally be carried off by the blood. Sodium builds up, and more fluid is retained, resulting in edema. In an attempt to compensate for this pumping deficit, the heart beats faster and enlarges. This adds to the heart's burden. In advanced cases when edema affects the lungs, death can occur.

With the inadequate circulation, body tissues do not receive sufficient amounts of nutrients. This insufficiency can cause malnutrition and underweight, although the edema can mask these problems. In some cases a fluid restriction may be ordered.

Diuretics to aid in the excretion of water and sodium and a sodium-restricted diet are typically prescribed. Because diuretics can cause an excessive loss of potassium, the patient's blood potassium should be carefully watched to prevent hypokalemia, which can upset the heartbeat. Fruits, especially oranges, bananas, and prunes, can be useful in such a situation because they are excellent sources of potassium and contain only negligible amounts of sodium (Table 18-4). When necessary, the physician will prescribe supplementary potassium.

TABLE 18-4 Potassium-Rich Foods

FRUITS		
Apricots	Dates	Kiwi fruit
Oranges	Figs	Peaches
Bananas	Raisins	Pineapple
Avocados	Honeydew melon	Prunes
Cantaloupe	Grapefruit	Strawberries
VEGETABLES		
Asparagus	Squash	
Broccoli	Tomatoes	
Cabbage	Spinach	
Green beans	Potatoes, sweet potatoes, yams	
Pumpkin		

hypertension

higher than normal blood
pressure

essential hypertension

high blood pressure with
unknown cause; also called primary hypertension

primary hypertension

high blood pressure resulting
from an unknown cause

secondary hypertension

high blood pressure caused by
another condition such as kidney
disease

HYPERTENSION

When blood pressure is chronically high, the condition is called hypertension (HT). In 90% of hypertension cases, the cause is unknown, and the condition is called essential, or primary hypertension. Ten percent of the cases are called secondary hypertension because the condition is caused by another problem. Some causes of secondary hypertension include kidney disease, problems of the adrenal glands, and use of oral contraceptives.

The blood pressure commonly measured is that of the artery in the upper arm. This measurement is made with an instrument called the sphygmomanometer. The top number is the systolic pressure, taken as the heart contracts. The lower number is the diastolic pressure, taken when the heart is resting. The pressure is measured in millimeters of mercury (mm Hg). Hypertension can be diagnosed when, on several occasions, the systolic pressure is 140 mm Hg or more and the diastolic pressure is 90 mm Hg or more.

Hypertension contributes to heart attack, stroke, heart failure, and kidney failure. It is sometimes called the *silent disease* because sufferers can be asymptomatic (without symptoms). Its frequency increases with age, and it is more prevalent among African Americans than others.

Heredity and obesity are predisposing factors in hypertension. Smoking and stress also contribute to hypertension. Weight loss usually lowers the blood pressure and, consequently, patients are often placed on weight-reduction diets.

Excessive use of ordinary table salt also is considered a contributory factor in hypertension. Table salt consists of over 40% sodium plus chloride. Both are essential in maintaining fluid balance and thus blood pressure. When consumed in normal quantities by healthy people, they are beneficial.

When the fluid balance is upset and sodium and fluid collect in body tissue, causing edema, extra pressure is placed on the blood vessels. A sodium-restricted diet, often accompanied by diuretics, can be prescribed to alleviate this condition. When the sodium content in the diet is reduced, the water and salts in the tissues flow back into the blood to be excreted by the kidneys. In this way, the edema is relieved. The amount of sodium restricted is determined by the physician, on the basis of the patient's condition.

Previous research focused primarily on sodium as a primary factor in the development of hypertension, but, as research continues, the effects of chloride also are receiving increasing scrutiny. In addition, the particular roles of calcium and magnesium in relation to hypertension are being studied. Recent research indicates that increasing intake of fruits and vegetables (especially those high in potassium) to 6 to 10 servings per day helps to lower blood pressure.

DIETARY TREATMENT FOR HYPERTENSION

As indicated above, weight loss for the obese patient with hypertension usually lowers blood pressure, and, thus, a kcal-restricted diet might be prescribed. A sodium-restricted diet frequently is prescribed for patients with hypertension. A discussion of this diet follows. When diuretics are prescribed together with a sodium-restricted diet, the patient may lose potassium via the urine and, thus, be advised to increase the amount of potassium-rich foods in the diet (see Table 18-4).

Sodium-Restricted Diets

A sodium-restricted diet is a regular diet in which the amount of sodium is limited. Such a diet is used to alleviate edema and hypertension. Most people obtain far too much sodium from their diets. It is estimated that the average adult consumes 7g of sodium a day. A committee of the Food and Nutrition Board recommends that the daily intake of sodium be limited to no more than 2,400 mg (2.4g), and the Board itself set a safe minimum at 500 mg/day for adults (see Table 8-5). Sodium is found in food, water, and medicine.

It is impossible to have a diet totally free of sodium. Meats, fish, poultry, dairy products, and eggs all contain substantial amounts of sodium naturally. Cereals, vegetables, fruits, and fats contain small amounts of sodium naturally. Water contains varying amounts of sodium. However, sodium often is added to foods during processing, cooking, and at the table. The food label should indicate the addition of sodium to commercial food products. In some of these foods, the addition of sodium is obvious because one can taste it, as in prepared dinners, potato chips, and canned soups. In others, it is not. The following are examples of sodium-containing products frequently added to foods that the consumer may not notice.

monosodium glutamate (MSG)

a form of spice containing large amounts of sodium

- Salt (sodium chloride)—used in cooking or at the table, and in canning and processing.
- Monosodium glutamate (called MSG and sold under several brand names)—a seasoning used in home, restaurant, and hotel cooking and in many packaged, canned, and frozen foods.
- Baking powder—used to leaven quick breads and cakes.
- Baking soda (sodium bicarbonate)—used to leaven breads and cakes; sometimes added to vegetables in cooking or used as an "alkalizer" for indigestion.
- Brine (table salt and water)—used in processing foods to inhibit growth of bacteria; in cleaning or blanching vegetables and fruits; in freezing and canning certain foods; and for flavor, as in corned beef, pickles, and sauerkraut.
- Disodium phosphate—present in some quick-cooking cereals and processed cheeses.
- Sodium alginate—used in many chocolate milks and ice creams for smooth texture.
- Sodium benzoate—used as a preservative in many condiments such as relishes, sauces, and salad dressings.
- Sodium hydroxide—used in food processing to soften and loosen skins of ripe olives, hominy, and certain fruits and vegetables.
- Sodium propionate—used in pasteurized cheeses and in some breads and cakes to inhibit growth of mold.
- Sodium sulfite—used to bleach certain fruits in which an artificial color is desired, such as maraschino cherries and glazed or crystallized fruit; also used as a preservative in some dried fruit, such as prunes.

Because the amount of sodium in tap water varies from one area to another, the local Department of Health or the American Heart Association affiliate should be consulted if this information is needed. Softened water always has additional sodium. If the sodium content of the water is high, the patient may have to use bottled water.

Some over-the-counter medicines contain sodium. A patient on a sodium-restricted diet should obtain the physician's permission before using any medication or salt substitute. Many salt substitutes contain potassium, which affects the heartbeat.

The amount of sodium allowed depends on the patient's condition and is prescribed by the physician. In extraordinary cases of fluid retention, a diet with 1g/day can be ordered. A mild restriction limits sodium to 2g a day. A moderate restriction limits sodium to 3–4g a day.

Adjustment to Sodium Restriction

Sodium-restricted diets range from "different" to "tasteless" because most people are accustomed to salt in their food. It can be difficult for the patient to understand the necessity for following such a diet, particularly if it must be followed for the remainder of his or her lifetime. If the physician allows, it will help the patient adjust if the sodium content of the diet can be reduced gradually.

It is helpful, too, to remind the patient of the numerous herbs, spices, and flavorings allowed on sodium-restricted diets (Table 18-5). Patients will also find it useful to practice ordering from a menu so as to learn to choose those foods lowest in sodium content.

TABLE 18-5 Foods to Allow and Foods to Avoid on 1–2g Sodium-Restricted Diets

FOODS PERMITTED ON MOST SODIUM-RESTRICTED DIETS	FOODS TO LIMIT OR AVOID
Fruit juices without additives	Tomato juice and vegetable cocktail
Fresh fruits	Canned vegetables
Fresh vegetables (except for those on "Avoid" list)	Sauerkraut
Dried peas or beans	Frozen vegetables if prepared with salt
Fat-free milk	Dried, breaded, smoked, or canned fish or meats
Puffed-type cereals	Cheeses; salted butter or margarine
Regular, cooked cereals without added salt, sugar, or flavorings	Salt-topped crackers or breads
Plain pasta	Salty foods such as potato chips, salted nuts, peanut butter, pretzels
Rice	Canned fish, meats, or soups
Unsalted, uncoated popcorn	Ham, salt pork, corned beef, luncheon meats, smoked or canned fish
Fresh fish	Prepared relishes, salad dressings, catsup, soy sauce
Fresh unsalted meats	Bouillon, baking soda, baking powder, MSG
Unsalted margarine	Commercially prepared meals
Oil	
Vinegar	
Spices containing no salt, herbs, lemon juice	
Unsalted nuts	
Hard candy	
Jams, jellies, honey	
Coffee, tea	

CONSIDERATIONS FOR THE HEALTH CARE PROFESSIONAL

Patients with heart conditions serious enough to require hospitalization can be frightened, depressed, or angry. Most will be told they must reduce the fats, sodium, and, sometimes, the amount of kcal in their diets, which could make them feel overwhelmed. The health care professional will find various moods among these patients. Most will need nutritional advice. Some will want it. Some will be against the new diets. The most important thing the health care professional can do is help the cardiac patient want to learn how to help himself or herself via nutrition.

● SUMMARY

Cardiovascular disease represents the leading cause of death in the United States. It may be acute, as in myocardial infarction, or chronic, as in hypertension and atherosclerosis. Hypertension may be a symptom of other disease. Weight loss, if the patient is overweight, and a salt-restricted diet are typically prescribed.

Atherosclerosis is a vascular disease in which the arteries are narrowed by fatty deposits, reducing blood flow. Angina pectoris, myocardial infarction, or stroke can result. Because cholesterol is associated with atherosclerosis, a low-cholesterol diet or a fat-restricted diet might be prescribed.

By maintaining one's weight and activities at a healthy level, limiting salt and fat intake, and avoiding smoking, one reduces the risks of heart disease.

● DISCUSSION TOPICS

1. Why are sodium-restricted diets prescribed for patients with hypertension or heart failure?

2. What precautions might one take to prevent hypertension? To prevent atherosclerosis? Explain your answers.

3. What may occur in severe myocardial infarction? What causes myocardial infarction?

4. What are diuretics? How could they be harmful? How could this danger be avoided?

5. What is edema? How is it related to cardiovascular disease?

6. Are sodium-restricted diets nutritious? Why?

7. Why is it impossible to prepare a diet absolutely free of salt?

8. Why might a sodium-restricted diet be unpleasant for a patient?

9. Why are potato chips and peanuts not allowed on sodium-restricted diets?

10. For what heart condition might a fat-controlled diet be ordered?

11. What is cholesterol? How is it associated with atherosclerosis?

12. Why is fat-free milk allowed on low-fat diets when whole milk is not?

13. What is hyperlipidemia? How is it related to atherosclerosis?

14. Discuss known risk factors for the development of atherosclerosis. Which could be avoided? Explain.

● SUGGESTED ACTIVITIES

1. Find recipes suitable for fat-controlled diets and for a low-cholesterol diet. Compare recipes and check one another's for correctness. Suggest alternate ingredients for any that are not suitable for these diets.

2. Make a list of the foods eaten yesterday. Circle those foods that would not be allowed on a low-cholesterol diet and suggest satisfactory substitutions. Underline those not allowed on moderate sodium-restricted diets. Are any both circled and underlined?

3. Visit a local supermarket. List the foods containing sodium compounds. Suggest substitutes for these foods for patients on sodium-restricted diets.

4. Find recipes suitable for sodium-restricted diets. Compare them with other students' recipes and discuss their appropriateness.

5. Mary Jones was placed on a fat-restricted diet containing no more than 70 grams fat. She wants to order the following breakfast. Would this be acceptable? Explain your answer and, if necessary, suggest alternate foods that would be acceptable.

Sliced Avocado
Poached Egg with Ham in Cheese Sauce
on English Muffin
Coffee with cream

6. John Brown has been told that he has atherosclerosis and must follow a low-cholesterol diet. He is visiting his aunt who is serving the following meal. Which of the foods can John eat and which must he avoid? Why? Can he eat certain parts of any of the foods? If so, which? Why?

Cream of Broccoli Soup
Roast Chicken
Mashed Potatoes with Gravy
Lima Beans with Butter
Green Salad with Vinegar and Oil Dressing
Rolls and Butter
Milk
Angel Food Cake with Whipped Cream
and Strawberries

7. Susan Smith has developed hypertension and has been placed on a mild sodium-restricted diet. She has planned the following dinner for her daughter's graduation party. Which of the foods can she eat and which must she avoid? Explain.

Fresh Fruit Cup
Baked Ham
Potato Chips
Fresh Frozen Broccoli Chunks Baked in
Canned Cream of Chicken Soup
Homemade Coleslaw
Rolls and Butter
Pickles and Olives
Chocolate Cake with Peppermint Ice Cream

● REVIEW

Multiple choice. Select the *letter* that precedes the best answer.

1. Sodium
   a. is an essential vitamin
   b. regulates metabolism
   c. adds flavor to foods
   d. is found in sugar

2. Sodium is commonly found in
   a. sugar
   b. fresh fruits
   c. baking soda and baking powder
   d. coffee and tea

3. A patient with angina pectoris might be advised to follow a diet
   a. that contains limited sodium
   b. in which the kcal are increased
   c. containing minimum amounts of proteins
   d. in which saturated fats are limited

4. Herbs, spices, and flavorings may
   a. be used in sodium-restricted diets
   b. never be used in sodium-restricted diets
   c. increase sodium in the diet
   d. be used only in the mild sodium-restricted diet

5. Lipoproteins
   a. carry proteins to the cells
   b. carry cholesterol to the liver
   c. always contribute to myocardial infarction
   d. are the major cause of hypertension

6. A sodium-restricted diet may be ordered for patients with
   a. angina pectoris   c. congestive heart failure
   b. lipidemia   d. atherosclerosis

7. When water accumulates in body tissues,
   a. the condition is called edema
   b. a fat-restricted diet may be prescribed
   c. it is a definite symptom of myocardial infarction
   d. salt is completely eliminated from the diet

8. It is thought that excessive fats in the blood over time contribute to
   a. congestive heart failure
   b. hypokalemia
   c. plaque
   d. edema

9. Table salt
   a. is 100% sodium
   b. is over 40% sodium
   c. contains only negligible amounts of sodium
   d. must be restricted in fat-restricted diets

10. In a low-cholesterol diet
   a. eggs are used freely
   b. fat-free milk is used instead of whole milk
   c. organ meats are permitted
   d. vegetable oils are not permitted

11. Cholesterol
   a. has no connection to lipoproteins
   b. is found in food and in body tissue
   c. is the primary cause of congestive heart failure
   d. is commonly found in fruits and vegetables

12. Persons on a low-fat diet will
   a. need to reduce their carbohydrate intake
   b. need information about cooking methods for their diets
   c. never be allowed butter or margarine
   d. find the diet quite pleasant

13. Foods allowed in a low-fat diet include
   a. cheese   c. sausage
   b. cooked vegetables   d. all soups

14. When preparing foods for the low-fat diet,
   a. small amounts of fat can be added
   b. visible fats must be removed from meats
   c. fat-free milk is never used
   d. butter is substituted for vegetable oil

15. On the low-cholesterol diet, saturated fats are
   a. reduced
   b. eliminated
   c. increased
   d. unchanged from the amount in the regular diet

16. Saturated fats are usually
   a. solid at room temperature
   b. liquid at room temperature
   c. found in fruits
   d. derived from plants

17. Polyunsaturated fats are usually
   a. solid at room temperature
   b. liquid at room temperature
   c. found in animal foods
   d. derived from dairy products

18. When the heart muscle reacts with pain because of inadequate blood supply after activity, the condition is called
a. cerebral accident
c. hypertension
b. edema
d. angina pectoris

19. Some examples of blood lipids are
a. triglycerides
c. diuretics
b. lumens
d. plaques

20. Examples of foods particularly rich in potassium are
a. milk and ice cream
b. beef and lamb
c. whole grain breads and cereals
d. bananas and oranges

C A S E   S T U D Y

Fred, a 68-year-old married lawyer, suffered an acute myocardial infarction (MI). It was noted that Fred had a cholesterol of 320 with elevated triglycerides and markedly elevated LDL. His tests indicated he had cardiovascular disease. While Fred was in the hospital, he was progressed to a low-cholesterol, low-fat diet. When Fred was ready for discharge the cardiologist discussed the need for Fred to follow the same diet he had in the hospital and to exercise and continue to monitor the status of his heart disease. The cardiologist wanted Fred to participate in a cardiac rehabilitation program to learn about how to exercise safely. The doctor ordered cardiac diet classes for Fred before his discharge from the hospital.

Fred was surprised by all the information. He and his wife, Arlene, considered themselves health nuts in regard to their diet. They avoided pesticides and preservatives in their foods. They always ate a balanced breakfast of bacon, eggs, and toast. They carried their lunches, which always included sandwiches, fruit, and whole milk. They enjoyed steaks, chops, or fish at dinner, especially shrimp or lobster that Fred bought at the health store. They felt fortunate that they could always purchase fresh vegetables to have with dinner. They used only real butter and whole milk purchased at the health food store. They did not indulge in sweets. They had ice cream before bedtime for a snack.

ASSESSMENT

1. What do you know about Fred? What does he value concerning the food he selects?
2. How significant is the problem?
3. What are the potential consequences if Fred decides to ignore the doctor's advice?

DIAGNOSIS

4. Write a statement about Fred's lack of knowledge regarding his cardiac condition and his new diet.
5. What education is needed to help achieve lower cholestorol?

PLAN/GOAL

6. What are several reasonable goals for Fred?

IMPLEMENTATION

7. What dietary issues does Fred need to learn to comply with his new diet?

8. What cardiac topics does Fred need to learn to understand his new diet? Who else needs to be in these classes with Fred?
9. Using the foods Fred described as typical of his diet, modify his old diet to reflect his new diet.
10. What two food categories can Fred use that have almost no restriction in his new diet?
11. What other risk factors does Fred have, and what does he need to do about them?
12. Why is it difficult for Fred to stick to the new health plan?

EVALUATION/OUTCOME CRITERIA

13. What changes will be measurable in 3 to 6 months?
14. What will the dietitian be able to assess in an interview with Fred?

C A S E   S T U D Y

Herbert and Irene M. have been married for 40 years. They haven't enjoyed much of their retirement yet because Herbert has been in and out of the hospital. Last year, he had a heart attack and required a coronary artery by-pass graft (CABG), also referred to as bypass surgery. Six months ago he had "a bout of congestive heart failure (CHF)" which, according to Irene, the doctor treated in the emergency room with diuretics. Herbert was told to take the salt shaker off the table at that time.

Now he is in the hospital with a serious episode of CHF. Recently, he woke up gasping for air and looking a little blue. The swelling in his ankles was up to his knees. Irene was frightened and called 911.

When he was in the emergency room 6 months ago, the doctor had told Herbert he has to follow a low-sodium diet. Now the dietitian has met with Herbert and has given him the assignment to write down what he eats on a typical day. Herbert's list follows.

Breakfast

Eggs, bacon, toast, and
    tomato juice
or
instant oatmeal with fruit
Coffee with cream

Lunch

Canned soup and crackers
    with coffee
or
a sandwich of luncheon meat
    with chips and a pickle
Coffee with cream

Dinner

Canned vegetables with butter
Ham steak with gravy
Potato with sour cream
Green salad with dressing
Dessert of ice cream or
    popcorn

Herbert also told the dietitian that, on Irene's bowling night, he just prepares a frozen dinner in the microwave.

ASSESSMENT

1. What do you know about Herbert's health?
2. How significant is his health problem?
3. What would the consequences be if Herbert decided to ignore the doctor's advice?
4. What do you know about Herbert's food choices?
5. What needs to be changed in his food choices?

DIAGNOSIS

6. Complete this statement. Herbert's alteration in cardiac output is related to _____.
7. What does Herbert not understand about CHF and his low-sodium diet?
8. Why does Herbert continue to retain fluid?

PLAN/GOAL

9. What are reasonable measurable goals for Herbert?

IMPLEMENTATION

10. What are the main topics to teach Herbert about his new diet? Who else needs to learn these topics with him?
11. Modify Herbert's food list to reflect a low-sodium diet.
12. What food categories can Herbert eat without restriction?
13. What else does Herbert need in order to control the edema?
14. What cooking tips would help Irene make the new diet more appealing?
15. What are the main topics that Irene and Herbert need to learn to manage his CHF?
16. Can this disease be cured?

EVALUATION/OUTCOME CRITERIA

17. At his 2-week doctor's appointment, what changes can the doctor observe and measure as evidence of the effectiveness of the diet?

Chapter
19

Diet and Renal Disease

Key Terms

acute renal failure
  (ARF)

chronic renal failure

creatinine

cystine

cysts

dialysis

end stage renal
  disease (ESRD)

glomerular filtration
  rate (GFR)

glomerulonephritis

glomerulus

hemodialysis

hyperkalemia

nephritis

nephrolithiasis

nephrons

nephrosclerosis

oliguria

peritoneal dialysis

polycystic kidney
  disease

purines

renal stones

urea

uremia

ureters

uric acid

nephron
unit of the kidney containing a
glomerulus

glomerulus
filtering unit in the kidneys

Objectives

After studying this chapter, you should be able to:

● Describe, in general terms, the work of the kidneys

● Explain why protein is restricted for renal patients

● Explain why sodium and water are sometimes
  restricted for renal patients

● Explain why potassium and phosphorus are sometimes restricted for renal patients

The kidneys are intricate and efficient processing systems that excrete wastes, maintain volume and composition of body fluids, and secrete certain hormones. To
accomplish these tasks, they filter the blood, cleansing it
of waste products, and recycle other, usable, substances
so that the necessary constituents of body fluids are constantly available (Figure 19-1).

Each kidney contains approximately 1 million working parts called **nephrons**. Each nephron contains a filtering unit, called a **glomerulus**, in which there is a
cluster of specialized capillaries (tiny blood vessels connecting veins and arteries). Approximately 180 liters of
ultrafiltrate is processed each day. As the filtrate passes
through the nephrons, it is concentrated or diluted to
meet the body's needs. In this way, the kidneys help
maintain both the composition and the volume of body

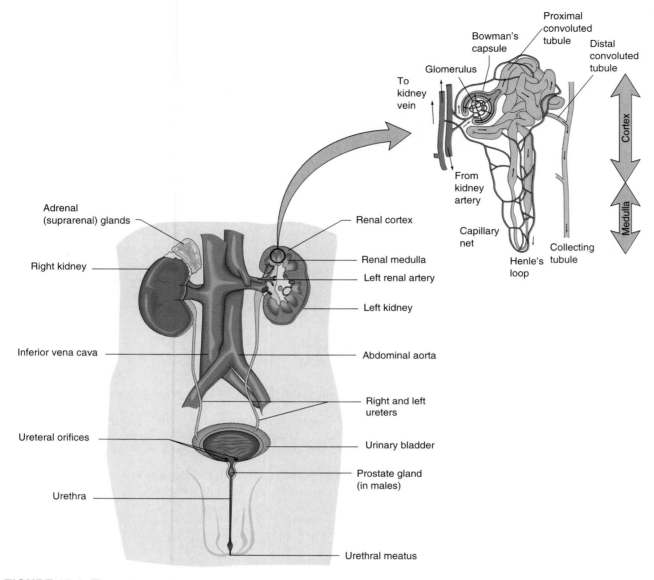

FIGURE 19-1 The urinary system with inset of a nephron.

ureters

tubes leading from the kidneys to the bladder

urea

chief nitrogenous waste product of protein metabolism

uric acid

one of the nitrogenous waste products of protein metabolism

fluids and, consequently, they maintain fluid balance, acid-base balance, and electrolyte balance.

The waste materials are sent via two tubes called **ureters** from the kidneys to the urinary bladder, from which they are excreted in approximately 1.5 liters of urine per day. These waste materials include end products of protein metabolism (**urea**, **uric acid**, **creatinine**, ammonia, and sulfates), excess water and nutrients, dead renal cells, and toxic substances. When the urinary output is less than 500 ml/day, it is impossible for all the daily wastes to be eliminated. This condition is called **oliguria**. When the kidneys are unable to adequately eliminate nitrogenous waste (end products of protein metabolism), renal failure can result. The recycled materials are reabsorbed (taken back) by the blood. They include amino acids, glucose, minerals, vitamins, and water.

The kidneys synthesize and secrete certain hormones as needed. For example, it is the kidneys that make the final conversion of vitamin D. Active vitamin D promotes the absorption of calcium and the metabolism of calcium and phosphorus. The kidneys indirectly stimulate the bone marrow to produce red blood cells.

TYPES OF RENAL DISORDERS

Kidney disorders can be initially caused by infection, degenerative changes, diabetes mellitus, cardiovascular disorders, **cysts**, **renal stones**, or trauma (surgery, burns, poisons). When they are severe, renal failure may develop. It may be acute or chronic. **Acute renal failure (ARF)** occurs suddenly and may last a few days or a few weeks. It is caused by another medical problem such as a serious burn, a crushing injury, or cardiac arrest. It can be expected in some of these situations, so preventive steps should be taken.

Chronic renal failure develops slowly, with the number of functioning nephrons constantly diminishing. When renal tissue has been destroyed to a point at which the kidneys are no longer able to filter the blood, excrete wastes, or recycle nutrients as needed, uremia occurs. **Uremia** is a condition in which protein wastes that should normally have been excreted are instead circulating in the blood. Symptoms include nausea, headache, coma, and convulsions. Severe renal failure will result in death unless **dialysis** is begun or a kidney transplant is performed.

Nephritis is a general term referring to the inflammatory diseases of the kidneys. Nephritis can be caused by infection, degenerative processes, or vascular disease.

Glomerulonephritis is a nephritis affecting the capillaries in the glomeruli. It may occur acutely in conjunction with another infection and be self-limiting, or it may lead to serious renal deterioration.

Nephrosclerosis is the hardening of renal arteries. It is caused by arteriosclerosis and hypertension. Although it usually occurs in older people, it sometimes develops in young diabetics.

Polycystic kidney disease is a relatively rare, hereditary disease. Cysts form and press on the kidneys. The kidneys enlarge and lose function. Although people with this condition have normal kidney function for many years, renal failure may develop near the age of 50.

Nephrolithiasis is a condition in which stones develop in the kidneys. The size of stones varies from that of a grain of sand to much larger. Some remain at their point of origin and others move. Although the condition is sometimes asymptomatic, symptoms include hematuria (blood in the urine), infection, obstruction, and, if the stones move, intense pain. The stones are classified according to their composition—calcium oxalate, uric acid, **cystine**, calcium phosphate, and magnesium ammonium phosphate (known as struvite). They are associated with metabolic disturbances and immobilization of the patient.

---

creatinine
an end (waste) product of protein metabolism

oliguria
decreased output of urine to less than 500 ml a day

cysts
growths

renal stones
kidney stones

acute renal failure (ARF)
suddenly occurring failure of the kidneys

chronic renal failure
slow development of kidney failure

uremia
condition in which protein wastes are circulating in the blood

dialysis
mechanical filtration of the blood; used when the kidneys are no longer able to perform normally

nephritis
inflammatory disease of the kidneys

glomerulonephritis
inflammation of the glomeruli of the kidneys

nephrosclerosis
hardening of renal arteries

polycystic kidney disease
rare, hereditary kidney disease causing cysts or growths on the kidneys that can ultimately cause kidney failure in middle age

nephrolithiasis
kidney, or renal, stones

NUTRITIONAL TREATMENT OF RENAL DISORDERS

Dietary Treatment of Renal Disease

The dietary treatment of renal disease can be extremely complicated. It is intended to reduce the amount of excretory work demanded of the kidneys while helping them maintain fluid, acid-base, and electrolyte balance. Patients require sufficient protein to prevent malnutrition and muscle wasting. Too much, however, can contribute to uremia. Typically, the patient with chronic renal failure will have protein and sodium, and possibly potassium and phosphorus, restricted.

It is essential that renal patients receive sufficient kcal—25 to 50 kcal per kilogram of body weight—unless they are overweight. Energy requirements should be fulfilled by carbohydrates and fat. The fats must be unsaturated to prevent or check hyperlipidemia. If the energy requirement is not met by carbohydrates and fat, ingested protein or body tissue will be metabolized for energy. Either would increase the work of the kidneys because protein increases the amount of nitrogen waste the kidneys must handle. The diet may limit protein to 40g. The specific amount of protein allowed is calculated according to the patient's glomerular filtration rate (GFR) and weight.

Sodium may be limited if the patient tends to retain it. Retained sodium and water could contribute to edema, hypertension, and congestive heart failure. Fluids are typically restricted for renal patients.

Calcium supplements may be prescribed. In addition, vitamin D may be added and phosphorus limited, to prevent osteomalacia (softening of the bones due to excessive loss of calcium). Phosphorus appears to be retained in patients with kidney disorders, and a disproportionately high ratio of phosphorus to calcium tends to increase calcium loss from bones.

Potassium may be restricted in some patients because hyperkalemia tends to occur in end stage renal disease (ESRD). Excess potassium can cause cardiac arrest. Because of this danger, renal patients should not use salt substitutes or low-sodium milk because the sodium in these products is replaced with potassium. Potassium restriction can be especially difficult for a renal patient, who probably must limit sodium intake. Potassium is particularly high in fruits—one of the few foods a patient on a sodium-restricted diet may eat without concern.

Renal patients often have an increased need for vitamins B, C, and D, and supplements are often given. Vitamin A should not be given because the blood level of vitamin A tends to be elevated in uremia. If a patient is receiving antibiotics, a vitamin K supplement may be given. Otherwise, supplements of vitamins E and K are not necessary. Iron is commonly prescribed because anemia frequently develops in renal patients. It is sometimes necessary to increase the amount of simple carbohydrates and fats to ensure sufficient kcal.

Dialysis

Dialysis is done by either hemodialysis or peritoneal dialysis. The most common is hemodialysis. Hemodialysis requires permanent access to the bloodstream through a fistula. Fistulas are unusual openings

---

cystine
a nonessential amino acid

glomerular filtration rate (GFR)
the rate at which the kidneys filter the blood

hyperkalemia
excessive amounts of potassium in the blood

end stage renal disease (ESRD)
the stage at which the kidneys have lost most or all of their ability to function

hemodialysis
cleansing the blood of wastes by circulating the blood through a machine that contains tubing of semipermeable membranes

peritoneal dialysis
removal of waste products from the blood by injecting the flushing solution into the abdomen and using the patient's peritoneum as the semipermeable membrane

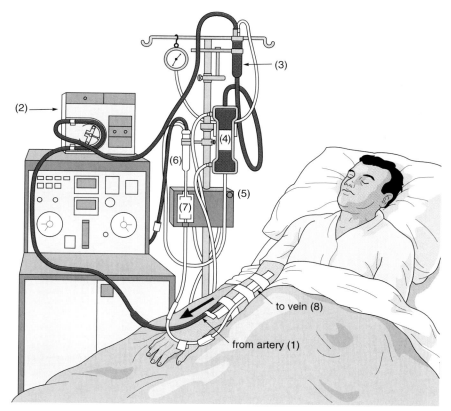

FIGURE 19-2 Hemodialysis. (1) Blood leaves the body via an artery. (2) Arterial blood passes through the blood pump. (3) Blood is filtered to remove any clots. (4) Blood passes through the dialyzer. (5) Blood passes into the venous blood line. (6) Blood is filtered to remove any clots. (7) Blood flows through the air detector. (8) Blood returns to the client through the venous blood line.

between two organs. They are often created near the wrist and connect an artery and a vein. Hemodialysis is done three times a week for approximately 3 to 5 hours (Figure 19-2).

Peritoneal dialysis makes use of the peritoneal cavity. Peritoneal dialysis is less efficient than hemodialysis, and treatments usually last about 10 to 12 hours a day, three times a week (Figure 19-3). Some patients also use continuous ambulatory peritoneal dialysis (CAPD). The dialysis fluid is exchanged four or five times daily, making this a 24-hour treatment. Patients on CAPD have a more normal lifestyle than do patients on either hemodialysis or peritoneal dialysis. Some complications associated with CAPD include peritonitis, hypotension, and weight gain.

Diet During Dialysis

Dialysis patients may need additional protein, but the amount must be carefully controlled to prevent the accumulation of protein waste between treatments.

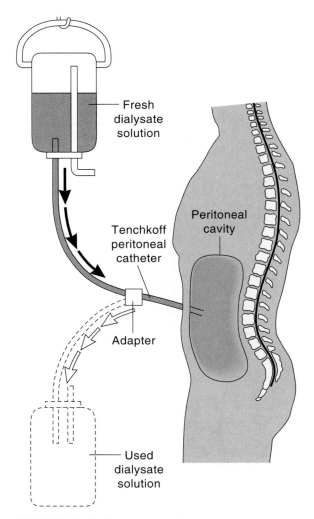

FIGURE 19-3 Peritoneal dialysis.

A patient on hemodialysis requires 1.0 to 1.2g of protein per kilogram of body weight to make up for losses during dialysis. A patient on peritoneal dialysis will require 1.2 to 1.5g of protein per kilogram body weight. The protein needs for patients on CAPD are 1.2g per kg of body weight. Seventy-five percent of this protein should be high biological value (HBV) protein, which is found in eggs, meat, fish, poultry, milk, and cheese.

Potassium is usually restricted for dialysis patients. Healthy people ingest from 2,000 to 6,000 mg per day. The daily intake allowed patients in renal failure is 3,000 to 4,000 mg. End stage renal disease (ESRD) further reduces intake allowed to 1500 to 2500 mg a day. The physician will prescribe the milligrams of potassium needed by the patient. Table 19-1 lists low, medium, and high-potassium fruits and vegetables.

Patients are taught to regulate their intake by making careful choices. Milk is normally restricted to one-half cup a day because it is high in potassium. A typical renal diet could be written as "80-3-3,"

TABLE 19-1 Potassium Content of Selected Fruits and Vegetables

LOW POTASSIUM (less than 150 mg/serving*)	MEDIUM POTASSIUM (150–250 mg/serving*)	HIGH POTASSIUM (over 250 mg/serving*)
Applesauce	Apple juice	Avocado, ½ fruit
Berries: blackberries, blueberries, boysenberries, gooseberries, raspberries, strawberries	Apple, raw, 1 large	Banana, ½ fruit
	Apricots, raw, 2 medium, canned	Dried fruits: figs, apricots, dates, prunes, raisins
Cranberries	Cherries, raw (15) or canned	Kiwi fruit
Cranberry sauce	Figs, raw, 2 medium	Mango
Figs, canned	Grapefruit juice	Melons: cantaloupe, ¼ medium; casaba, ¾ cubed; honeydew ⅛ medium; watermelon, 2 cups, cubed
Fruit cocktail, canned	Peach, raw, 1 medium	
Grapes, canned or raw	Pear, raw, 1 medium	
Grape juice	Pineapple juice, raw or canned	Nectarine, 1 medium
Lemon or lime, 1 medium	Plums, raw, 2 medium	Orange, naval
Nectors: peach, pear, or apricot	Tangerine	Orange juice, fresh, frozen, canned
Mandarin oranges, canned	Grapefruit sections	Prune juice, canned or bottled
Peaches, canned	Pineapple spears	Tangelo
Pears, canned		Papaya
Plums, canned		Raisins, seedless
Rhubarb		
Bamboo shoots	Asparagus	Artichoke
Bean sprouts	Beets	Beet greens
Beans, green, wax, snap	Brussels sprouts	Broccoli
Cabbage	Carrots, cooked	Dried beans and peas: kidney, lima, garbanzo, navy, and pinto beans; blackeye peas
Cauliflower	Corn, canned or 1 small ear	
Celery	Greens: collard, mustard, kale, dandelion, beet, turnip greens	
Cucumber		Potato, ½ cup baked, boiled, or fried
Eggplant cooked	Mixed vegetables	Pumpkin
Hominy grits, cooked	Okra	Spinach
Leek	Peas, green	Sweet potato or yams
Lettuce: cos, romaine, iceburg, leaf, endive, watercress (1 cup shredded)	Rutabaga	Tomato, raw or canned
	Summer squash: yellow crookneck, white scallop, zucchini	Unsalted tomato juice
Mushrooms		Winter squash: acorn, butternut, hubbard, spaghetti
Onion: green, red, yellow, white		
Peppers, sweet or hot		
Radishes, raw		
Turnips		
Waterchestnuts, canned		
Watercress, chopped		

*All portions are ½ cup unless otherwise noted.

which means 80g of protein, 3g sodium, and 3g potassium a day. There may be a phosphorus restriction also. And there is often a need for supplements of water-soluble vitamins, vitamin D, calcium, and iron.

The ability of the kidney to handle sodium and water in ESRD must be assessed often. Usually, the diet contains 3g of sodium, which is the equivalent of a "no added salt" diet. Sodium and fluid needs may increase with perspiration, vomiting, fever, and diarrhea. The fluid content of foods, other than liquids, is not counted in fluid restriction. Patients on fluid restriction must be taught to measure their fluid intake and urine output, examine their ankles for edema, and weigh themselves regularly.

Diet After Kidney Transplant

After kidney transplant, there may be a need for extra protein or for the restriction of protein. Carbohydrates and sodium may be restricted. The appropriate amounts of these nutrients will depend largely on the medications given at that time.

Additional calcium and phosphorus may be necessary if there was substantial bone loss before the transplant. There may be an increase in appetite after transplants. Fats and simple carbohydrates may be limited to prevent excessive weight gain.

Dietary Treatment of Renal Stones

Because the causes of renal stones have not been confirmed, treatment of them may vary. In general, however, large amounts of fluid—at least half of it water—are helpful in diluting the urine, as is a well-balanced diet. Once the stones have been analyzed, specific diet modifications may be indicated.

Calcium Oxalate Stones.   About 80% of the renal stones formed contain calcium oxalate. Recent studies provide no support for the theory that a diet low in calcium can reduce the risk of calcium oxalate renal stones. In fact, higher dietary calcium intake may decrease the incidence of renal stones for most people. Dietary intake of excessive animal protein has been shown to be a risk factor for stone formation in some patients.

Stones containing oxalate are thought to be partially caused by a diet especially rich in oxalate, which is found in beets, wheat bran, chocolate, tea, rhubarb, strawberries, and spinach. Evidence also indicates that deficiencies of pyridoxine, thiamin, and magnesium may contribute to the formation of oxalate renal stones.

Uric Acid Stones.   When the stones contain uric acid, purine-rich foods are restricted (see Table 19-2). **Purines** are the end products of nucleoprotein metabolism and are found in all meats, fish, and poultry. Organ meats, anchovies, sardines, meat extracts, and broths are especially rich sources of them. Uric acid stones are usually associated with gout, GI diseases that cause diarrhea, and malignant disease.

purines

end products of nucleoprotein metabolism

TABLE 19-2 Purine-Rich Foods

AVOID	LIMIT
Liver	Meats
Kidneys	Fish
Sweetbreads	Poultry
Brains	Meat soups
Heart	
Anchovies	
Sardines	
Meat extracts	
Bouillon	
Broth	

Cystine Stones. Cystine is an amino acid. Cystine stones may form when the cystine concentration in the urine becomes excessive because of a hereditary metabolic disorder. The usual practice is to increase fluids and recommend an alkaline-ash diet.

Struvite Stones. Struvite stones are composed of magnesium ammonium phosphate. They are sometimes called infection stones because they develop following urinary tract infections caused by certain microorganisms.

CONSIDERATIONS FOR THE HEALTH CARE PROFESSIONAL

The patient with renal disease has a lifelong challenge. Anger and depression are common among these patients. These feelings complicate management of the disease if they contribute to the patient's unwillingness to learn about his or her nutritional needs. These complications then add to the patient's problems.

The health care professional can be extremely helpful if he or she can develop a trusting relationship with the patient. Such a relationship can be established by listening to the patient's complaints, needs, and concerns and responding with sincere understanding and sympathy. This approach can help motivate patients to learn how to manage their nutritional requirements and help the dietitian assist them.

● SUMMARY

The kidneys rid the body of wastes, maintain fluid, electrolyte, and acid-base balance, and secrete hormones. When they are damaged by disease or injury, the entire body is affected. Diet therapy for renal disorders can be extremely complex because of the multifaceted nature of the kidneys' functions. Untreated severe kidney disease can result in death unless dialysis or kidney transplant is undertaken.

● DISCUSSION TOPICS

1. Discuss the three main tasks of the kidneys.
2. Define nephrons, and explain what they do.
3. Discuss some causes of kidney disease.
4. What is nephritis? Glomerulonephritis? Nephrosclerosis?
5. Why is diet therapy for renal disease so complex?
6. Discuss why protein is typically decreased for patients with renal disease.
7. Why are sodium and water sometimes restricted in renal disease?
8. Why is potassium sometimes restricted in renal disease? What is hyperkalemia?
9. Why is phosphorus sometimes restricted in renal disease?
10. Why might kcal be restricted in renal disease?
11. What is nephrolithiasis? How is it treated?

● SUGGESTED ACTIVITIES

1. Invite a registered nurse or renal dietitian to discuss renal disease with your class.
2. Invite a dialysis patient to discuss her or his condition and reactions to dialysis.
3. Using outside sources, prepare a short report on the functions of the circulatory system, the liver, and the kidneys in eliminating nitrogenous waste products from the body.
4. List the foods you ate yesterday. Compute the amount of protein by using Table A-4 in the Appendix. Compare the total protein with the RDA of protein for someone your age and sex as listed on the inside front cover. Discuss ways of reducing the protein to 30g.
5. Role-play a discussion between a renal dietitian and a 150-lb hemodialysis patient (requiring 1.2g of protein per kilogram of body weight) who is a vegetarian.

● REVIEW

Multiple choice. Select the *letter* that precedes the best answer.

1. The kidneys maintain the body's
   a. acid-base balance
   b. electrolyte balance
   c. fluid balance
   d. all of these

2. The specialized part within each nephron that actually filters the blood is called the
   a. ureter
   b. filter
   c. glomerulus
   d. capillary bunch

3. Kidney disorders may be caused by
   a. diabetes
   b. infections
   c. burns
   d. all of these

4. When renal tissue has been destroyed to a point at which it can no longer filter the blood, the following occurs:
   a. nephritis
   b. nephrosclerosis
   c. uremia
   d. nephrolithiasis

5. The general term referring to the inflammatory diseases of the kidneys is
   a. nephritis
   b. nephrosclerosis
   c. uremia
   d. nephrolithiasis

6. The term referring to the hardening of renal arteries is
   a. nephritis
   b. nephrosclerosis
   c. uremia
   d. nephrolithiasis

7. The rare hereditary disease causing cysts to develop on the kidneys is called
   a. nephritis
   b. glomerulonephritis
   c. renal stones
   d. polycystic kidney disease

8. The condition in which stones develop in the kidneys, ureters, or bladder is called
   a. nephritis
   b. nephrolithiasis
   c. polycystic kidney disease
   d. glomerulonephritis

9. Because its nitrogenous wastes contribute to uremia, the following nutrient may be restricted in diets of renal patients.
   a. carbohydrate
   b. saturated fat
   c. protein
   d. vitamin A

10. Kidney dialysis
    a. is a means of filtering all protein from the blood
    b. is a means of removing toxic substances from the blood
    c. always requires the patient be on a low-protein diet
    d. requires the patient to increase his or her sodium intake

11. Sodium and water may be restricted in the diets of renal patients because they
    a. contribute to uremia
    b. increase hypercalcemia
    c. contribute to hyperlipidemia
    d. contribute to hypertension

12. If osteomalacia occurs in renal patients, the following nutrient may be prescribed
    a. potassium
    b. protein
    c. calcium
    d. phosphorus

13. In a case of hyperkalemia, the following nutrient may be restricted
    a. potassium
    b. protein
    c. calcium
    d. phosphorus

14. Fruits are an especially rich source of
    a. potassium
    b. protein
    c. calcium
    d. phosphorus

15. The vitamins renal patients may have an increased need for are
    a. the water-soluble vitamins
    b. the fat-soluble vitamins
    c. vitamins B, C, and D
    d. vitamins E and A

16. An excess of the following nutrient can compound bone loss in renal patients
   a. phosphorus
   b. carbohydrate
   c. calcium
   d. iron

17. Purine-rich foods include
   a. meats
   b. dairy foods
   c. vegetables, except corn and lentils
   d. fruits, except cranberries, plums, and prunes

18. An example of nitrogenous waste found in the urine is
   a. ureter
   b. uremia
   c. urea
   d. all of these

C A S E   S T U D Y

Shantelle, a 23-year-old black female, was admitted to the hospital with nausea, vomiting, and a severe headache. In the emergency room, her blood pressure was very high. With intravenous medication, her blood pressure was decreased to a safer level within 24 hours. Shantelle had about 200 ml of urine output in 12 hours.

A nephrologist was consulted, and he ordered a renal ultrasound and dialysis for the following day. The renal ultrasound showed decreased kidney size. The nephrologist told Shantelle and her parents that it was possible that Shantelle would need dialysis for the rest of her life, unless her kidneys started functioning again. Her blood pressure would have to be controlled very carefully with medication. Shantelle would have to stay on a 1–2g sodium, low-potassium, 30g protein diet. He would prescribe a special vitamin with iron for renal patients and refer her to a dietitian who would teach her about her diet.

Shantelle and her parents were shocked at the news. They cried and yet were glad that Shantelle was alive. Her parents resolved to help her in any way they could.

ASSESSMENT

1. What do you know about Shantelle that put her at risk for this problem?
2. How significant is her health problem?
3. How will it alter her life?

DIAGNOSIS

4. Write a statement about what Shantelle needs to know about high blood pressure and renal failure.
5. Write a statement about the risk of excess fluid in the body.

PLAN/GOAL

6. Write a plan for Shantelle's new diet.
7. What goals are important for Shantelle?

IMPLEMENTATION

8. What major topics would be important for the dietitian to discuss with Shantelle?
9. Create a day's menu for Shantelle using her new diet. Spread the protein out throughout the day.
10. What teaching aids could the dietitian give Shantelle to help her remember her new diet?
11. What other agencies or resources may be helpful to Shantelle to adapt to this change?
12. What impact will this condition have on her ability to be employed? What impact will it have on her physical condition and psychological status?

EVALUATION/OUTCOME CRITERIA

13. At her next dialysis treatment, how will the nephrologist know if she has been compliant with her diet and medications?

C A S E   S T U D Y

Alfred was a third-generation farmer and was proud to say he lived off the land. He raised wheat, corn, sheep, cattle, and chickens. He proudly pointed out that they used every part of the animals they slaughtered. His wife, Hilda, put out a 1-acre garden each year and canned enough to provide for most of their winter fruit and vegetable needs.

Alfred had not felt well lately. He had a sharp stabbing pain in his left side and down his left leg. Sometimes it was so sharp, he would stop in his tracks and double up. He finally got scared enough to go to the doctor. The doctor did some tests and found that Alfred had a renal stone. Once Alfred passed the stone, the doctor was able to determine it was a uric acid stone. He told Alfred he would have to be on a low-purine diet and drink at least 10 glasses of water a day.

Alfred was relieved to know what the problem was. But Alfred wasn't sure about this "diet business" and how it was going to work out. Alfred had an appointment with a dietitian to learn about it.

ASSESSMENT

1. What do you know about Alfred that put him at risk for the renal stones?

2. What were Alfred's symptoms?

3. How will this condition affect Alfred for the rest of his life?

4. How significant is this dietary change?

DIAGNOSIS

5. What is the cause of uric acid stones?

6. Fill in the rest of the diagnostic statement. Alfred's knowledge deficit is related to _____.

PLAN/GOAL

7. What are reasonable measurable goals for Alfred's change in health?

IMPLEMENTATION

8. What changes does Alfred need to make in his diet?

9. What would the consequences be if Alfred ignored the doctor's advice?

10. Could Alfred have another stone?

EVALUATION/OUTCOME CRITERIA

11. How will the doctor know if the plan is effective?

Chapter 20

Diet and Gastrointestinal Problems

Key Terms

Objectives

After studying this chapter, you should be able to:

● Explain the uses of diet therapy in the gastrointestinal disturbances discussed here

● Identify the foods allowed and disallowed in the therapeutic diets discussed

● Adapt normal diets to meet the requirements of patients with these conditions

The gastrointestinal (GI) tract is where digestion and absorption of food occurs. The primary organs include the mouth, esophagus, stomach, and the small and large intestine. The liver, gallbladder, and pancreas are accessory organs that are also involved in these processes.

Numerous disorders of the gastrointestinal system cause countless individuals distress and consequently affect the nation's economy because they keep so many people home from work. Some problems are physiologically caused; others can be psychological in origin. It is sometimes difficult to determine the cause or causes of a GI problem. Consequently, controversy exists in some cases about proper treatment.

DISORDERS OF THE PRIMARY ORGANS
Dyspepsia

dyspepsia
gastrointestinal discomfort of
vague origin

Dyspepsia, or indigestion, is a condition of discomfort in the digestive tract that can be physical or psychological in origin. Symptoms include "heartburn," bloating, pain and, sometimes, regurgitation. If the cause is physical, it can be due to rushed eating or over-rich foods, or it may be a symptom of another problem, such as appendicitis or a kidney, gallbladder, or colon disease or, possibly cancer. If the problem is organic in origin, treatment of the underlying cause will be the normal procedure.

Psychological stress can affect stomach secretions and trigger dyspepsia. Treatment should include counseling to help the patient

- find relief from the underlying stress
- allow sufficient time to relax and enjoy meals
- learn to improve eating habits.

Esophagitis

esophagitis
inflammation of mucosal lining
of esophagus

**gastroesophageal reflux
(GER)**
backflow of stomach contents
into the esophagus

Esophagitis is caused by the irritating effect of acidic gastric reflux on the mucosa of the esophagus. Heartburn, regurgitation, and dysphagia (difficulty swallowing) are common symptoms. Acute esophagitis is caused by ingesting an irritating agent, by intubation, or by an infection. Chronic, or reflux esophagitis is caused by recurrent **gastroesophageal reflux (GER)**. This can be caused by a hiatal hernia, reduced lower esophogeal sphincter (LES) pressure, abdominal pressure, or recurrent vomiting. Gastroesophageal reflux can be life-threatening, particularly for patients with chronic lung disease who aspirate while sleeping.

Hiatal Hernia

hiatal hernia
condition wherein part of the
stomach protrudes through the
diaphragm into the chest cavity

diaphragm
thin membrane or partition

Hiatal hernia is a condition in which a part of the stomach protrudes through the **diaphragm** into the thoracic cavity (Figure 20-1). The hernia prevents the food from moving normally along the digestive tract, although the food does mix somewhat with the gastric juices. Sometimes the food will move back into the esophagus, creating a burning sensation (heartburn), and sometimes food will be regurgitated into the mouth. This condition can be very uncomfortable.

Medical Nutrition Therapy.   The symptoms can sometimes be alleviated by serving small, frequent meals (from a well-balanced diet) so that the amount of food in the stomach is never large. Avoid irritants to the esophagus such as carbonated beverages, citrus fruits and juices, tomato products, spicy foods, coffee, pepper, and some herbs. Some foods can cause the lower esophageal sphincter to relax, and these should be avoided. Examples are alcohol, garlic, onion, oil of peppermint and spearmint, chocolate, cream sauces, gravies, margarine, butter, and oil. If the patient is obese, weight loss may be recommended to reduce pressure on the abdomen. It may also be helpful if patients

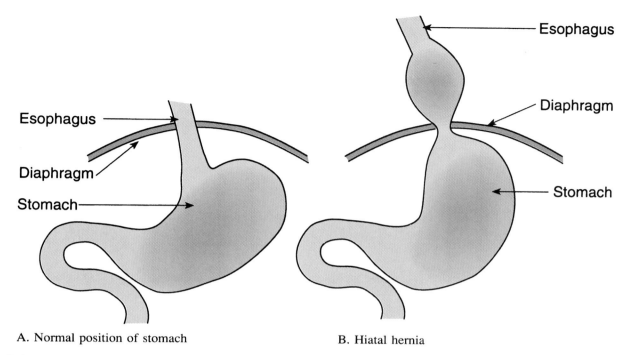

A. Normal position of stomach   B. Hiatal hernia

FIGURE 20-1 A hiatal hernia prevents food from moving through the diaphragm into the thoracic cavity.

avoid lying down for 2–3 hours after eating. When they do lie down, they may be more comfortable sleeping with their heads and upper torso somewhat elevated. If discomfort cannot be controlled, surgery may be necessary.

Peptic Ulcers

An ulcer is an erosion of the mucous membrane. **Peptic ulcers** may occur in the stomach (**gastric ulcer**) or the duodenum (**duodenal ulcer**). The specific cause of ulcers is not clear, but some physicians believe that a number of factors including genetic predisposition, abnormally high secretion of hydrochloric acid by the stomach, stress, excessive use of aspirin or ibuprofen (analgesics), cigarette smoking, and, in some cases, a bacterium called **Helicobacter Pylori** may contribute to their development.

Symptoms include gastric pain that is sometimes described as burning and, in some cases, hemorrhage. The pain is typically relieved with food or antacids. A hemorrhage usually requires surgery.

Ulcers are generally treated with drugs such as antibiotics and cimetidine. The antibiotics kill the bacteria and cimetidine inhibits acid secretion in the stomach and thus helps to heal the ulcer. Antacids containing calcium carbonate can also be prescribed to neutralize any excess acid. Rest and counseling to help the patient learn to deal with pressure and stress are also useful in the treatment of ulcers.

Sufficient low-fat protein should be provided, but not in excess because of its ability to stimulate gastric acid secretion. It is recommended that patients receive no less than 0.8g of protein per kilogram

peptic ulcers
ulcer of the stomach or duodenum

gastric ulcer
ulcer in the stomach

duodenal ulcer
ulcer occurring in the duodenum

Heliobacter Pylori
bacteria that can cause peptic ulcer

of body weight. However, if there has been blood loss, protein may be increased to 1 or 1.5g per kilogram of body weight. Vitamin and mineral supplements, especially iron if there has been hemorrhage, may be prescribed.

Although fat inhibits gastric secretions, because of the danger of atherosclerosis, the amount of fat in the diet should not be excessive. Carbohydrates have little effect on gastric acid secretion.

Spicy foods may be eaten as tolerated. Coffee, tea, anything containing caffeine, or that seems to cause indigestion in the patient or stimulates gastric secretion should be avoided. Alcohol and aspirin irritate the mucous membrane of the stomach, and cigarette smoking decreases the secretion of the pancreas that buffers gastric acid in the duodenum. Currently, a well-balanced diet of three meals a day consisting of foods that do not irritate the patient is generally recommended.

Diverticulosis/Diverticulitis

diverticulosis
intestinal disorder characterized by little pockets forming in the sides of the intestines; pockets are called diverticula

diverticulitis
inflammation of the diverticula

Diverticulosis is an intestinal disorder characterized by little pockets in the sides of the large intestine (colon). When fecal matter collects in these pockets instead of moving on through the colon, bacteria may breed, and inflammation and pain can result, causing **diverticulitis**. If a diverticulum ruptures, surgery may be needed. This condition is thought to be caused by a diet lacking sufficient fiber. A high-fiber diet is commonly recommended for patients with diverticulosis.

Along with antibiotics, diet therapy for diverticulitis may begin with a clear liquid diet, followed by a low-residue diet and, very gradually (over several weeks), progress to a high-fiber diet. The bulk provided by the high-fiber diet increases stool volume, reduces the pressure in the colon, and shortens the time the food is in the intestine, giving bacteria less time to grow.

RESIDUE-CONTROLLED DIETS

dietary fiber
indigestible parts of plants; absorbs water in large intestine, helping to create soft, bulky stool; some is believed to bind cholesterol in the colon, helping to rid cholesterol from the body; some is believed to lower blood glucose levels

Fiber is that part of food that is not broken down by digestive enzymes. It is called **dietary fiber**. Most dietary fiber is found in plant foods. Some is soluble and some is insoluble (see Chapter 4). Examples of dietary fiber in plants include the outer shells of corn kernels, strings of celery, seeds of strawberries, and the connective tissue of citrus fruits.

Residue is the solid part of feces. Residue is made up of all the undigested and unabsorbed parts of food (including fiber), connective tissue in animal foods, dead cells, and intestinal bacteria and their products. Most of this residue is composed of fiber.

Diets can be adjusted to increase or decrease fiber and residue. The specific names of these diets vary among health care facilities. The specific foods allowed and, thus, the amount of fiber and residue allowed will depend on the physician's experience and the patient's condition.

The High-Fiber Diet

High-fiber diets containing 30g or more of dietary fiber are believed to help prevent diverticulosis, constipation, hemorrhoids, and colon cancer. They also are helpful in the treatment of diabetes mellitus (see Chapter 17) and atherosclerosis (see Chapter 18).

It is currently estimated that the normal diet in the United States contains about 11g of dietary fiber each day. A high-fiber diet is often 25 to 35g and can be as much as 50g a day. The recommended foods for this diet include coarse and whole grain breads and cereals, bran, all fruits, vegetables (especially raw), and legumes. Milk, meats, and fats do not contain fiber (Table 20-1). The diet is nutritionally adequate. High-fiber diets must be introduced gradually to prevent the formation of gas and the discomfort that accompanies it. Eight 8-oz glasses of water also must be consumed along with the increased fiber.

TABLE 20-1 Sample Menus for a High-Fiber Diet

BREAKFAST	DINNER	LUNCH OR SUPPER
Stewed prunes	Baked pork chops	Fresh fruit cup
Bran cereal with milk and sugar	Baked potato	Roast beef sandwich on cracked wheat bread
Whole wheat toast with marmalade	Fresh corn	Coleslaw
Coffee	Green salad with oil and vinegar dressing	Carrot cake
	Whole grain bread with margarine	Fat-free milk
	Fresh pineapple	Coffee or tea
	Fat-free milk	
	Tea	

The Low-Residue Diet

The low-residue diet of 5 to 10g of fiber a day is intended to reduce the normal work of the intestines by restricting the amount of dietary fiber and reducing food residue. Low-fiber or residue-restricted diets may be used in cases of severe diarrhea, diverticulitis, ulcerative colitis, and intestinal blockage and in preparation for and immediately after intestinal surgery.

In some facilities, these diets consist of foods that provide no more than 3g of fiber a day and that do not increase fecal residue (Tables 20-2 and 20-3). Some foods that do not actually leave residue in the colon are considered "high-residue" foods because they increase stool volume or provide a laxative effect. Milk and prune juice are examples. Milk increases stool volume, and prune juice acts as a laxative.

TABLE 20-2 Foods to Allow and to Avoid on Low-Residue Diets

FOODS TO ALLOW	FOODS TO AVOID
Milk, buttermilk (limited to 2 cups daily) if physician allows	Fresh or dried fruits and vegetables
Cottage cheese and some mild cheeses as flavorings in small amounts	Whole grain breads and cereals
Butter and margarine	Nuts, seeds, legumes, coconut, and marmalade
Eggs, except fried	Tough meats
Tender chicken, fish, sweetbreads, ground beef, and ground lamb (meats must be baked, boiled, or broiled)	Rich pastries
Soup broth	Milk, unless physician allows
Cooked, mild-flavored vegetables without coarse fibers; strained fruit juices (except for prune); applesauce; canned fruits including white cherries, peaches, and pears; pureed apricots; ripe bananas	Meats and fish with tough connective tissue
Refined breads and cereals, white crackers, macaroni, spaghetti, and noodles	
Custard, sherbet, vanilla ice cream, junket and *cereal puddings* when considered as part of the 2-cup milk allowance and if physician allows; plain gelatin; angel food cake, sponge cake; and plain cookies	
Coffee, tea, cocoa, carbonated beverage	
Salt, sugar, small amount of spices as permitted by physician	

TABLE 20-3 Sample Menus for a Low-Residue Diet

BREAKFAST	DINNER	LUNCH OR SUPPER
Strained orange juice	Chicken broth	Tomato juice
Cream of rice cereal with milk and sugar	Ground beef patty	Macaroni and cheese
White toast with margarine and jelly	Boiled potato, no skin	Green beans
Coffee with cream and sugar	Baked squash	White bread and butter
	Gelatin dessert	Lemon sherbet
	Milk	Tea with milk and sugar

The Minimum-Residue Diet

The minimum-residue diet is extremely restrictive and can contain no more than 1g of fiber a day. In general, fruits and vegetables are not allowed except for limited amounts of fruit and vegetable juices (other than prune). Whole grain breads and cereals are not allowed, and milk may be prohibited (Table 20-4).

TABLE 20-4 Mimimum-Residue Foods

FOODS TO ALLOW		FOODS TO AVOID
1 cup or less milk, if allowed	Refined breads and cereals, white crackers	Fruits and vegetables
Cottage cheese, if tolerated and in small amounts	Macaroni, spaghetti, and noodles	Fried foods
Margarine	Sherbet, gelatin, plain cake and plain cookies	Coarse, whole grain breads and cereals, quick breads
Eggs, except fried	Tea, coffee (if physician permits)	Fibrous meats
Tender chicken and fish; ground beef and lamb	Small amounts of salt and sugar	Milk, unless permitted by physician
Soup broth		Nuts, seeds, legumes
Vegetable juice		
Fruit juice except prune		

Because of the severe limitations on foods allowed, this diet is nutritionally inadequate and should be used for only a short time. If this diet must be used for a long period of time, the physician may prescribe an oral elemental formula along with vitamin and mineral supplements. The modifications made for the minimum-residue diet can be seen in Table 20-5. This diet is seldom used.

TABLE 20-5 Sample Menus for a Minimum-Residue Diet

BREAKFAST	DINNER	LUNCH OR SUPPER
Strained orange juice	Pineapple juice	Tomato juice
Poached egg on white toast	Ground beef	Minced white poached fish
Coffee or tea	Buttered noodles	Macaroni with butter
	Toast with butter	White bread and butter
	Plain gelatin	Lemon sherbet
	Tea	Tea

Inflammatory Bowel Disease

Inflammatory bowel diseases (IBDs) are chronic conditions causing inflammation in the gastrointestinal tract. The inflammation causes malabsorption that often leads to malnutrition. The acute phases of these diseases occur at irregular intervals and are followed by periods in which patients are relatively free of symptoms. Neither cause nor cure for these conditions is known.

Two examples are **ulcerative colitis** and **Crohn's disease** (Table 20-6). Ulcerative colitis causes inflammation and ulceration of the colon, the rectum or, sometimes, the entire large intestine. Crohn's disease is a chronic progressive disorder that can affect both the small and large intestines. The ulcers can penetrate the entire intestinal wall,

inflammatory bowel disease
chronic condition causing inflammation in the gastrointestinal tract

ulcerative colitis
disease characterized by inflammation and ulceration of the colon, rectum, and sometimes entire large intestine

Crohn's disease
a chronic progressive disorder that causes inflammation, ulcers, and thickening of intestinal walls, sometimes causing obstruction

TABLE 20-6 Crohn's Disease and Ulcerative Colitis

	CROHN'S DISEASE	ULCERATIVE COLITIS
Involvement	Patchy areas; can involve small and large intestines	Starts in lower colon and spreads progressively throughout colon
Tissue affected	Entire thickness of bowel	Mucosal lining of the bowel
Major complication	Malabsorption	Toxic megacolon
Long-term complications	Intestinal obstruction, fistulas, abscesses, perforations; cancer risk increases with age	Fissures, abscesses, increased risk for colorectal cancer
Surgical intervention	Usually needed at some point to repair structural damage; does not cure or limit the progress of the disease	Colostomy performed in approximately 20% of cases to remove the colon; cures the disease
Cause	Unknown; possibly altered immune state	Unknown; possibly enteric bacterium *Escherichia coli*
Stools	3 to 4 semisoft/day; rarely blood; steatorrhea (fat in stool), mucus	15 to 20 liquid/day; blood present; no steatorrhea (fat in stool)

Source: From *Medical-Surgical Nursing* (p. 987), by L. White and G. Duncan, 1998, Albany, NY: Delmar.

and the chronic inflammation can thicken the intestinal wall, causing obstruction.

Both conditions cause bloody diarrhea, cramps, fatigue, nausea, anorexia, malnutrition, and weight loss. Electrolytes, fluids, vitamins, and other minerals are lost in the diarrhea, and the bleeding can cause loss of iron and protein.

Treatment may involve anti-inflammatory drugs plus medical nutrition therapy. Usually a low-residue diet is required to avoid irritating the inflamed area and to avoid the danger of obstruction. When tolerated, the diet should include about 100g of protein, additional kcal, vitamins, and minerals.

In severe cases, **total parenteral nutrition (TPN)**; (a process in which nutrients are delivered directly into the superior vena cava; see Chapter 22) may be necessary for a period. As the patient begins to regain health, the diet may be increasingly liberalized to suit the patient's tastes while maintaining good nutrition.

Ileostomy or Colostomy

Patients with severe ulcerative colitis or Crohn's disease frequently require a surgical opening from the body surface to the intestine for the purpose of defecation. The opening that is created is called a **stoma** and is about the size of a nickel. An **ileostomy** (from the ileum to abdomen surface) is required when the entire colon, rectum, and anus must be removed. A **colostomy** (from the colon to abdomen surface) can provide entrance into the colon if the rectum and anus are removed. This can be a temporary or a permanent procedure.

total parenteral nutrition (TPN)
process of providing all nutrients intravenously

stoma
surgically created opening in the abdominal wall

ileostomy
opening from ileum to abdomen surface

colostomy
opening from colon to abdomen surface

Patients with ileostomies have a greater than normal need for salt and water because of excess losses. A vitamin C supplement is recommended, and, in some cases, a B_{12} supplement may be needed. Eating a well-balanced individualized diet will prevent a nutritional deficiency for patients with ileostomies and colostomies.

Celiac Disease

Celiac disease, also called nontopical sprue or gluten sensitivity, is a disorder characterized by malabsorption of virtually all nutrients. It is thought to be due to heredity.

Symptoms include diarrhea, weight loss, and malnutrition. Stools are usually foul-smelling, light-colored, and bulky. The cause is unknown, but it has been found that the elimination of gluten from the diet gives relief. Untreated, it is life-threatening because of the severe malnutrition and weight loss it can cause.

A gluten-controlled diet (Table 20-7) is used in the treatment of celiac disease. Gluten is a protein found in barley, oats, rye, and wheat. All products containing these grains are disallowed. Rice and corn may be used. A reduction in the fiber content is also frequently recommended. If the patient is underweight, the diet should also be high in kcal, carbohydrates, and protein (Table 20-8). Fat may be restricted until bowel function is normalized. Vitamin and mineral supplements may be prescribed. Lactose intolerance sometimes develops with celiac disease.

nontropical sprue
a disorder of the gastrointestinal tract characterized by malabsorption; also called gluten sensitivity

gluten
protein found in grains

TABLE 20-7 Sources of Gluten

FOOD GROUP	FOODS THAT DO NOT CONTAIN GLUTEN	FOODS THAT CONTAIN GLUTEN	FOODS THAT MAY CONTAIN GLUTEN
Beverage	Coffee; tea; decaffeinated coffee; carbonated beverages; chocolate drinks made with pure cocoa powder; wine; distilled liquor	Cereal beverages (e.g., Postum), malt, Ovaltine, beer, ale	Commercial chocolate milk; cocoa mixes; other beverage mixes; dietary supplements
Meat and meat substitutes	Pure meat, fish, fowl, eggs, cottage cheese, and peanut butter	Commercially breaded meats	Meat loaf and patties, cold cuts and prepared meats, stuffing, cheese foods and spreads; commercial souffles, omelets, and fondue; soy protein meat substitutes
Fat and oil	Butter, margarine, vegetable oil	Commercial gravies, white and cream sauces	Commercial salad dressing and mayonnaise, nondairy creamer
Milk	Whole, low-fat, fat-free milk; buttermilk	Milk beverages that contain malt	Commercial chocolate milk
Grains and grain products	Specially prepared breads made with wheat starch, rice, potato, or soybean flour or cornmeal; pure corn or rice cereals; hominy grits; white, brown, and wild rice; popcorn; low-protein pasta made from wheat starch	Bread, crackers, cereal and pasta that contain wheat, oats, rye, malt, malt flavoring, graham flour, durham flour, pastry flour, bran, or wheat germ; barley; millet; pretzels; communion wafers	Commercially seasoned rice and potato mixes

(continued)

TABLE 20-7 *continued*

FOOD GROUP	FOODS THAT DO NOT CONTAIN GLUTEN	FOODS THAT CONTAIN GLUTEN	FOODS THAT MAY CONTAIN GLUTEN
Vegetable	All fresh vegetables; plain commercially frozen or canned vegetables	Commercially breaded vegetables or vegetables with a cream or cheese sauce	Commercial seasoned vegetable mixes; canned baked beans
Fruit	All plain or sweetened fruits; fruit thickened with tapioca or cornstarch		Commercial pie fillings
Soup	Soup thickened with cornstarch, wheat starch, or potato, rice, or soybean flour; pure broth	Most commercial soup and soup mixes; soup that contains barley, wheat pasta; soup thickened with wheat flour or other gluten-containing grains	
Desserts	Gelatin; custard; fruit ice; specially prepared cakes, cookies, and pastries made with gluten-free flour or starch; pudding and fruit filling thickened with tapioca, cornstarch, or arrowroot flour	Commercial cakes, cookies and pastries; commercial dessert mixes	Commercial ice cream and sherbet, puddings
Sweets			Commercial candies, especially chocolates
Miscellaneous	Monosodium glutamate; salt; pepper; pure spices and herbs; yeast; pure baking chocolate or cocoa powder; carob; flavoring extracts; artificial flavoring; cider and wine vinegar		Ketchup; prepared mustard; soy sauce; commercially prepared meat sauces and pickles; white vinegar; flavoring syrups (syrups for pancakes or ice cream)

Source: Used with permission of Mayo Clinic.

TABLE 20-8 High-kcal, High-Protein, Low-Residue Diet Menus

BREAKFAST	LUNCH	DINNER
Orange juice	Baked chicken	Ground beef patty
Poached egg	Rice	Mashed potato
Rice toast	Pureed green beans	Mashed acorn squash
Butter and jelly	Rolls made from wheat starch and butter	Rice bread and butter
Coffee with milk and sugar	Lemon chiffon pudding	Applesauce with sponge cake made from wheat starch
	Tea with milk and sugar	Coffee with milk and sugar

SNACK	SNACK	SNACK
Eggnog, if tolerated	Sugar cookies baked with gluten-free flour	Beef broth
	Pineapple juice	Rice cakes

It is not easy to avoid food products containing wheat. Breads, cereals, crackers, pasta products, desserts, gravies, white sauces, and beer contain wheat or other cereal grains with gluten. The patient will have to learn to read food labels carefully and to avoid restaurant foods such as breaded meats or fish, meat loaf, creamed vegetables, and cream soups.

DISORDERS OF THE ACCESSORY ORGANS

Cirrhosis and Hepatitis. The liver is of major importance to, and plays many roles in, metabolism. Except for a few of the fatty acids, all nutrients that are absorbed in the intestines are transported to the liver. The liver dismantles some of these nutrients, stores others, and uses some to synthesize other substances.

The liver determines where amino acids are needed and synthesizes some proteins, enzymes, and urea. It changes the simple sugars to glycogen, provides glucose to body cells, and synthesizes glucose from amino acids if needed. It converts fats to lipoproteins and synthesizes cholesterol. It stores iron, copper, zinc, and magnesium as well as the fat-soluble vitamins and B vitamins. The liver synthesizes bile and stores it in the gallbladder. It detoxifies many substances such as barbiturates and morphine.

Liver disease may be acute or chronic. Early treatment can usually lead to recovery. Cirrhosis is a general term referring to all types of liver disease characterized by cell loss. Alcohol abuse is the most common cause of cirrhosis, but it can also be caused by congenital defects, infections, or other toxic chemicals.

Although the liver does regenerate, the replacement during cirrhosis does not match the loss. In addition to the cell loss during cirrhosis, there is fatty infiltration and fibrosis. These developments prevent the liver from functioning normally. Blood flow through the liver is upset and a form of hypertension, anemia, and hemorrhage in the esophagus can occur. The normal metabolic processes will also be disturbed to such a degree that, in severe cases, death may result.

The dietary treatment of cirrhosis provides at least 25 to 35 kcal or more, and 0.8 to 1.0g of protein per kilogram of weight each day, depending on the patient's condition. If hepatic coma appears imminent, the lower amount is advocated. Supplements of vitamins and minerals are usually needed. In advanced cirrhosis, 50 to 60% of the kcal should be from carbohydrates.

In some forms of cirrhosis, patients cannot tolerate fat well, so it is restricted. In another form, protein may not be well tolerated, so it is restricted to 35 to 40g a day. Sometimes cirrhosis causes ascites. In such a case, sodium and fluids may be restricted. If there is bleeding in the esophagus, fiber can be restricted to prevent irritation of the tissue. Smaller feedings will be better accepted than larger ones. No alcohol is allowed.

cirrhosis
generic term for liver disease characterized by cell loss

fibrosis
development of tough, stringy tissue

ascites
abnormal collection of fluid in the abdomen

Hepatitis

Hepatitis is an inflammation of the liver. It is caused by viruses or toxic agents such as drugs and alcohol. **Necrosis** occurs, and the liver's normal metabolic activities are constricted. Hepatitis may be acute or chronic.

Hepatitis A virus (HAV) is contracted through contaminated drinking water, food, and sewage via a fecal-oral route. Hepatitis B virus (HBV) and hepatitis C virus (HCV) are transmitted through blood, blood products, semen, and saliva. Hepatitis B and C can lead to chronic active hepatitis (CAH), which is diagnosed by live biopsy. Chronic active hepatitis can lead to liver failure and end stage liver disease (ESLD).

In mild cases, the cells can be replaced. In severe cases, the damage can be so extensive that the necrosis leads to liver failure and death. There can be bile **stasis** and decreased blood albumin levels. Patients experience nausea, headache, fever, fatigue, tender and enlarged liver, anorexia, and **jaundice**. Weight loss can be pronounced.

Treatment is usually bed rest, plenty of fluids, and diet therapy. The diet should provide 35 to 40 kcal per kilogram of body weight. Most of the kcal should be provided by carbohydrates; there should be moderate amounts of fat; and, if the necrosis has not been severe, up to 70 to 80g of protein for cell regeneration. If the necrosis has been severe and the proteins cannot be properly metabolized, they must be limited to prevent the accumulation of ammonia in the blood. Patients may prefer frequent, small meals rather than three large ones.

Patients with liver disease require a great deal of encouragement because their anorexia and consequent feelings of general malaise can be severe. Their recovery takes patience, rest, and time.

Cholecystitis and Cholelithiasis

The dual function of the gallbladder is the concentration and storage of bile. After bile is formed in the liver, the gallbladder concentrates it to several times its original strength and stores it until needed. Fat in the duodenum triggers the gallbladder to contract and release bile into the common duct for the digestion of fat in the small intestine. If this flow is hindered, there may be pain.

The precise etiology of gallbladder disease is unknown, but heredity factors may be involved. Women develop gallbladder disease more often than men do. Obesity, total parenteral nutrition (TPN), very-low-calorie diets for rapid weight loss, the use of estrogen, and various diseases of the small intestine are frequently associated.

Cholecystitis (inflammation) and **cholelithiasis** (gallstones) may inhibit the flow of bile and cause pain. Cholecystitis can cause changes in the gallbladder tissue, which in turn can affect the cholesterol (a constituent of bile), causing it to harden and form stones. It is also thought that chronic overindulgence in fats may contribute to gallstones because the fat stimulates the liver to produce more cholesterol for the bile, which is necessary for the digestion of fat. In addition to pain, which can be severe, there may be indigestion and vomiting, particularly after the ingestion of fatty foods.

Treatment may include medication to dissolve the stones and diet therapy. If medication does not succeed, surgery to remove the gallbladder (**cholecystectomy**) may be indicated.

Diet therapy includes abstinence during the acute phase. This is followed by a clear liquid diet and, gradually, a regular but fat-restricted diet. Amounts of fats allowed run from 40 to 45g a day. In chronic cases, fat may be restricted on a permanent basis. For obese patients, weight loss is recommended in addition to a fat-restricted diet. (For information on fat-restricted diets, see Chapter 18.) Patients with chronic gallbladder conditions may require the water-soluble forms of fat-soluble vitamins.

cholecystectomy
removal of the gallbladder

Pancreatitis

In addition to the hormone insulin, the pancreas produces other hormones and enzymes that are important in the digestion of protein, fats, and carbohydrates. When food reaches the duodenum, the pancreas sends its enzymes to the small intestine to aid in digestion.

Pancreatitis is an inflammation of the pancreas. It may be caused by infections, surgery, alcoholism, biliary tract (includes bile ducts and gallbladder) disease, or certain drugs. It may be acute or chronic.

Abdominal pain, nausea and steatorrhea are symptoms. Malabsorption (particularly of fat-soluble vitamins) and weight loss occur, and, in cases in which the islets of Langerhans are destroyed, diabetes mellitus may result.

pancreatitis
inflammation of the pancreas

steatorrhea
abnormal amounts of fat in the feces

Diet therapy is intended to reduce pancreatic secretions and bile. Just as fat stimulates the gallbladder to secrete bile, protein and hydrochloric acid stimulate the pancreas to secrete its juices and enzymes. During acute pancreatitis, the patient is nourished strictly parenterally. Later, when the patient can tolerate oral feedings, a liquid diet consisting mainly of carbohydrates is given because, of these three nutrients, carbohydrates have the least stimulatory effect on pancreatic secretions.

As recovery progresses, small, frequent feedings of carbohydrates and protein with little fat or fiber are given. The fat is restricted because of deficiencies of pancreatic lipase. The patient is gradually returned to a less-restricted diet as tolerated. Vitamin supplements may be given. Alcohol is forbidden in all cases.

CONSIDERATIONS FOR THE HEALTH CARE PROFESSIONAL

Patients with gastrointestinal problems can be frustrated and irritable. Their problems can be psychologically caused; they may fear surgery or cancer; and they may suffer nausea, pain, or both. Some will want to eat foods that are disallowed; others will refuse foods they need.

Health care professionals who show respect and understanding for their patients will have the most success in helping them learn what they should and should not eat and why.

In teaching these patients, it is helpful to group foods by types, to draw diagrams or pictures, or use colored paper, and, most of all, to maintain a sense of humor.

● SUMMARY

Disturbances of the gastrointestinal tract require a wide variety of therapeutic diets. Peptic ulcers are treated with drugs, and diet therapy generally involves only the avoidance of alcohol and caffeine. Diverticulosis may be treated with a high-fiber diet, whereas diverticulitis is treated with a gradual progression from clear liquid to the high-fiber diet. Ulcerative colitis may require a low-residue diet combined with high protein and high kcal. Cirrhosis requires a substantial, balanced diet, with occasional restrictions of fat, protein, salt, or fluids. Diet therapy for hepatitis may include a full, well-balanced diet, although protein may be restricted, depending upon the patient's condition. Cholescystitis and cholelithiasis patients require a fat-restricted diet and, in cases of overweight, a kcal-restricted diet as well. Pancreatitis diet therapy ranges from TPN to an individualized diet as tolerated.

● DISCUSSION TOPICS

1. Name the accessory organs in the gastrointestinal system and explain their roles in digestion and metabolism.
2. Discuss dyspepsia. Include its probable causes and the suggested therapy for it.
3. Describe hiatal hernia. Name its symptoms and possible treatment.
4. Define ulcers. Where are they found in the gastrointestinal system, and how are they treated? What substances should not be allowed an ulcer patient? Why?
5. Explain the difference between diverticulosis and diverticulitis. How are these conditions treated?
6. Discuss the high-fiber diet. For what conditions might it be used? Compare it with the low-fiber diet. Why is corn on the cob not allowed on the low-fiber diet? Name other foods that are not allowed on the low-fiber diet and tell why they would not be allowed.
7. Discuss ulcerative colitis. What is it? What causes it? How is it treated?

● SUGGESTED ACTIVITIES

1. Write a report on one or more of the gastrointestinal disturbances included in this chapter and the dietary treatment of them.
2. Make a list of foods eaten yesterday. Circle the foods that would be allowed on a restricted-residue diet.
3. Adapt the following menu to suit a patient on a minimum-residue diet:

Orange Juice	Whole Wheat Toast with
Fried Egg	Butter and Marmalade
Bacon	Coffee
Milk	

4. List ten of your favorite foods. Circle those foods that would not be allowed on a low-residue diet.

● REVIEW

Multiple choice. Select the *letter* that precedes the best answer.

1. Dyspepsia
  a. may be an indication of serious gastrointestinal disturbance
  b. is always psychological in origin
  c. cannot be overcome with improved eating habits
  d. is caused by high-fiber foods

2. Hiatal hernia
  a. occurs only in the small intestine
  b. is a typical sign of colon cancer
  c. causes weight loss in all patients
  d. patients may be more comfortable with small, frequent meals

3. Peptic ulcers
  a. can occur in the stomach or the duodenum
  b. cannot be caused by stress
  c. are always treated with aspirin and a low-carbohydrate diet
  d. are usually treated with a low protein diet

4. Protein foods may be somewhat restricted in cases of peptic ulcers because they
  a. contribute to uremia
  b. contain large amounts of vitamin C
  c. neutralize gastric acid secretions
  d. stimulate gastric acid secretions

5. The following should not be allowed an ulcer patient:
  a. cola drinks   c. antacids
  b. milkshakes   d. protein-rich foods

6. Diverticulosis
  a. is the inflammation of diverticula
  b. may be initially treated with a clear-liquid diet
  c. may be prevented with a high-fiber diet
  d. occurs in the liver

7. Food residue
  a. is ultimately evacuated in the feces
  b. never leaves the stomach
  c. never leaves the intestines
  d. results from incorrect cooking methods

8. Large amounts of food residue cause
  a. a decrease in fecal matter
  b. an increase in fecal matter
  c. weight gain
  d. diverticulosis

9. The following would be recommended for the high-fiber diet:
  a. pureed pears   c. rice pudding
  b. mashed potatoes   d. bran cereal

10. The following would be allowed on a low-residue diet:

a. fresh oranges   c. macaroni and cheese

b. corn on the cob   d. fresh fruit cup

11. Ulcerative colitis

a. affects the small intestine

b. always requires parenteral feedings

c. may be treated with a high-residue diet that is also high in kcal and protein

d. patients may be malnourished

12. The following foods would be recommended for an ulcerative colitis patient, provided the patient tolerates milk:

a. fresh grapefruit

b. chicken salad with chopped celery

c. mashed potatoes with minced onion

d. cream of tomato soup with crackers

13. The liver

a. has no role in metabolism

b. secretes insulin

c. converts glucose to glycogen

d. stores water-soluble vitamins

14. Cirrhosis

a. is a liver disease characterized by cell loss

b. is always caused by alcoholism

c. inevitably results in death

d. occurs only in the large intestine

15. Ascites

a. is necessary for regeneration of liver cells

b. is an accumulation of fluid in the abdomen

c. requires the addition of sodium and water to the diet

d. is caused by a shortage of iron

16. Hepatitis

a. only occurs following exposure to HIV

b. patients must have very low-carbohydrate diets

c. is always fatal

d. may be caused by viruses or toxic agents

17. Gallbladder problems may require

a. the dietary restriction of dairy products

b. cholecystectomy

c. additional fat in the diet

d. additional protein in the diet

18. Inflammation of the pancreas

a. is called pancreatitis

b. is asymptomatic

c. can require a low-carbohydrate diet

d. always signifies cancer

C A S E   S T U D Y

Martin F. was a 48-year-old male who had a very successful computer company. His company was his life. He put in long hours when he was working on an important contract and seldom took even a Sunday off. He was ecstatic when a deal came together, and he celebrated his successes at his favorite Mexican restaurant. When he worked 10–12 hours at a stretch, he just ordered Chinese or deli take-out, which frequently gave him bouts of diarrhea. The latest episode was very bad. Besides the diarrhea, he was nauseated and had cramps for two nights in a row. He was sure he had a temperature, but he felt too bad to get up and check it. On the second night that he saw blood in the toilet, he resolved to call the doctor.

After 3 days of treatment in the hospital, his doctor suggested that Martin plan to follow a low-residue diet when he went home, to help prevent further episodes of ulcerative colitis. The doctor requested a consult with a registered dietitian to teach Martin about his new diet.

ASSESSMENT

1. What do you know about Martin that puts him at risk for ulcerative colitis?
2. What symptoms did Martin have?
3. How will the disease alter his life?
4. How significant is this disease?

DIAGNOSIS

5. What probably caused Martin's problems with diarrhea?
6. Were Martin's eating habits entirely to blame for his colitis?

PLAN/GOAL

7. What dietary goals are measurable and appropriate for Martin?
8. What education goals are specific and measurable for Martin?

IMPLEMENTATION

9. What dietary changes does Martin need to learn to decrease or eliminate the symptoms?
10. What types of foods are going to be a problem for Martin?
11. What major topics about ulcerative colitis does Martin need to learn to understand the dietary changes?
12. What alternatives does Martin have if he doesn't change his diet?

EVALUATION/OUTCOME CRITERIA

13. At his follow-up doctor's appointment, what is his doctor likely to ask to see if the plan was successful?

C A S E   S T U D Y

Irina D. was a 28-year-old Russian-born ballerina with long slender arms and dark expressive eyes. She was the star of the traveling company from Moscow. She had dreamed of the opportunity to tour the United States. Her mother was traveling with her. Her mother was worried that Irina's ulcer would act up with the traveling, strange foods, and the pressure Irina put on herself to be perfect. Irina was also nursing an ankle injury and using ice packs and aspirin after each practice.

After rave reviews on opening night, Irina and her mother were able to relax a little. During the second week of the tour, Irina complained of burning pain in her chest and abdomen. Irina was in the emergency room that night. The doctor determined it was not a heart attack, as Irina had thought, but it was her ulcer bleeding again. She was admitted to the hospital. When she was discharged, the doctor prescribed Pepcid, Prilosec, and a low-residue diet with no stimulants, spices, or alcohol.

ASSESSMENT

1. What put Irina at risk for her ulcer to bleed?
2. What symptoms did she have?
3. What could have been done to prevent this problem?
4. What impact did this health problem have on Irina?

DIAGNOSIS

5. What could have caused Irina's bleeding ulcer?

PLAN/GOAL

6. What goals would be appropriate for Irina's education and nutrition?

IMPLEMENTATION

7. What does Irina need to learn about her new diet?
8. What does she need to learn about her ulcer and her new medications?
9. What challenges will she face in complying with the diet while on tour?

EVALUATION/OUTCOME CRITERIA

10. How will Irina's mother, who is supervising her health, know this plan is effective?

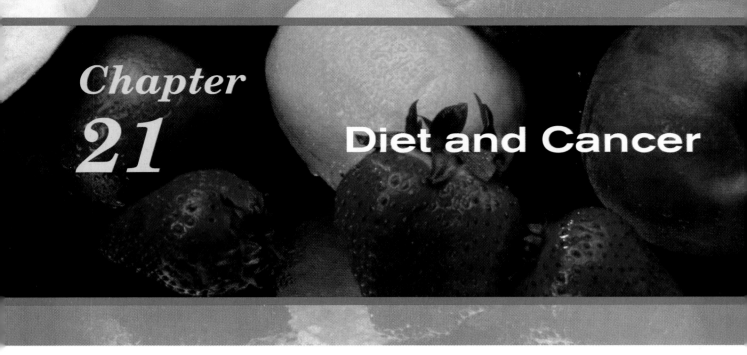

Chapter 21

Diet and Cancer

Key Terms

cachexia

carcinogens

chemotherapy

dysphagia

endometrium

genetic predisposition

hyperglycemia

hypoalbuminemia

malignant

metastasize

neoplasia

neoplasm

oncologist

oncology

phytochemicals

resection

xerostomia

neoplasm
abnormal growth of new tissue

neoplasia
abnormal development of cells

Objectives

After studying this chapter, you should be able to:

● Discuss how nutrition can be related to the development or the prevention of cancer

● State the effects of cancer on the nutritional status of the host

● Describe nutritional problems resulting from the medical treatment of cancer

● Describe nutritional therapy for cancer patients

THE NATURE OF CANCER

Cancer is the second leading cause of death in the United States. It is a disease characterized by abnormal cell growth and can occur in any organ. In some way the genes lose control of cell growth, and reproduction becomes unstructured and excessive. The developing mass caused by the abnormal growth is called a tumor, or **neoplasm**. Cancer is also called **neoplasia**. Cancerous tumors are **malignant**, affecting the structure and consequently the function of organs. When cancer cells break away from their original site, move through the blood, and spread to a new site, they are said to **metastasize**. The mortality rate for cancer patients is high,

malignant
life-threatening

metastasize
spread of cancer cells from one organ to another

oncology
the study of cancer

oncologist
doctor specializing in the study of cancer

carcinogen
cancer-causing substance

genetic predisposition
inherited tendency

but cancer does not always cause death. When it is found early in its development, prompt treatment can eradicate it. Oncology is the study of cancer, and a physician who specializes in cancer cases is called an oncologist.

THE CAUSES OF CANCER

The precise etiology of cancer is not known, but it is thought that heredity, viruses, environmental carcinogens, and possibly emotional stress contribute to its development. Cancer is not inherited, but some families appear to have a genetic predisposition for it. When such seems to be the case, environmental carcinogens should be carefully avoided and medical checkups made regularly. Environmental carcinogens include radiation (whether from X-rays, sun, or nuclear wastes), certain chemicals ingested in food or water, some chemicals that touch the skin regularly, and certain substances that are breathed in, such as tobacco smoke and asbestos.

Carcinogens are not known to cause cancer from one or even a few exposures, but after prolonged exposure. For example, skin cancer does not develop after one sunburn.

RELATIONSHIPS OF FOOD AND CANCER

Although the relationships of food and cancer have not been proved, there appear to be associations between them—both good and bad. Certain substances in foods, for example, are thought to be carcinogenic. Nitrites in cured and smoked foods such as bacon and ham can be changed to nitrosamines (carcinogens) during cooking. Regular ingestion of these foods is associated with cancers of the stomach and esophagus. High-fat diets have been associated with cancers of the uterus, breast, prostate, and colon. The regular, excessive intake of kcal is associated with cancers of the gallbladder and endometrium. People who smoke and drink alcohol immoderately appear to be at greater risk of cancers of the mouth, pharynx, and esophagus than those who do not.

endometrium
mucous membrane of uterus

phytochemicals
substances occurring naturally in plant foods

On the positive side, it is thought that diets high in fiber help to protect against colorectal cancer. Diets containing sufficient amounts of vitamin C–rich foods may protect against cancers of the stomach and esophagus. Diets containing sufficient carotene and vitamin A–rich foods may protect against cancers of the lung, bladder, and larynx. Phytochemicals, substances that occur naturally in plant foods, are thought to be anticarcinogenic agents. Examples include flavonoids, phenols, and indoles, and fruits and vegetables appear to have an abundance of them. It is advisable to eat five or more servings of fruits and vegetables each day. Legumes such as soybeans, dried beans, and lentils contain vitamins, minerals, protein, and fiber and may protect against cancer. High intakes of soy foods are associated with a decreased risk of breast and colon cancer.

Appropriate amounts of protein foods are essential for the maintenance of a healthy immune system. An immune system that has been damaged—possibly through malnutrition—may be a contributing factor in the development of cancer. Excessive protein and fat intake, however, may be a factor in the development of cancer of the colon.

The most important principle is *moderation*. An occasional serving of bacon or buttered popcorn or wine is not likely to cause cancer, but the regular, excessive use of carcinogenic foods may contribute to cancer. Vitamins that are thought to prevent cancer should be ingested *in foods* that naturally contain them. Excessive intake of vitamin supplements can be harmful. For example, abnormally large amounts of vitamin A can cause bone pain and fragility, hair loss, headaches, and liver and skin problems.

THE EFFECTS OF CANCER

One of the first indications of cancer may be unexplained weight loss because the tumor cells use for their own metabolism and development the nutrients the host has taken in. The host may suffer from weakness, and anorexia may occur, which compounds the weight loss. The weight loss includes the loss of muscle tissue and **hypoalbuminemia** and anemia may develop. The sense of taste and of smell may become abnormal in cancer patients, possibly because of nutrient deficiency. Foods may taste less sweet and more bitter than they would to healthy people.

hypoalbuminemia
abnormally low amounts of protein in the blood

Cancer patients become satiated earlier than normal, possibly because of decreased digestive secretions. Insulin production may be abnormal and **hyperglycemia** can delay the stomach's emptying and dull the appetite. Some cancers cause hypercalcemia. If this is chronic, renal stones and impaired kidney function can occur.

hyperglycemia
excessive amounts of sugar in the blood

The effects of cancer on the host are particularly determined by the location of a tumor. For example, an esophageal or intestinal tumor can cause blockage in the gastrointestinal tract, causing malabsorption. If the cancer is untreated, the continued anorexia and weight loss will create a state of malnutrition, which in turn can lead to **cachexia** and, ultimately, death.

cachexia
severe malnutrition and body wasting caused by chronic disease

THE TREATMENT OF CANCER

Medical treatment of cancer can include surgical removal, radiation, **chemotherapy**, or a combination of these methods. These treatments, unfortunately, have side effects that can further undermine the nutritional status of the patient. The nutritional effects of surgery in general are discussed in Chapter 22. Cancer surgery, however, can have some additional effects. Surgery on the mouth, for example, might well affect the ability to chew or swallow. Gastric or intestinal **resection** can affect absorption and result in nutritional deficiencies. The removal of the pancreas will result in diabetes mellitus.

chemotherapy
treatment of diseased tissue with chemicals

resection
reduction

Radiation can change the senses of taste and smell, particularly if it is done for cancer of the head or neck. It also can cause a decrease in salivary secretions, which causes dry mouth (**xerostomia**) and difficulty in swallowing (**dysphagia**). This reduction in saliva also causes

xerostomia
sore, dry mouth caused by a reduction of salivary secretions; may be caused by radiation for treatment of cancer

dysphagia
difficulty swallowing

tooth decay and sometimes the loss of teeth. Radiation reduces the amount of absorptive tissue in the small intestine. In addition, it can cause bowel obstruction or diarrhea.

Chemotherapy reduces the ability of the small intestine to regenerate absorptive cells, and it can cause hemorrhagic colitis. Both radiation and chemotherapy depress appetite. They may cause nausea, vomiting, and diarrhea leading to fluid and electrolyte imbalances, which can lead to fluid retention. However, when the therapy is completed and the patient is able to return to a well-balanced diet, these problems may disappear.

NUTRITIONAL CARE OF THE CANCER PATIENT

The nutrient and kcal needs of the cancer patient are actually greater than they were before the onset of the disease. The cancer causes an increase in the metabolic rate; tissue must be rebuilt; and the nutrients lost to the cancer must be replaced. Patients who can maintain their weight or minimize its loss increase their chances of responding to treatment and, thus, their survival. Patients on high-protein and high-kcal diets tolerate the side effects of therapy and higher doses of drugs better than those who cannot eat normally. And those patients who can eat will feel better than those who cannot.

Despite their nutritional needs, however, anorexia is a major problem for cancer patients. It is particularly difficult to combat because cancer patients tend to develop strong food aversions that are thought to be caused by the effects of chemotherapy. Patients receiving chemotherapy near mealtime associate the foods at that meal with the nausea caused by the chemotherapy and often form aversions to those particular foods. These aversions result in limited acceptance of food and contribute further to the patient's malnutrition. It is preferable that chemotherapy be withheld for 2 to 3 hours before and after meals. The appetite and absorption usually improve after chemotherapy, so the patient can improve nutritional status between chemotherapy treatments.

Obviously, diet plans for cancer patients require special attention. The patient's diet history should be taken, as usual, at the outset of hospitalization. Nutrient and kcal needs must be determined by the dietitian, and the patient's diet plan made in consultation with the patient. It is essential that favorite foods, prepared in familiar ways and served attractively, be included. Nutritious food beautifully served is useless if the patient refuses it.

If chewing is a problem, a soft diet may be helpful. If diarrhea is a problem, a low-residue diet may help (see Chapter 20). Patients should be evaluated inconspicuously.

If the patient is scheduled to undergo radiation or chemotherapy, these factors must be included in the diet planning. High-protein and high-kcal diets may be recommended. Energy demands are high because of the hypermetabolic state often caused by cancer. Kcal needs will vary from patient to patient, but 45 to 50 kcal per kilogram of body weight may be recommended.

Carbohydrates and fat will be needed to provide this energy and spare protein for tissue building and the immune system. Patients with good nutritional status will need from 1.0 to 1.2g of protein per kilogram of body weight a day. Malnourished patients may need from 1.3 to 2.0g of protein per kilogram of body weight a day. Vitamins and minerals are essential for metabolism, tissue maintenance, and appetite, and they may be supplied in supplemental form. Fluids are important to help the kidneys eliminate the metabolic wastes and the toxins from drugs.

The patient's food habits may require change if, before the illness, the patient had scrupulously avoided desserts and high-kcal foods to maintain normal weight.

Sometimes patients may be willing to eat foods that are brought from home. Some may find cold foods more appealing than hot foods. Meats may taste bitter so milk, cheese, eggs, and fish may be more appealing. If foods taste less sweet to the cancer patient than to the well person, sugar may be added to juices and fruits. The added sweetness may please the patient and make it easier to add kcal to the diet.

Supplementation with high-kcal, high-protein, liquid foods between meals may be useful but should not be used if their consumption reduces the patient's appetite at meals.

If the patient suffers from dry mouth, salad dressings, gravies, sauces, and syrups appropriately served on foods can be helpful. Several small meals may be better tolerated than three large meals. It is preferable to serve the nutritionally richer meals early in the day because the patient is less tired and may have a better appetite at that time. If nausea or pain are a continuous problem, drugs to control them, particularly at mealtimes, may be helpful. Although oral feedings are definitely preferred, enteral or total parenteral feedings may become necessary if cachexia is extreme. Sometimes an oral diet with a nutritional supplement may be used in conjunction with total parenteral feeding (see Chapter 22). As the patient improves, kcal and nutritional content of the diet should be gradually increased.

CONSIDERATIONS FOR THE HEALTH CARE PROFESSIONAL

It is important that the dietitian establish a good relationship with the patient and that constant reminders to eat be avoided. The patient usually understands the situation and such comments are only depressing reminders of the cancer. When appropriate, however, it may be helpful to:

1. explain why it is important that the patient eat

2. encourage him or her to eat foods he or she enjoys

3. recommend that he or she avoid eating at the time of day when nausea typically occurs

4. refrain from serving foods that give off odors that contribute to nausea

If the prognosis for the patient is not good, nutritional care will not be as important as the patient's feelings and immediate comfort.

● SUMMARY

Cancer is a disease characterized by abnormal cell growth. It can strike any body tissue. Energy needs increase because of the hypermetabolic state and the tumor's needs for energy nutrients. At the same time anorexia occurs in the patient. Its cause is not known. It causes severe wasting, blockages, anemia, and various metabolic problems. Treatment of cancer includes surgery, radiation, and chemotherapy. Improving the patient's nutritional state is difficult because of the illness and anorexia. Parenteral or enteral nutrition may be necessary.

● DISCUSSION TOPICS

1. Discuss cancer, telling what it is and how it affects body functions and nutritional status.
2. Discuss the etiology of cancer. Include any current news items that are related to the subject, including their accuracy.
3. Explain why cancer patients lose weight.
4. Why is the anorexia of cancer patients especially difficult to combat? What causes it? Are there any ways it can be prevented?
5. Are supplemental feedings of liquid foods useful in the nutritional rehabilitation of a cancer patient? Explain?
6. Discuss enteral and parenteral nutrition in relation to cancer patients.

● SUGGESTED ACTIVITIES

1. Invite an oncologist to speak to the class.
2. Role play a situation where a nurse is attempting to help a cancer patient with lunch. The patient had chemotherapy an hour after yesterday's lunch and was quite ill afterward.
3. Write an essay about how you might feel if you had just been told that you had a malignant tumor.
4. Plan a day's menus for a cancer patient who will eat only the following foods.

sweetened orange juice	soda crackers
bananas	milkshakes
applesauce	eggnog
cooked pears	cottage cheese
puffed rice cereal	cream of chicken soup
rice pudding	poached eggs
white toast with currant jelly	bouillon

● REVIEW

Multiple choice. Select the *letter* that precedes the best answer.

1. Cancer
    a. is characterized by reduced cell growth
    b. growth called a tumor can also be called a neoplasm
    c. inevitably causes death
    d. can metastasize only in patients 50 years and older

2. Carcinogens may include
    a. viruses
    b. certain green vegetables
    c. gluten-containing foods
    d. salmonella

3. Carcinogens
    a. cause cancer after only limited exposure
    b. include some chemical substances
    c. are never found in food or water
    d. are found only in meats and fish

4. Cancer patients
    a. seldom experience weight loss
    b. usually experience an increase in appetite
    c. seldom suffer from anorexia
    d. may suffer from cachexia

5. Radiation and chemotherapy
    a. seldom affect cancer patients' nutritional status
    b. may increase appetite
    c. have no connection to electrolyte imbalance
    d. may create food aversions

6. It is thought that cancer may be caused by
    a. frequent ingestion of smoked meats over a long period
    b. moderate use of alcohol
    c. high-fiber diets
    d. excessive use of vitamin A–rich foods

7. High-fat diets
    a. usually are harmless
    b. have been associated with breast and prostate cancer
    c. provide large amounts of fiber and vitamin C
    d. contribute to the health of the immune system

8. Phytochemicals are
    a. abundantly supplied in fruits and vegetables
    b. widely known carcinogens
    c. most prevalent in carbohydrates and fats
    d. plentifully supplied in proteins

9. High intakes of soy foods
    a. are associated with increased risk of endometrial cancer
    b. are associated with decreased risk of breast and colon cancer
    c. may increase the risk of prostate cancer
    d. are unrelated to the development of cancer

10. Cachexia
    a. is the result of continued anorexia and weight loss
    b. is inevitable in all cancer patients
    c. occurs only in patients with mouth and throat cancers
    d. does not seem to appear in untreated cancer

C A S E   S T U D Y

Edwin H. was a 54-year-old male receiving chemotherapy for cancer. He was about to begin round four of seven rounds of chemotherapy. He was pleased that he had been able to control the nausea and to maintain his weight so far. The oncologist warned Edwin that it was common that round four was "a little bit rougher" than the previous three rounds. The doctor ordered Zofran, an appetite stimulant, and a liquid supplement between meals. He requested a daily assessment by a registered dietitian to help Edwin maintain his weight.

ASSESSMENT

1. What has Edwin's response to the chemotherapy been so far?

2. What does the doctor suspect will happen to Edwin's nutrition during round four?

3. What can the dietitian assess to measure how Edwin is eating?

DIAGNOSIS

4. Write a statement describing the nutrition problems Edwin could have with chemotherapy.

PLAN/GOAL

5. What is the major nutrition goal for Edwin?

IMPLEMENTATION

6. List four strategies the dietitian can use to encourage Edwin to eat.

7. List three strategies that his family can use to help him eat.

8. If Edwin eats only 5–10% of his normal food volume, what foods should be a priority?

9. In preparation for round five of chemotherapy, what could Edwin do to enhance his nutrition once his appetite returns?

EVALUATION/OUTCOME CRITERIA

10. What criteria would the doctor use to evaluate the success of the diet plan?

C A S E   S T U D Y

Betty had just been discharged from the hospital after having had her left breast removed because of breast cancer. She still had drains in place and a large bulky dressing. She had consumed only 7-Up and some clear liquids in the hospital. Her husband, Harvey, and her daughter, Susan, were very concerned about her appetite. The doctor ordered a home health nurse to assist Betty in her recovery at home. Betty also knows she will have chemotherapy and radiation in the near future.

Betty was still having a lot of incisional pain on her day of discharge. It hurt to take a deep breath or to walk and it was hard to get comfortable in any position. She had some relief with the oral pain medications. She felt as if she hadn't slept in 3 days and she was looking forward to being in her own bed.

ASSESSMENT

1. What do you know about Betty?
2. What barriers does she have to balanced nutrition?
3. What resources does she have to overcome these barriers?
4. How important is her nutrition to her current health?

DIAGNOSIS

5. Write a statement about the effects of Betty's discomfort.
6. Write a diagnosis about potential nutrition problems for Betty.
7. Describe how a lack of knowledge about nutrition might affect her recovery.

PLAN/GOAL

8. What goal is a priority for Betty's nutrition?

IMPLEMENTATION

9. What can the home health nurse do to enhance Betty's nutrition?
10. What could a dietitian do?
11. What could her husband do?
12. What does Betty need to learn?
13. List four strategies to encourage Betty to eat at home.

EVALUATION/OUTCOME CRITERIA

14. What can the home health nurse observe and measure as evidence of the success of the plan?

Chapter 22

Diet and Surgery, Enteral and Parenteral Nutrition, Burns, Infections, and AIDS

Key Terms

acquired immune
 deficiency syndrome
 (AIDS)
antibodies
aspirated
continuous infusion
dumping syndrome
elemental formulas
enteral nutrition
gastrostomy
hemorrhage
homeostasis
human immuno-
 deficiency virus
 (HIV)
hydrolyzed formulas
hypermetabolic

hypoalbuminemia
jejunostomy
Kaposi's sarcoma
modular formulas
nasogastric (NG)
 tube
opportunistic
 infections
osmolality
parenteral nutrition
peripheral vein
phlebitis
polymeric formulas
sepsis
thrombosis
tube feeding (TF)

Objectives

After studying this chapter, you should be able to:

● Describe the body's reactions to stress and relate
 them to nutrition

● Explain the special dietary needs of surgical and
 burn patients

● Discuss enteral and parenteral nutrition

● Explain the special dietary needs of patients with
 fever and infection

● Explain the special dietary needs of AIDS patients

Normally, the human body operates in a state of **homeostasis**. When the body experiences the trauma of surgery, severe burns, or infections, this balance is upset. The body reacts in an attempt to restore itself to homeostasis.

During its response to physical stress, the body signals the endocrine system, which activates a self-protective, **hypermetabolic** response. This increases energy output. The intensity of the response depends on the severity of the condition.

Catabolism occurs, causing the rapid breakdown of energy reserves to provide glucose and other substances necessary for the anabolic phase of wound healing and tissue maintenance. Proteins, fats, and minerals are lost in the catabolic phase just when there is an increased need for them to rebuild tissue. When the condition includes hemorrhage and vomiting, these losses are compounded.

Sufficient nutrients, fluids, and kcal are required as soon as possible to replace the losses, build and repair tissue, and return the body to homeostasis. Obviously, nutrition plays an important role in the lives of patients undergoing surgery or of those who suffer from burns or infections.

NUTRITIONAL CARE OF SURGERY PATIENTS

Presurgery Nutritional Care

Surgery stresses the patient regardless of whether it is elective or not. If the surgery is elective, the patient's nutritional status should be evaluated before surgery, and if improvement is needed, it should be undertaken immediately. A good nutritional status before surgery

homeostasis
state of physical balance; stable condition

hypermetabolic
higher than normal rate of metabolism

hemorrhage
unusually heavy bleeding

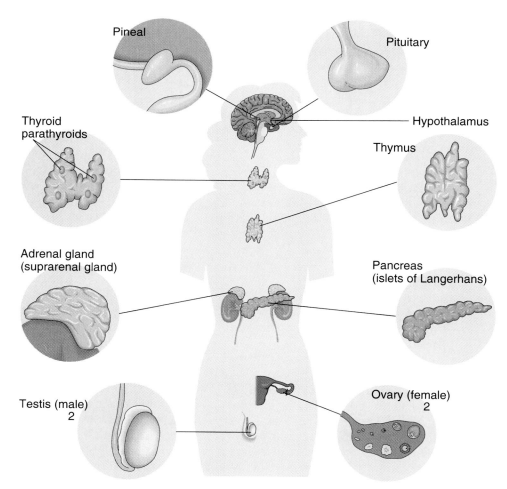

FIGURE 22-1 The structures of the endocrine system. (Courtesy of Delmar Publishers, Albany, NY)

enhances recovery. A nutritional assessment of the patient before surgery will be helpful to the dietitian in providing foods that will be accepted by the patient after surgery, when appetite is poor.

Improvement of nutritional status will usually mean providing extra protein, carbohydrates, vitamins, and minerals. The extra protein is needed for wound healing, tissue building, and blood regeneration. Extra carbohydrates will be converted to glycogen and stored to help provide energy after surgery, when needs are high and when patients may be unable to eat normally. The B vitamins are needed for the increased metabolism, vitamins A and C and zinc for wound healing, vitamin D for the absorption of calcium, and vitamin K for proper clotting of the blood. Iron is necessary for blood building, calcium and phosphorus for bones, and the other minerals for maintenance of acid-base, electrolyte, and fluid balance in the body.

In cases of overweight, improved nutritional status includes weight reduction before surgery whenever possible. Excess fat is a surgical hazard because the extra tissue increases the chances of infection, and fatty tissue tends to retain the anesthetic longer than other tissue.

Many physicians order their patients to be NPO (nothing by mouth) after midnight the night before surgery. Withholding food ensures that the stomach contains no food, which could be regurgitated and then **aspirated** during surgery. If there is to be gastrointestinal surgery, a low-residue diet may be ordered for a few days before surgery (see Chapter 20). This is intended to reduce intestinal residue.

Postsurgery Nutritional Care

The postsurgery diet is intended to provide kcal and nutrients in amounts sufficient to fulfill the patient's increased metabolic needs and to promote healing and subsequent recovery. In general, during the 24 hours immediately following major surgery, most patients will be given intravenous solutions only. These solutions will contain water, 5 to 10% dextrose, electrolytes, vitamins, and medications as needed. The maximum kcal supplied by them is about 400 to 500 kcal per 24-hour period. The estimated daily kcal requirement for adults after surgery is 35 to 45 kcal per kilogram of body weight. A 110-pound individual would require at least 2,000 kcal a day. Obviously, until the patient can take food, there will be a considerable kcal deficit each day. Body fat will be used to provide energy and to spare body protein, but the kcal intake must be increased to meet energy demands as soon as possible.

Because protein losses following surgery can be significant and because protein is especially needed then to rebuild tissue, control edema, avoid shock, resist infection, and transport fats, a high-protein diet of 80 to 100g a day may be recommended. In addition, extra minerals and vitamins are needed. When peristalsis returns, ice chips may be given and, if they are tolerated, a clear liquid diet can follow. (Peristalsis is evidenced by the presence of bowel sounds.)

Normally in postoperative cases, patients proceed from the clear-liquid diet to the regular diet. Sometimes this change is done directly, and sometimes by way of the full-liquid diet, depending on the patient

aspirated

inhaled or suctioned

and the type of surgery. The average patient will be able to take food within 1 to 4 days after surgery. If the patient cannot take food then, parenteral or enteral feeding may be necessary.

Sometimes following gastric surgery, dumping syndrome occurs within 15 to 30 minutes after eating. This is characterized by dizziness, weakness, cramps, vomiting, and diarrhea. It is caused by food moving too quickly from the stomach into the small intestine.

To prevent dumping syndrome, the diet should be high in protein and fat, and carbohydrates should be restricted. Foods should contain little fiber or concentrated sugars and only limited amounts of starch. Complex carbohydrates are gradually reintroduced. Gradual reintroduction is recommended because carbohydrates leave the stomach faster than do proteins and fats. Fluids should be limited to 4 ounces at meals, or restricted completely. They can be taken 30 minutes after meals. The total daily food intake may be divided and served as several small meals rather than the usual three meals, in an attempt to avoid overloading the stomach. Some patients do not tolerate milk well after gastric surgery, so its inclusion in the diet will depend on the patient's tolerance.

The food habits of the postoperative patient should be closely observed because they will affect recovery. When the patient's appetite fails to improve, the physician and the dietitian should be notified and efforts should be made to offer nutritious foods that the patient will eat. The patient should be encouraged to eat and to eat slowly to avoid swallowing air, which can cause abdominal distension and pain.

TUBE FEEDING

The term **enteral nutrition** means the forms of feeding that bring nutrients directly into the digestive tract (Figure 22-2). Oral feeding is the usual method and should be used whenever possible. When patients cannot or will not take food by mouth, but their gastrointestinal tract is working, they will be given **tube feedings** (TF). Sometimes this may be necessary because of unconsciousness, surgery, stroke, severe malnutrition, or extensive burns.

Usually, for periods that do not exceed 6 weeks, tube feeding is administered through a **nasogastric (NG) tube** inserted through the nose and into the stomach or small intestine. When the tube cannot be placed in the nose or when tube feedings will be required for more than 6 weeks, an opening called an ostomy is surgically created into the esophagus (an esophagostomy), the stomach (**gastrostomy**), or the intestine (**jejunostomy**).

The tubes used for these feedings are soft, flexible, and as small as they can be and still allow the feeding to pass through. Although some tubes are weighted to keep them in place in the stomach or intestine, the use of weighted tubes is controversial.

Numerous commercial formulas are available, with varying types and amounts of nutrients. Patients who are able to digest and absorb nutrients can be given **polymeric formulas** (1–2 kcal/ml) containing intact proteins, carbohydrates, and fats that require digestion. Patients

dumping syndrome
nausea and diarrhea caused by food moving too quickly from the stomach to the small intestine

enteral nutrition
feeding by tube directly into the patient's digestive tract

tube feeding
feeding by tube directly into the stomach or intestine or via a vein

nasogastric (NG) tube
tube leading from the nose to the stomach for tube feeding

gastrostomy
opening created by the surgeon directly into the stomach for enteral nutrition

jejunostomy
opening created by the surgeon in the intestine for enteral nutrition

polymeric formulas
commercially prepared formulas for tube feedings that contain intact proteins, carbohydrates, and fats that require digestion

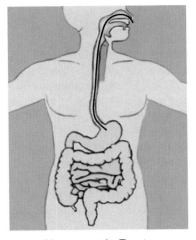

Nasogastric Route

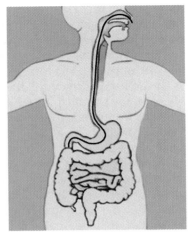

Nasoduodenal Route

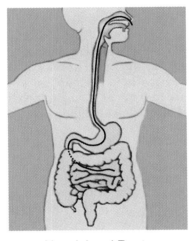

Nasojejunal Route

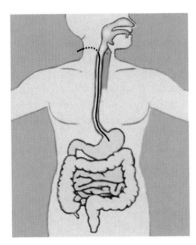

Esophagostomy Route

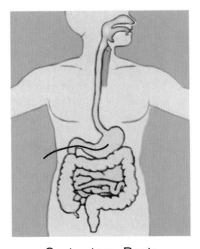

Gastrostomy Route

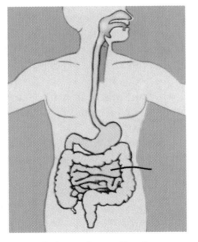

Jejunostomy Route

FIGURE 22-2 Enteral feeding routes. (Courtesy of Delmar Publishers, Albany, NY)

who have limited ability to digest or absorb nutrients may be given **elemental**, or **hydrolyzed**, **formulas** (1.0 kcal/ml) that contain the products of digestion of proteins, carbohydrates, and fats, and are lactose-free. **Modular formulas** (3.8–4.0 kcal/ml) can be used as supplements to other formulas or for developing customized formulas for certain patients. They are not nutritionally complete by themselves.

There are three methods for administering tube feedings: continuous, intermittent, and bolus. Intermittent can mean to only administer tube feeding at night, with solid foods eaten during the day. If there is a food/drug interaction, such as with Dilantin, the TF should be stopped 1 hr before and be restarted 1 hr after administration of the medication by mouth.

Daily kcal needs of the patient are usually divided into 6 servings per day (not to exceed 400 cc at a time). These feedings are given over a 15-minute time span and followed by 25 to 60 ml of water, hence the term *bolus*. This method is usually done when a patient has a percutaneous endoscopic gastrostomy (PEG) tube, but it could also be done with an NG tube.

Usually they are administered by the **continuous infusion** method, preferably with a pump. This means the feeding is continuous during a 16- to 24-hour period. Sometimes the formula is given at half strength at a rate of from 30 to 50 ml per hour. This rate may be increased by about 25 ml every 4 hours until tolerance has been established. Once the patient tolerates the half-strength formula, a full-strength formula is initiated at the appropriate rate. When patients are ready to return to oral feedings, the transfer must be done gradually.

Problems Associated with Tube Feeding

The **osmolality** of a liquid substance means the number of particles per kilogram of solution. Solutions with more particles (high osmolality) exert more pressure than solutions with fewer particles. Solutions with high osmolality attract water from nearby fluids that contain lower osmolality. When a formula with high osmolality reaches the intestine, the body may draw fluid from the blood to dilute the formula. This process can cause weakness and diarrhea in the patient. However, diarrhea should be attributed to the tube feeding only when all other causes have been ruled out. Liquid medications containing sorbitol or *Clostridium difficile* (the bacterium that causes dysentery) are two possible causes of diarrhea.

Aspiration can occur (some of the formula enters the lung), causing the patient to develop pneumonia. The tube may become clogged, or the patient may pull the tube out. The placement of the feeding tube should be checked with an X-ray to decrease the possibility of aspiration. Before beginning the tube feeding, the nurse must administer the flush solution according to the physician's order and raise the head of the bed. If the feeding is continuous, then the head of the bed needs to remain elevated.

Obviously, patients requiring tube feeding need a great deal of patience and understanding. They have been deprived of a basic pleasure of life—eating. They may also be uncomfortable and apprehensive.

elemental formulas
those formulas containing products of digestion of proteins, carbohydrates, and fats; also called hydrolyzed formulas

hydrolyzed formulas
contain products of digestion of proteins, carbohydrates, and fats; also called elemental formulas; used for patients who have difficulty digesting food

modular formulas
made by combining specific nutrients

continuous infusion
enteral nutrition administered continuously during a 16- to 24-hour period

osmolality
number of particles per kilogram of solution; solutions with high osmolality exert more pressure than do those with fewer particles

parenteral nutrition
nutrition provided via a vein

peripheral vein
a vein that is near the surface of the skin

phlebitis
inflammation of a vein

thrombosis
blockage, as a blood clot

sepsis
infection of the blood

PARENTERAL NUTRITION

Parenteral nutrition is the provision of nutrients intravenously. It is used if the gastrointestinal tract is not functional or if normal feeding is not adequate for the patient's needs. It can be used alone or as part of a dietary plan that includes oral or tube feeding as well. When parenteral nutrition is used to provide total nutrition, it is called total parenteral nutrition (TPN) or hyperalimentation.

Nutrient solutions are prescribed by the physician and dietitian and are prepared by a pharmacist. They can be administered via a central vein or, for a period of 2 weeks or less, a **peripheral vein**. Typically, a dextrose-amino acid-fat solution is given. This solution is not combined until just before entry into the vein because the components do not form a stable solution.

Total parenteral nutrition that is required for an extended period is provided via a central vein. A catheter is surgically inserted, under sterile conditions, by a physician. It is inserted into a subclavian vein or the superior vena cava. The vena cava is used because the high blood flow there facilitates the quick dilution of the highly concentrated TPN solution. Dilution reduces the possibility of **phlebitis** and **thrombosis**.

When parenteral nutrition is no longer necessary, the patient must be transferred gradually to an oral diet. Sometimes patients are given tube feeding before oral feeding as they are weaned from TPN.

Possible Complications Associated with Parenteral Nutrition

Infection can occur at the site of the catheter and enter the bloodstream, causing an infection of the blood called **sepsis**. Bacterial or fungal infections can develop in the solution if it is unrefrigerated for over 24 hours. Abnormal electrolyte levels may develop, as can phlebitis or blood clots. Careful monitoring of the patient is essential.

MEDICAL NUTRITION THERAPY FOR BURN PATIENTS

In cases of serious burns, the loss of skin surface leads to enormous losses of fluids, electrolytes, and proteins. Water moves from other tissues to the burn site in an effort to compensate for the loss, but this only compounds the problem. This fluid loss can reduce the blood volume and thus blood pressure, as well as urine output.

Fluids and electrolytes are replaced by intravenous therapy immediately to prevent shock. Glucose is not included in these fluids for the first 2 or 3 days after the burn, because it could cause hyperglycemia.

The hypermetabolic state after a serious burn continues until the skin is largely healed, so there is an enormous increase in energy needed for the healing process. Kcal requirements are based on weight (size) and the total burned surface, including depth of burns. Protein needs can be as high as 1.5 to 3.0 or more grams per kilogram of weight, and fat intake, 15 to 20% of nonprotein calories. A high-protein, high-kcal diet is used. There is an increased need for vitamin C for healing and B vitamins for the metabolism of the extra nutrients. Vitamin A is important for the immune system and the epithelial tissues.

Also, it is essential that badly burned patients have sufficient fluids to help the kidneys hold the unusual load of wastes in solution and to replace those lost.

If the patient can and will eat, oral feedings are advisable. Liquid commercial formulas may be used at first, and solid food may be added during the second week after the burn. If the patient cannot or will not eat, tube feedings should be started immediately. In some cases, parenteral feeding is required. The foods served should be those the patient likes, and service should be as attractive as possible. To accommodate these needs, a registered dietitian must perform an individualized assessment for each burn victim. The best assessment of the adequacy of the nutrients provided is wound healing.

Burn patients need a great deal of encouragement. They are in pain, worried about disfigurement, and know they face a long, costly, and painful hospital stay with the possibility of surgery.

MEDICAL NUTRITION THERAPY DURING FEVERS AND INFECTIONS

Fever typically accompanies an infection. Fevers and infections may be acute or chronic. Fever is a hypermetabolic state in which each degree of fever on the Fahrenheit scale raises the basal metabolic rate (BMR) 7%. If extra kcal are not provided during fever, the body first uses its supply of glycogen, then its stored fat, and finally its own muscle tissue for energy.

Protein intake should be increased because of infections (sepsis). Amounts required need to be individualized. Protein is needed to replace body tissue and to produce **antibodies** to fight the infection. Minerals are needed to help build and repair body tissue and to maintain acid-base, electrolyte, and fluid balance. Extra kcal are needed for the increased metabolic rate. Extra vitamins are also necessary for the increased metabolic rate and to help fight the infection causing the fever. Extra liquid is needed to replace that lost through perspiration and possibly vomiting and diarrhea, which can accompany infection.

antibodies
substances produced by body in reaction to foreign substance; neutralize toxins from foreign bodies

Patients with fever usually have very poor appetites, but they will often accept ice water, fruit juice, and carbonated beverages. Some will accept bouillon or consommé.

Usually, the diet during fever and infection progresses from the liquid to the regular diet, with frequent, small meals recommended. It should be high in protein, kcal, and vitamins. In some cases, parenteral and enteral feedings are necessary.

NUTRITION AND THE AIDS PATIENT

A virus is a microscopic parasite that invades and lives in or on, and thus infects, another organism called the host. The virus obtains nourishment from the host and duplicates itself countless times. There are many viruses that infect humans. Some, like those of the common cold,

human immunodeficiency virus (HIV)

a virus that weakens the body's immune system and ultimately leads to AIDS

opportunistic infections

caused by microorganisms that are present but that do not normally affect people with healthy immune systems

acquired immune deficiency syndrome (AIDS)

caused by the human immunodeficiency virus (HIV) which weakens the body's immune system leaving it susceptible to fatal infections

make the host only mildly ill. Others are deadly, and the human immunodeficiency virus (HIV) is among the latter.

HIV invades the T cells, which are white blood cells that protect the body from infections. When the T cells cannot function normally, the body has no resistance to opportunistic infections. Opportunistic infections are caused by other microorganisms that are present but do not affect people with healthy immune systems.

Persons infected with HIV are said to be HIV-positive. HIV infection ultimately leads to acquired immune deficiency syndrome (AIDS), which is incurable and fatal.

HIV can affect anyone exposed to it, regardless of age, sex, or physical condition. HIV infection cannot be cured, but it can be prevented. The virus is not transmitted through casual contact, such as shaking hands. It is transmitted via body fluids, specifically:

- through sexual contact
- by transfusions of contaminated blood
- by use of contaminated needles during ear piercing, tattooing, acupuncture, or injection of illegal drugs
- by infected mothers to their fetuses during pregnancy or to their infants during lactation

Progression from HIV Infection to AIDS

There are essentially three stages in the progress of AIDS. The first stage begins soon after exposure to HIV, when the body produces antibodies in an attempt to destroy the virus. At that time, some people may experience a few days' of symptoms resembling mild flu. Others may have no symptoms. At this point and thereafter, the infected person will test positive to HIV and will be among those called HIV-positive. Unless tested, the individual will feel normal and will have no idea that he or she is HIV-positive for a period ranging from a few months to 10 years.

During this period, the virus is incubating. Viral cells are multiplying in the tonsils, adenoid glands, and spleen, gradually taking over the body's T cells.

Anyone suspecting that he or she has been exposed to HIV should be tested as soon as possible. An ever-growing number of medications are available that may increase the time the virus needs to multiply and, thus, may prolong the life of the host.

The second stage of HIV is known as the *ARC period. ARC* stands for AIDS-related complex. The body's immune system has by this point grown weaker, and symptoms and opportunistic infections occur. There may be fatigue, skin rashes, headache, night sweats, diarrhea, weight loss, oral lesions or thrush (candidiasis, a fungal infection of the mouth), cough, sore throat, fevers, or shortness of breath (Table 22-1).

The third and end stage of HIV infection is known as AIDS (acquired immune deficiency syndrome). It is manifested by a very low T-cell count, which makes it impossible for the body to fight off infections. Tuberculosis or Kaposi's sarcoma commonly develops at this point. As the T-cell count continues to diminish, other parasites invade and, ultimately, overwhelm the body, causing death.

Kaposi's sarcoma

type of cancer common to AIDS patients

TABLE 22-1 Causes of Nutrient Loss in AIDS Patients

- Anorexia
- Cancer
- Diarrhea
- Increased metabolism due to fever
- Certain medications
- Malabsorption caused by cancer or diarrhea
- Protein energy malnutrition

The Relationship of HIV Infection and Nutrition

A healthful diet is essential for a healthy immune system, which may delay the onset of AIDS. Persons diagnosed as being HIV-positive should have a baseline nutrition and diet assessment by a registered dietitian. Unhealthful eating habits can be corrected at an early stage of the disease, and future nutritional needs explained.

As the condition progresses, the patient begins to experience the physical problems previously listed. Infections increase the metabolic rate and nutrient and kcal needs and, at the same time, decrease the appetite and often the body's ability to absorb nutrients. Medications may further reduce the appetite and cause nausea. When there are oral infections, taste may change, and swallowing can become painful. Anorexia commonly occurs (Table 22-2).

AIDS patients experience serious protein-energy malnutrition (PEM) and thus, body wasting. This may be referred to as HIV wasting syndrome, which results in **hypoalbuminemia** and weight loss. The immune system is further damaged by insufficient amounts of protein and kcal, thus hastening death.

hypoalbuminemia
abnormally low amounts of protein in the blood

TABLE 22-2 Causes of Anorexia among AIDS Patients

Medications	Cause nausea, vomiting
Oral infections	Diminish saliva, alter taste, cause mouth pain
Altered taste	Changes or exaggerates flavors
Fever	Depresses appetite
Pain	Depresses appetite
Depression	Depresses appetite
Dysphagia	Makes swallowing difficult
Dementia	May cause patient to forget to eat

Problems Related to Feeding AIDS Patients

Just when an AIDS patient most needs a nutrient- and kcal-rich diet, he or she is most apt to refuse it. In some cases, it may be useful to discuss nutritional care with the patient. When possible, medications should be given after meals to reduce the chance of nausea. Sores in the mouth or esophagus can make eating painful, and soft foods may be better tolerated than others. Taste can be affected by the disease, so spicy, highly acidic, extremely hot or extremely cold foods may be rejected. Frequent small meals and, sometimes, liquid supplements may be helpful. Additional sugar and flavoring may increase the acceptability of liquid supplements. Because of the nausea and diarrhea, sufficient fluids are essential. If the patient has difficulty swallowing or simply cannot eat, tube feeding may be imperative. If the tube causes pain, parenteral nutrition may be necessary.

The patient should be helped to eat as much as possible, especially on "good" days. Patients may suffer from pain and depression, and they may worry about finances and what people think of them. These factors can further diminish their appetites, but positive discussions can help (Table 22-3).

Neurological impairment usually occurs in varying degrees in AIDS patients and may cause confusion and dysphagia. In such cases, meal trays should be kept simple, the consistency of food modified to best suit the patient, and special utensils provided if needed.

Some patients may want to try nontraditional diets, thinking they will help or even cure them. These patients need to be made aware of any potentially harmful effects from such diets. In some cases, the *idea* of improvement may help the patient's appetite.

Those patients who will benefit no further from either medication or nutrition can still be comforted by the health care professional who shows support, understanding, and respect for them.

TABLE 22-3 Methods To Improve the Appetite of an AIDS Patient

- Give medications *after* meals
- Offer soft food
- Avoid spicy, acidic, and extremely hot or cold foods
- Serve frequent, small meals
- Add sugar and flavorings to liquid supplements
- Take advantage of the "good" days and offer any food the patient tolerates
- Talk with the patient to help ease concerns about finances, family, and friends

CONSIDERATIONS FOR THE HEALTH CARE PROFESSIONAL

Patients who fall within the categories of conditions discussed in this chapter can be a challenge for the health care professional. Those recovering from surgery may seem to complain a great deal. Those suffering from burns will pull at one's heartstrings. Patients suffering from fatal infections can require extra attention. Patients receiving tube feedings or some medications may suffer from frequent diarrhea and require total patient care.

In each of these cases, the health care professional can help herself or himself as well as the patient by thinking positively and being cheerful. Cheerfulness can be contagious, but it is never harmful.

● SUMMARY

Surgery, burns, fevers, and infections are traumas that cause the body to respond hypermetabolically. This response creates the need for additional nutrients at the same time that the injury causes a loss of nutrients. Care must be taken to provide extra fluid, proteins, kcal, vitamins, minerals, and carbohydrates as needed in these situations. When surgery is elective, nutritional status should be improved before surgery, if necessary. When food cannot be taken orally, enteral or parenteral nutrition should be used.

● DISCUSSION TOPICS

1. Describe the body's reaction to trauma and how nutrition is related to it.
2. Why are extra nutrients needed during trauma?
3. When might surgery be elective?
4. In what ways might a diet history of a presurgical patient be helpful?
5. Explain why a burn patient needs extra protein. What happens when the extra protein is not provided?
6. Why does a surgical patient need extra minerals?
7. Why must a patient's stomach be empty at the time of surgery?
8. Explain why intravenous dextrose solutions are not sufficient to fulfill nutritional requirements after surgery.
9. Describe dumping syndrome, and tell how it may be alleviated.
10. Describe parenteral nutrition. What is it? How is it delivered? What are some dangers related to it?
11. Could parenteral nutrition be used in the treatment of anorexia nervosa? Explain.

● SUGGESTED ACTIVITIES

1. Ask a certified nutrition support dietitian (CNSD) to visit the class and discuss tube feedings, telling why and when they are used and problems associated with them.

2. Invite a nurse from a local hospital to discuss burns and their treatment.

3. If a class member has experienced any of the traumas discussed in this chapter, ask that person to describe it, her or his reactions, appetite, and recovery.

4. Role-play a situation in which a patient is 9 days postsurgery and cannot eat, and the nurse is trying to convince her to eat.

5. Role-play a situation between a 10-year-old child and a nurse. The child has rheumatic fever, a temperature of 100°F, and refuses most food.

● REVIEW

Multiple choice. Select the *letter* that precedes the best answer.

1. Trauma
   a. can be described as injury
   b. causes a hypometabolic response in the body
   c. usually decreases the body's need for protein
   d. has no relation to nutrition

2. During trauma, there is usually
   a. reduced need for protein and minerals
   b. a hypermetabolic response in the body
   c. only minor changes in nutritional requirements
   d. a decreased need for kcal

3. Wound healing, tissue building, and blood regeneration all require
   a. extra fat
   b. extra cholesterol
   c. reduced kcal intake
   d. protein

4. Intravenous solutions
   a. rarely contain vitamins
   b. usually contain cellulose
   c. are usually given after surgery
   d. provide 2,000 kcal per day

5. Protein is needed to
   a. provide kcal
   b. resist infection
   c. control fat metabolism during trauma
   d. kill bacteria

6. It would not be surprising for TPN to be used in the treatment of
   a. fractured hip
   b. third-degree burns over a large part of the patient's body
   c. broken leg
   d. appendicitis

7. Dumping syndrome is characterized by
   a. migraine headache
   b. hypertension and tremors
   c. reduced clotting time
   d. dizziness and cramps

8. TPN for more than 2 weeks is given through
   a. a nasogastric tube
   b. a peripheral vein in the ankle
   c. the superior vena cava
   d. an esophagostomy

9. Severely burned patients will need
   a. to replace protein and fluids
   b. extra amounts of glucose the first 2–3 days after the burn
   c. reduced amounts of liquid
   d. a low-protein, low-kcal diet

10. Fever
    a. creates a need for extra kcal
    b. patients have enormous appetites
    c. patients experience reduced metabolic rate
    d. patients should be kept on a low-kcal diet

C A S E   S T U D Y

Irving W. was an 83-year-old male who lived in an assisted-living apartment in a nursing home complex. Irving was admitted to the hospital for chest pain. Within 2 days, the doctors had determined that he had a myocardial infarction (MI). During the following 3 days in the hospital, Irving had complications with his MI. The gastroenterologist determined that Irving had a bowel obstruction. Irving was made NPO and started on TPN through his IV.

After Irving's bowel resection, when he had active bowel sounds, he was allowed to have clear liquids. The doctors were anxious to stop the TPN and advance him to a regular diet. When Irving progressed to soft foods the TPN was stopped.

Irving's appetite started to drop. He only ate half of his meals and complained that nothing looked good. He missed his wife, Matilda, and worried about her even though he spoke to her every day. When Matilda was there, Irving was so glad to see her that he talked up a storm and his appetite seemed to improve. The doctor told Irving he had lost 10 pounds since he had been in the hospital and he couldn't afford to lose any more weight. The doctor told him if he couldn't maintain his weight a feeding tube would have to be inserted and tube feedings started.

ASSESSMENT

1. What do you know about Irving and his diet?
2. What are some reasons that Irving was not eating 100% of his meals?
3. How significant is this problem?

DIAGNOSIS

4. What were Irving's diagnoses?

PLAN/GOAL

5. What is the overall nutritional goal for Irving?

IMPLEMENTATION

6. What are some natural strategies that the nurse can use to stimulate bowel activity in Irving?
7. What strategies can the dietitian use to increase Irving's food intake?
8. What categories of food are a priority for Irving right now?
9. What can his family do to help?
10. What could an appetite stimulant do?

EVALUATION/OUTCOME CRITERIA

11. What criteria would the doctor use to evaluate the above plan?

C A S E   S T U D Y

Peter was a 30-year-old grade school teacher. He was 5 feet 9 inches tall and weighed about 165 pounds. He liked teaching, and his students enjoyed his classes. When he was diagnosed as HIV-positive, he was devastated. For the first time, he felt ashamed of his lifestyle.

He was the only child of his widowed mother. He grew up in a small rural community. His mother always boasted of his teaching success and her pride in his career. He didn't want to embarrass or hurt his mother. When he finally told her about his HIV status, she just cried and hugged him and told him she loved him.

Within months of his revelation to his mother, his T-cell counts dropped to the lowest level yet. He was having a hard time shaking his third episode of pneumonia. His mother came to take care of him. She cooked all his favorite foods, sometimes serving him four desserts for dinner. She always watched that he took his medications as prescribed.

When he refused to go back to the hospital anymore and just wanted to die at home, she consulted with the hospital dietitian to learn how she could help him. She told the dietitian he weighed about 120 pounds now.

ASSESSMENT

1. What do you know about Peter and his nutrition?
2. What barriers to good nutrition does he have?
3. What resources does he have?
4. Why would his mother talk to a dietitian?
5. How important is nutrition to health maintenance in HIV-positive persons?

DIAGNOSIS

6. Write a statement describing the reasons why Peter was unable to remain well-nourished.

PLAN/GOAL

7. What is the priority goal for Peter?

IMPLEMENTATION

8. What strategies can the dietitian suggest?
9. What can she teach the mother about HIV and nutrition?
10. What foods are a priority during his active infection?
11. Who else can help?

EVALUATION/OUTCOME CRITERIA

12. What criteria can the mother use to see if her plan is successful?

Chapter

23

Nutritional Care of Patients

Key Terms

iatrogenic malnutrition
pressure ulcer

Objectives

After studying this chapter, you should be able to:

- Describe how illness and surgery can affect the nutrition of patients

- Identify and describe three or more nutrition-related health problems that are common among elderly patients needing long-term care

- Demonstrate correct procedures for feeding a bedridden patient

- Explain the importance of adapting the family's meal to suit the patient's nutritional requirements

HOSPITALIZED PATIENTS

Illness and surgery can have devastating effects on nutritional status. Fever, nausea, fear, depression, chemotherapy, and radiation can destroy appetite. Vomiting, diarrhea, chemotherapy, radiation, and some medications can reduce or prevent absorption of nutrients. In addition, food is restricted before surgery and some diagnostic tests. Ironically, this reduced nutrient and kcal intake occurs just at a time when requirements are increased.

Protein Energy Malnutrition

When the increased needs for energy and protein are not met by food intake, the body must use its stores of glycogen and fat. When they have been used, the body breaks down its own tissues to provide protein for energy. It has no other "stores" of protein. Protein-energy malnutrition, commonly called PEM, can be a problem among hospitalized patients. It can delay wound healing, contribute to anemia, depress the immune system, and, because of the depressed immune system, increase susceptibility to infections. Symptoms of PEM include weight loss and dry, pale skin. When malnutrition occurs as a result of hospitalization, it is called **iatrogenic malnutrition**.

iatrogenic malnutrition
caused by treatment or diagnostic procedures

Improving the Patient's Nutritional Status

The importance of improving a patient's nutritional status is obvious. Formal nutritional assessments of patients should be made on a regular basis, but all members of the health care team should be alert to signs of malnutrition every day. The nurse or nursing assistant who sees the patient regularly is in the best position to help the patient. This person will be most familiar to the patient and will hear the patient's complaints about and see the reactions to the food served. She or he can bring problems to the attention of the dietitian responsible for the patient's nutrition. The patient may

1. need reassurance about his or her condition
2. need information about nutritional needs
3. need personal attention
4. want other foods

If approved by the dietitian, it can be helpful to invite friends and relatives to bring the patient some of his or her favorite foods.

FEEDING THE PATIENT

In the home, the family menu should serve as the basis of the patient's meal whenever possible. This usually pleases the patient because it makes her or him feel a part of the family. It also reduces food preparation time and costs.

Family meals are easily adapted for the patient by omitting or adding certain foods or by varying the method of preparation. Suppose the patient was to limit fat intake and the family menu was the following:

> Fried hamburgers
> Mashed potatoes with butter
> Buttered peas
> Lettuce with French dressing
> Ice cream with fresh strawberries
> Whole milk

Broiling the hamburgers for everyone instead of frying would help limit the fat content. The patient's mashed potatoes might be served with little or no butter, and the peas with only salt and pepper and perhaps a suitable spice, herb, or lemon. The patient could be served lettuce with fat-free dressing and, for dessert, strawberries with low-fat ice cream. Fat-free milk is a simple substitute for whole milk.

Serving the Meal

When a meal is served at the bedside, the tray should be lined with a pretty cloth or paper liner. Attractive dishes that fit the tray conveniently without crowding it should be used. The food should be arranged attractively on the plate, with a colorful garnish such as a slice of fruit, parsley, or vegetable stick. The garnish must fit into the patient's diet plan, however. Utensils must be arranged conveniently. Water should be served as well as another beverage (unless it is prohibited by the physician). Foods must be served at proper temperatures.

When the patient is on complete bed rest, special preparations are required before the meal is served. The patient should be given the opportunity to use the bedpan and to wash before the meal is served. The room can be ventilated and the bedcovers straightened. The patient should be helped to a comfortable position, and any unpleasant sights should be removed before the meal is served. Pleasant conversation during the preparations can improve the patient's mood considerably. Certain topics of conversation can help stimulate the patient's interest in eating. The patient might be told that the family is anticipating the same meal. Perhaps the recipes used will interest some patients. Appropriate remarks on the patient's progress, whenever possible, are helpful.

When the meal preparations are complete, the tray should be placed so that it is easy for the patient to feed herself or himself or, if necessary, convenient for someone else to do the feeding. If the patient needs help, the napkin should be opened and placed, the bread spread, the meat cut, the eggs shelled, and the straw offered. The patient should be encouraged to eat and be allowed sufficient time. If the meal is interrupted by the physician, the tray should be reheated and served again as soon as the physician leaves.

The tray should be removed and the patient helped to brush her or his teeth when the meal is finished. The kinds and amounts of food refused, the time, type of diet, and patient's appetite should be recorded on the patient's chart after each meal. At times, the doctor may request a calorie and protein count, which is an accurate report of the types and amounts of food eaten.

Feeding the Patient with Disability

If the patient is unable to feed herself or himself, the person doing the feeding should sit near the side of the bed. Small amounts of food should be placed toward the back of the mouth with a slight pressure on the tongue with the spoon or fork. Patients should not be fed with a syringe. If the patient is suffering from one-sided paralysis, the food and drinking straw must be placed in the nonparalyzed side of the mouth (Figure 23-1). The patient must be allowed to help herself or himself as much as possible. If the patient begins to choke, help her or him sit up straight. Do not give food or water while the patient is choking. The patient's mouth should be wiped as needed. A patient with dysphagia will require thickened liquids to prevent aspiration.

Feeding the Blind Patient

Special care must be taken in serving a meal to a blind patient. An appetizing description of it can help create a desire to eat. To help the blind patient feed herself or himself, arrange the food as if the plate were the face of a clock (Figure 23-2). The meat might be put at 6 o'clock, vegetables at 9 o'clock, salad at 12, and bread at 3 o'clock. The person who regularly arranges the meal should remember to use the same pattern for all meals. Blind people usually feel better when they can help themselves.

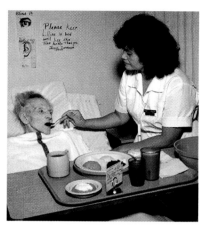

FIGURE 23-1 Some patients require assistance when eating.

LONG-TERM CARE OF THE ELDERLY

Because of increasing longevity (length of life), the number of elderly people requiring long-term care is expected to increase. The changes people undergo with age that can affect their nutritional status were discussed in Chapter 15.

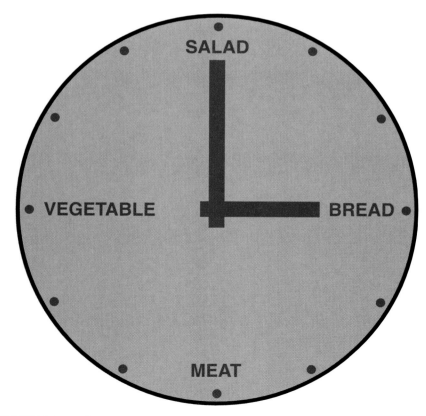

FIGURE 23-2 To a blind patient, a plate of food can be pictured as the face of a clock.

Physical Problems of the Institutionalized Elderly

It is estimated that the majority of people 85 and over have at least one chronic disease such as arthritis, osteoporosis, diabetes mellitus, cardiovascular disease, or mental disorder. These conditions affect their attitudes, physical activities, appetites and, thus, nutritional status. PEM is a major problem for this population.

Anemia can develop if the patient has too little animal protein in the diet. It can contribute to confusion and depression but may go unnoticed because one of its major symptoms, fatigue, may be simply thought to be a characteristic of old age. It is helpful to make sure there is sufficient animal protein and vitamin C (an iron enhancer) in the patient's diet.

pressure ulcers
bedsores

Pressure ulcers (bedsores) can develop in bedridden patients. They develop in areas where unrelieved pressure on the skin prevents the blood from bringing nutrients and oxygen and removing wastes. Healing requires treatment of the ulcer, relief of the pressure, a high-kcal diet with sufficient protein, and vitamin C and zinc supplements.

Constipation can be caused by inadequate fiber, fluid, or exercise; by medication; by reduced peristalsis; or by former abuse of laxatives. It can be relieved by increased fluid, fiber, and exercise (if possible).

Diarrhea can be caused by lack of muscle tone in the colon. It will reduce the absorption of nutrients and can contribute to dehydration. An increase of fiber in the diet combined with supplemental vitamins and minerals may be helpful.

The sense of smell declines with age and the appetite diminishes. A reduced sense of taste can be caused by medications, disease, mineral deficiencies, or xerostomia (dry mouth). The addition of spices, herbs, salt, and sugar (if allowed) can be helpful. Xerostomia can be caused by disease or medications. Drinking water, eating frequent small meals, and chewing sugar-free gums or candies may be helpful. The inadequate amount of saliva in these patients contributes to increased tooth decay.

Dysphagia (difficulty swallowing) can result from a stroke, closed head trauma, head or neck cancer, surgery, or Alzheimer's and other diseases. A swallow study needs to be done to determine the consistency of diet needed by patients with dysphagia. A swallow study is done by a speech therapist using a video fluoroscope. While being videotaped, the patient is given liquids, semi-liquids, pureed food, and solid food to determine the consistency of the bolus (food mass) that he or she is able to swallow without aspirating. Many dysphagia patients must have thickened liquids. Dysphagia patients should always be in an upright position when eating.

CONSIDERATIONS FOR THE HEALTH CARE PROFESSIONAL

The needs of bedridden patients are nearly total. They are unable to walk, use the bathroom, brush their teeth, or wash their hands without help. The feelings of helplessness they endure are terrible. In addition, they may be embarrassed by their appearance, or by needing a bedpan when only a thin curtain separates them from their neighbor's guests.

It is helpful to the patient if the health care professional can imagine himself or herself in the place of the patient.

The needs of many elderly patients in nursing homes are also total. They may be arthritic and unable to walk; some may be incontinent; others may forget their names and how to dress; they may wander off the premises unless they are constantly watched; they may need to be fed. Each remains an individual. They all need, respond to, and deserve warmth and respect from their caregivers.

● SUMMARY

Illness and surgery can have devastating effects on patients' nutritional status. PEM can be a significant problem in hospitals. The health care team should work together to improve patients' nutritional status.

Once a patient is at home, her or his meals should be adapted from the family's meals. This saves time and expense and allows the patient to feel less of a burden and more a part of the family.

A bedridden patient should be given the bedpan and allowed to wash her or his hands before the meal. Patients should be encouraged to feed themselves. However, help should be offered if it is needed. The blind patient can eat more easily if food is arranged in a set pattern on the plate. Pleasant conversation and cheerfulness on the part of the nurse can improve the patient's appetite. The type of diet, time of meal, patient's appetite, and type and amount of food eaten should all be recorded on the patient's chart. Elderly patients requiring long-term care may suffer from several nutrition-related health problems that, with proper treatment, can sometimes be relieved.

● DISCUSSION TOPICS

1. How do illness and surgery affect one's nutrition?

2. What is iatrogenic malnutrition? How might it develop?

3. In what ways might the nurse help improve the patient's nutrition?

4. When might it be unwise to invite a patient's friends and family to bring foods to the patient? When might it be appropriate? Who would decide?

5. Discuss the importance of proper preparation of the patient and room before the meal. What could disturb a patient and affect appetite?

6. How may the appearance of the tray affect the patient's appetite?

7. Why should the patient be encouraged to feed herself or himself?

8. Why is it important to remove the tray as soon as the patient has finished the meal?

9. How can the behavior and attitude of the attending person affect the appetite of the patient?

10. Why is anemia so easily overlooked in elderly patients?

11. Discuss how a diminished sense of smell might affect one's appetite.

● SUGGESTED ACTIVITIES

1. Have two students participate in the following role-playing situation. The class should evaluate and discuss the "nurse's" tact and skill in dealing with the "patient."

   Mrs. Jones is a young, active woman with a family. She is recovering from viral pneumonia. Although she is allowed out of bed, she is not supposed to prepare meals or do housework until her condition improves. Dr. Malcolm has told Miss Wilson, the nurse, that it is important for Mrs. Jones to regain her lost weight. One day, before her dinner was served, Mrs. Jones complained to Miss Wilson. She was discouraged about her lack of energy and stated that her family needed her. Miss Wilson noticed that Mrs. Jones had eaten very little for breakfast and lunch. What should she say to Mrs. Jones?

2. Invite a gerontologist to speak to the class on nutrition and the elderly.

3. Invite a nurse who works in a nursing home to talk to the class. Ask him or her to describe how these patients are fed.

4. Visit a local nursing home in groups of two or three. Talk to some of the patients. Write a report on your visit.

● REVIEW

Multiple choice. Select the *letter* that precedes the best answer.

1. Surgery
   a. reduces the number of kcal normally needed
   b. has only a slight effect on appetite
   c. is always followed by TPN
   d. can temporarily devastate a patient's nutritional status

2. Normal absorption of nutrients
   a. is not affected by chemotherapy
   b. is unaffected by diarrhea
   c. can be decreased after surgery
   d. is unaffected by PEM

3. When energy and protein needs are not met by food intake, the body will
   a. first use its stores of fat and second its glycogen
   b. first use its stores of glycogen and second its fat
   c. first use its stores of protein
   d. increase its metabolic rate

4. PEM
   a. can delay wound healing
   b. has no relationship to the development of anemia
   c. strengthens the immune system
   d. decreases the risk of infection

5. Surgery may
   a. reduce nutritional requirements
   b. decrease one's kcal requirement
   c. contribute to the development of PEM
   d. increase one's fat requirements

6. Favorite foods brought to hospital patients from home
   a. should not be allowed
   b. have no effect on the patient's nutritional status
   c. should be approved by the dietitian before being given to the patient
   d. are neither helpful nor harmful

7. Iatrogenic malnutrition
   a. is the inevitable result of surgery
   b. is commonly caused by low-grade fevers
   c. can be a result of hospitalization
   d. has no effect on wound healing

8. Dysphagia
   a. means memory loss
   b. is common following bone surgery
   c. can safely be ignored
   d. patients should not be in a supine position when eating

9. Anemia
   a. can result from insufficient fat intake
   b. can contribute to hyperthyroidism
   c. occurs only in males over 50
   d. can be helped by the addition of vitamin C and iron

10. Pressure ulcers
   a. occur only in the stomach
   b. can occur in the duodenum
   c. do not affect bedridden patients
   d. develop in areas where, because of pressure, blood cannot get to the tissue

C A S E   S T U D Y

Jessie was a thin, 30-year-old black man who had been a paraplegic for 5 years. He lived in a house with his three brothers who helped take care of him. Harold did the cooking. He made fried eggs, grits, bacon, and coffee for breakfast. Pork and potatoes with greens were a typical dinner. Jessie didn't like milk; it gave him gas.

Jessie loved to play basketball, or wheelchair ball as he called it, with the neighborhood kids. He'd have his boom box blasting on the side of the court and play for hours. The kids loved the attention, and Jessie loved to be outside. During the school year, Jessie took classes at the local college and tried to sell his drawings to any admirer. He felt most alive when he was just wheeling around the neighborhood in the warmer months.

Jessie wasn't good at limiting the amount of time he was in his wheelchair. He was even worse at staying in bed, off his bottom. He had a tendency to develop pressure ulcers.

This time Jessie had the worst problem yet. His doctor said he had to go into the hospital for skin flap surgery to close the decubiti. He would have to stay off his back at least 3 weeks, possibly 6 weeks until the incision lines had healed. Jessie couldn't smoke in the hospital. The doctor was willing to let him use a nicotine patch if needed.

Initially, Jessie did well after surgery. He made the transition to regular food. Within 2 weeks, he was complaining of dry itchy skin, and the doctor was worried about his 5-pound weight loss. The doctor ordered a dietary assessment.

ASSESSMENT

1. What do you know about Jessie and his nutrition? Did he eat a balanced diet?

2. What barriers were there to his healing?

3. What foods are a priority to healing?

4. How significant is nutrition to this problem?

DIAGNOSIS

5. Write at least two diagnoses that apply to Jessie's problems.

PLAN/GOAL

6. What is the priority goal for Jessie?

IMPLEMENTATION

7. If Jessie is unable to eat enough food to maintain his weight, what alternatives does the doctor have?

8. Who else can help?

9. What does the dietitian need to know about Jessie to help?

10. What is the dietitian likely to recommend?

11. What strategies could be helpful?

12. How could supplemental vitamins help?

EVALUATION/OUTCOME CRITERIA

13. What needs to happen for Jessie to avoid having a feeding tube?

14. What criteria will the doctor use to determine if the plan is effective?

CASE STUDY

When Connie's husband died, her only daughter insisted that Connie move to a nursing home near her. Connie, who was only 75 years old, felt fine at the time and didn't want to move away from her only brother and her friends. She agreed reluctantly to try it. Her daughter was worried about Connie being alone.

When Connie saw the assisted-living area and the tiny room she had, she cried. The food was bad, and there weren't too many people she could play cards with or have a conversation with. When her brother came to visit her, he was shocked at Connie's appearance. She looked thin and pale. She was still in her pajamas at noon. She seemed withdrawn and sullen.

Her brother wanted to take her back home with him. The daughter sheepishly agreed. Her brother's wife, Viola, was a wonderful cook and enjoyed Connie's company. Within a month, Connie had regained some weight, was out walking every day with Viola, and was alert enough to play cards again. Connie even said she felt like her old self again. Connie returned to her own home after 2 months at her brother's home.

When her daughter visited her at the end of the 2 months, she readily admitted that she had made a mistake. She was pleased to see that Connie had returned to her old self.

ASSESSMENT

1. What do you know about Connie?
2. What caused the change in her health?
3. How significant was the problem?

DIAGNOSIS

4. Write two diagnoses about Connie.

PLAN/GOAL

5. What was her brother's goal when he took Connie out of assisted living?

IMPLEMENTATION

6. What factors contributed to her return to her old self?
7. How significant is maintaining independence in elders?
8. What are nutritional priorities for elders?

EVALUATION/OUTCOME CRITERIA

9. What had the daughter and Viola observed that deemed the plan successful?

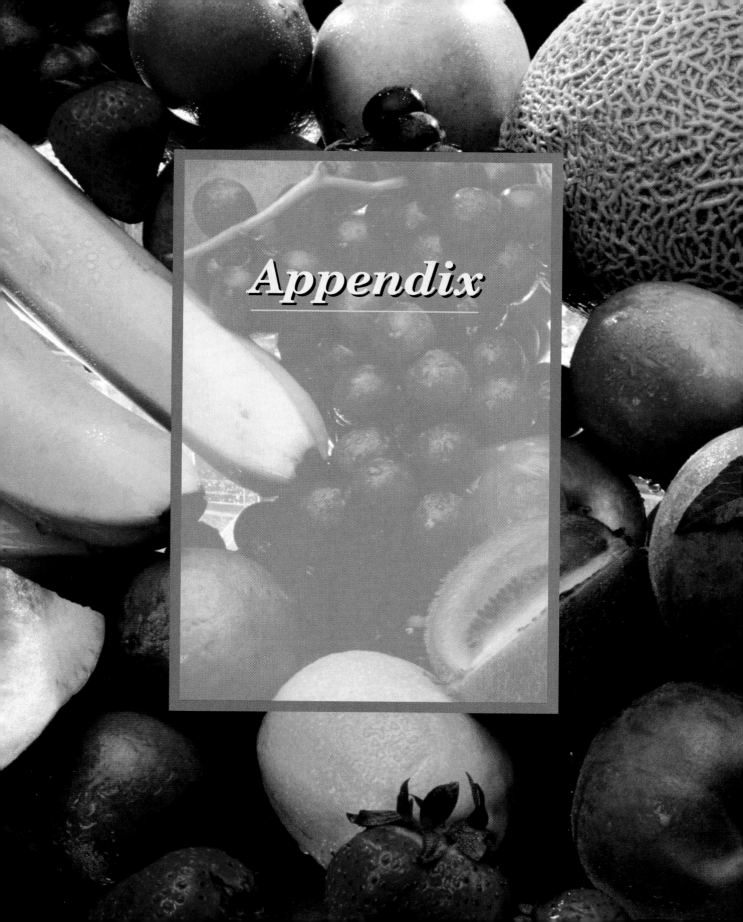

Appendix

Table A-1 1983 Metropolitan Height and Weight Tables. Weights at ages 25–59 based on lowest mortality. Weight in pounds according to frame (in indoor clothing weighing 5 lbs. for men and 3 lbs. for women; shoes with 1″ heels).

Men					Women				
Height Feet	Inches	Small Frame	Medium Frame	Large Frame	Height Feet	Inches	Small Frame	Medium Frame	Large Frame
5	2	128–134	131–141	138–150	4	10	102–111	109–121	118–131
5	3	130–136	133–143	140–153	4	11	103–113	111–123	120–134
5	4	132–138	135–145	142–156	5	0	104–115	113–126	122–137
5	5	134–140	137–148	144–160	5	1	106–118	115–129	125–140
5	6	136–142	139–151	146–164	5	2	108–121	118–132	128–143
5	7	138–145	142–154	149–168	5	3	111–124	121–135	131–147
5	8	140–148	145–157	152–172	5	4	114–127	124–138	134–151
5	9	142–151	148–160	155–176	5	5	117–130	127–141	137–155
5	10	144–154	151–163	158–180	5	6	120–133	130–144	140–159
5	11	146–157	154–166	161–184	5	7	123–136	133–147	143–163
6	0	149–160	157–170	164–188	5	8	126–139	136–150	146–167
6	1	152–164	160–174	168–192	5	9	129–142	139–153	149–170
6	2	155–168	164–178	172–197	5	10	132–145	142–156	152–173
6	3	158–172	167–182	176–202	5	11	135–148	145–159	155–176
6	4	162–176	171–187	181–207	6	0	138–151	148–162	158–179

Source: *Metropolitan Life Insurance Company* Source of basic data 1979 Build Study Society of Actuaries and Association of Life Insurance Medical Directors of America 1980.

Table A-2 Drug-Nutrient Interactions

Drug	Effect
Alcohol	Decreased absorption of thiamin, folic acid, and vitamin B_{12}; increased urinary excretion of magnesium and zinc
Analgesics	
Aspirin (salicylates)	Decreased serum folate level; increased excretion of vitamin C
Colchicine	Decreased absorption of vitamin B_{12}, carotene, fat, lactose, sodium, potassium, protein, and cholesterol
Amphetamines	Decreased appetite and caloric intake; possibly reduced growth
Antacids	
Aluminum hydroxide	Decreased absorption of phosphate
Other antacids	Decreased thiamin and fatty acid absorption
Anticonvulsants	
Barbiturates	Decreased vitamin B_{12} and thiamin absorption; increased excretion of vitamin C; deficiency of folate and vitamin D
Hydantoins	Decreased serum folate, vitamin B_{12}, pyridoxine, calcium, and vitamin D levels; increased excretion of vitamin C
Antidepressants	Increased appetite; weight gain
Antimetabolites	General absorptive decrease secondary to intestinal wall damage and oral mucus break-down; specific malabsorption of B_{12}, folate, fat, and xylose
Antimicrobials	
Chloramphenicol	Increased riboflavin, pyridoxine, and B_{12} requirements
Neomycin	Decreased absorption of fat; carbohydrate; protein; vitamin A, B_{12}, D, and E; calcium; iron; sugar; potassium; sodium; and nitrogen
Penicillin	Increased potassium excretion; inhibition of glutathione
Sulfonamides	Decreased synthesis of folic acid, vitamin K, and B vitamins
Tetracyclines	Decreased absorption of calcium, iron, magnesium, and fat; increased excretion of vitamin C, riboflavin, nitrogen, folic acid, and niacin; decreased vitamin K synthesis
Cathartics	Decreased absorption of calcium, vitamin D, potassium, protein, glucose, and fat
Chelating agents	Increased excretion of zinc, copper, and pyridoxine; depression of appetite
Corticosteroids	Decreased absorption of calcium, phosphorus, and iron; increased excretion of vitamin C, calcium, potassium, zinc, and nitrogen; decreased tolerance of glucose; increased triglyceride and cholesterol absorption; increased vitamin D metabolism; increased appetite
Diuretics	
Furosemide	Increased excretion of calcium, magnesium, and potassium
Mercurials	Increased excretion of thiamin, magnesium, calcium, and potassium
Thiazides	Increased excretion of potassium, magnesium, zinc, and riboflavin
Triamterence	Decreased serum folate and vitamin B_{12} levels
Hypocholesterolemic agent	
Cholestyramine	Decreased absorption of cholesterol; potassium; vitamins A, D, K, and B_{12}; folate, fat; glucose; and iron
Clofibrate	Decreased absorption of vitamin B_{12}, iron, glucose, potassium, and sodium; decreased taste acuity; aftertaste
Hypotensive agents	Increased excretion of pyridoxine
Laxatives	
Mineral oil	Decreased absorption of vitamins A, D, E, and K; calcium; and phosphate
Phenolphthalein	Increased excretion of potassium
Levodopa	Decreased absorption of amino acids; increased use of ascorbic acid and pyridoxine; increased excretion of sodium and potassium
Oral contraceptives	Decreased serum levels of vitamin C, vitamin B_{12}, folate, pyridoxine, riboflavin, magnesium, and zinc; increased absorption of iron; increased serum lipid levels; increased appetite
Potassium chloride	Decreased absorption of vitamin B_{12}
Sedatives	
Glutethimide	Increased metabolism of vitamin D
Sulfonamides	
Azulfidine	Decreased absorption of folate; decreased serum iron level
Other sulfonamides	Decreased synthesis of folate and vitamins B and K
Surfactants	Decreased absorption of fat
Tranquilizers	Increased appetite; weight gain

Source: Green, Marilyn L. and Harry, Joann. *Nutrition in Contemporary Nursing Practice*, Second Edition. New York; John Wiley & Sons, 1987.

Table A-3 English and Metric Units and Conversions

Units of Measure in the English System

Unit	Abbreviation	Equivalent
dash		less than $\frac{1}{8}$ teaspoon
few grains	f.g.	less than $\frac{1}{8}$ teaspoon
drop		—
15 drops		—
1 teaspoon	tsp	$\frac{1}{3}$ tablespoon
1 tablespoon	Tbsp	3 teaspoons
1 fluid ounce	oz	2 tablespoons
1 cup	c	8 fluid ounces or 16 tablespoons
1 pint	pt	2 cups
1 quart	qt	2 pints or 4 cups
1 gallon	gal	4 quarts
1 peck	pk	2 gallons
1 bushel	bu	4 pecks
1 pound	lb	16 ounces

Units of Measure in the Metric System

Basic unit of *weight* is the *gram* (g)
Basic unit of *volume* is the *liter* (1)
Basic unit of *length* is the *meter* (m)
Temperature is measured in degrees *Celsius* (°C)

kilo: (*key*–low) = 1,000
deci: (*dess*–ee) = 0.1 (1/10)
centi: (*sent*–ee) = 0.01 (1/100)
milli: (*mill*–ee) = 0.001 (1/1000)

Unit Relationships within the Metric System

Weight		Volume	
1000 grams =	1 *kilo*gram	1000 liters =	1 *kilo*liter*
100 grams =	1 *hecto*gram*	100 liters =	1 *hecto*liter*
10 grams =	1 *deka*gram*	10 liters =	1 *deka*liter*
	1 gram		1 liter
.1 gram =	1 *deci*gram*	.1 liter =	1 *deci*liter*
.01 gram =	1 *centi*gram*	.01 liter =	1 *centi*liter*
.001 gram =	1 *milli*gram	.001 liter =	1 *milli*liter
.000001 gram =	1 *micro*gram*	.000001 liter =	1 *micro*liter*

*Units not commonly used.

Table A-3 (continued)

Converting from the English System to the Metric System

Convert to Metric	When You Know	Multiply By	To Find
Weight	ounces (oz) pounds (lb)	28 0.45	grams (g) kilograms (kg)
Volume	teaspoons (tsp) tablespoons (Tbsp) fluid ounces (fl oz) cups (c) pints (pt) quarts (qt) gallons (gal) cubic feet (ft³) cubic yards (yd³)	5 15 30 0.24 0.47 0.95 3.8 0.03 0.76	milliliters (ml) milliliters milliliters liters (1) liters liters liters cubic meters (m³) cubic meters
Temperature	Fahrenheit (°F) temperature	5/9 (after subtracting 32)	Celsius (°C) temperature

Source: Adapted from "Some References on Metric Information" by U.S. Dept. of Commerce, National Bureau of Standards.

Converting from the Metric System to the English System

Convert to English	When You Know	Multiply By	To Find
Weight	grams (g) kilograms (kg) metric tons (1000 kg)	0.035 2.2 1.1	ounces (oz) pounds (lb) short tons
Volume	milliliters (ml) liters (1) liters liters cubic meters (m³) cubic meters	0.03 2.1 1.06 0.26 35 1.3	fluid ounces (fl oz) pints (pt) quarts (qt) gallons (gal) cubic feet (ft³) cubic yards (yd³)
Temperature	Celsius (°C) temperature	9/5 (then add 32)	Fahrenheit (°F) temperature

Source: Adapted from "Some References on Metric Information" by U.S. Dept. of Commerce, National Bureau of Standards.

Weight Equivalents

	Milligram	Gram	Kilogram	Grain	Ounce	Pound
1 microgram (µg)	0.001	0.000001				
1 milligram (mg)	1.0	0.001		0.0154		
1 gram (g)	1,000.0	1.0	0.001	15.4	0.035	0.0022
1 kilogram (kg)	1,000,000.0	1,000.0	1.0	15,400.0	35.2	2.2
1 grain (gr)	64.8	0.065		1.0		
1 ounce (oz)		28.3		437.5	1.0	0.063
1 pound (lb)		453.6	0.454		16.0	1.0

Volume Equivalents

	Cubic Millimeter	Cubic Centimeter	Liter	Fluid Ounce	Pint	Quart
1 cubic millimeter (mm³)	1.0	0.001				
1 cubic centimeter (cm³)	1,000.0	1.0	0.001			
1 liter (1)	1,000,000.0	1,000.0	1.0	33.8	2.1	1.06
1 fluid ounce (fl oz)		30.(29.57)	0.03	1.0		
1 pint (pt)		473.0	0.473	16.0	1.0	
1 quart (qt)		946.0	0.946	32.0	2.0	1.0

Table A-4 Nutritive Value of the Edible Part of Food

(Tr indicates nutrient present in trace amount.)

Item No.	Foods, approximate measures, units, and weight (weight of edible portion only)		Water	Food energy	Pro-tein	Fat	Fatty acids		
							Satu-rated	Mono-unsatu-rated	Poly-unsatu-rated
		Grams	Per-cent	Cal-ories	Grams	Grams	Grams	Grams	Grams
	Beverages								
	Alcoholic:								
	Beer:								
1	Regular----------------------	12 fl oz--------	360	92	150	1	0	0.0	0.0	0.0
2	Light------------------------	12 fl oz--------	355	95	95	1	0	0.0	0.0	0.0
	Gin, rum, vodka, whiskey:								
3	80-proof---------------------	1-1/2 fl oz-----	42	67	95	0	0	0.0	0.0	0.0
4	86-proof---------------------	1-1/2 fl oz-----	42	64	105	0	0	0.0	0.0	0.0
5	90-proof---------------------	1-1/2 fl oz-----	42	62	110	0	0	0.0	0.0	0.0
	Wines:								
6	Dessert----------------------	3-1/2 fl oz-----	103	77	140	Tr	0	0.0	0.0	0.0
	Table:								
7	Red--------------------------	3-1/2 fl oz-----	102	88	75	Tr	0	0.0	0.0	0.0
8	White------------------------	3-1/2 fl oz-----	102	87	80	Tr	0	0.0	0.0	0.0
	Carbonated:[2]								
9	Club soda--------------------	12 fl oz--------	355	100	0	0	0	0.0	0.0	0.0
	Cola type:								
10	Regular----------------------	12 fl oz--------	369	89	160	0	0	0.0	0.0	0.0
11	Diet, artificially sweetened	12 fl oz--------	355	100	Tr	0	0	0.0	0.0	0.0
12	Ginger ale-------------------	12 fl oz--------	366	91	125	0	0	0.0	0.0	0.0
13	Grape------------------------	12 fl oz--------	372	88	180	0	0	0.0	0.0	0.0
14	Lemon-lime--------------------	12 fl oz--------	372	89	155	0	0	0.0	0.0	0.0
15	Orange-----------------------	12 fl oz--------	372	88	180	0	0	0.0	0.0	0.0
16	Pepper type------------------	12 fl oz--------	369	89	160	0	0	0.0	0.0	0.0
17	Root beer--------------------	12 fl oz--------	370	89	165	0	0	0.0	0.0	0.0
	Cocoa and chocolate-flavored beverages. See Dairy Products (items 95-98).								
	Coffee:								
18	Brewed-----------------------	6 fl oz--------	180	100	Tr	Tr	Tr	Tr	Tr	Tr
19	Instant, prepared (2 tsp powder plus 6 fl oz water)----------	6 fl oz--------	182	99	Tr	Tr	Tr	Tr	Tr	Tr
	Fruit drinks, noncarbonated:								
	Canned:								
20	Fruit punch drink-----------	6 fl oz--------	190	88	85	Tr	0	0.0	0.0	0.0
21	Grape drink------------------	6 fl oz--------	187	86	100	Tr	0	0.0	0.0	0.0
22	Pineapple-grapefruit juice drink----------------------	6 fl oz--------	187	87	90	Tr	Tr	Tr	Tr	Tr
	Frozen:								
	Lemonade concentrate:								
23	Undiluted-------------------	6-fl-oz can-----	219	49	425	Tr	Tr	Tr	Tr	Tr
24	Diluted with 4-1/3 parts water by volume----------	6 fl oz--------	185	89	80	Tr	Tr	Tr	Tr	Tr
	Limeade concentrate:								
25	Undiluted-------------------	6-fl-oz can-----	218	50	410	Tr	Tr	Tr	Tr	Tr
26	Diluted with 4-1/3 parts water by volume----------	6 fl oz--------	185	89	75	Tr	Tr	Tr	Tr	Tr
	Fruit juices. See type under Fruits and Fruit Juices.								
	Milk beverages. See Dairy Products (items 92-105).								
	Tea:								
27	Brewed-----------------------	8 fl oz--------	240	100	Tr	Tr	Tr	Tr	Tr	Tr
	Instant, powder, prepared:								
28	Unsweetened (1 tsp powder plus 8 fl oz water)--------	8 fl oz--------	241	100	Tr	Tr	Tr	Tr	Tr	Tr
29	Sweetened (3 tsp powder plus 8 fl oz water)-------------	8 fl oz--------	262	91	85	Tr	Tr	Tr	Tr	Tr

[1]Value not determined.
[2]Mineral content varies depending on water source.

Table A-4 Nutritive Value of the Edible Part of Food (Continued)

Cholesterol	Carbohydrate	Calcium	Phosphorus	Iron	Potassium	Sodium	Vitamin A value		Thiamin	Riboflavin	Niacin	Ascorbic acid	Item No
							(IU)	(RE)					
Milligrams	Grams	Milligrams	Milligrams	Milligrams	Milligrams	Milligrams	International units	Retinol equivalents	Milligrams	Milligrams	Milligrams	Milligrams	
0	13	14	50	0.1	115	18	0	0	0.02	0.09	1.8	0	1
0	5	14	43	0.1	64	11	0	0	0.03	0.11	1.4	0	2
0	Tr	Tr	Tr	Tr	1	Tr	0	0	Tr	Tr	Tr	0	3
0	Tr	Tr	Tr	Tr	1	Tr	0	0	Tr	Tr	Tr	0	4
0	Tr	Tr	Tr	Tr	1	Tr	0	0	Tr	Tr	Tr	0	5
0	8	8	9	0.2	95	9	(1)	(1)	0.01	0.02	0.2	0	6
0	3	8	18	0.4	113	5	(1)	(1)	0.00	0.03	0.1	0	7
0	3	9	14	0.3	83	5	(1)	(1)	0.00	0.01	0.1	0	8
0	0	18	0	Tr	0	78	0	0	0.00	0.00	0.0	0	9
0	41	11	52	0.2	7	18	0	0	0.00	0.00	0.0	0	10
0	Tr	14	39	0.2	7	[3]32	0	0	0.00	0.00	0.0	0	11
0	32	11	0	0.1	4	29	0	0	0.00	0.00	0.0	0	12
0	46	15	0	0.4	4	48	0	0	0.00	0.00	0.0	0	13
0	39	7	0	0.4	4	33	0	0	0.00	0.00	0.0	0	14
0	46	15	4	0.3	7	52	0	0	0.00	0.00	0.0	0	15
0	41	11	41	0.1	4	37	0	0	0.00	0.00	0.0	0	16
0	42	15	0	0.2	4	48	0	0	0.00	0.00	0.0	0	17
0	Tr	4	2	Tr	124	2	0	0	0.00	0.02	0.4	0	18
0	1	2	6	0.1	71	Tr	0	0	0.00	0.03	0.6	0	19
0	22	15	2	0.4	48	15	20	2	0.03	0.04	Tr	[4]61	20
0	26	2	2	0.3	9	11	Tr	Tr	0.01	0.01	Tr	[4]64	21
0	23	13	7	0.9	97	24	60	6	0.06	0.04	0.5	[4]110	22
0	112	9	13	0.4	153	4	40	4	0.04	0.07	0.7	66	23
0	21	2	2	0.1	30	1	10	1	0.01	0.02	0.2	13	24
0	108	11	13	0.2	129	Tr	Tr	Tr	0.02	0.02	0.2	26	25
0	20	2	2	Tr	24	Tr	Tr	Tr	Tr	Tr	Tr	4	26
0	Tr	0	2	Tr	36	1	0	0	0.00	0.03	Tr	0	27
0	1	1	4	Tr	61	1	0	0	0.00	0.02	0.1	0	28
0	22	1	3	Tr	49	Tr	0	0	0.00	0.04	0.1	0	29

[3]Blend of aspartame and saccharin; if only sodium saccharin is used, sodium is 75 mg; if only aspartame is used, sodium is 23 mg.
[4]With added ascorbic acid.

Table A-4 Nutritive Value of the Edible Part of Food *(Continued)*

(Tr indicates nutrient present in trace amount.)

Item No.	Foods, approximate measures, units, and weight (weight of edible portion only)		Water	Food energy	Pro-tein	Fat	Fatty acids		
							Satu-rated	Mono-unsatu-rated	Poly-unsatu-rated
		Grams	Per-cent	Cal-ories	Grams	Grams	Grams	Grams	Grams

Dairy Products

	Butter. See Fats and Oils (items 128-130).								
	Cheese:								
	Natural:								
30	Blue	1 oz	28	42	100	6	8	5.3	2.2	0.2
31	Camembert (3 wedges per 4-oz container)	1 wedge	38	52	115	8	9	5.8	2.7	0.3
	Cheddar:								
32	Cut pieces	1 oz	28	37	115	7	9	6.0	2.7	0.3
33		1 in³	17	37	70	4	6	3.6	1.6	0.2
34	Shredded	1 cup	113	37	455	28	37	23.8	10.6	1.1
	Cottage (curd not pressed down):								
	Creamed (cottage cheese, 4% fat):								
35	Large curd	1 cup	225	79	235	28	10	6.4	2.9	0.3
36	Small curd	1 cup	210	79	215	26	9	6.0	2.7	0.3
37	With fruit	1 cup	226	72	280	22	8	4.9	2.2	0.2
38	Lowfat (2%)	1 cup	226	79	205	31	4	2.8	1.2	0.1
39	Uncreamed (cottage cheese dry curd, less than 1/2% fat)	1 cup	145	80	125	25	1	0.4	0.2	Tr
40	Cream	1 oz	28	54	100	2	10	6.2	2.8	0.4
41	Feta	1 oz	28	55	75	4	6	4.2	1.3	0.2
	Mozzarella, made with:								
42	Whole milk	1 oz	28	54	80	6	6	3.7	1.9	0.2
43	Part skim milk (low moisture)	1 oz	28	49	80	8	5	3.1	1.4	0.1
44	Muenster	1 oz	28	42	105	7	9	5.4	2.5	0.2
	Parmesan, grated:								
45	Cup, not pressed down	1 cup	100	18	455	42	30	19.1	8.7	0.7
46	Tablespoon	1 tbsp	5	18	25	2	2	1.0	0.4	Tr
47	Ounce	1 oz	28	18	130	12	9	5.4	2.5	0.2
48	Provolone	1 oz	28	41	100	7	8	4.8	2.1	0.2
	Ricotta, made with:								
49	Whole milk	1 cup	246	72	430	28	32	20.4	8.9	0.9
50	Part skim milk	1 cup	246	74	340	28	19	12.1	5.7	0.6
51	Swiss	1 oz	28	37	105	8	8	5.0	2.1	0.3
	Pasteurized process cheese:								
52	American	1 oz	28	39	105	6	9	5.6	2.5	0.3
53	Swiss	1 oz	28	42	95	7	7	4.5	2.0	0.2
54	Pasteurized process cheese food, American	1 oz	28	43	95	6	7	4.4	2.0	0.2
55	Pasteurized process cheese spread, American	1 oz	28	48	80	5	6	3.8	1.8	0.2
	Cream, sweet:								
56	Half-and-half (cream and milk)	1 cup	242	81	315	7	28	17.3	8.0	1.0
57		1 tbsp	15	81	20	Tr	2	1.1	0.5	0.1
58	Light, coffee, or table	1 cup	240	74	470	6	46	28.8	13.4	1.7
59		1 tbsp	15	74	30	Tr	3	1.8	0.8	0.1
	Whipping, unwhipped (volume about double when whipped):								
60	Light	1 cup	239	64	700	5	74	46.2	21.7	2.1
61		1 tbsp	15	64	45	Tr	5	2.9	1.4	0.1
62	Heavy	1 cup	238	58	820	5	88	54.8	25.4	3.3
63		1 tbsp	15	58	50	Tr	6	3.5	1.6	0.2
64	Whipped topping, (pressurized)	1 cup	60	61	155	2	13	8.3	3.9	0.5
65		1 tbsp	3	61	10	Tr	1	0.4	0.2	Tr
66	Cream, sour	1 cup	230	71	495	7	48	30.0	13.9	1.8
67		1 tbsp	12	71	25	Tr	3	1.6	0.7	0.1

Table A-4 Nutritive Value of the Edible Part of Food (Continued)

Cholesterol	Carbohydrate	Calcium	Phosphorus	Iron	Potassium	Sodium	Vitamin A value (IU)	(RE)	Thiamin	Riboflavin	Niacin	Ascorbic acid	Item No.
Milligrams	Grams	Milligrams	Milligrams	Milligrams	Milligrams	Milligrams	International units	Retinol equivalents	Milligrams	Milligrams	Milligrams	Milligrams	
21	1	150	110	0.1	73	396	200	65	0.01	0.11	0.3	0	30
27	Tr	147	132	0.1	71	320	350	96	0.01	0.19	0.2	0	31
30	Tr	204	145	0.2	28	176	300	86	0.01	0.11	Tr	0	32
18	Tr	123	87	0.1	17	105	180	52	Tr	0.06	Tr	0	33
119	1	815	579	0.8	111	701	1,200	342	0.03	0.42	0.1	0	34
34	6	135	297	0.3	190	911	370	108	0.05	0.37	0.3	Tr	35
31	6	126	277	0.3	177	850	340	101	0.04	0.34	0.3	Tr	36
25	30	108	236	0.2	151	915	280	81	0.04	0.29	0.2	Tr	37
19	8	155	340	0.4	217	918	160	45	0.05	0.42	0.3	Tr	38
10	3	46	151	0.3	47	19	40	12	0.04	0.21	0.2	0	39
31	1	23	30	0.3	34	84	400	124	Tr	0.06	Tr	0	40
25	1	140	96	0.2	18	316	130	36	0.04	0.24	0.3	0	41
22	1	147	105	0.1	19	106	220	68	Tr	0.07	Tr	0	42
15	1	207	149	0.1	27	150	180	54	0.01	0.10	Tr	0	43
27	Tr	203	133	0.1	38	178	320	90	Tr	0.09	Tr	0	44
79	4	1,376	807	1.0	107	1,861	700	173	0.05	0.39	0.3	0	45
4	Tr	69	40	Tr	5	93	40	9	Tr	0.02	Tr	0	46
22	1	390	229	0.3	30	528	200	49	0.01	0.11	0.1	0	47
20	1	214	141	0.1	39	248	230	75	0.01	0.09	Tr	0	48
124	7	509	389	0.9	257	207	1,210	330	0.03	0.48	0.3	0	49
76	13	669	449	1.1	307	307	1,060	278	0.05	0.46	0.2	0	50
26	1	272	171	Tr	31	74	240	72	0.01	0.10	Tr	0	51
27	Tr	174	211	0.1	46	406	340	82	0.01	0.10	Tr	0	52
24	1	219	216	0.2	61	388	230	65	Tr	0.08	Tr	0	53
18	2	163	130	0.2	79	337	260	62	0.01	0.13	Tr	0	54
16	2	159	202	0.1	69	381	220	54	0.01	0.12	Tr	0	55
89	10	254	230	0.2	314	98	1,050	259	0.08	0.36	0.2	2	56
6	1	16	14	Tr	19	6	70	16	0.01	0.02	Tr	Tr	57
159	9	231	192	0.1	292	95	1,730	437	0.08	0.36	0.1	2	58
10	1	14	12	Tr	18	6	110	27	Tr	0.02	Tr	Tr	59
265	7	166	146	0.1	231	82	2,690	705	0.06	0.30	0.1	1	60
17	Tr	10	9	Tr	15	5	170	44	Tr	0.02	Tr	Tr	61
326	7	154	149	0.1	179	89	3,500	1,002	0.05	0.26	0.1	1	62
21	Tr	10	9	Tr	11	6	220	63	Tr	0.02	Tr	Tr	63
46	7	61	54	Tr	88	78	550	124	0.02	0.04	Tr	0	64
2	Tr	3	3	Tr	4	4	30	6	Tr	Tr	Tr	0	65
102	10	268	195	0.1	331	123	1,820	448	0.08	0.34	0.2	2	66
5	1	14	10	Tr	17	6	90	23	Tr	0.02	Tr	Tr	67

Table A-4 Nutritive Value of the Edible Part of Food *(Continued)*

(Tr indicates nutrient present in trace amount.)

Item No.	Foods, approximate measures, units, and weight (weight of edible portion only)		Water	Food energy	Pro-tein	Fat	Fatty acids		
							Satu-rated	Mono-unsatu-rated	Poly-unsatu-rated
		Grams	Per-cent	Cal-ories	Grams	Grams	Grams	Grams	Grams
	Dairy Products—Con.								
	Cream products, imitation (made with vegetable fat):									
	Sweet:									
	Creamers:									
68	Liquid (frozen)----------- 1 tbsp----------	15	77	20	Tr	1	1.4	Tr	Tr
69	Powdered------------------ 1 tsp-----------	2	2	10	Tr	1	0.7	Tr	Tr
	Whipped topping:									
70	Frozen-------------------- 1 cup-----------	75	50	240	1	19	16.3	1.2	0.4
71	1 tbsp----------	4	50	15	Tr	1	0.9	0.1	Tr
	Powdered, made with whole milk------------------------									
72	1 cup-----------	80	67	150	3	10	8.5	0.7	0.2
73	1 tbsp----------	4	67	10	Tr	Tr	0.4	Tr	Tr
74	Pressurized--------------- 1 cup-----------	70	60	185	1	16	13.2	1.3	0.2
75	1 tbsp----------	4	60	10	Tr	1	0.8	0.1	Tr
76	Sour dressing (filled cream type product, nonbutterfat)-- 1 cup-----------	235	75	415	8	39	31.2	4.6	1.1
77	1 tbsp----------	12	75	20	Tr	2	1.6	0.2	0.1
	Ice cream. See Milk desserts, frozen (items 106-111).									
	Ice milk. See Milk desserts, frozen (items 112-114).									
	Milk:									
	Fluid:									
78	Whole (3.3% fat)------------- 1 cup-----------	244	88	150	8	8	5.1	2.4	0.3
	Lowfat (2%):									
79	No milk solids added------- 1 cup-----------	244	89	120	8	5	2.9	1.4	0.2
80	Milk solids added, label claim less than 10 g of protein per cup---------- 1 cup-----------	245	89	125	9	5	2.9	1.4	0.2
	Lowfat (1%):									
81	No milk solids added------- 1 cup-----------	244	90	100	8	3	1.6	0.7	0.1
82	Milk solids added, label claim less than 10 g of protein per cup---------- 1 cup-----------	245	90	105	9	2	1.5	0.7	0.1
	Nonfat (skim):									
83	No milk solids added------- 1 cup-----------	245	91	85	8	Tr	0.3	0.1	Tr
84	Milk solids added, label claim less than 10 g of protein per cup---------- 1 cup-----------	245	90	90	9	1	0.4	0.2	Tr
85	Buttermilk---------------- 1 cup-----------	245	90	100	8	2	1.3	0.6	0.1
	Canned:									
86	Condensed, sweetened--------- 1 cup-----------	306	27	980	24	27	16.8	7.4	1.0
	Evaporated:									
87	Whole milk---------------- 1 cup-----------	252	74	340	17	19	11.6	5.9	0.6
88	Skim milk----------------- 1 cup-----------	255	79	200	19	1	0.3	0.2	Tr
	Dried:									
89	Buttermilk---------------- 1 cup-----------	120	3	465	41	7	4.3	2.0	0.3
	Nonfat, instantized:									
90	Envelope, 3.2 oz, net wt.[6] 1 envelope------	91	4	325	32	1	0.4	0.2	Tr
91	Cup---------------- 1 cup-------------	68	4	245	24	Tr	0.3	0.1	Tr
	Milk beverages:									
	Chocolate milk (commercial):									
92	Regular------------------- 1 cup-----------	250	82	210	8	8	5.3	2.5	0.3
93	Lowfat (2%)--------------- 1 cup-----------	250	84	180	8	5	3.1	1.5	0.2
94	Lowfat (1%)--------------- 1 cup-----------	250	85	160	8	3	1.5	0.8	0.1

[5] Vitamin A value is largely from beta-carotene used for coloring.
[6] Yields 1 qt of fluid milk when reconstituted according to package directions.

Table A-4 Nutritive Value of the Edible Part of Food *(Continued)*

Nutrients in Indicated Quantity

Cholesterol	Carbohydrate	Calcium	Phosphorus	Iron	Potassium	Sodium	Vitamin A value		Thiamin	Riboflavin	Niacin	Ascorbic acid	Item No
							(IU)	(RE)					
Milligrams	Grams	Milligrams	Milligrams	Milligrams	Milligrams	Milligrams	International units	Retinol equivalents	Milligrams	Milligrams	Milligrams	Milligrams	
0	2	1	10	Tr	29	12	⁵10	⁵1	0.00	0.00	0.0	0	68
0	1	Tr	8	Tr	16	4	Tr	Tr	0.00	Tr	0.0	0	69
0	17	5	6	0.1	14	19	⁵650	⁵65	0.00	0.00	0.0	0	70
0	1	Tr	Tr	Tr	1	1	⁵30	⁵3	0.00	0.00	0.0	0	71
8	13	72	69	Tr	121	53	⁵290	⁵39	0.02	0.09	Tr	1	72
Tr	1	4	3	Tr	6	3	⁵10	⁵2	Tr	Tr	Tr	Tr	73
0	11	4	13	Tr	13	43	⁵330	⁵33	0.00	0.00	0.0	0	74
0	1	Tr	1	Tr	1	2	⁵20	⁵2	0.00	0.00	0.0	0	75
13	11	266	205	0.1	380	113	20	5	0.09	0.38	0.2	2	76
1	1	14	10	Tr	19	6	Tr	Tr	Tr	0.02	Tr	Tr	77
33	11	291	228	0.1	370	120	310	76	0.09	0.40	0.2	2	78
18	12	297	232	0.1	377	122	500	139	0.10	0.40	0.2	2	79
18	12	313	245	0.1	397	128	500	140	0.10	0.42	0.2	2	80
10	12	300	235	0.1	381	123	500	144	0.10	0.41	0.2	2	81
10	12	313	245	0.1	397	128	500	145	0.10	0.42	0.2	2	82
4	12	302	247	0.1	406	126	500	149	0.09	0.34	0.2	2	83
5	12	316	255	0.1	418	130	500	149	0.10	0.43	0.2	2	84
9	12	285	219	0.1	371	257	80	20	0.08	0.38	0.1	2	85
104	166	868	775	0.6	1,136	389	1,000	248	0.28	1.27	0.6	8	86
74	25	657	510	0.5	764	267	610	136	0.12	0.80	0.5	5	87
9	29	738	497	0.7	845	293	1,000	298	0.11	0.79	0.4	3	88
83	59	1,421	1,119	0.4	1,910	621	260	65	0.47	1.89	1.1	7	89
17	47	1,120	896	0.3	1,552	499	⁷2,160	⁷646	0.38	1.59	0.8	5	90
12	35	837	670	0.2	1,160	373	⁷1,610	⁷483	0.28	1.19	0.6	4	91
31	26	280	251	0.6	417	149	300	73	0.09	0.41	0.3	2	92
17	26	284	254	0.6	422	151	500	143	0.09	0.41	0.3	2	93
7	26	287	256	0.6	425	152	500	148	0.10	0.42	0.3	2	94

⁷With added vitamin A.

Table A-4 Nutritive Value of the Edible Part of Food (Continued)

(Tr indicates nutrient present in trace amount.)

Item No.	Foods, approximate measures, units, and weight (weight of edible portion only)			Water	Food energy	Pro-tein	Fat	Fatty acids		
								Satu-rated	Mono-unsatu-rated	Poly-unsatu-rated
			Grams	Per-cent	Cal-ories	Grams	Grams	Grams	Grams	Grams
	Dairy Products—Con.									
	Milk beverages:									
	Cocoa and chocolate-flavored beverages:									
95	Powder containing nonfat dry milk	1 oz	28	1	100	3	1	0.6	0.3	Tr
96	Prepared (6 oz water plus 1 oz powder)	1 serving	206	86	100	3	1	0.6	0.3	Tr
97	Powder without nonfat dry milk	3/4 oz	21	1	75	1	1	0.3	0.2	Tr
98	Prepared (8 oz whole milk plus 3/4 oz powder)	1 serving	265	81	225	9	9	5.4	2.5	0.3
99	Eggnog (commercial)	1 cup	254	74	340	10	19	11.3	5.7	0.9
	Malted milk:									
	Chocolate:									
100	Powder	3/4 oz	21	2	85	1	1	0.5	0.3	0.1
101	Prepared (8 oz whole milk plus 3/4 oz powder)	1 serving	265	81	235	9	9	5.5	2.7	0.4
	Natural:									
102	Powder	3/4 oz	21	3	85	3	2	0.9	0.5	0.3
103	Prepared (8 oz whole milk plus 3/4 oz powder)	1 serving	265	81	235	11	10	6.0	2.9	0.6
	Shakes, thick:									
104	Chocolate	10-oz container	283	72	335	9	8	4.8	2.2	0.3
105	Vanilla	10-oz container	283	74	315	11	9	5.3	2.5	0.3
	Milk desserts, frozen:									
	Ice cream, vanilla:									
	Regular (about 11% fat):									
106	Hardened	1/2 gal	1,064	61	2,155	38	115	71.3	33.1	4.3
107		1 cup	133	61	270	5	14	8.9	4.1	0.5
108		3 fl oz	50	61	100	2	5	3.4	1.6	0.2
109	Soft serve (frozen custard)	1 cup	173	60	375	7	23	13.5	6.7	1.0
110	Rich (about 16% fat), hardened	1/2 gal	1,188	59	2,805	33	190	118.3	54.9	7.1
111		1 cup	148	59	350	4	24	14.7	6.8	0.9
	Ice milk, vanilla:									
112	Hardened (about 4% fat)	1/2 gal	1,048	69	1,470	41	45	28.1	13.0	1.7
113		1 cup	131	69	185	5	6	3.5	1.6	0.2
114	Soft serve (about 3% fat)	1 cup	175	70	225	8	5	2.9	1.3	0.2
115	Sherbet (about 2% fat)	1/2 gal	1,542	66	2,160	17	31	19.0	8.8	1.1
116		1 cup	193	66	270	2	4	2.4	1.1	0.1
	Yogurt:									
	With added milk solids:									
	Made with lowfat milk:									
117	Fruit-flavored[8]	8-oz container	227	74	230	10	2	1.6	0.7	0.1
118	Plain	8-oz container	227	85	145	12	4	2.3	1.0	0.1
119	Made with nonfat milk	8-oz container	227	85	125	13	Tr	0.3	0.1	Tr
	Without added milk solids:									
120	Made with whole milk	8-oz container	227	88	140	8	7	4.8	2.0	0.2
	Eggs									
	Eggs, large (24 oz per dozen):									
	Raw:									
121	Whole, without shell	1 egg	50	75	80	6	6	1.7	2.2	0.7
122	White	1 white	33	88	15	3	Tr	0.0	0.0	0.0
123	Yolk	1 yolk	17	49	65	3	6	1.7	2.2	0.7
	Cooked:									
124	Fried in butter	1 egg	46	68	95	6	7	2.7	2.7	0.8
125	Hard-cooked, shell removed	1 egg	50	75	80	6	6	1.7	2.2	0.7
126	Poached	1 egg	50	74	80	6	6	1.7	2.2	0.7
127	Scrambled (milk added) in butter. Also omelet	1 egg	64	73	110	7	8	3.2	2.9	0.8

[8]Carbohydrate content varies widely because of amount of sugar added and amount and solids content of added flavoring. Consult the label if more precise values for carbohydrate and calories are needed.

Table A-4 Nutritive Value of the Edible Part of Food *(Continued)*

Nutrients in Indicated Quantity

Cho-les-terol	Carbo-hydrate	Calcium	Phos-phorus	Iron	Potas-sium	Sodium	Vitamin A value (IU)	(RE)	Thiamin	Ribo-flavin	Niacin	Ascorbic acid	Item No
Milli-grams	Grams	Milli-grams	Milli-grams	Milli-grams	Milli-grams	Milli-grams	Inter-national units	Retinol equiva-lents	Milli-grams	Milli-grams	Milli-grams	Milli-grams	
1	22	90	88	0.3	223	139	Tr	Tr	0.03	0.17	0.2	Tr	95
1	22	90	88	0.3	223	139	Tr	Tr	0.03	0.17	0.2	Tr	96
0	19	7	26	0.7	136	56	Tr	Tr	Tr	0.03	0.1	Tr	97
33	30	298	254	0.9	508	176	310	76	0.10	0.43	0.3	3	98
149	34	330	278	0.5	420	138	890	203	0.09	0.48	0.3	4	99
1	18	13	37	0.4	130	49	20	5	0.04	0.04	0.4	0	100
34	29	304	265	0.5	500	168	330	80	0.14	0.43	0.7	2	101
4	15	56	79	0.2	159	96	70	17	0.11	0.14	1.1	0	102
37	27	347	307	0.3	529	215	380	93	0.20	0.54	1.3	2	103
30	60	374	357	0.9	634	314	240	59	0.13	0.63	0.4	0	104
33	50	413	326	0.3	517	270	320	79	0.08	0.55	0.4	0	105
476	254	1,406	1,075	1.0	2,052	929	4,340	1,064	0.42	2.63	1.1	6	106
59	32	176	134	0.1	257	116	540	133	0.05	0.33	0.1	1	107
22	12	66	51	Tr	96	44	200	50	0.02	0.12	0.1	Tr	108
153	38	236	199	0.4	338	153	790	199	0.08	0.45	0.2	1	109
703	256	1,213	927	0.8	1,771	868	7,200	1,758	0.36	2.27	0.9	5	110
88	32	151	115	0.1	221	108	900	219	0.04	0.28	0.1	1	111
146	232	1,409	1,035	1.5	2,117	836	1,710	419	0.61	2.78	0.9	6	112
18	29	176	129	0.2	265	105	210	52	0.08	0.35	0.1	1	113
13	38	274	202	0.3	412	163	175	44	0.12	0.54	0.2	1	114
113	469	827	594	2.5	1,585	706	1,480	308	0.26	0.71	1.0	31	115
14	59	103	74	0.3	198	88	190	39	0.03	0.09	0.1	4	116
10	43	345	271	0.2	442	133	100	25	0.08	0.40	0.2	1	117
14	16	415	326	0.2	531	159	150	36	0.10	0.49	0.3	2	118
4	17	452	355	0.2	579	174	20	5	0.11	0.53	0.3	2	119
29	11	274	215	0.1	351	105	280	68	0.07	0.32	0.2	1	120
274	1	28	90	1.0	65	69	260	78	0.04	0.15	Tr	0	121
0	Tr	4	4	Tr	45	50	0	0	Tr	0.09	Tr	0	122
272	Tr	26	86	0.9	15	8	310	94	0.04	0.07	Tr	0	123
278	1	29	91	1.1	66	162	320	94	0.04	0.14	Tr	0	124
274	1	28	90	1.0	65	69	260	78	0.04	0.14	Tr	0	125
273	1	28	90	1.0	65	146	260	78	0.03	0.13	Tr	0	126
282	2	54	109	1.0	97	176	350	102	0.04	0.18	Tr	Tr	127

Table A-4 Nutritive Value of the Edible Part of Food (Continued)

(Tr indicates nutrient present in trace amount.)

Item No.	Foods, approximate measures, units, and weight (weight of edible portion only)		Grams	Water Per-cent	Food energy Cal-ories	Pro-tein Grams	Fat Grams	Fatty acids Satu-rated Grams	Mono-unsatu-rated Grams	Poly-unsatu-rated Grams
	Fats and Oils									
	Butter (4 sticks per lb):									
128	Stick	1/2 cup	113	16	810	1	92	57.1	26.4	3.4
129	Tablespoon (1/8 stick)	1 tbsp	14	16	100	Tr	11	7.1	3.3	0.4
130	Pat (1 in square, 1/3 in high; 90 per lb)	1 pat	5	16	35	Tr	4	2.5	1.2	0.2
131	Fats, cooking (vegetable shortenings)	1 cup	205	0	1,810	0	205	51.3	91.2	53.5
132		1 tbsp	13	0	115	0	13	3.3	5.8	3.4
133	Lard	1 cup	205	0	1,850	0	205	80.4	92.5	23.0
134		1 tbsp	13	0	115	0	13	5.1	5.9	1.5
	Margarine:									
135	Imitation (about 40% fat), soft	8-oz container	227	58	785	1	88	17.5	35.6	31.3
136		1 tbsp	14	58	50	Tr	5	1.1	2.2	1.9
	Regular (about 80% fat): Hard (4 sticks per lb):									
137	Stick	1/2 cup	113	16	810	1	91	17.9	40.5	28.7
138	Tablespoon (1/8 stick)	1 tbsp	14	16	100	Tr	11	2.2	5.0	3.6
139	Pat (1 in square, 1/3 in high; 90 per lb)	1 pat	5	16	35	Tr	4	0.8	1.8	1.3
140	Soft	8-oz container	227	16	1,625	2	183	31.3	64.7	78.5
141		1 tbsp	14	16	100	Tr	11	1.9	4.0	4.8
	Spread (about 60% fat): Hard (4 sticks per lb):									
142	Stick	1/2 cup	113	37	610	1	69	15.9	29.4	20.5
143	Tablespoon (1/8 stick)	1 tbsp	14	37	75	Tr	9	2.0	3.6	2.5
144	Pat (1 in square, 1/3 in high; 90 per lb)	1 pat	5	37	25	Tr	3	0.7	1.3	0.9
145	Soft	8-oz container	227	37	1,225	1	138	29.1	71.5	31.3
146		1 tbsp	14	37	75	Tr	9	1.8	4.4	1.9
	Oils, salad or cooking:									
147	Corn	1 cup	218	0	1,925	0	218	27.7	52.8	128.0
148		1 tbsp	14	0	125	0	14	1.8	3.4	8.2
149	Olive	1 cup	216	0	1,910	0	216	29.2	159.2	18.1
150		1 tbsp	14	0	125	0	14	1.9	10.3	1.2
151	Peanut	1 cup	216	0	1,910	0	216	36.5	99.8	69.1
152		1 tbsp	14	0	125	0	14	2.4	6.5	4.5
153	Safflower	1 cup	218	0	1,925	0	218	19.8	26.4	162.4
154		1 tbsp	14	0	125	0	14	1.3	1.7	10.4
155	Soybean oil, hydrogenated (partially hardened)	1 cup	218	0	1,925	0	218	32.5	93.7	82.0
156		1 tbsp	14	0	125	0	14	2.1	6.0	5.3
157	Soybean-cottonseed oil blend, hydrogenated	1 cup	218	0	1,925	0	218	39.2	64.3	104.9
158		1 tbsp	14	0	125	0	14	2.5	4.1	6.7
159	Sunflower	1 cup	218	0	1,925	0	218	22.5	42.5	143.2
160		1 tbsp	14	0	125	0	14	1.4	2.7	9.2
	Salad dressings: Commercial:									
161	Blue cheese	1 tbsp	15	32	75	1	8	1.5	1.8	4.2
	French:									
162	Regular	1 tbsp	16	35	85	Tr	9	1.4	4.0	3.5
163	Low calorie	1 tbsp	16	75	25	Tr	2	0.2	0.3	1.0
	Italian:									
164	Regular	1 tbsp	15	34	80	Tr	9	1.3	3.7	3.2
165	Low calorie	1 tbsp	15	86	5	Tr	Tr	Tr	Tr	Tr
	Mayonnaise:									
166	Regular	1 tbsp	14	15	100	Tr	11	1.7	3.2	5.8
167	Imitation	1 tbsp	15	63	35	Tr	3	0.5	0.7	1.6
168	Mayonnaise type	1 tbsp	15	40	60	Tr	5	0.7	1.4	2.7
169	Tartar sauce	1 tbsp	14	34	75	Tr	8	1.2	2.6	3.9
	Thousand island:									
170	Regular	1 tbsp	16	46	60	Tr	6	1.0	1.3	3.2
171	Low calorie	1 tbsp	15	69	25	Tr	2	0.2	0.4	0.9

[9]For salted butter; unsalted butter contains 12 mg sodium per stick, 2 mg per tbsp, or 1 mg per pat.
[10]Values for vitamin A are year-round average.

Table A-4 Nutritive Value of the Edible Part of Food (Continued)

Nutrients in Indicated Quantity

Cholesterol	Carbohydrate	Calcium	Phosphorus	Iron	Potassium	Sodium	Vitamin A value (IU)	Vitamin A value (RE)	Thiamin	Riboflavin	Niacin	Ascorbic acid	Item No.
Milligrams	Grams	Milligrams	Milligrams	Milligrams	Milligrams	Milligrams	International units	Retinol equivalents	Milligrams	Milligrams	Milligrams	Milligrams	
247	Tr	27	26	0.2	29	[9]933	[10]3,460	[10]852	0.01	0.04	Tr	0	128
31	Tr	3	3	Tr	4	[9]116	[10]430	[10]106	Tr	Tr	Tr	0	129
11	Tr	1	1	Tr	1	[9]41	[10]150	[10]38	Tr	Tr	Tr	0	130
0	0	0	0	0.0	0	0	0	0	0.00	0.00	0.0	0	131
0	0	0	0	0.0	0	0	0	0	0.00	0.00	0.0	0	132
195	0	0	0	0.0	0	0	0	0	0.00	0.00	0.0	0	133
12	0	0	0	0.0	0	0	0	0	0.00	0.00	0.0	0	134
0	1	40	31	0.0	57	[11]2,178	[12]7,510	[12]2,254	0.01	0.05	Tr	Tr	135
0	Tr	2	2	0.0	4	[11]134	[12]460	[12]139	Tr	Tr	Tr	Tr	136
0	1	34	26	0.1	48	[11]1,066	[12]3,740	[12]1,122	0.01	0.04	Tr	Tr	137
0	Tr	4	3	Tr	6	[11]132	[12]460	[12]139	Tr	0.01	Tr	Tr	138
0	Tr	1	1	Tr	2	[11]47	[12]170	[12]50	Tr	Tr	Tr	Tr	139
0	1	60	46	0.0	86	[11]2,449	[12]7,510	[12]2,254	0.02	0.07	Tr	Tr	140
0	Tr	4	3	0.0	5	[11]151	[12]460	[12]139	Tr	Tr	Tr	Tr	141
0	0	24	18	0.0	34	[11]1,123	[12]3,740	[12]1,122	0.01	0.03	Tr	Tr	142
0	0	3	2	0.0	4	[11]139	[12]460	[12]139	Tr	Tr	Tr	Tr	143
0	0	1	1	0.0	1	[11]50	[12]170	[12]50	Tr	Tr	Tr	Tr	144
0	0	47	37	0.0	68	[11]2,256	[12]7,510	[12]2,254	0.02	0.06	Tr	Tr	145
0	0	3	2	0.0	4	[11]139	[12]460	[12]139	Tr	Tr	Tr	Tr	146
0	0	0	0	0.0	0	0	0	0	0.00	0.00	0.0	0	147
0	0	0	0	0.0	0	0	0	0	0.00	0.00	0.0	0	148
0	0	0	0	0.0	0	0	0	0	0.00	0.00	0.0	0	149
0	0	0	0	0.0	0	0	0	0	0.00	0.00	0.0	0	150
0	0	0	0	0.0	0	0	0	0	0.00	0.00	0.0	0	151
0	0	0	0	0.0	0	0	0	0	0.00	0.00	0.0	0	152
0	0	0	0	0.0	0	0	0	0	0.00	0.00	0.0	0	153
0	0	0	0	0.0	0	0	0	0	0.00	0.00	0.0	0	154
0	0	0	0	0.0	0	0	0	0	0.00	0.00	0.0	0	155
0	0	0	0	0.0	0	0	0	0	0.00	0.00	0.0	0	156
0	0	0	0	0.0	0	0	0	0	0.00	0.00	0.0	0	157
0	0	0	0	0.0	0	0	0	0	0.00	0.00	0.0	0	158
0	0	0	0	0.0	0	0	0	0	0.00	0.00	0.0	0	159
0	0	0	0	0.0	0	0	0	0	0.00	0.00	0.0	0	160
3	1	12	11	Tr	6	164	30	10	Tr	0.02	Tr	Tr	161
0	1	2	1	Tr	2	188	Tr	Tr	Tr	Tr	Tr	Tr	162
0	2	6	5	Tr	3	306	Tr	Tr	Tr	Tr	Tr	Tr	163
0	1	1	1	Tr	5	162	30	3	Tr	Tr	Tr	Tr	164
0	2	1	1	Tr	4	136	Tr	Tr	Tr	Tr	Tr	Tr	165
8	Tr	3	4	0.1	5	80	40	12	0.00	0.00	Tr	0	166
4	2	Tr	Tr	0.0	2	75	0	0	0.00	0.00	0.0	0	167
4	4	2	4	Tr	1	107	30	13	Tr	Tr	Tr	0	168
4	1	3	4	0.1	11	182	30	9	Tr	Tr	0.0	Tr	169
4	2	2	3	0.1	18	112	50	15	Tr	Tr	Tr	0	170
2	2	2	3	0.1	17	150	50	14	Tr	Tr	Tr	0	171

[11]For salted margarine.
[12]Based on average vitamin A content of fortified margarine. Federal specifications for fortified margarine require a minimum of 15,000 IU per pound.

Table A-4 Nutritive Value of the Edible Part of Food (Continued)

(Tr indicates nutrient present in trace amount.)

Item No.	Foods, approximate measures, units, and weight (weight of edible portion only)		Grams	Water Per-cent	Food energy Cal-ories	Pro-tein Grams	Fat Grams	Fatty acids Satu-rated Grams	Mono-unsatu-rated Grams	Poly-unsatu-rated Grams
	Fats and Oils—Con.									
	Salad dressings:									
	Prepared from home recipe:									
172	Cooked type[13]	1 tbsp	16	69	25	1	2	0.5	0.6	0.3
173	Vinegar and oil	1 tbsp	16	47	70	0	8	1.5	2.4	3.9
	Fish and Shellfish									
	Clams:									
174	Raw, meat only	3 oz	85	82	65	11	1	0.3	0.3	0.3
175	Canned, drained solids	3 oz	85	77	85	13	2	0.5	0.5	0.4
176	Crabmeat, canned	1 cup	135	77	135	23	3	0.5	0.8	1.4
177	Fish sticks, frozen, reheated, (stick, 4 by 1 by 1/2 in)	1 fish stick	28	52	70	6	3	0.8	1.4	0.8
	Flounder or Sole, baked, with lemon juice:									
178	With butter	3 oz	85	73	120	16	6	3.2	1.5	0.5
179	With margarine	3 oz	85	73	120	16	6	1.2	2.3	1.9
180	Without added fat	3 oz	85	78	80	17	1	0.3	0.2	0.4
181	Haddock, breaded, fried[14]	3 oz	85	61	175	17	9	2.4	3.9	2.4
182	Halibut, broiled, with butter and lemon juice	3 oz	85	67	140	20	6	3.3	1.6	0.7
183	Herring, pickled	3 oz	85	59	190	17	13	4.3	4.6	3.1
184	Ocean perch, breaded, fried[14]	1 fillet	85	59	185	16	11	2.6	4.6	2.8
	Oysters:									
185	Raw, meat only (13-19 medium Selects)	1 cup	240	85	160	20	4	1.4	0.5	1.4
186	Breaded, fried[14]	1 oyster	45	65	90	5	5	1.4	2.1	1.4
	Salmon:									
187	Canned (pink), solids and liquid	3 oz	85	71	120	17	5	0.9	1.5	2.1
188	Baked (red)	3 oz	85	67	140	21	5	1.2	2.4	1.4
189	Smoked	3 oz	85	59	150	18	8	2.6	3.9	0.7
190	Sardines, Atlantic, canned in oil, drained solids	3 oz	85	62	175	20	9	2.1	3.7	2.9
191	Scallops, breaded, frozen, reheated	6 scallops	90	59	195	15	10	2.5	4.1	2.5
	Shrimp:									
192	Canned, drained solids	3 oz	85	70	100	21	1	0.2	0.2	0.4
193	French fried (7 medium)[16]	3 oz	85	55	200	16	10	2.5	4.1	2.6
194	Trout, broiled, with butter and lemon juice	3 oz	85	63	175	21	9	4.1	2.9	1.6
	Tuna, canned, drained solids:									
195	Oil pack, chunk light	3 oz	85	61	165	24	7	1.4	1.9	3.1
196	Water pack, solid white	3 oz	85	63	135	30	1	0.3	0.2	0.3
197	Tuna salad[17]	1 cup	205	63	375	33	19	3.3	4.9	9.2
	Fruits and Fruit Juices									
	Apples:									
	Raw:									
	Unpeeled, without cores:									
198	2-3/4-in diam. (about 3 per lb with cores)	1 apple	138	84	80	Tr	Tr	0.1	Tr	0.1
199	3-1/4-in diam. (about 2 per lb with cores)	1 apple	212	84	125	Tr	1	0.1	Tr	0.2
200	Peeled, sliced	1 cup	110	84	65	Tr	Tr	0.1	Tr	0.1
201	Dried, sulfured	10 rings	64	32	155	1	Tr	Tr	Tr	0.1
202	Apple juice, bottled or canned[19]	1 cup	248	88	115	Tr	Tr	Tr	Tr	0.1
	Applesauce, canned:									
203	Sweetened	1 cup	255	80	195	Tr	Tr	0.1	Tr	0.1
204	Unsweetened	1 cup	244	88	105	Tr	Tr	Tr	Tr	Tr

[13] Fatty acid values apply to product made with regular margarine.
[14] Dipped in egg, milk, and breadcrumbs; fried in vegetable shortening.
[15] If bones are discarded, value for calcium will be greatly reduced.
[16] Dipped in egg, breadcrumbs, and flour; fried in vegetable shortening.

Table A-4 Nutritive Value of the Edible Part of Food (Continued)

Cholesterol (Milligrams)	Carbohydrate (Grams)	Calcium (Milligrams)	Phosphorus (Milligrams)	Iron (Milligrams)	Potassium (Milligrams)	Sodium (Milligrams)	Vitamin A value (IU) (International units)	Vitamin A value (RE) (Retinol equivalents)	Thiamin (Milligrams)	Riboflavin (Milligrams)	Niacin (Milligrams)	Ascorbic acid (Milligrams)	Item No.
9	2	13	14	0.1	19	117	70	20	0.01	0.02	Tr	Tr	172
0	Tr	0	0	0.0	1	Tr	0	0	0.00	0.00	0.0	0	173
43	2	59	138	2.6	154	102	90	26	0.09	0.15	1.1	9	174
54	2	47	116	3.5	119	102	90	26	0.01	0.09	0.9	3	175
135	1	61	246	1.1	149	1,350	50	14	0.11	0.11	2.6	0	176
26	4	11	58	0.3	94	53	20	5	0.03	0.05	0.6	0	177
68	Tr	13	187	0.3	272	145	210	54	0.05	0.08	1.6	1	178
55	Tr	14	187	0.3	273	151	230	69	0.05	0.08	1.6	1	179
59	Tr	13	197	0.3	286	101	30	10	0.05	0.08	1.7	1	180
75	7	34	183	1.0	270	123	70	20	0.06	0.10	2.9	0	181
62	Tr	14	206	0.7	441	103	610	174	0.06	0.07	7.7	1	182
85	0	29	128	0.9	85	850	110	33	0.04	0.18	2.8	0	183
66	7	31	191	1.2	241	138	70	20	0.10	0.11	2.0	0	184
120	8	226	343	15.6	290	175	740	223	0.34	0.43	6.0	24	185
35	5	49	73	3.0	64	70	150	44	0.07	0.10	1.3	4	186
34	0	[15]167	243	0.7	307	443	60	18	0.03	0.15	6.8	0	187
60	0	26	269	0.5	305	55	290	87	0.18	0.14	5.5	0	188
51	0	12	208	0.8	327	1,700	260	77	0.17	0.17	6.8	0	189
85	0	[15]371	424	2.6	349	425	190	56	0.03	0.17	4.6	0	190
70	10	39	203	2.0	369	298	70	21	0.11	0.11	1.6	0	191
128	1	98	224	1.4	104	1,955	50	15	0.01	0.03	1.5	0	192
168	11	61	154	2.0	189	384	90	26	0.06	0.09	2.8	0	193
71	Tr	26	259	1.0	297	122	230	60	0.07	0.07	2.3	1	194
55	0	7	199	1.6	298	303	70	20	0.04	0.09	10.1	0	195
48	0	17	202	0.6	255	468	110	32	0.03	0.10	13.4	0	196
80	19	31	281	2.5	531	877	230	53	0.06	0.14	13.3	6	197
0	21	10	10	0.2	159	Tr	70	7	0.02	0.02	0.1	8	198
0	32	15	15	0.4	244	Tr	110	11	0.04	0.03	0.2	12	199
0	16	4	8	0.1	124	Tr	50	5	0.02	0.01	0.1	4	200
0	42	9	24	0.9	288	[18]56	0	0	0.00	0.10	0.6	2	201
0	29	17	17	0.9	295	7	Tr	Tr	0.05	0.04	0.2	[20]2	202
0	51	10	18	0.9	156	8	30	3	0.03	0.07	0.5	[20]4	203
0	28	7	17	0.3	183	5	70	7	0.03	0.06	0.5	[20]3	204

[17] Made with drained chunk light tuna, celery, onion, pickle relish, and mayonnaise-type salad dressing.
[18] Sodium bisulfite used to preserve color; unsulfited product would contain less sodium.
[19] Also applies to pasteurized apple cider.
[20] Without added ascorbic acid. For value with added ascorbic acid, refer to label.

Table A-4 Nutritive Value of the Edible Part of Food *(Continued)*

(Tr indicates nutrient present in trace amount.)

Item No.	Foods, approximate measures, units, and weight (weight of edible portion only)		Water	Food energy	Pro-tein	Fat	Fatty acids		
							Satu-rated	Mono-unsatu-rated	Poly-unsatu-rated
		Grams	Per-cent	Cal-ories	Grams	Grams	Grams	Grams	Grams
	Fruits and Fruit Juices—Con.								
	Apricots:								
205	Raw, without pits (about 12 per lb with pits)	3 apricots	106	86	50	1	Tr	Tr	0.2	0.1
	Canned (fruit and liquid):								
206	Heavy syrup pack	1 cup	258	78	215	1	Tr	Tr	0.1	Tr
207		3 halves	85	78	70	Tr	Tr	Tr	Tr	Tr
208	Juice pack	1 cup	248	87	120	2	Tr	Tr	Tr	Tr
209		3 halves	84	87	40	1	Tr	Tr	Tr	Tr
	Dried:								
210	Uncooked (28 large or 37 medium halves per cup)	1 cup	130	31	310	5	1	Tr	0.3	0.1
211	Cooked, unsweetened, fruit and liquid	1 cup	250	76	210	3	Tr	Tr	0.2	0.1
212	Apricot nectar, canned	1 cup	251	85	140	1	Tr	Tr	0.1	Tr
	Avocados, raw, whole, without skin and seed:								
213	California (about 2 per lb with skin and seed)	1 avocado	173	73	305	4	30	4.5	19.4	3.5
214	Florida (about 1 per lb with skin and seed)	1 avocado	304	80	340	5	27	5.3	14.8	4.5
	Bananas, raw, without peel:								
215	Whole (about 2-1/2 per lb with peel)	1 banana	114	74	105	1	1	0.2	Tr	0.1
216	Sliced	1 cup	150	74	140	2	1	0.3	0.1	0.1
217	Blackberries, raw	1 cup	144	86	75	1	1	0.2	0.1	0.1
	Blueberries:								
218	Raw	1 cup	145	85	80	1	1	Tr	0.1	0.3
219	Frozen, sweetened	10-oz container	284	77	230	1	Tr	Tr	0.1	0.2
220		1 cup	230	77	185	1	Tr	Tr	Tr	0.1
	Cantaloup. See Melons (item 251).								
	Cherries:								
221	Sour, red, pitted, canned, water pack	1 cup	244	90	90	2	Tr	0.1	0.1	0.1
222	Sweet, raw, without pits and stems	10 cherries	68	81	50	1	1	0.1	0.2	0.2
223	Cranberry juice cocktail, bottled, sweetened	1 cup	253	85	145	Tr	Tr	Tr	Tr	0.1
224	Cranberry sauce, sweetened, canned, strained	1 cup	277	61	420	1	Tr	Tr	0.1	0.2
	Dates:								
225	Whole, without pits	10 dates	83	23	230	2	Tr	0.1	0.1	Tr
226	Chopped	1 cup	178	23	490	4	1	0.3	0.2	Tr
227	Figs, dried	10 figs	187	28	475	6	2	0.4	0.5	1.0
	Fruit cocktail, canned, fruit and liquid:								
228	Heavy syrup pack	1 cup	255	80	185	1	Tr	Tr	Tr	0.1
229	Juice pack	1 cup	248	87	115	1	Tr	Tr	Tr	Tr
	Grapefruit:								
230	Raw, without peel, membrane and seeds (3-3/4-in diam., 1 lb 1 oz, whole, with refuse)	1/2 grapefruit	120	91	40	1	Tr	Tr	Tr	Tr
231	Canned, sections with syrup	1 cup	254	84	150	1	Tr	Tr	Tr	0.1
	Grapefruit juice:								
232	Raw	1 cup	247	90	95	1	Tr	Tr	Tr	0.1
	Canned:								
233	Unsweetened	1 cup	247	90	95	1	Tr	Tr	Tr	0.1
234	Sweetened	1 cup	250	87	115	1	Tr	Tr	Tr	0.1
	Frozen concentrate, unsweetened								
235	Undiluted	6-fl-oz can	207	62	300	4	1	0.1	0.1	0.2
236	Diluted with 3 parts water by volume	1 cup	247	89	100	1	Tr	Tr	Tr	0.1

[20] Without added ascorbic acid. For value with added ascorbic acid, refer to label.
[21] With added ascorbic acid.

Table A-4 Nutritive Value of the Edible Part of Food (Continued)

							Nutrients in Indicated Quantity						
Cholesterol	Carbohydrate	Calcium	Phosphorus	Iron	Potassium	Sodium	Vitamin A value (IU)	Vitamin A value (RE)	Thiamin	Riboflavin	Niacin	Ascorbic acid	Item No
Milligrams	Grams	Milligrams	Milligrams	Milligrams	Milligrams	Milligrams	International units	Retinol equivalents	Milligrams	Milligrams	Milligrams	Milligrams	
0	12	15	20	0.6	314	1	2,770	277	0.03	0.04	0.6	11	205
0	55	23	31	0.8	361	10	3,170	317	0.05	0.06	1.0	8	206
0	18	8	10	0.3	119	3	1,050	105	0.02	0.02	0.3	3	207
0	31	30	50	0.7	409	10	4,190	419	0.04	0.05	0.9	12	208
0	10	10	17	0.3	139	3	1,420	142	0.02	0.02	0.3	4	209
0	80	59	152	6.1	1,791	13	9,410	941	0.01	0.20	3.9	3	210
0	55	40	103	4.2	1,222	8	5,910	591	0.02	0.08	2.4	4	211
0	36	18	23	1.0	286	8	3,300	330	0.02	0.04	0.7	[20]2	212
0	12	19	73	2.0	1,097	21	1,060	106	0.19	0.21	3.3	14	213
0	27	33	119	1.6	1,484	15	1,860	186	0.33	0.37	5.8	24	214
0	27	7	23	0.4	451	1	90	9	0.05	0.11	0.6	10	215
0	35	9	30	0.5	594	2	120	12	0.07	0.15	0.8	14	216
0	18	46	30	0.8	282	Tr	240	24	0.04	0.06	0.6	30	217
0	20	9	15	0.2	129	9	150	15	0.07	0.07	0.5	19	218
0	62	17	20	1.1	170	3	120	12	0.06	0.15	0.7	3	219
0	50	14	16	0.9	138	2	100	10	0.05	0.12	0.6	2	220
0	22	27	24	3.3	239	17	1,840	184	0.04	0.10	0.4	5	221
0	11	10	13	0.3	152	Tr	150	15	0.03	0.04	0.3	5	222
0	38	8	3	0.4	61	10	10	1	0.01	0.04	0.1	[21]108	223
0	108	11	17	0.6	72	80	60	6	0.04	0.06	0.3	6	224
0	61	27	33	1.0	541	2	40	4	0.07	0.08	1.8	0	225
0	131	57	71	2.0	1,161	5	90	9	0.16	0.18	3.9	0	226
0	122	269	127	4.2	1,331	21	250	25	0.13	0.16	1.3	1	227
0	48	15	28	0.7	224	15	520	52	0.05	0.05	1.0	5	228
0	29	20	35	0.5	236	10	760	76	0.03	0.04	1.0	7	229
0	10	14	10	0.1	167	Tr	[22]10	[22]1	0.04	0.02	0.3	41	230
0	39	36	25	1.0	328	5	Tr	Tr	0.10	0.05	0.6	54	231
0	23	22	37	0.5	400	2	20	2	0.10	0.05	0.5	94	232
0	22	17	27	0.5	378	2	20	2	0.10	0.05	0.6	72	233
0	28	20	28	0.9	405	5	20	2	0.10	0.06	0.8	67	234
0	72	56	101	1.0	1,002	6	60	6	0.30	0.16	1.6	248	235
0	24	20	35	0.3	336	2	20	2	0.10	0.05	0.5	83	236

[22]For white grapefruit; pink grapefruit have about 310 IU or 31 RE.

Table A-4 Nutritive Value of the Edible Part of Food *(Continued)*

(Tr indicates nutrient present in trace amount.)

Item No.	Foods, approximate measures, units, and weight (weight of edible portion only)		Water	Food energy	Protein	Fat	Fatty acids		
							Saturated	Monounsaturated	Polyunsaturated
		Grams	Percent	Calories	Grams	Grams	Grams	Grams	Grams
	Fruits and Fruit Juices—Con.								
	Grapes, European type (adherent skin), raw:								
237	Thompson Seedless--------------- 10 grapes-------	50	81	35	Tr	Tr	0.1	Tr	0.1
238	Tokay and Emperor, seeded types 10 grapes-------	57	81	40	Tr	Tr	0.1	Tr	0.1
	Grape juice:								
239	Canned or bottled-------------- 1 cup-----------	253	84	155	1	Tr	0.1	Tr	0.1
	Frozen concentrate, sweetened:								
240	Undiluted--------------------- 6-fl-oz can-----	216	54	385	1	1	0.2	Tr	0.2
241	Diluted with 3 parts water by volume--------------------- 1 cup-----------	250	87	125	Tr	Tr	0.1	Tr	0.1
242	Kiwifruit, raw, without skin (about 5 per lb with skin)----- 1 kiwifruit-----	76	83	45	1	Tr	Tr	0.1	0.1
243	Lemons, raw, without peel and seeds (about 4 per lb with peel and seeds)--------------------- 1 lemon---------	58	89	15	1	Tr	Tr	Tr	0.1
	Lemon juice:								
244	Raw------------------------- 1 cup-----------	244	91	60	1	Tr	Tr	Tr	Tr
245	Canned or bottled, unsweetened 1 cup-----------	244	92	50	1	1	0.1	Tr	0.2
246	1 tbsp----------	15	92	5	Tr	Tr	Tr	Tr	Tr
247	Frozen, single-strength, unsweetened------------------ 6-fl-oz can-----	244	92	55	1	1	0.1	Tr	0.2
	Lime juice:								
248	Raw------------------------- 1 cup-----------	246	90	65	1	Tr	Tr	Tr	0.1
249	Canned, unsweetened----------- 1 cup-----------	246	93	50	1	1	0.1	0.1	0.2
250	Mangos, raw, without skin and seed (about 1-1/2 per lb with skin and seed)---------------- 1 mango---------	207	82	135	1	1	0.1	0.2	0.1
	Melons, raw, without rind and cavity contents:								
251	Cantaloup, orange-fleshed (5-in diam., 2-1/3 lb, whole, with rind and cavity contents)---- 1/2 melon-------	267	90	95	2	1	0.1	0.1	0.3
252	Honeydew (6-1/2-in diam., 5-1/4 lb, whole, with rind and cavity contents)---------------- 1/10 melon------	129	90	45	1	Tr	Tr	Tr	0.1
253	Nectarines, raw, without pits (about 3 per lb with pits)----- 1 nectarine-----	136	86	65	1	1	0.1	0.2	0.3
	Oranges, raw:								
254	Whole, without peel and seeds (2-5/8-in diam., about 2-1/2 per lb, with peel and seeds) 1 orange--------	131	87	60	1	Tr	Tr	Tr	Tr
255	Sections without membranes----- 1 cup-----------	180	87	85	2	Tr	Tr	Tr	Tr
	Orange juice:								
256	Raw, all varieties------------- 1 cup-----------	248	88	110	2	Tr	0.1	0.1	0.1
257	Canned, unsweetened----------- 1 cup-----------	249	89	105	1	Tr	Tr	0.1	0.1
258	Chilled----------------------- 1 cup-----------	249	88	110	2	1	0.1	0.1	0.2
	Frozen concentrate:								
259	Undiluted--------------------- 6-fl-oz can-----	213	58	340	5	Tr	0.1	0.1	0.1
260	Diluted with 3 parts water by volume--------------------- 1 cup-----------	249	88	110	2	Tr	Tr	Tr	Tr
261	Orange and grapefruit juice, canned------------------------ 1 cup-----------	247	89	105	1	Tr	Tr	Tr	Tr
262	Papayas, raw, 1/2-in cubes------- 1 cup-----------	140	86	65	1	Tr	0.1	0.1	Tr
	Peaches:								
	Raw:								
263	Whole, 2-1/2-in diam., peeled, pitted (about 4 per lb with peels and pits)---- 1 peach---------	87	88	35	1	Tr	Tr	Tr	Tr
264	Sliced----------------------- 1 cup-----------	170	88	75	1	Tr	Tr	0.1	0.1
	Canned, fruit and liquid:								
265	Heavy syrup pack------------- 1 cup-----------	256	79	190	1	Tr	Tr	0.1	0.1
266	1 half----------	81	79	60	Tr	Tr	Tr	Tr	Tr
267	Juice pack------------------- 1 cup-----------	248	87	110	2	Tr	Tr	Tr	Tr
268	1 half----------	77	87	35	Tr	Tr	Tr	Tr	Tr

[20]Without added ascorbic acid. For value with added ascorbic acid, refer to label.
[21]With added ascorbic acid.

Table A-4 Nutritive Value of the Edible Part of Food *(Continued)*

Nutrients in Indicated Quantity

Cho-les-terol	Carbo-hydrate	Calcium	Phos-phorus	Iron	Potas-sium	Sodium	Vitamin A value		Thiamin	Ribo-flavin	Niacin	Ascorbic acid	Item No.
							(IU)	(RE)					
Milli-grams	Grams	Milli-grams	Milli-grams	Milli-grams	Milli-grams	Milli-grams	Inter-national units	Retinol equiva-lents	Milli-grams	Milli-grams	Milli-grams	Milli-grams	
0	9	6	7	0.1	93	1	40	4	0.05	0.03	0.2	5	237
0	10	6	7	0.1	105	1	40	4	0.05	0.03	0.2	6	238
0	38	23	28	0.6	334	8	20	2	0.07	0.09	0.7	[20]Tr	239
0	96	28	32	0.8	160	15	60	6	0.11	0.20	0.9	[21]179	240
0	32	10	10	0.3	53	5	20	2	0.04	0.07	0.3	[21]60	241
0	11	20	30	0.3	252	4	130	13	0.02	0.04	0.4	74	242
0	5	15	9	0.3	80	1	20	2	0.02	0.01	0.1	31	243
0	21	17	15	0.1	303	2	50	5	0.07	0.02	0.2	112	244
0	16	27	22	0.3	249	[23]51	40	4	0.10	0.02	0.5	61	245
0	1	2	1	Tr	15	[23]3	Tr	Tr	0.01	Tr	Tr	4	246
0	16	20	20	0.3	217	2	30	3	0.14	0.03	0.3	77	247
0	22	22	17	0.1	268	2	20	2	0.05	0.02	0.2	72	248
0	16	30	25	0.6	185	[23]39	40	4	0.08	0.01	0.4	16	249
0	35	21	23	0.3	323	4	8,060	806	0.12	0.12	1.2	57	250
0	22	29	45	0.6	825	24	8,610	861	0.10	0.06	1.5	113	251
0	12	8	13	0.1	350	13	50	5	0.10	0.02	0.8	32	252
0	16	7	22	0.2	288	Tr	1,000	100	0.02	0.06	1.3	7	253
0	15	52	18	0.1	237	Tr	270	27	0.11	0.05	0.4	70	254
0	21	72	25	0.2	326	Tr	370	37	0.16	0.07	0.5	96	255
0	26	27	42	0.5	496	2	500	50	0.22	0.07	1.0	124	256
0	25	20	35	1.1	436	5	440	44	0.15	0.07	0.8	86	257
0	25	25	27	0.4	473	2	190	19	0.28	0.05	0.7	82	258
0	81	68	121	0.7	1,436	6	590	59	0.60	0.14	1.5	294	259
0	27	22	40	0.2	473	2	190	19	0.20	0.04	0.5	97	260
0	25	20	35	1.1	390	7	290	29	0.14	0.07	0.8	72	261
0	17	35	12	0.3	247	9	400	40	0.04	0.04	0.5	92	262
0	10	4	10	0.1	171	Tr	470	47	0.01	0.04	0.9	6	263
0	19	9	20	0.2	335	Tr	910	91	0.03	0.07	1.7	11	264
0	51	8	28	0.7	236	15	850	85	0.03	0.06	1.6	7	265
0	16	2	9	0.2	75	5	270	27	0.01	0.02	0.5	2	266
0	29	15	42	0.7	317	10	940	94	0.02	0.04	1.4	9	267
0	9	5	13	0.2	99	3	290	29	0.01	0.01	0.4	3	268

[23]Sodium benzoate and sodium bisulfite added as preservatives.

Table A-4 Nutritive Value of the Edible Part of Food *(Continued)*

(Tr indicates nutrient present in trace amount.)

Item No.	Foods, approximate measures, units, and weight (weight of edible portion only)			Water	Food energy	Pro-tein	Fat	Fatty acids		
								Satu-rated	Mono-unsatu-rated	Poly-unsatu-rated
	Fruits and Fruit Juices—Con.		Grams	Per-cent	Cal-ories	Grams	Grams	Grams	Grams	Grams
	Peaches:									
	Dried:									
269	Uncooked---------------------	1 cup-----------	160	32	380	6	1	0.1	0.4	0.6
270	Cooked, unsweetened, fruit and liquid-----------------	1 cup-----------	258	78	200	3	1	0.1	0.2	0.3
271	Frozen, sliced, sweetened------	10-oz container	284	75	265	2	Tr	Tr	0.1	0.2
272		1 cup-----------	250	75	235	2	Tr	Tr	0.1	0.2
	Pears:									
	Raw, with skin, cored:									
273	Bartlett, 2-1/2-in diam. (about 2-1/2 per lb with cores and stems)------------	1 pear----------	166	84	100	1	1	Tr	0.1	0.2
274	Bosc, 2-1/2-in diam. (about 3 per lb with cores and stems)--------------------	1 pear----------	141	84	85	1	1	Tr	0.1	0.1
275	D'Anjou, 3-in diam. (about 2 per lb with cores and stems)--------------------	1 pear----------	200	84	120	1	1	Tr	0.2	0.2
	Canned, fruit and liquid:									
276	Heavy syrup pack-------------	1 cup-----------	255	80	190	1	Tr	Tr	0.1	0.1
277		1 half----------	79	80	60	Tr	Tr	Tr	Tr	Tr
278	Juice pack-------------------	1 cup-----------	248	86	125	1	Tr	Tr	Tr	Tr
279		1 half----------	77	86	40	Tr	Tr	Tr	Tr	Tr
	Pineapple:									
280	Raw, diced-------------------	1 cup-----------	155	87	75	1	1	Tr	0.1	0.2
	Canned, fruit and liquid:									
	Heavy syrup pack:									
281	Crushed, chunks, tidbits---	1 cup-----------	255	79	200	1	Tr	Tr	Tr	0.1
282	Slices---------------------	1 slice--------	58	79	45	Tr	Tr	Tr	Tr	Tr
	Juice pack:									
283	Chunks or tidbits----------	1 cup-----------	250	84	150	1	Tr	Tr	Tr	0.1
284	Slices---------------------	1 slice--------	58	84	35	Tr	Tr	Tr	Tr	Tr
285	Pineapple juice, unsweetened, canned----------------------	1 cup-----------	250	86	140	1	Tr	Tr	Tr	0.1
	Plantains, without peel:									
286	Raw-------------------------	1 plantain------	179	65	220	2	1	0.3	0.1	0.1
287	Cooked, boiled, sliced---------	1 cup-----------	154	67	180	1	Tr	0.1	Tr	0.1
	Plums, without pits:									
	Raw:									
288	2-1/8-in diam. (about 6-1/2 per lb with pits)---------	1 plum----------	66	85	35	1	Tr	Tr	0.3	0.1
289	1-1/2-in diam. (about 15 per lb with pits)--------------	1 plum----------	28	85	15	Tr	Tr	Tr	0.1	Tr
	Canned, purple, fruit and liquid:									
290	Heavy syrup pack-------------	1 cup-----------	258	76	230	1	Tr	Tr	0.2	0.1
291		3 plums--------	133	76	120	Tr	Tr	Tr	0.1	Tr
292	Juice pack-------------------	1 cup-----------	252	84	145	1	Tr	Tr	Tr	Tr
293		3 plums--------	95	84	55	Tr	Tr	Tr	Tr	Tr
	Prunes, dried:									
294	Uncooked----------------------	4 extra large or 5 large prunes	49	32	115	1	Tr	Tr	0.2	0.1
295	Cooked, unsweetened, fruit and liquid----------------------	1 cup-----------	212	70	225	2	Tr	Tr	0.3	0.1
296	Prune juice, canned or bottled---	1 cup-----------	256	81	180	2	Tr	Tr	0.1	Tr
	Raisins, seedless:									
297	Cup, not pressed down----------	1 cup-----------	145	15	435	5	1	0.2	Tr	0.2
298	Packet, 1/2 oz (1-1/2 tbsp)----	1 packet-------	14	15	40	Tr	Tr	Tr	Tr	Tr
	Raspberries:									
299	Raw-------------------------	1 cup-----------	123	87	60	1	1	Tr	0.1	0.4
300	Frozen, sweetened--------------	10-oz container	284	73	295	2	Tr	Tr	Tr	0.3
301		1 cup-----------	250	73	255	2	Tr	Tr	Tr	0.2

[21] With added ascorbic acid.

Table A-4 Nutritive Value of the Edible Part of Food (Continued)

							Vitamin A value						
Choles-terol	Carbo-hydrate	Calcium	Phos-phorus	Iron	Potas-sium	Sodium	(IU)	(RE)	Thiamin	Ribo-flavin	Niacin	Ascorbic acid	Item No
Milli-grams	Grams	Milli-grams	Milli-grams	Milli-grams	Milli-grams	Milli-grams	Inter-national units	Retinol equiva-lents	Milli-grams	Milli-grams	Milli-grams	Milli-grams	
0	98	45	190	6.5	1,594	11	3,460	346	Tr	0.34	7.0	8	269
0	51	23	98	3.4	826	5	510	51	0.01	0.05	3.9	10	270
0	68	9	31	1.1	369	17	810	81	0.04	0.10	1.9	[21]268	271
0	60	8	28	0.9	325	15	710	71	0.03	0.09	1.6	[21]236	272
0	25	18	18	0.4	208	Tr	30	3	0.03	0.07	0.2	7	273
0	21	16	16	0.4	176	Tr	30	3	0.03	0.06	0.1	6	274
0	30	22	22	0.5	250	Tr	40	4	0.04	0.08	0.2	8	275
0	49	13	18	0.6	166	13	10	1	0.03	0.06	0.6	3	276
0	15	4	6	0.2	51	4	Tr	Tr	0.01	0.02	0.2	1	277
0	32	22	30	0.7	238	10	10	1	0.03	0.03	0.5	4	278
0	10	7	9	0.2	74	3	Tr	Tr	0.01	0.01	0.2	1	279
0	19	11	11	0.6	175	2	40	4	0.14	0.06	0.7	24	280
0	52	36	18	1.0	265	3	40	4	0.23	0.06	0.7	19	281
0	12	8	4	0.2	60	1	10	1	0.05	0.01	0.2	4	282
0	39	35	15	0.7	305	3	100	10	0.24	0.05	0.7	24	283
0	9	8	3	0.2	71	1	20	2	0.06	0.01	0.2	6	284
0	34	43	20	0.7	335	3	10	1	0.14	0.06	0.6	27	285
0	57	5	61	1.1	893	7	2,020	202	0.09	0.10	1.2	33	286
0	48	3	43	0.9	716	8	1,400	140	0.07	0.08	1.2	17	287
0	9	3	7	0.1	114	Tr	210	21	0.03	0.06	0.3	6	288
0	4	1	3	Tr	48	Tr	90	9	0.01	0.03	0.1	3	289
0	60	23	34	2.2	235	49	670	67	0.04	0.10	0.8	1	290
0	31	12	17	1.1	121	25	340	34	0.02	0.05	0.4	1	291
0	38	25	38	0.9	388	3	2,540	254	0.06	0.15	1.2	7	292
0	14	10	14	0.3	146	1	960	96	0.02	0.06	0.4	3	293
0	31	25	39	1.2	365	2	970	97	0.04	0.08	1.0	2	294
0	60	49	74	2.4	708	4	650	65	0.05	0.21	1.5	6	295
0	45	31	64	3.0	707	10	10	1	0.04	0.18	2.0	10	296
0	115	71	141	3.0	1,089	17	10	1	0.23	0.13	1.2	5	297
0	11	7	14	0.3	105	2	Tr	Tr	0.02	0.01	0.1	Tr	298
0	14	27	15	0.7	187	Tr	160	16	0.04	0.11	1.1	31	299
0	74	43	48	1.8	324	3	170	17	0.05	0.13	0.7	47	300
0	65	38	43	1.6	285	3	150	15	0.05	0.11	0.6	41	301

Table A-4 Nutritive Value of the Edible Part of Food (Continued)

(Tr indicates nutrient present in trace amount.)

Item No.	Foods, approximate measures, units, and weight (weight of edible portion only)		Grams	Water Percent	Food energy Calories	Protein Grams	Fat Grams	Saturated Grams	Monounsaturated Grams	Polyunsaturated Grams
	Fruits and Fruit Juices—Con.									
302	Rhubarb, cooked, added sugar	1 cup	240	68	280	1	Tr	Tr	Tr	0.1
	Strawberries:									
303	Raw, capped, whole	1 cup	149	92	45	1	1	Tr	0.1	0.3
304	Frozen, sweetened, sliced	10-oz container	284	73	275	2	Tr	Tr	0.1	0.2
305		1 cup	255	73	245	1	Tr	Tr	Tr	0.2
	Tangerines:									
306	Raw, without peel and seeds (2-3/8-in diam., about 4 per lb, with peel and seeds)	1 tangerine	84	88	35	1	Tr	Tr	Tr	Tr
307	Canned, light syrup, fruit and liquid	1 cup	252	83	155	1	Tr	Tr	Tr	0.1
308	Tangerine juice, canned, sweetened	1 cup	249	87	125	1	Tr	Tr	Tr	0.1
	Watermelon, raw, without rind and seeds:									
309	Piece (4 by 8 in wedge with rind and seeds; 1/16 of 32-2/3-lb melon, 10 by 16 in)	1 piece	482	92	155	3	2	0.3	0.2	1.0
310	Diced	1 cup	160	92	50	1	1	0.1	0.1	0.3
	Grain Products									
311	Bagels, plain or water, enriched, 3-1/2-in diam.[24]	1 bagel	68	29	200	7	2	0.3	0.5	0.7
312	Barley, pearled, light, uncooked	1 cup	200	11	700	16	2	0.3	0.2	0.9
	Biscuits, baking powder, 2-in diam. (enriched flour, vegetable shortening):									
313	From home recipe	1 biscuit	28	28	100	2	5	1.2	2.0	1.3
314	From mix	1 biscuit	28	29	95	2	3	0.8	1.4	0.9
315	From refrigerated dough	1 biscuit	20	30	65	1	2	0.6	0.9	0.6
	Breadcrumbs, enriched:									
316	Dry, grated	1 cup	100	7	390	13	5	1.5	1.6	1.0
	Soft. See White bread (item 351).									
	Breads:									
317	Boston brown bread, canned, slice, 3-1/4 in by 1/2 in[25]	1 slice	45	45	95	2	1	0.3	0.1	0.1
	Cracked-wheat bread (3/4 enriched wheat flour, 1/4 cracked wheat flour):[25]									
318	Loaf, 1 lb	1 loaf	454	35	1,190	42	16	3.1	4.3	5.7
319	Slice (18 per loaf)	1 slice	25	35	65	2	1	0.2	0.2	0.3
320	Toasted	1 slice	21	26	65	2	1	0.2	0.2	0.3
	French or vienna bread, enriched:[25]									
321	Loaf, 1 lb	1 loaf	454	34	1,270	43	18	3.8	5.7	5.9
	Slice:									
322	French, 5 by 2-1/2 by 1 in	1 slice	35	34	100	3	1	0.3	0.4	0.5
323	Vienna, 4-3/4 by 4 by 1/2 in	1 slice	25	34	70	2	1	0.2	0.3	0.3
	Italian bread, enriched:									
324	Loaf, 1 lb	1 loaf	454	32	1,255	41	4	0.6	0.3	1.6
325	Slice, 4-1/2 by 3-1/4 by 3/4 in	1 slice	30	32	85	3	Tr	Tr	Tr	0.1
	Mixed grain bread, enriched:[25]									
326	Loaf, 1 lb	1 loaf	454	37	1,165	45	17	3.2	4.1	6.5
327	Slice (18 per loaf)	1 slice	25	37	65	2	1	0.2	0.2	0.4
328	Toasted	1 slice	23	27	65	2	1	0.2	0.2	0.4

[24] Egg bagels have 44 mg cholesterol and 22 IU or 7 RE vitamin A per bagel.
[25] Made with vegetable shortening.

Table A-4 Nutritive Value of the Edible Part of Food (Continued)

Nutrients in Indicated Quantity

Cholesterol	Carbohydrate	Calcium	Phosphorus	Iron	Potassium	Sodium	Vitamin A value		Thiamin	Riboflavin	Niacin	Ascorbic acid	Item No
							(IU)	(RE)					
Milligrams	Grams	Milligrams	Milligrams	Milligrams	Milligrams	Milligrams	International units	Retinol equivalents	Milligrams	Milligrams	Milligrams	Milligrams	
0	75	348	19	0.5	230	2	170	17	0.04	0.06	0.5	8	302
0	10	21	28	0.6	247	1	40	4	0.03	0.10	0.3	84	303
0	74	31	37	1.7	278	9	70	7	0.05	0.14	1.1	118	304
0	66	28	33	1.5	250	8	60	6	0.04	0.13	1.0	106	305
0	9	12	8	0.1	132	1	770	77	0.09	0.02	0.1	26	306
0	41	18	25	0.9	197	15	2,120	212	0.13	0.11	1.1	50	307
0	30	45	35	0.5	443	2	1,050	105	0.15	0.05	0.2	55	308
0	35	39	43	0.8	559	10	1,760	176	0.39	0.10	1.0	46	309
0	11	13	14	0.3	186	3	590	59	0.13	0.03	0.3	15	310
0	38	29	46	1.8	50	245	0	0	0.26	0.20	2.4	0	311
0	158	32	378	4.2	320	6	0	0	0.24	0.10	6.2	0	312
Tr	13	47	36	0.7	32	195	10	3	0.08	0.08	0.8	Tr	313
Tr	14	58	128	0.7	56	262	20	4	0.12	0.11	0.8	Tr	314
1	10	4	79	0.5	18	249	0	0	0.08	0.05	0.7	0	315
5	73	122	141	4.1	152	736	0	0	0.35	0.35	4.8	0	316
3	21	41	72	0.9	131	113	[26]0	[26]0	0.06	0.04	0.7	0	317
0	227	295	581	12.1	608	1,966	Tr	Tr	1.73	1.73	15.3	Tr	318
0	12	16	32	0.7	34	106	Tr	Tr	0.10	0.09	0.8	Tr	319
0	12	16	32	0.7	34	106	Tr	Tr	0.07	0.09	0.8	Tr	320
0	230	499	386	14.0	409	2,633	Tr	Tr	2.09	1.59	18.2	Tr	321
0	18	39	30	1.1	32	203	Tr	Tr	0.16	0.12	1.4	Tr	322
0	13	28	21	0.8	23	145	Tr	Tr	0.12	0.09	1.0	Tr	323
0	256	77	350	12.7	336	2,656	0	0	1.80	1.10	15.0	0	324
0	17	5	23	0.8	22	176	0	0	0.12	0.07	1.0	0	325
0	212	472	962	14.8	990	1,870	Tr	Tr	1.77	1.73	18.9	Tr	326
0	12	27	55	0.8	56	106	Tr	Tr	0.10	0.10	1.1	Tr	327
0	12	27	55	0.8	56	106	Tr	Tr	0.08	0.10	1.1	Tr	328

[26] Made with white cornmeal. If made with yellow cornmeal, value is 32 IU or 3 RE.

Table A-4 Nutritive Value of the Edible Part of Food *(Continued)*

(Tr indicates nutrient present in trace amount.)

Item No.	Foods, approximate measures, units, and weight (weight of edible portion only)		Grams	Water Per-cent	Food energy Cal-ories	Pro-tein Grams	Fat Grams	Fatty acids Satu-rated Grams	Mono-unsatu-rated Grams	Poly-unsatu-rated Grams
	Grain Products—Con.									
	Breads:									
	Oatmeal bread, enriched:[25]									
329	Loaf, 1 lb	1 loaf	454	37	1,145	38	20	3.7	7.1	8.2
330	Slice (18 per loaf)	1 slice	25	37	65	2	1	0.2	0.4	0.5
331	Toasted	1 slice	23	30	65	2	1	0.2	0.4	0.5
332	Pita bread, enriched, white, 6-1/2-in diam.	1 pita	60	31	165	6	1	0.1	0.1	0.4
	Pumpernickel (2/3 rye flour, 1/3 enriched wheat flour):[25]									
333	Loaf, 1 lb	1 loaf	454	37	1,160	42	16	2.6	3.6	6.4
334	Slice, 5 by 4 by 3/8 in	1 slice	32	37	80	3	1	0.2	0.3	0.5
335	Toasted	1 slice	29	28	80	3	1	0.2	0.3	0.5
	Raisin bread, enriched:[25]									
336	Loaf, 1 lb	1 loaf	454	33	1,260	37	18	4.1	6.5	6.7
337	Slice (18 per loaf)	1 slice	25	33	65	2	1	0.2	0.3	0.4
338	Toasted	1 slice	21	24	65	2	1	0.2	0.3	0.4
	Rye bread, light (2/3 enriched wheat flour, 1/3 rye flour):[25]									
339	Loaf, 1 lb	1 loaf	454	37	1,190	38	17	3.3	5.2	5.5
340	Slice, 4-3/4 by 3-3/4 by 7/16 in	1 slice	25	37	65	2	1	0.2	0.3	0.3
341	Toasted	1 slice	22	28	65	2	1	0.2	0.3	0.3
	Wheat bread, enriched:[25]									
342	Loaf, 1 lb	1 loaf	454	37	1,160	43	19	3.9	7.3	4.5
343	Slice (18 per loaf)	1 slice	25	37	65	2	1	0.2	0.4	0.3
344	Toasted	1 slice	23	28	65	3	1	0.2	0.4	0.3
	White bread, enriched:[25]									
345	Loaf, 1 lb	1 loaf	454	37	1,210	38	18	5.6	6.5	4.2
346	Slice (18 per loaf)	1 slice	25	37	65	2	1	0.3	0.4	0.2
347	Toasted	1 slice	22	28	65	2	1	0.3	0.4	0.2
348	Slice (22 per loaf)	1 slice	20	37	55	2	1	0.2	0.3	0.2
349	Toasted	1 slice	17	28	55	2	1	0.2	0.3	0.2
350	Cubes	1 cup	30	37	80	2	1	0.4	0.4	0.4
351	Crumbs, soft	1 cup	45	37	120	4	2	0.6	0.6	0.4
	Whole-wheat bread:[25]									
352	Loaf, 1 lb	1 loaf	454	38	1,110	44	20	5.8	6.8	5.2
353	Slice (16 per loaf)	1 slice	28	38	70	3	1	0.4	0.4	0.3
354	Toasted	1 slice	25	29	70	3	1	0.4	0.4	0.3
	Bread stuffing (from enriched bread), prepared from mix:									
355	Dry type	1 cup	140	33	500	9	31	6.1	13.3	9.6
356	Moist type	1 cup	203	61	420	9	26	5.3	11.3	8.0
	Breakfast cereals:									
	Hot type, cooked:									
	Corn (hominy) grits:									
357	Regular and quick, enriched	1 cup	242	85	145	3	Tr	Tr	0.1	0.2
358	Instant, plain	1 pkt	137	85	80	2	Tr	Tr	Tr	0.1
	Cream of Wheat®:									
359	Regular, quick, instant	1 cup	244	86	140	4	Tr	0.1	Tr	0.2
360	Mix'n Eat, plain	1 pkt	142	82	100	3	Tr	Tr	Tr	0.1
361	Malt-O-Meal®	1 cup	240	88	120	4	Tr	Tr	Tr	0.1
	Oatmeal or rolled oats:									
362	Regular, quick, instant, nonfortified	1 cup	234	85	145	6	2	0.4	0.8	1.0
	Instant, fortified:									
363	Plain	1 pkt	177	86	105	4	2	0.3	0.6	0.7
364	Flavored	1 pkt	164	76	160	5	2	0.3	0.7	0.8

[25] Made with vegetable shortening.
[27] Nutrient added.
[28] Cooked without salt. If salt is added according to label recommendations, sodium content is 540 mg.
[29] For white corn grits. Cooked yellow grits contain 145 IU or 14 RE.
[30] Value based on label declaration for added nutrients.

Table A-4 Nutritive Value of the Edible Part of Food (Continued)

Nutrients in Indicated Quantity

Cholesterol	Carbohydrate	Calcium	Phosphorus	Iron	Potassium	Sodium	Vitamin A value (IU) International units	Vitamin A value (RE) Retinol equivalents	Thiamin	Riboflavin	Niacin	Ascorbic acid	Item No.
Milligrams	Grams	Milligrams	Milligrams	Milligrams	Milligrams	Milligrams			Milligrams	Milligrams	Milligrams	Milligrams	
0	212	267	563	12.0	707	2,231	0	0	2.09	1.20	15.4	0	329
0	12	15	31	0.7	39	124	0	0	0.12	0.07	0.9	0	330
0	12	15	31	0.7	39	124	0	0	0.09	0.07	0.9	0	331
0	33	49	60	1.4	71	339	0	0	0.27	0.12	2.2	0	332
0	218	322	990	12.4	1,966	2,461	0	0	1.54	2.36	15.0	0	333
0	16	23	71	0.9	141	177	0	0	0.11	0.17	1.1	0	334
0	16	23	71	0.9	141	177	0	0	0.09	0.17	1.1	0	335
0	239	463	395	14.1	1,058	1,657	Tr	Tr	1.50	2.81	18.6	Tr	336
0	13	25	22	0.8	59	92	Tr	Tr	0.08	0.15	1.0	Tr	337
0	13	25	22	0.8	59	92	Tr	Tr	0.06	0.15	1.0	Tr	338
0	218	363	658	12.3	926	3,164	0	0	1.86	1.45	15.0	0	339
0	12	20	36	0.7	51	175	0	0	0.10	0.08	0.8	0	340
0	12	20	36	0.7	51	175	0	0	0.08	0.08	0.8	0	341
0	213	572	835	15.8	627	2,447	Tr	Tr	2.09	1.45	20.5	Tr	342
0	12	32	47	0.9	35	138	Tr	Tr	0.12	0.08	1.2	Tr	343
0	12	32	47	0.9	35	138	Tr	Tr	0.10	0.08	1.2	Tr	344
0	222	572	490	12.9	508	2,334	Tr	Tr	2.13	1.41	17.0	Tr	345
0	12	32	27	0.7	28	129	Tr	Tr	0.12	0.08	0.9	Tr	346
0	12	32	27	0.7	28	129	Tr	Tr	0.09	0.08	0.9	Tr	347
0	10	25	21	0.6	22	101	Tr	Tr	0.09	0.06	0.7	Tr	348
0	10	25	21	0.6	22	101	Tr	Tr	0.07	0.06	0.7	Tr	349
0	15	38	32	0.9	34	154	Tr	Tr	0.14	0.09	1.1	Tr	350
0	22	57	49	1.3	50	231	Tr	Tr	0.21	0.14	1.7	Tr	351
0	206	327	1,180	15.5	799	2,887	Tr	Tr	1.59	0.95	17.4	Tr	352
0	13	20	74	1.0	50	180	Tr	Tr	0.10	0.06	1.1	Tr	353
0	13	20	74	1.0	50	180	Tr	Tr	0.08	0.06	1.1	Tr	354
0	50	92	136	2.2	126	1,254	910	273	0.17	0.20	2.5	0	355
67	40	81	134	2.0	118	1,023	850	256	0.10	0.18	1.6	0	356
0	31	0	29	[27]1.5	53	[28]0	[29]0	[29]0	[27]0.24	[27]0.15	[27]2.0	0	357
0	18	7	16	[27]1.0	29	343	0	0	[27]0.18	[27]0.08	[27]1.3	0	358
0	29	[30]54	[31]43	[30]10.9	46	[31,32]5	0	0	[30]0.24	[30]0.07	[30]1.5	0	359
0	21	[30]20	[30]20	[30]8.1	38	241	[30]1,250	[30]376	[30]0.43	[30]0.28	[30]5.0	0	360
0	26	5	[30]24	[30]9.6	31	[33]2	0	0	[30]0.48	[30]0.24	[30]5.8	0	361
0	25	19	178	1.6	131	[34]2	40	4	0.26	0.05	0.3	0	362
0	18	[27]163	133	[27]6.3	99	[27]285	[27]1,510	[27]453	[27]0.53	[27]0.28	[27]5.5	0	363
0	31	[27]168	148	[27]6.7	137	[27]254	[27]1,530	[27]460	[27]0.53	[27]0.38	[27]5.9	Tr	364

[31] For regular and instant cereal. For quick cereal, phosphorus is 102 mg and sodium is 142 mg.
[32] Cooked without salt. If salt is added according to label recommendations, sodium content is 390 mg.
[33] Cooked without salt. If salt is added according to label recommendations, sodium content is 324 mg.
[34] Cooked without salt. If salt is added according to label recommendations, sodium content is 374 mg.

Table A-4 Nutritive Value of the Edible Part of Food *(Continued)*

(Tr indicates nutrient present in trace amount.)

Item No.	Foods, approximate measures, units, and weight (weight of edible portion only)			Water	Food energy	Pro-tein	Fat	Fatty acids		
								Satu-rated	Mono-unsatu-rated	Poly-unsatu-rated
			Grams	Per-cent	Cal-ories	Grams	Grams	Grams	Grams	Grams
	Grain Products—Con.									
	Breakfast cereals:									
	Ready to eat:									
365	All-Bran® (about 1/3 cup)----	1 oz------------	28	3	70	4	1	0.1	0.1	0.3
366	Cap'n Crunch® (about 3/4 cup)	1 oz------------	28	3	120	1	3	1.7	0.3	0.4
367	Cheerios® (about 1-1/4 cup)--	1 oz------------	28	5	110	4	2	0.3	0.6	0.7
	Corn Flakes (about 1-1/4 cup):									
368	Kellogg's® ----------------	1 oz------------	28	3	110	2	Tr	Tr	Tr	Tr
369	Toasties® -----------------	1 oz------------	28	3	110	2	Tr	Tr	Tr	Tr
	40% Bran Flakes:									
370	Kellogg's® (about 3/4 cup)	1 oz------------	28	3	90	4	1	0.1	0.1	0.3
371	Post® (about 2/3 cup)------	1 oz------------	28	3	90	3	Tr	0.1	0.1	0.2
372	Froot Loops® (about 1 cup)---	1 oz------------	28	3	110	2	1	0.2	0.1	0.1
373	Golden Grahams® (about 3/4 cup)---------------------	1 oz------------	28	2	110	2	1	0.7	0.1	0.2
374	Grape-Nuts® (about 1/4 cup)--	1 oz------------	28	3	100	3	Tr	Tr	Tr	0.1
375	Honey Nut Cheerios® (about 3/4 cup)-------------------	1 oz------------	28	3	105	3	1	0.1	0.3	0.3
376	Lucky Charms® (about 1 cup)--	1 oz------------	28	3	110	3	1	0.2	0.4	0.4
377	Nature Valley® Granola (about 1/3 cup)-------------------	1 oz------------	28	4	125	3	5	3.3	0.7	0.7
378	100% Natural Cereal (about 1/4 cup)-------------------	1 oz------------	28	2	135	3	6	4.1	1.2	0.5
379	Product 19® (about 3/4 cup)--	1 oz------------	28	3	110	3	Tr	Tr	Tr	0.1
	Raisin Bran:									
380	Kellogg's® (about 3/4 cup)-	1 oz------------	28	8	90	3	1	0.1	0.1	0.3
381	Post® (about 1/2 cup)------	1 oz------------	28	9	85	3	1	0.1	0.1	0.3
382	Rice Krispies® (about 1 cup)	1 oz------------	28	2	110	2	Tr	Tr	Tr	0.1
383	Shredded Wheat (about 2/3 cup)---------------------	1 oz------------	28	5	100	3	1	0.1	0.1	0.3
384	Special K® (about 1-1/3 cup)	1 oz------------	28	2	110	6	Tr	Tr	Tr	Tr
385	Super Sugar Crisp® (about 7/8 cup)---------------------	1 oz------------	28	2	105	2	Tr	Tr	Tr	0.1
386	Sugar Frosted Flakes, Kellogg's® (about 3/4 cup)	1 oz------------	28	3	110	1	Tr	Tr	Tr	Tr
387	Sugar Smacks® (about 3/4 cup)	1 oz------------	28	3	105	2	1	0.1	0.1	0.2
388	Total® (about 1 cup)-------	1 oz------------	28	4	100	3	1	0.1	0.1	0.3
389	Trix® (about 1 cup)---------	1 oz------------	28	3	110	2	Tr	0.2	0.1	0.1
390	Wheaties® (about 1 cup)------	1 oz------------	28	5	100	3	Tr	0.1	Tr	0.2
391	Buckwheat flour, light, sifted---	1 cup----------	98	12	340	6	1	0.2	0.4	0.4
392	Bulgur, uncooked-----------------	1 cup----------	170	10	600	19	3	1.2	0.3	1.2
	Cakes prepared from cake mixes with enriched flour:[35]									
	Angelfood:									
393	Whole cake, 9-3/4-in diam. tube cake------------------	1 cake----------	635	38	1,510	38	2	0.4	0.2	1.0
394	Piece, 1/12 of cake----------	1 piece--------	53	38	125	3	Tr	Tr	Tr	0.1
	Coffeecake, crumb:									
395	Whole cake, 7-3/4 by 5-5/8 by 1-1/4 in------------	1 cake----------	430	30	1,385	27	41	11.8	16.7	9.6
396	Piece, 1/6 of cake----------	1 piece--------	72	30	230	5	7	2.0	2.8	1.6
	Devil's food with chocolate frosting:									
397	Whole, 2-layer cake, 8- or 9-in diam.-----------------	1 cake----------	1,107	24	3,755	49	136	55.6	51.4	19.7
398	Piece, 1/16 of cake----------	1 piece--------	69	24	235	3	8	3.5	3.2	1.2
399	Cupcake, 2-1/2-in diam.------	1 cupcake-------	35	24	120	2	4	1.8	1.6	0.6
	Gingerbread:									
400	Whole cake, 8 in square------	1 cake----------	570	37	1,575	18	39	9.6	16.4	10.5
401	Piece, 1/9 of cake-----------	1 piece--------	63	37	175	2	4	1.1	1.8	1.2

[27] Nutrient added.
[30] Value based on label declaration for added nutrients.

Table A-4 Nutritive Value of the Edible Part of Food (Continued)

Nutrients in Indicated Quantity

Cholesterol (Milligrams)	Carbohydrate (Grams)	Calcium (Milligrams)	Phosphorus (Milligrams)	Iron (Milligrams)	Potassium (Milligrams)	Sodium (Milligrams)	Vitamin A value (IU) International units	Vitamin A value (RE) Retinol equivalents	Thiamin (Milligrams)	Riboflavin (Milligrams)	Niacin (Milligrams)	Ascorbic acid (Milligrams)	Item No
0	21	23	264	[30]4.5	350	320	[30]1,250	[30]375	[30]0.37	[30]0.43	[30]5.0	[30]15	365
0	23	5	36	[27]7.5	37	213	40	[30]4	[27]0.50	[27]0.55	[27]6.6	[30]0	366
0	20	48	134	[30]4.5	101	307	[30]1,250	[30]375	[30]0.37	[30]0.43	[30]5.0	[30]15	367
0	24	1	18	[30]1.8	26	351	[30]1,250	[30]375	[30]0.37	[30]0.43	[30]5.0	[30]15	368
0	24	1	12	[27]0.7	33	297	[30]1,250	[30]375	[30]0.37	[30]0.43	[30]5.0	0	369
0	22	14	139	[30]8.1	180	264	[30]1,250	[30]375	[30]0.37	[30]0.43	[30]5.0	0	370
0	22	12	179	[30]4.5	151	260	[30]1,250	[30]375	[30]0.37	[30]0.43	[30]5.0	0	371
0	25	3	24	[30]4.5	26	145	[30]1,250	[30]375	[30]0.37	[30]0.43	[30]5.0	[30]15	372
Tr	24	17	41	[30]4.5	63	346	[30]1,250	[30]375	[30]0.37	[30]0.43	[30]5.0	[30]15	373
0	23	11	71	1.2	95	197	[30]1,250	[30]375	[30]0.37	[30]0.43		0	374
0	23	20	105	[30]4.5	99	257	[30]1,250	[30]375	[30]0.37	[30]0.43	[30]5.0	[30]15	375
0	23	32	79	[30]4.5	59	201	[30]1,250	[30]375	[30]0.37	[30]0.43	[30]5.0	[30]15	376
0	19	18	89	0.9	98	58	20	2	0.10	0.05	0.2	0	377
Tr	18	49	104	0.8	140	12	20	2	0.09	0.15	0.6	0	378
0	24	3	40	[30]18.0	44	325	[30]5,000	[30]1,501	[30]1.50	[30]1.70	[30]20.0	[30]60	379
0	21	10	105	[30]3.5	147	207	[30]960	[30]288	[30]0.28	[30]0.34	[30]3.9	0	380
0	21	13	119	[30]4.5	175	185	[30]1,250	[30]375	[30]0.37	[30]0.43	[30]5.0	0	381
0	25	4	34	[30]1.8	29	340	[30]1,250	[30]375	[30]0.37	[30]0.43	[30]5.0	[30]15	382
0	23	11	100	1.2	102	3	0	0	0.07	0.08	1.5	0	383
Tr	21	8	55	[30]4.5	49	265	[30]1,250	[30]375	[30]0.37	[30]0.43	[30]5.0	[30]15	384
0	26	6	52	[30]1.8	105	25	[30]1,250	[30]375	[30]0.37	[30]0.43	[30]5.0	0	385
0	26	1	21	[30]1.8	18	230	[30]1,250	[30]375	[30]0.37	[30]0.43	[30]5.0	[30]15	386
0	25	3	31	[30]1.8	42	75	[30]1,250	[30]375	[30]0.37	[30]0.43	[30]5.0	[30]15	387
0	22	48	118	[30]18.0	106	352	[30]5,000	[30]1,501	[30]1.50	[30]1.70	[30]20.0	[30]60	388
0	25	6	19	[30]4.5	27	181	[30]1,250	[30]375	[30]0.37	[30]0.43	[30]5.0	[30]15	389
0	23	43	98	[30]4.5	106	354	[30]1,250	[30]375	[30]0.37	[30]0.43	[30]5.0	[30]15	390
0	78	11	86	1.0	314	2	0	0	0.08	0.04	0.4	0	391
0	129	49	575	9.5	389	7	0	0	0.48	0.24	7.7	0	392
0	342	527	1,086	2.7	845	3,226	0	0	0.32	1.27	1.6	0	393
0	29	44	91	0.2	71	269	0	0	0.03	0.11	0.1	0	394
279	225	262	748	7.3	469	1,853	690	194	0.82	0.90	7.7	1	395
47	38	44	125	1.2	78	310	120	32	0.14	0.15	1.3	Tr	396
598	645	653	1,162	22.1	1,439	2,900	1,660	498	1.11	1.66	10.0	1	397
37	40	41	72	1.4	90	181	100	31	0.07	0.10	0.6	Tr	398
19	20	21	37	0.7	46	92	50	16	0.04	0.05	0.3	Tr	399
6	291	513	570	10.8	1,562	1,733	0	0	0.86	1.03	7.4	1	400
1	32	57	63	1.2	173	192	0	0	0.09	0.11	0.8	Tr	401

[35] Excepting angelfood cake, cakes were made from mixes containing vegetable shortening and frostings were made with margarine.

Table A-4 Nutritive Value of the Edible Part of Food (Continued)

(Tr indicates nutrient present in trace amount.)

Item No.	Foods, approximate measures, units, and weight (weight of edible portion only)			Water	Food energy	Protein	Fat	Fatty acids		
								Saturated	Monounsaturated	Polyunsaturated
	Grain Products—Con.		Grams	Percent	Calories	Grams	Grams	Grams	Grams	Grams
	Cakes prepared from cake mixes with enriched flour:[35]									
	Yellow with chocolate frosting:									
402	Whole, 2-layer cake, 8- or 9-in diam.	1 cake	1,108	26	3,735	45	125	47.8	48.8	21.8
403	Piece, 1/16 of cake	1 piece	69	26	235	3	8	3.0	3.0	1.4
	Cakes prepared from home recipes using enriched flour:									
	Carrot, with cream cheese frosting:[36]									
404	Whole cake, 10-in diam. tube cake	1 cake	1,536	23	6,175	63	328	66.0	135.2	107.5
405	Piece, 1/16 of cake	1 piece	96	23	385	4	21	4.1	8.4	6.7
	Fruitcake, dark:[36]									
406	Whole cake, 7-1/2-in diam., 2-1/4-in high tube cake	1 cake	1,361	18	5,185	74	228	47.6	113.0	51.7
407	Piece, 1/32 of cake, 2/3-in arc	1 piece	43	18	165	2	7	1.5	3.6	1.6
	Plain sheet cake:[37]									
	Without frosting:									
408	Whole cake, 9-in square	1 cake	777	25	2,830	35	108	29.5	45.1	25.6
409	Piece, 1/9 of cake	1 piece	86	25	315	4	12	3.3	5.0	2.8
	With uncooked white frosting:									
410	Whole cake, 9-in square	1 cake	1,096	21	4,020	37	129	41.6	50.4	26.3
411	Piece, 1/9 of cake	1 piece	121	21	445	4	14	4.6	5.6	2.9
	Pound:[38]									
412	Loaf, 8-1/2 by 3-1/2 by 3-1/4 in	1 loaf	514	22	2,025	33	94	21.1	40.9	26.7
413	Slice, 1/17 of loaf	1 slice	30	22	120	2	5	1.2	2.4	1.6
	Cakes, commercial, made with enriched flour:									
	Pound:									
414	Loaf, 8-1/2 by 3-1/2 by 3 in	1 loaf	500	24	1,935	26	94	52.0	30.0	4.0
415	Slice, 1/17 of loaf	1 slice	29	24	110	2	5	3.0	1.7	0.2
	Snack cakes:									
416	Devil's food with creme filling (2 small cakes per pkg)	1 small cake	28	20	105	1	4	1.7	1.5	0.6
417	Sponge with creme filling (2 small cakes per pkg)	1 small cake	42	19	155	1	5	2.3	2.1	0.5
	White with white frosting:									
418	Whole, 2-layer cake, 8- or 9-in diam.	1 cake	1,140	24	4,170	43	148	33.1	61.6	42.2
419	Piece, 1/16 of cake	1 piece	71	24	260	3	9	2.1	3.8	2.6
	Yellow with chocolate frosting:									
420	Whole, 2-layer cake, 8- or 9-in diam.	1 cake	1,108	23	3,895	40	175	92.0	58.7	10.0
421	Piece, 1/16 of cake	1 piece	69	23	245	2	11	5.7	3.7	0.6
	Cheesecake:									
422	Whole cake, 9-in diam.	1 cake	1,110	46	3,350	60	213	119.9	65.5	14.4
423	Piece, 1/12 of cake	1 piece	92	46	280	5	18	9.9	5.4	1.2
	Cookies made with enriched flour:									
	Brownies with nuts:									
424	Commercial, with frosting, 1-1/2 by 1-3/4 in	1 brownie	25	13	100	1	4	1.6	2.0	0.6
425	From home recipe, 1-3/4 by 1-3/4 by 7/8 in[36]	1 brownie	20	10	95	1	6	1.4	2.8	1.2
	Chocolate chip:									
426	Commercial, 2-1/4-in diam., 3/8 in thick	4 cookies	42	4	180	2	9	2.9	3.1	2.6

[35] Excepting angelfood cake, cakes were made from mixes containing vegetable shortening and frostings were made with margarine.
[36] Made with vegetable oil.

Table A-4 Nutritive Value of the Edible Part of Food (Continued)

							Vitamin A value						
Cho-les-terol	Carbo-hydrate	Calcium	Phos-phorus	Iron	Potas-sium	Sodium	(IU)	(RE)	Thiamin	Ribo-flavin	Niacin	Ascorbic acid	Item No
Milli-grams	Grams	Milli-grams	Milli-grams	Milli-grams	Milli-grams	Milli-grams	Inter-national units	Retinol equiva-lents	Milli-grams	Milli-grams	Milli-grams	Milli-grams	
576	638	1,008	2,017	15.5	1,208	2,515	1,550	465	1.22	1.66	11.1	1	402
36	40	63	126	1.0	75	157	100	29	0.08	0.10	0.7	Tr	403
1183	775	707	998	21.0	1,720	4,470	2,240	246	1.83	1.97	14.7	23	404
74	48	44	62	1.3	108	279	140	15	0.11	0.12	0.9	1	405
640	783	1,293	1,592	37.6	6,138	2,123	1,720	422	2.41	2.55	17.0	504	406
20	25	41	50	1.2	194	67	50	13	0.08	0.08	0.5	16	407
552	434	497	793	11.7	614	2,331	1,320	373	1.24	1.40	10.1	2	408
61	48	55	88	1.3	68	258	150	41	0.14	0.15	1.1	Tr	409
636	694	548	822	11.0	669	2,488	2,190	647	1.21	1.42	9.9	2	410
70	77	61	91	1.2	74	275	240	71	0.13	0.16	1.1	Tr	411
555	265	339	473	9.3	483	1,645	3,470	1,033	0.93	1.08	7.8	1	412
32	15	20	28	0.5	28	96	200	60	0.05	0.06	0.5	Tr	413
1100	257	146	517	8.0	443	1,857	2,820	715	0.96	1.12	8.1	0	414
64	15	8	30	0.5	26	108	160	41	0.06	0.06	0.5	0	415
15	17	21	26	1.0	34	105	20	4	0.06	0.09	0.7	0	416
7	27	14	44	0.6	37	155	30	9	0.07	0.06	0.6	0	417
46	670	536	1,585	15.5	832	2,827	640	194	3.19	2.05	27.6	0	418
3	42	33	99	1.0	52	176	40	12	0.20	0.13	1.7	0	419
609	620	366	1,884	19.9	1,972	3,080	1,850	488	0.78	2.22	10.0	0	420
38	39	23	117	1.2	123	192	120	30	0.05	0.14	0.6	0	421
2053	317	622	977	5.3	1,088	2,464	2,820	833	0.33	1.44	5.1	56	422
170	26	52	81	0.4	90	204	230	69	0.03	0.12	0.4	5	423
14	16	13	26	0.6	50	59	70	18	0.08	0.07	0.3	Tr	424
18	11	9	26	0.4	35	51	20	6	0.05	0.05	0.3	Tr	425
5	28	13	41	0.8	68	140	50	15	0.10	0.23	1.0	Tr	426

[37] Cake made with vegetable shortening; frosting with margarine.
[38] Made with margarine.

Table A-4 Nutritive Value of the Edible Part of Food *(Continued)*

(Tr indicates nutrient present in trace amount.)

Item No.	Foods, approximate measures, units, and weight (weight of edible portion only)		Water	Food energy	Pro-tein	Fat	Fatty acids		
							Satu-rated	Mono-unsatu-rated	Poly-unsatu-rated
		Grams	Per-cent	Cal-ories	Grams	Grams	Grams	Grams	Grams
	Grain Products—Con.								
	Cookies made with enriched flour:								
	Chocolate chip:								
427	From home recipe, 2-1/3-in diam.[25]	4 cookies	40	3	185	2	11	3.9	4.3	2.0
428	From refrigerated dough, 2-1/4-in diam., 3/8 in thick	4 cookies	48	5	225	2	11	4.0	4.4	2.0
429	Fig bars, square, 1-5/8 by 1-5/8 by 3/8 in or rectangu-lar, 1-1/2 by 1-3/4 by 1/2 in	4 cookies	56	12	210	2	4	1.0	1.5	1.0
430	Oatmeal with raisins, 2-5/8-in diam., 1/4 in thick	4 cookies	52	4	245	3	10	2.5	4.5	2.8
431	Peanut butter cookie, from home recipe, 2-5/8-in diam.[25]	4 cookies	48	3	245	4	14	4.0	5.8	2.8
432	Sandwich type (chocolate or vanilla), 1-3/4-in diam., 3/8 in thick	4 cookies	40	2	195	2	8	2.0	3.6	2.2
	Shortbread:								
433	Commercial	4 small cookies	32	6	155	2	8	2.9	3.0	1.1
434	From home recipe[38]	2 large cookies	28	3	145	2	8	1.3	2.7	3.4
435	Sugar cookie, from refrigerated dough, 2-1/2-in diam., 1/4 in thick	4 cookies	48	4	235	2	12	2.3	5.0	3.6
436	Vanilla wafers, 1-3/4-in diam., 1/4 in thick	10 cookies	40	4	185	2	7	1.8	3.0	1.8
437	Corn chips	1-oz package	28	1	155	2	9	1.4	2.4	3.7
	Cornmeal:								
438	Whole-ground, unbolted, dry form	1 cup	122	12	435	11	5	0.5	1.1	2.5
439	Bolted (nearly whole-grain), dry form	1 cup	122	12	440	11	4	0.5	0.9	2.2
	Degermed, enriched:								
440	Dry form	1 cup	138	12	500	11	2	0.2	0.4	0.9
441	Cooked	1 cup	240	88	120	3	Tr	Tr	0.1	0.2
	Crackers:[39]								
	Cheese:								
442	Plain, 1 in square	10 crackers	10	4	50	1	3	0.9	1.2	0.3
443	Sandwich type (peanut butter)	1 sandwich	8	3	40	1	2	0.4	0.8	0.3
444	Graham, plain, 2-1/2 in square	2 crackers	14	5	60	1	1	0.4	0.6	0.4
445	Melba toast, plain	1 piece	5	4	20	1	Tr	0.1	0.1	0.1
446	Rye wafers, whole-grain, 1-7/8 by 3-1/2 in	2 wafers	14	5	55	1	1	0.3	0.4	0.3
447	Saltines[40]	4 crackers	12	4	50	1	1	0.5	0.4	0.2
448	Snack-type, standard	1 round cracker	3	3	15	Tr	1	0.2	0.4	0.1
449	Wheat, thin	4 crackers	8	3	35	1	1	0.5	0.5	0.4
450	Whole-wheat wafers	2 crackers	8	4	35	1	2	0.5	0.6	0.4
451	Croissants, made with enriched flour, 4-1/2 by 4 by 1-3/4 in	1 croissant	57	22	235	5	12	3.5	6.7	1.4
	Danish pastry, made with enriched flour:								
	Plain without fruit or nuts:								
452	Packaged ring, 12 oz	1 ring	340	27	1,305	21	71	21.8	28.6	15.6
453	Round piece, about 4-1/4-in diam., 1 in high	1 pastry	57	27	220	4	12	3.6	4.8	2.6
454	Ounce	1 oz	28	27	110	2	6	1.8	2.4	1.3
455	Fruit, round piece	1 pastry	65	30	235	4	13	3.9	5.2	2.9
	Doughnuts, made with enriched flour:								
456	Cake type, plain, 3-1/4-in diam., 1 in high	1 doughnut	50	21	210	3	12	2.8	5.0	3.0
457	Yeast-leavened, glazed, 3-3/4-in diam., 1-1/4 in high	1 doughnut	60	27	235	4	13	5.2	5.5	0.9
458	English muffins, plain, enriched	1 muffin	57	42	140	5	1	0.3	0.2	0.3
459	Toasted	1 muffin	50	29	140	5	1	0.3	0.2	0.3

[25]Made with vegetable shortening.
[38]Made with margarine.

Table A-4 Nutritive Value of the Edible Part of Food (Continued)

							Vitamin A value						
Cho-les-terol	Carbo-hydrate	Calcium	Phos-phorus	Iron	Potas-sium	Sodium	(IU)	(RE)	Thiamin	Ribo-flavin	Niacin	Ascorbic acid	Item No.
Milli-grams	Grams	Milli-grams	Milli-grams	Milli-grams	Milli-grams	Milli-grams	Inter-national units	Retinol equiva-lents	Milli-grams	Milli-grams	Milli-grams	Milli-grams	
18	26	13	34	1.0	82	82	20	5	0.06	0.06	0.6	0	427
22	32	13	34	1.0	62	173	30	8	0.06	0.10	0.9	0	428
27	42	40	34	1.4	162	180	60	6	0.08	0.07	0.7	Tr	429
2	36	18	58	1.1	90	148	40	12	0.09	0.08	1.0	0	430
22	28	21	60	1.1	110	142	20	5	0.07	0.07	1.9	0	431
0	29	12	40	1.4	66	189	0	0	0.09	0.07	0.8	0	432
27	20	13	39	0.8	38	123	30	8	0.10	0.09	0.9	0	433
0	17	6	31	0.6	18	125	300	89	0.08	0.06	0.7	Tr	434
29	31	50	91	0.9	33	261	40	11	0.09	0.06	1.1	0	435
25	29	16	36	0.8	50	150	50	14	0.07	0.10	1.0	0	436
0	16	35	52	0.5	52	233	110	11	0.04	0.05	0.4	1	437
0	90	24	312	2.2	346	1	620	62	0.46	0.13	2.4	0	438
0	91	21	272	2.2	303	1	590	59	0.37	0.10	2.3	0	439
0	108	8	137	5.9	166	1	610	61	0.61	0.36	4.8	0	440
0	26	2	34	1.4	38	0	140	14	0.14	0.10	1.2	0	441
6	6	11	17	0.3	17	112	20	5	0.05	0.04	0.4	0	442
1	5	7	25	0.3	17	90	Tr	Tr	0.04	0.03	0.6	0	443
0	11	6	20	0.4	36	86	0	0	0.02	0.03	0.6	0	444
0	4	6	10	0.1	11	44	0	0	0.01	0.01	0.1	0	445
0	10	7	44	0.5	65	115	0	0	0.06	0.03	0.5	0	446
4	9	3	12	0.5	17	165	0	0	0.06	0.05	0.6	0	447
0	2	3	6	0.1	4	30	Tr	Tr	0.01	0.01	0.1	0	448
0	5	3	15	0.3	17	69	Tr	Tr	0.04	0.03	0.4	0	449
0	5	3	22	0.2	31	59	0	0	0.02	0.03	0.4	0	450
13	27	20	64	2.1	68	452	50	13	0.17	0.13	1.3	0	451
292	152	360	347	6.5	316	1,302	360	99	0.95	1.02	8.5	Tr	452
49	26	60	58	1.1	53	218	60	17	0.16	0.17	1.4	Tr	453
24	13	30	29	0.5	26	109	30	8	0.08	0.09	0.7	Tr	454
56	28	17	80	1.3	57	233	40	11	0.16	0.14	1.4	Tr	455
20	24	22	111	1.0	58	192	20	5	0.12	0.12	1.1	Tr	456
21	26	17	55	1.4	64	222	Tr	Tr	0.28	0.12	1.8	0	457
0	27	96	67	1.7	331	378	0	0	0.26	0.19	2.2	0	458
0	27	96	67	1.7	331	378	0	0	0.23	0.19	2.2	0	459

[39] Crackers made with enriched flour except for rye wafers and whole-wheat wafers.
[40] Made with lard.

Table A-4 Nutritive Value of the Edible Part of Food (Continued)

(Tr indicates nutrient present in trace amount.)

Item No.	Foods, approximate measures, units, and weight (weight of edible portion only)		Grams	Water Percent	Food energy Calories	Protein Grams	Fat Grams	Fatty acids		
								Saturated Grams	Mono-unsaturated Grams	Poly-unsaturated Grams
	Grain Products—Con.									
460	French toast, from home recipe---	1 slice---------	65	53	155	6	7	1.6	2.0	1.6
	Macaroni, enriched, cooked (cut lengths, elbows, shells):									
461	Firm stage (hot)--------------	1 cup-----------	130	64	190	7	1	0.1	0.1	0.3
	Tender stage:									
462	Cold-------------------------	1 cup-----------	105	72	115	4	Tr	0.1	0.1	0.2
463	Hot--------------------------	1 cup-----------	140	72	155	5	1	0.1	0.1	0.2
	Muffins made with enriched flour, 2-1/2-in diam., 1-1/2 in high:									
	From home recipe:									
464	Blueberry [25]---------------	1 muffin--------	45	37	135	3	5	1.5	2.1	1.2
465	Bran [36]--------------------	1 muffin--------	45	35	125	3	6	1.4	1.6	2.3
466	Corn (enriched, degermed cornmeal and flour) [25]------	1 muffin--------	45	33	145	3	5	1.5	2.2	1.4
	From commercial mix (egg and water added):									
467	Blueberry--------------------	1 muffin--------	45	33	140	3	5	1.4	2.0	1.2
468	Bran-------------------------	1 muffin--------	45	28	140	3	4	1.3	1.6	1.0
469	Corn-------------------------	1 muffin--------	45	30	145	3	6	1.7	2.3	1.4
470	Noodles (egg noodles), enriched, cooked------------------------	1 cup-----------	160	70	200	7	2	0.5	0.6	0.6
471	Noodles, chow mein, canned-------	1 cup-----------	45	11	220	6	11	2.1	7.3	0.4
	Pancakes, 4-in diam.:									
472	Buckwheat, from mix (with buckwheat and enriched flours), egg and milk added-----------	1 pancake-------	27	58	55	2	2	0.9	0.9	0.5
	Plain:									
473	From home recipe using enriched flour-------------	1 pancake-------	27	50	60	2	2	0.5	0.8	0.5
474	From mix (with enriched flour), egg, milk, and oil added---------------------	1 pancake-------	27	54	60	2	2	0.5	0.9	0.5
	Piecrust, made with enriched flour and vegetable shortening, baked:									
475	From home recipe, 9-in diam.---	1 pie shell-----	180	15	900	11	60	14.8	25.9	15.7
476	From mix, 9-in diam.----------	Piecrust for 2-crust pie-----	320	19	1,485	20	93	22.7	41.0	25.0
	Pies, piecrust made with enriched flour, vegetable shortening, 9-in diam.:									
	Apple:									
477	Whole-----------------------	1 pie----------	945	48	2,420	21	105	27.4	44.4	26.5
478	Piece, 1/6 of pie------------	1 piece--------	158	48	405	3	18	4.6	7.4	4.4
	Blueberry:									
479	Whole-----------------------	1 pie----------	945	51	2,285	23	102	25.5	44.4	27.4
480	Piece, 1/6 of pie------------	1 piece--------	158	51	380	4	17	4.3	7.4	4.6
	Cherry:									
481	Whole-----------------------	1 pie----------	945	47	2,465	25	107	28.4	46.3	27.4
482	Piece, 1/6 of pie------------	1 piece--------	158	47	410	4	18	4.7	7.7	4.6
	Creme:									
483	Whole-----------------------	1 pie----------	910	43	2,710	20	139	90.1	23.7	6.4
484	Piece, 1/6 of pie------------	1 piece--------	152	43	455	3	23	15.0	4.0	1.1
	Custard:									
485	Whole-----------------------	1 pie----------	910	58	1,985	56	101	33.7	40.0	19.1
486	Piece, 1/6 of pie------------	1 piece--------	152	58	330	9	17	5.6	6.7	3.2
	Lemon meringue:									
487	Whole-----------------------	1 pie----------	840	47	2,140	31	86	26.0	34.4	17.6
488	Piece, 1/6 of pie------------	1 piece--------	140	47	355	5	14	4.3	5.7	2.9
	Peach:									
489	Whole-----------------------	1 pie----------	945	48	2,410	24	101	24.6	43.5	26.5
490	Piece, 1/6 of pie------------	1 piece--------	158	48	405	4	17	4.1	7.3	4.4

[25] Made with vegetable shortening.

Table A-4 Nutritive Value of the Edible Part of Food (Continued)

Choles-terol	Carbo-hydrate	Calcium	Phos-phorus	Iron	Potas-sium	Sodium	Vitamin A value		Thiamin	Ribo-flavin	Niacin	Ascorbic acid	Item No.
							(IU)	(RE)					
Milli-grams	Grams	Milli-grams	Milli-grams	Milli-grams	Milli-grams	Milli-grams	Inter-national units	Retinol equiva-lents	Milli-grams	Milli-grams	Milli-grams	Milli-grams	
112	17	72	85	1.3	86	257	110	32	0.12	0.16	1.0	Tr	460
0	39	14	85	2.1	103	1	0	0	0.23	0.13	1.8	0	461
0	24	8	53	1.3	64	1	0	0	0.15	0.08	1.2	0	462
0	32	11	70	1.7	85	1	0	0	0.20	0.11	1.5	0	463
19	20	54	46	0.9	47	198	40	9	0.10	0.11	0.9	1	464
24	19	60	125	1.4	99	189	230	30	0.11	0.13	1.3	3	465
23	21	66	59	0.9	57	169	80	15	0.11	0.11	0.9	Tr	466
45	22	15	90	0.9	54	225	50	11	0.10	0.17	1.1	Tr	467
28	24	27	182	1.7	50	385	100	14	0.08	0.12	1.9	0	468
42	22	30	128	1.3	31	291	90	16	0.09	0.09	0.8	Tr	469
50	37	16	94	2.6	70	3	110	34	0.22	0.13	1.9	0	470
5	26	14	41	0.4	33	450	0	0	0.05	0.03	0.6	0	471
20	6	59	91	0.4	66	125	60	17	0.04	0.05	0.2	Tr	472
16	9	27	38	0.5	33	115	30	10	0.06	0.07	0.5	Tr	473
16	8	36	71	0.7	43	160	30	7	0.09	0.12	0.8	Tr	474
0	79	25	90	4.5	90	1,100	0	0	0.54	0.40	5.0	0	475
0	141	131	272	9.3	179	2,602	0	0	1.06	0.80	9.9	0	476
0	360	76	208	9.5	756	2,844	280	28	1.04	0.76	9.5	9	477
0	60	13	35	1.6	126	476	50	5	0.17	0.13	1.6	2	478
0	330	104	217	12.3	945	2,533	850	85	1.04	0.85	10.4	38	479
0	55	17	36	2.1	158	423	140	14	0.17	0.14	1.7	6	480
0	363	132	236	9.5	992	2,873	4,160	416	1.13	0.85	9.5	0	481
0	61	22	40	1.6	166	480	700	70	0.19	0.14	1.6	0	482
46	351	273	919	6.8	796	2,207	1,250	391	0.36	0.89	6.4	0	483
8	59	46	154	1.1	133	369	210	65	0.06	0.15	1.1	0	484
1010	213	874	1,028	9.1	1,247	2,612	2,090	573	0.82	1.91	5.5	0	485
169	36	146	172	1.5	208	436	350	96	0.14	0.32	0.9	0	486
857	317	118	412	8.4	420	2,369	1,430	395	0.59	0.84	5.0	25	487
143	53	20	69	1.4	70	395	240	66	0.10	0.14	0.8	4	488
0	361	95	274	11.3	1,408	2,533	6,900	690	1.04	0.95	14.2	28	489
0	60	16	46	1.9	235	423	1,150	115	0.17	0.16	2.4	5	490

[36] Made with vegetable oil.

Table A-4 Nutritive Value of the Edible Part of Food *(Continued)*

(Tr indicates nutrient present in trace amount.)

Item No.	Foods, approximate measures, units, and weight (weight of edible portion only)		Grams	Water	Food energy	Protein	Fat	Fatty acids		
								Saturated	Mono-unsaturated	Poly-unsaturated
			Grams	Percent	Calories	Grams	Grams	Grams	Grams	Grams
	Grain Products—Con.									
	Pies, piecrust made with enriched flour, vegetable shortening, 9-inch diam.:									
	Pecan:									
491	Whole	1 pie	825	20	3,450	42	189	28.1	101.5	47.0
492	Piece, 1/6 of pie	1 piece	138	20	575	7	32	4.7	17.0	7.9
	Pumpkin:									
493	Whole	1 pie	910	59	1,920	36	102	38.2	40.0	18.2
494	Piece, 1/6 of pie	1 piece	152	59	320	6	17	6.4	6.7	3.0
	Pies, fried:									
495	Apple	1 pie	85	43	255	2	14	5.8	6.6	0.6
496	Cherry	1 pie	85	42	250	2	14	5.8	6.7	0.6
	Popcorn, popped:									
497	Air-popped, unsalted	1 cup	8	4	30	1	Tr	Tr	0.1	0.2
498	Popped in vegetable oil, salted	1 cup	11	3	55	1	3	0.5	1.4	1.2
499	Sugar syrup coated	1 cup	35	4	135	2	1	0.1	0.3	0.6
	Pretzels, made with enriched flour:									
500	Stick, 2-1/4 in long	10 pretzels	3	3	10	Tr	Tr	Tr	Tr	Tr
501	Twisted, dutch, 2-3/4 by 2-5/8 in	1 pretzel	16	3	65	2	1	0.1	0.2	0.2
502	Twisted, thin, 3-1/4 by 2-1/4 by 1/4 in	10 pretzels	60	3	240	6	2	0.4	0.8	0.6
	Rice:									
503	Brown, cooked, served hot	1 cup	195	70	230	5	1	0.3	0.3	0.4
	White, enriched:									
	Commercial varieties, all types:									
504	Raw	1 cup	185	12	670	12	1	0.2	0.2	0.3
505	Cooked, served hot	1 cup	205	73	225	4	Tr	0.1	0.1	0.1
506	Instant, ready-to-serve, hot	1 cup	165	73	180	4	0	0.1	0.1	0.1
	Parboiled:									
507	Raw	1 cup	185	10	685	14	1	0.1	0.1	0.2
508	Cooked, served hot	1 cup	175	73	185	4	Tr	Tr	Tr	0.1
	Rolls, enriched:									
	Commercial:									
509	Dinner, 2-1/2-in diam., 2 in high	1 roll	28	32	85	2	2	0.5	0.8	0.6
510	Frankfurter and hamburger (8 per 11-1/2-oz pkg.)	1 roll	40	34	115	3	2	0.5	0.8	0.6
511	Hard, 3-3/4-in diam., 2 in high	1 roll	50	25	155	5	2	0.4	0.5	0.6
512	Hoagie or submarine, 11-1/2 by 3 by 2-1/2 in	1 roll	135	31	400	11	8	1.8	3.0	2.2
	From home recipe:									
513	Dinner, 2-1/2-in diam., 2 in high	1 roll	35	26	120	3	3	0.8	1.2	0.9
	Spaghetti, enriched, cooked:									
514	Firm stage, "al dente," served hot	1 cup	130	64	190	7	1	0.1	0.1	0.3
515	Tender stage, served hot	1 cup	140	73	155	5	1	0.1	0.1	0.2
516	Toaster pastries	1 pastry	54	13	210	2	6	1.7	3.6	0.4
517	Tortillas, corn	1 tortilla	30	45	65	2	1	0.1	0.3	0.6
	Waffles, made with enriched flour, 7-in diam.:									
518	From home recipe	1 waffle	75	37	245	7	13	4.0	4.9	2.6
519	From mix, egg and milk added	1 waffle	75	42	205	7	8	2.7	2.9	1.5
	Wheat flours:									
	All-purpose or family flour, enriched:									
520	Sifted, spooned	1 cup	115	12	420	12	1	0.2	0.1	0.5
521	Unsifted, spooned	1 cup	125	12	455	13	1	0.2	0.1	0.5
522	Cake or pastry flour, enriched, sifted, spooned	1 cup	96	12	350	7	1	0.1	0.1	0.3
523	Self-rising, enriched, unsifted, spooned	1 cup	125	12	440	12	1	0.2	0.1	0.5
524	Whole-wheat, from hard wheats, stirred	1 cup	120	12	400	16	2	0.3	0.3	1.1

Table A-4 Nutritive Value of the Edible Part of Food *(Continued)*

Cholesterol (Milligrams)	Carbohydrate (Grams)	Calcium (Milligrams)	Phosphorus (Milligrams)	Iron (Milligrams)	Potassium (Milligrams)	Sodium (Milligrams)	Vitamin A value (IU) International units	Vitamin A value (RE) Retinol equivalents	Thiamin (Milligrams)	Riboflavin (Milligrams)	Niacin (Milligrams)	Ascorbic acid (Milligrams)	Item No
569	423	388	850	27.2	1,015	1,823	1,320	322	1.82	0.99	6.6	0	491
95	71	65	142	4.6	170	305	220	54	0.30	0.17	1.1	0	492
655	223	464	628	8.2	1,456	1,947	22,480	2,493	0.82	1.27	7.3	0	493
109	37	78	105	1.4	243	325	3,750	416	0.14	0.21	1.2	0	494
14	31	12	34	0.9	42	326	30	3	0.09	0.06	1.0	1	495
13	32	11	41	0.7	61	371	190	19	0.06	0.06	0.6	1	496
0	6	1	22	0.2	20		10	1	0.03	0.01	0.2	0	497
0	6	3	31	0.3	19	86	20	2	0.01	0.02	0.1	0	498
	30	2	47	0.5	90	Tr	30	3	0.13	0.02	0.4	0	499
0	2	1	3	0.1	3	48	0	0	0.01	0.01	0.1	0	500
0	13	4	15	0.3	16	258	0	0	0.05	0.04	0.7	0	501
0	48	16	55	1.2	61	966	0	0	0.19	0.15	2.6	0	502
0	50	23	142	1.0	137	0	0	0	0.18	0.04	2.7	0	503
0	149	44	174	5.4	170	9	0	0	0.81	0.06	6.5	0	504
0	50	21	57	1.8	57	0	0	0	0.23	0.02	2.1	0	505
0	40	5	31	1.3	0	0	0	0	0.21	0.02	1.7	0	506
0	150	111	370	5.4	278	17	0	0	0.81	0.07	6.5	0	507
0	41	33	100	1.4	75	0	0	0	0.19	0.02	2.1	0	508
Tr	14	33	44	0.8	36	155	Tr	Tr	0.14	0.09	1.1	Tr	509
Tr	20	54	44	1.2	56	241	Tr	Tr	0.20	0.13	1.6	Tr	510
Tr	30	24	46	1.4	49	313	0	0	0.20	0.12	1.7	0	511
Tr	72	100	115	3.8	128	683	0	0	0.54	0.33	4.5	0	512
12	20	16	36	1.1	41	98	30	8	0.12	0.12	1.2	0	513
0	39	14	85	2.0	103	1	0	0	0.23	0.13	1.8	0	514
0	32	11	70	1.7	85	1	0	0	0.20	0.11	1.5	0	515
0	38	104	104	2.2	91	248	520	52	0.17	0.18	2.3	4	516
0	13	42	55	0.6	43	1	80	8	0.05	0.03	0.4	0	517
102	26	154	135	1.5	129	445	140	39	0.18	0.24	1.5	Tr	518
59	27	179	257	1.2	146	515	170	49	0.14	0.23	0.9	Tr	519
0	88	18	100	5.1	109	2	0	0	0.73	0.46	6.1	0	520
0	95	20	109	5.5	119	3	0	0	0.80	0.50	6.6	0	521
0	76	16	70	4.2	91	2	0	0	0.58	0.38	5.1	0	522
0	93	331	583	5.5	113	1,349	0	0	0.80	0.50	6.6	0	523
0	85	49	446	5.2	444	4	0	0	0.66	0.14	5.2	0	524

Table A-4 Nutritive Value of the Edible Part of Food *(Continued)*

(Tr indicates nutrient present in trace amount.)

Item No.	Foods, approximate measures, units, and weight (weight of edible portion only)		Grams	Water Percent	Food energy Calories	Protein Grams	Fat Grams	Saturated Grams	Monounsaturated Grams	Polyunsaturated Grams
	Legumes, Nuts, and Seeds									
	Almonds, shelled:									
525	Slivered, packed	1 cup	135	4	795	27	70	6.7	45.8	14.8
526	Whole	1 oz	28	4	165	6	15	1.4	9.6	3.1
	Beans, dry:									
	Cooked, drained:									
527	Black	1 cup	171	66	225	15	1	0.1	0.1	0.5
528	Great Northern	1 cup	180	69	210	14	1	0.1	0.1	0.6
529	Lima	1 cup	190	64	260	16	1	0.2	0.1	0.5
530	Pea (navy)	1 cup	190	69	225	15	1	0.1	0.1	0.7
531	Pinto	1 cup	180	65	265	15	1	0.1	0.1	0.5
	Canned, solids and liquid:									
	White with:									
532	Frankfurters (sliced)	1 cup	255	71	365	19	18	7.4	8.8	0.7
533	Pork and tomato sauce	1 cup	255	71	310	16	7	2.4	2.7	0.7
534	Pork and sweet sauce	1 cup	255	66	385	16	12	4.3	4.9	1.2
535	Red kidney	1 cup	255	76	230	15	1	0.1	0.1	0.6
536	Black-eyed peas, dry, cooked (with residual cooking liquid)	1 cup	250	80	190	13	1	0.2	Tr	0.3
537	Brazil nuts, shelled	1 oz	28	3	185	4	19	4.6	6.5	6.8
538	Carob flour	1 cup	140	3	255	6	Tr	Tr	0.1	0.1
	Cashew nuts, salted:									
539	Dry roasted	1 cup	137	2	785	21	63	12.5	37.4	10.7
540		1 oz	28	2	165	4	13	2.6	7.7	2.2
541	Roasted in oil	1 cup	130	4	750	21	63	12.4	36.9	10.6
542		1 oz	28	4	165	5	14	2.7	8.1	2.3
543	Chestnuts, European (Italian), roasted, shelled	1 cup	143	40	350	5	3	0.6	1.1	1.2
544	Chickpeas, cooked, drained	1 cup	163	60	270	15	4	0.4	0.9	1.9
	Coconut:									
	Raw:									
545	Piece, about 2 by 2 by 1/2 in	1 piece	45	47	160	1	15	13.4	0.6	0.2
546	Shredded or grated	1 cup	80	47	285	3	27	23.8	1.1	0.3
547	Dried, sweetened, shredded	1 cup	93	13	470	3	33	29.3	1.4	0.4
548	Filberts (hazelnuts), chopped	1 cup	115	5	725	15	72	5.3	56.5	6.9
549		1 oz	28	5	180	4	18	1.3	13.9	1.7
550	Lentils, dry, cooked	1 cup	200	72	215	16	1	0.1	0.2	0.5
551	Macadamia nuts, roasted in oil, salted	1 cup	134	2	960	10	103	15.4	80.9	1.8
552		1 oz	28	2	205	2	22	3.2	17.1	0.4
	Mixed nuts, with peanuts, salted:									
553	Dry roasted	1 oz	28	2	170	5	15	2.0	8.9	3.1
554	Roasted in oil	1 oz	28	2	175	5	16	2.5	9.0	3.8
555	Peanuts, roasted in oil, salted	1 cup	145	2	840	39	71	9.9	35.5	22.6
556		1 oz	28	2	165	8	14	1.9	6.9	4.4
557	Peanut butter	1 tbsp	16	1	95	5	8	1.4	4.0	2.5
558	Peas, split, dry, cooked	1 cup	200	70	230	16	1	0.1	0.1	0.3
559	Pecans, halves	1 cup	108	5	720	8	73	5.9	45.5	18.1
560		1 oz	28	5	190	2	19	1.5	12.0	4.7
561	Pine nuts (pinyons), shelled	1 oz	28	6	160	3	17	2.7	6.5	7.3
562	Pistachio nuts, dried, shelled	1 oz	28	4	165	6	14	1.7	9.3	2.1
563	Pumpkin and squash kernels, dry, hulled	1 oz	28	7	155	7	13	2.5	4.0	5.9
564	Refried beans, canned	1 cup	290	72	295	18	3	0.4	0.6	1.4
565	Sesame seeds, dry, hulled	1 tbsp	8	5	45	2	4	0.6	1.7	1.9
566	Soybeans, dry, cooked, drained	1 cup	180	71	235	20	10	1.3	1.9	5.3
	Soy products:									
567	Miso	1 cup	276	53	470	29	13	1.8	2.6	7.3
568	Tofu, piece 2-1/2 by 2-3/4 by 1 in	1 piece	120	85	85	9	5	0.7	1.0	2.9
569	Sunflower seeds, dry, hulled	1 oz	28	5	160	6	14	1.5	2.7	9.3
570	Tahini	1 tbsp	15	3	90	3	8	1.1	3.0	3.5

[41] Cashews without salt contain 21 mg sodium per cup or 4 mg per oz.
[42] Cashews without salt contain 22 mg sodium per cup or 5 mg per oz.
[43] Macadamia nuts without salt contain 9 mg sodium per cup or 2 mg per oz.

Table A-4 Nutritive Value of the Edible Part of Food *(Continued)*

Cholesterol	Carbohydrate	Calcium	Phosphorus	Iron	Potassium	Sodium	Vitamin A value (IU) International units	Vitamin A value (RE) Retinol equivalents	Thiamin	Riboflavin	Niacin	Ascorbic acid	Item No.
Milligrams	Grams	Milligrams	Milligrams	Milligrams	Milligrams	Milligrams	International units	Retinol equivalents	Milligrams	Milligrams	Milligrams	Milligrams	
0	28	359	702	4.9	988	15	0	0	0.28	1.05	4.5	1	525
0	6	75	147	1.0	208	3	0	0	0.06	0:22	1.0	Tr	526
0	41	47	239	2.9	608	1	Tr	Tr	0.43	0.05	0.9	0	527
0	38	90	266	4.9	749	13	0	0	0.25	0.13	1.3	0	528
0	49	55	293	5.9	1,163	4	0	0	0.25	0.11	1.3	0	529
0	40	95	281	5.1	790	13	0	0	0.27	0.13	1.3	0	530
0	49	86	296	5.4	882	3	Tr	Tr	0.33	0.16	0.7	0	531
30	32	94	303	4.8	668	1,374	330	33	0.18	0.15	3.3	Tr	532
10	48	138	235	4.6	536	1,181	330	33	0.20	0.08	1.5	5	533
10	54	161	291	5.9	536	969	330	33	0.15	0.10	1.3	5	534
0	42	74	278	4.6	673	968	10	1	0.13	0.10	1.5	0	535
0	35	43	238	3.3	573	20	30	3	0.40	0.10	1.0	0	536
0	4	50	170	1.0	170	1	Tr	Tr	0.28	0.03	0.5	Tr	537
0	126	390	102	5.7	1,275	24	Tr	Tr	0.07	0.07	2.2	Tr	538
0	45	62	671	8.2	774	[41]877	0	0	0.27	0.27	1.9	0	539
0	9	13	139	1.7	160	[41]181	0	0	0.06	0.06	0.4	0	540
0	37	53	554	5.3	689	[42]814	0	0	0.55	0.23	2.3	0	541
0	8	12	121	1.2	150	[42]177	0	0	0.12	0.05	0.5	0	542
0	76	41	153	1.3	847	3	30	3	0.35	0.25	1.9	37	543
0	45	80	273	4.9	475	11	Tr	Tr	0.18	0.09	0.9	0	544
0	7	6	51	1.1	160	9	0	0	0.03	0.01	0.2	1	545
0	12	11	90	1.9	285	16	0	0	0.05	0.02	0.4	3	546
0	44	14	99	1.8	313	244	0	0	0.03	0.02	0.4	1	547
0	18	216	359	3.8	512	3	80	8	0.58	0.13	1.3	1	548
0	4	53	88	0.9	126	1	20	2	0.14	0.03	0.3	Tr	549
0	38	50	238	4.2	498	26	40	4	0.14	0.12	1.2	0	550
0	17	60	268	2.4	441	[43]348	10	1	0.29	0.15	2.7	0	551
0	4	13	57	0.5	93	[43]74	Tr	Tr	0.06	0.03	0.6	0	552
0	7	20	123	1.0	169	[44]190	Tr	Tr	0.06	0.06	1.3	0	553
0	6	31	131	0.9	165	[44]185	10	1	0.14	0.06	1.4	Tr	554
0	27	125	734	2.8	1,019	[45]626	0	0	0.42	0.15	21.5	0	555
0	5	24	143	0.5	199	[45]122	0	0	0.08	0.03	4.2	0	556
0	3	5	60	0.3	110	75	0	0	0.02	0.02	2.2	0	557
0	42	22	178	3.4	592	26	80	8	0.30	0.18	1.8	0	558
0	20	39	314	2.3	423	1	140	14	0.92	0.14	1.0	2	559
0	5	10	83	0.6	111	Tr	40	4	0.24	0.04	0.3	1	560
0	5	2	10	0.9	178	20	10	1	0.35	0.06	1.2	1	561
0	7	38	143	1.9	310	2	70	7	0.23	0.05	0.3	Tr	562
0	5	12	333	4.2	229	5	110	11	0.06	0.09	0.5	Tr	563
0	51	141	245	5.1	1,141	1,228	0	0	0.14	0.16	1.4	17	564
0	1	11	62	0.6	33	3	10	1	0.06	0.01	0.4	0	565
0	19	131	322	4.9	972	4	50	5	0.38	0.16	1.1	0	566
0	65	188	853	4.7	922	8,142	110	11	0.17	0.28	0.8	0	567
0	3	108	151	2.3	50	8	0	0	0.07	0.04	0.1	0	568
0	5	33	200	1.9	195	1	10	1	0.65	0.07	1.3	Tr	569
0	3	21	119	0.7	69	5	10	1	0.24	0.02	0.8	1	570

[44]Mixed nuts without salt contain 3 mg sodium per oz.
[45]Peanuts without salt contain 22 mg sodium per cup or 4 mg per oz.

Table A-4 Nutritive Value of the Edible Part of Food *(Continued)*

(Tr indicates nutrient present in trace amount.)

Item No.	Foods, approximate measures, units, and weight (weight of edible portion only)		Grams	Water Per-cent	Food energy Cal-ories	Pro-tein Grams	Fat Grams	Fatty acids		
								Satu-rated Grams	Mono-unsatu-rated Grams	Poly-unsatu-rated Grams
	Legumes, Nuts, and Seeds—Con.									
	Walnuts:									
571	Black, chopped-----------------	1 cup----------	125	4	760	30	71	4.5	15.9	46.9
572		1 oz-----------	28	4	170	7	16	1.0	3.6	10.6
573	English or Persian, pieces or chips------------------------	1 cup----------	120	4	770	17	74	6.7	17.0	47.0
574		1 oz-----------	28	4	180	4	18	1.6	4.0	11.1
	Meat and Meat Products									
	Beef, cooked:[46]									
	Cuts braised, simmered, or pot roasted:									
	Relatively fat such as chuck blade:									
575	Lean and fat, piece, 2-1/2 by 2-1/2 by 3/4 in-------	3 oz-----------	85	43	325	22	26	10.8	11.7	0.9
576	Lean only from item 575----	2.2 oz----------	62	53	170	19	9	3.9	4.2	0.3
	Relatively lean, such as bottom round:									
577	Lean and fat, piece, 4-1/8 by 2-1/4 by 1/2 in-------	3 oz-----------	85	54	220	25	13	4.8	5.7	0.5
578	Lean only from item 577----	2.8 oz----------	78	57	175	25	8	2.7	3.4	0.3
	Ground beef, broiled, patty, 3 by 5/8 in:									
579	Lean------------------------	3 oz-----------	85	56	230	21	16	6.2	6.9	0.6
580	Regular---------------------	3 oz-----------	85	54	245	20	18	6.9	7.7	0.7
581	Heart, lean, braised-----------	3 oz-----------	85	65	150	24	5	1.2	0.8	1.6
582	Liver, fried, slice, 6-1/2 by 2-3/8 by 3/8 in[47]-----------	3 oz-----------	85	56	185	23	7	2.5	3.6	1.3
	Roast, oven cooked, no liquid added:									
	Relatively fat, such as rib:									
583	Lean and fat, 2 pieces, 4-1/8 by 2-1/4 by 1/4 in	3 oz-----------	85	46	315	19	26	10.8	11.4	0.9
584	Lean only from item 583----	2.2 oz----------	61	57	150	17	9	3.6	3.7	0.3
	Relatively lean, such as eye of round:									
585	Lean and fat, 2 pieces, 2-1/2 by 2-1/2 by 3/8 in	3 oz-----------	85	57	205	23	12	4.9	5.4	0.5
586	Lean only from item 585----	2.6 oz----------	75	63	135	22	5	1.9	2.1	0.2
	Steak:									
	Sirloin, broiled:									
587	Lean and fat, piece, 2-1/2 by 2-1/2 by 3/4 in-------	3 oz-----------	85	53	240	23	15	6.4	6.9	0.6
588	Lean only from item 587----	2.5 oz----------	72	59	150	22	6	2.6	2.8	0.3
589	Beef, canned, corned------------	3 oz-----------	85	59	185	22	10	4.2	4.9	0.4
590	Beef, dried, chipped------------	2.5 oz----------	72	48	145	24	4	1.8	2.0	0.2
	Lamb, cooked:									
	Chops, (3 per lb with bone):									
	Arm, braised:									
591	Lean and fat----------------	2.2 oz----------	63	44	220	20	15	6.9	6.0	0.9
592	Lean only from item 591----	1.7 oz----------	48	49	135	17	7	2.9	2.6	0.4
	Loin, broiled:									
593	Lean and fat----------------	2.8 oz----------	80	54	235	22	16	7.3	6.4	1.0
594	Lean only from item 593----	2.3 oz----------	64	61	140	19	6	2.6	2.4	0.4
	Leg, roasted:									
595	Lean and fat, 2 pieces, 4-1/8 by 2-1/4 by 1/4 in---------	3 oz-----------	85	59	205	22	13	5.6	4.9	0.8
596	Lean only from item 595------	2.6 oz----------	73	64	140	20	6	2.4	2.2	0.4
	Rib, roasted:									
597	Lean and fat, 3 pieces, 2-1/2 by 2-1/2 by 1/4 in---------	3 oz-----------	85	47	315	18	26	12.1	10.6	1.5
598	Lean only from item 597------	2 oz-----------	57	60	130	15	7	3.2	3.0	0.5

[46]Outer layer of fat was removed to within approximately 1/2 inch of the lean. Deposits of fat within the cut were not removed.
[47]Fried in vegetable shortening.

Table A-4 Nutritive Value of the Edible Part of Food (Continued)

							Nutrients in Indicated Quantity						
Cho-les-terol	Carbo-hydrate	Calcium	Phos-phorus	Iron	Potas-sium	Sodium	Vitamin A value		Thiamin	Ribo-flavin	Niacin	Ascorbic acid	Item No
							(IU)	(RE)					
Milli-grams	Grams	Milli-grams	Milli-grams	Milli-grams	Milli-grams	Milli-grams	Inter-national units	Retinol equiva-lents	Milli-grams	Milli-grams	Milli-grams	Milli-grams	
0	15	73	580	3.8	655	1	370	37	0.27	0.14	0.9	Tr	571
0	3	16	132	0.9	149	Tr	80	8	0.06	0.03	0.2	Tr	572
0	22	113	380	2.9	602	12	150	15	0.46	0.18	1.3	4	573
0	5	27	90	0.7	142	3	40	4	0.11	0.04	0.3	1	574
87	0	11	163	2.5	163	53	Tr	Tr	0.06	0.19	2.0	0	575
66	0	8	146	2.3	163	44	Tr	Tr	0.05	0.17	1.7	0	576
81	0	5	217	2.8	248	43	Tr	Tr	0.06	0.21	3.3	0	577
75	0	4	212	2.7	240	40	Tr	Tr	0.06	0.20	3.0	0	578
74	0	9	134	1.8	256	65	Tr	Tr	0.04	0.18	4.4	0	579
76	0	9	144	2.1	248	70	Tr	Tr	0.03	0.16	4.9	0	580
164	0	5	213	6.4	198	54	Tr	Tr	0.12	1.31	3.4	5	581
410	7	9	392	5.3	309	90	[48]30,690	[48]9,120	0.18	3.52	12.3	23	582
72	0	8	145	2.0	246	54	Tr	Tr	0.06	0.16	3.1	0	583
49	0	5	127	1.7	218	45	Tr	Tr	0.05	0.13	2.7	0	584
62	0	5	177	1.6	308	50	Tr	Tr	0.07	0.14	3.0	0	585
52	0	3	170	1.5	297	46	Tr	Tr	0.07	0.13	2.8	0	586
77	0	9	186	2.6	306	53	Tr	Tr	0.10	0.23	3.3	0	587
64	0	8	176	2.4	290	48	Tr	Tr	0.09	0.22	3.1	0	588
80	0	17	90	3.7	51	802	Tr	Tr	0.02	0.20	2.9	0	589
46	0	14	287	2.3	142	3,053	Tr	Tr	0.05	0.23	2.7	0	590
77	0	16	132	1.5	195	46	Tr	Tr	0.04	0.16	4.4	0	591
59	0	12	111	1.3	162	36	Tr	Tr	0.03	0.13	3.0	0	592
78	0	16	162	1.4	272	62	Tr	Tr	0.09	0.21	5.5	0	593
60	0	12	145	1.3	241	54	Tr	Tr	0.08	0.18	4.4	0	594
78	0	8	162	1.7	273	57	Tr	Tr	0.09	0.24	5.5	0	595
65	0	6	150	1.5	247	50	Tr	Tr	0.08	0.20	4.6	0	596
77	0	19	139	1.4	224	60	Tr	Tr	0.08	0.18	5.5	0	597
50	0	12	111	1.0	179	46	Tr	Tr	0.05	0.13	3.5	0	598

[48] Value varies widely.

Table A-4 Nutritive Value of the Edible Part of Food *(Continued)*

(Tr indicates nutrient present in trace amount.)

Item No.	Foods, approximate measures, units, and weight (weight of edible portion only)		Grams	Water Per-cent	Food energy Cal-ories	Pro-tein Grams	Fat Grams	Fatty acids Satu-rated Grams	Mono-unsatu-rated Grams	Poly-unsatu-rated Grams
	Meat and Meat Products—Con.									
	Pork, cured, cooked:									
	Bacon:									
599	Regular----------------------	3 medium slices	19	13	110	6	9	3.3	4.5	1.1
600	Canadian-style----------------	2 slices--------	46	62	85	11	4	1.3	1.9	0.4
	Ham, light cure, roasted:									
601	Lean and fat, 2 pieces, 4-1/8 by 2-1/4 by 1/4 in---------	3 oz------------	85	58	205	18	14	5.1	6.7	1.5
602	Lean only from item 601------	2.4 oz----------	68	66	105	17	4	1.3	1.7	0.4
603	Ham, canned, roasted, 2 pieces, 4-1/8 by 2-1/4 by 1/4 in-----	3 oz------------	85	67	140	18	7	2.4	3.5	0.8
	Luncheon meat:									
604	Canned, spiced or unspiced, slice, 3 by 2 by 1/2 in----	2 slices--------	42	52	140	5	13	4.5	6.0	1.5
605	Chopped ham (8 slices per 6 oz pkg)--------------------	2 slices--------	42	64	95	7	7	2.4	3.4	0.9
	Cooked ham (8 slices per 8-oz pkg):									
606	Regular------------------	2 slices--------	57	65	105	10	6	1.9	2.8	0.7
607	Extra lean--------------	2 slices--------	57	71	75	11	3	0.9	1.3	0.3
	Pork, fresh, cooked:									
	Chop, loin (cut 3 per lb with bone):									
	Broiled:									
608	Lean and fat----------------	3.1 oz----------	87	50	275	24	19	7.0	8.8	2.2
609	Lean only from item 608----	2.5 oz----------	72	57	165	23	8	2.6	3.4	0.9
	Pan fried:									
610	Lean and fat----------------	3.1 oz----------	89	45	335	21	27	9.8	12.5	3.1
611	Lean only from item 610----	2.4 oz----------	67	54	180	19	11	3.7	4.8	1.3
	Ham (leg), roasted:									
612	Lean and fat, piece, 2-1/2 by 2-1/2 by 3/4 in-----------	3 oz------------	85	53	250	21	18	6.4	8.1	2.0
613	Lean only from item 612------	2.5 oz----------	72	60	160	20	8	2.7	3.6	1.0
	Rib, roasted:									
614	Lean and fat, piece, 2-1/2 by 3/4 in--------------------	3 oz------------	85	51	270	21	20	7.2	9.2	2.3
615	Lean only from item 614------	2.5 oz----------	71	57	175	20	10	3.4	4.4	1.2
	Shoulder cut, braised:									
616	Lean and fat, 3 pieces, 2-1/2 by 2-1/2 by 1/4 in---------	3 oz------------	85	47	295	23	22	7.9	10.0	2.4
617	Lean only from item 616------	2.4 oz------	67	54	165	22	8	2.8	3.7	1.0
	Sausages (See also Luncheon meats, items 604-607):									
618	Bologna, slice (8 per 8-oz pkg)	2 slices--------	57	54	180	7	16	6.1	7.6	1.4
619	Braunschweiger, slice (6 per 6-oz pkg)--------------------	2 slices--------	57	48	205	8	18	6.2	8.5	2.1
620	Brown and serve (10-11 per 8-oz pkg), browned-----------	1 link---------	13	45	50	2	5	1.7	2.2	0.5
621	Frankfurter (10 per 1-lb pkg), cooked (reheated)------------	1 frankfurter---	45	54	145	5	13	4.8	6.2	1.2
622	Pork link (16 per 1-lb pkg), cooked[50] --------------------	1 link---------	13	45	50	3	4	1.4	1.8	0.5
	Salami:									
623	Cooked type, slice (8 per 8-oz pkg)------------------	2 slices--------	57	60	145	8	11	4.6	5.2	1.2
624	Dry type, slice (12 per 4-oz pkg)--------------------	2 slices--------	20	35	85	5	7	2.4	3.4	0.6
625	Sandwich spread (pork, beef)---	1 tbsp----------	15	60	35	1	3	0.9	1.1	0.4
626	Vienna sausage (7 per 4-oz can)	1 sausage-------	16	60	45	2	4	1.5	2.0	0.3
	Veal, medium fat, cooked, bone removed:									
627	Cutlet, 4-1/8 by 2-1/4 by 1/2 in, braised or broiled-------	3 oz------------	85	60	185	23	9	4.1	4.1	0.6
628	Rib, 2 pieces, 4-1/8 by 2-1/4 by 1/4 in, roasted----------	3 oz------------	85	55	230	23	14	6.0	6.0	1.0

[49]Contains added sodium ascorbate. If sodium ascorbate is not added, ascorbic acid content is negligible.

Table A-4 Nutritive Value of the Edible Part of Food *(Continued)*

							Vitamin A value						
Cholesterol	Carbohydrate	Calcium	Phosphorus	Iron	Potassium	Sodium	(IU)	(RE)	Thiamin	Riboflavin	Niacin	Ascorbic acid	Item No.
Milligrams	Grams	Milligrams	Milligrams	Milligrams	Milligrams	Milligrams	International units	Retinol equivalents	Milligrams	Milligrams	Milligrams	Milligrams	
16	Tr	2	64	0.3	92	303	0	0	0.13	0.05	1.4	6	599
27	1	5	136	0.4	179	711	0	0	0.38	0.09	3.2	10	600
53	0	6	182	0.7	243	1,009	0	0	0.51	0.19	3.8	0	601
37	0	5	154	0.6	215	902	0	0	0.46	0.17	3.4	0	602
35	Tr	6	188	0.9	298	908	0	0	0.82	0.21	4.3	[49]19	603
26	1	3	34	0.3	90	541	0	0	0.15	0.08	1.3	Tr	604
21	0	3	65	0.3	134	576	0	0	0.27	0.09	1.6	[49]8	605
32	2	4	141	0.6	189	751	0	0	0.49	0.14	3.0	[49]16	606
27	1	4	124	0.4	200	815	0	0	0.53	0.13	2.8	[49]15	607
84	0	3	184	0.7	312	61	10	3	0.87	0.24	4.3	Tr	608
71	0	4	176	0.7	302	56	10	1	0.83	0.22	4.0	Tr	609
92	0	4	190	0.7	323	64	10	3	0.91	0.24	4.6	Tr	610
72	0	3	178	0.7	305	57	10	1	0.84	0.22	4.0	Tr	611
79	0	5	210	0.9	280	50	10	2	0.54	0.27	3.9	Tr	612
68	0	5	202	0.8	269	46	10	1	0.50	0.25	3.6	Tr	613
69	0	9	190	0.8	313	37	10	3	0.50	0.24	4.2	Tr	614
56	0	8	182	0.7	300	33	10	2	0.45	0.22	3.8	Tr	615
93	0	6	162	1.4	286	75	10	3	0.46	0.26	4.4	Tr	616
76	0	5	151	1.3	271	68	10	1	0.40	0.24	4.0	Tr	617
31	2	7	52	0.9	103	581	0	0	0.10	0.08	1.5	[49]12	618
89	2	5	96	5.3	113	652	8,010	2,405	0.14	0.87	4.8	[49]6	619
9	Tr	1	14	0.1	25	105	0	0	0.05	0.02	0.4	0	620
23	1	5	39	0.5	75	504	0	0	0.09	0.05	1.2	[49]12	621
11	Tr	4	24	0.2	47	168	0	0	0.10	0.03	0.6	Tr	622
37	1	7	66	1.5	113	607	0	0	0.14	0.21	2.0	[49]7	623
16	1	2	28	0.3	76	372	0	0	0.12	0.06	1.0	[49]5	624
6	2	2	9	0.1	17	152	10	1	0.03	0.02	0.3	0	625
8	Tr	2	8	0.1	16	152	0	0	0.01	0.02	0.3	0	626
109	0	9	196	0.8	258	56	Tr	Tr	0.06	0.21	4.6	0	627
109	0	10	211	0.7	259	57	Tr	Tr	0.11	0.26	6.6	0	628

[50] One patty (8 per pound) of bulk sausage is equivalent to 2 links.

Table A-4 Nutritive Value of the Edible Part of Food *(Continued)*

(Tr indicates nutrient present in trace amount.)

Item No.	Foods, approximate measures, units, and weight (weight of edible portion only)		Water	Food energy	Pro-tein	Fat	Fatty acids		
							Satu-rated	Mono-unsatu-rated	Poly-unsatu-rated
		Grams	Per-cent	Cal-ories	Grams	Grams	Grams	Grams	Grams
	Mixed Dishes and Fast Foods								
	Mixed dishes:								
629	Beef and vegetable stew, from home recipe	1 cup	245	82	220	16	11	4.4	4.5	0.5
630	Beef potpie, from home recipe, baked, piece, 1/3 of 9-in diam. pie[51]	1 piece	210	55	515	21	30	7.9	12.9	7.4
631	Chicken a la king, cooked, from home recipe	1 cup	245	68	470	27	34	12.9	13.4	6.2
632	Chicken and noodles, cooked, from home recipe	1 cup	240	71	365	22	18	5.1	7.1	3.9
	Chicken chow mein:								
633	Canned	1 cup	250	89	95	7	Tr	0.1	0.1	0.8
634	From home recipe	1 cup	250	78	255	31	10	4.1	4.9	3.5
635	Chicken potpie, from home recipe, baked, piece, 1/3 of 9-in diam. pie[51]	1 piece	232	57	545	23	31	10.3	15.5	6.6
636	Chili con carne with beans, canned	1 cup	255	72	340	19	16	5.8	7.2	1.0
637	Chop suey with beef and pork, from home recipe	1 cup	250	75	300	26	17	4.3	7.4	4.2
	Macaroni (enriched) and cheese:								
638	Canned[52]	1 cup	240	80	230	9	10	4.7	2.9	1.3
639	From home recipe[38]	1 cup	200	58	430	17	22	9.8	7.4	3.6
640	Quiche Lorraine, 1/8 of 8-in diam. quiche[51]	1 slice	176	47	600	13	48	23.2	17.8	4.1
	Spaghetti (enriched) in tomato sauce with cheese:								
641	Canned	1 cup	250	80	190	6	2	0.4	0.4	0.5
642	From home recipe	1 cup	250	77	260	9	9	3.0	3.6	1.2
	Spaghetti (enriched) with meat-balls and tomato sauce:								
643	Canned	1 cup	250	78	260	12	10	2.4	3.9	3.1
644	From home recipe	1 cup	248	70	330	19	12	3.9	4.4	2.2
	Fast food entrees:								
	Cheeseburger:								
645	Regular	1 sandwich	112	46	300	15	15	7.3	5.6	1.0
646	4 oz patty	1 sandwich	194	46	525	30	31	15.1	12.2	1.4
	Chicken, fried. See Poultry and Poultry Products (items 656-659).								
647	Enchilada	1 enchilada	230	72	235	20	16	7.7	6.7	0.6
648	English muffin, egg, cheese, and bacon	1 sandwich	138	49	360	18	18	8.0	8.0	0.7
	Fish sandwich:								
649	Regular, with cheese	1 sandwich	140	43	420	16	23	6.3	6.9	7.7
650	Large, without cheese	1 sandwich	170	48	470	18	27	6.3	8.7	9.5
	Hamburger:								
651	Regular	1 sandwich	98	46	245	12	11	4.4	5.3	0.5
652	4 oz patty	1 sandwich	174	50	445	25	21	7.1	11.7	0.6
653	Pizza, cheese, 1/8 of 15-in diam. pizza[51]	1 slice	120	46	290	15	9	4.1	2.6	1.3
654	Roast beef sandwich	1 sandwich	150	52	345	22	13	3.5	6.9	1.8
655	Taco	1 taco	81	55	195	9	11	4.1	5.5	0.8

[38]Made with margarine.
[51]Crust made with vegetable shortening and enriched flour.

Table A-4 Nutritive Value of the Edible Part of Food (Continued)

Nutrients in Indicated Quantity

Cho-les-terol	Carbo-hydrate	Calcium	Phos-phorus	Iron	Potas-sium	Sodium	Vitamin A value (IU)	(RE)	Thiamin	Ribo-flavin	Niacin	Ascorbic acid	Item No.
Milli-grams	Grams	Milli-grams	Milli-grams	Milli-grams	Milli-grams	Milli-grams	Inter-national units	Retinol equiva-lents	Milli-grams	Milli-grams	Milli-grams	Milli-grams	
71	15	29	184	2.9	613	292	5,690	568	0.15	0.17	4.7	17	629
42	39	29	149	3.8	334	596	4,220	517	0.29	0.29	4.8	6	630
221	12	127	358	2.5	404	760	1,130	272	0.10	0.42	5.4	12	631
103	26	26	247	2.2	149	600	430	130	0.05	0.17	4.3	Tr	632
8	18	45	85	1.3	418	725	150	28	0.05	0.10	1.0	13	633
75	10	58	293	2.5	473	718	280	50	0.08	0.23	4.3	10	634
56	42	70	232	3.0	343	594	7,220	735	0.32	0.32	4.9	5	635
28	31	82	321	4.3	594	1,354	150	15	0.08	0.18	3.3	8	636
68	13	60	248	4.8	425	1,053	600	60	0.28	0.38	5.0	33	637
24	26	199	182	1.0	139	730	260	72	0.12	0.24	1.0	Tr	638
44	40	362	322	1.8	240	1,086	860	232	0.20	0.40	1.8	1	639
285	29	211	276	1.0	283	653	1,640	454	0.11	0.32	Tr	Tr	640
3	39	40	88	2.8	303	955	930	120	0.35	0.28	4.5	10	641
8	37	80	135	2.3	408	955	1,080	140	0.25	0.18	2.3	13	642
23	29	53	113	3.3	245	1,220	1,000	100	0.15	0.18	2.3	5	643
89	39	124	236	3.7	665	1,009	1,590	159	0.25	0.30	4.0	22	644
44	28	135	174	2.3	219	672	340	65	0.26	0.24	3.7	1	645
104	40	236	320	4.5	407	1,224	670	128	0.33	0.48	7.4	3	646
19	24	97	198	3.3	653	1,332	2,720	352	0.18	0.26	Tr	Tr	647
213	31	197	290	3.1	201	832	650	160	0.46	0.50	3.7	1	648
56	39	132	223	1.8	274	667	160	25	0.32	0.26	3.3	2	649
91	41	61	246	2.2	375	621	110	15	0.35	0.23	3.5	1	650
32	28	56	107	2.2	202	463	80	14	0.23	0.24	3.8	1	651
71	38	75	225	4.8	404	763	160	28	0.38	0.38	7.8	1	652
56	39	220	216	1.6	230	699	750	106	0.34	0.29	4.2	2	653
55	34	60	222	4.0	338	757	240	32	0.40	0.33	6.0	2	654
21	15	109	134	1.2	263	456	420	57	0.09	0.07	1.4	1	655

[52]Made with corn oil.

Table A-4 Nutritive Value of the Edible Part of Food *(Continued)*

(Tr indicates nutrient present in trace amount.)

Item No.	Foods, approximate measures, units, and weight (weight of edible portion only)		Water	Food energy	Pro-tein	Fat	Fatty acids		
							Satu-rated	Mono-unsatu-rated	Poly-unsatu-rated
		Grams	Per-cent	Cal-ories	Grams	Grams	Grams	Grams	Grams
	Poultry and Poultry Products								
	Chicken:								
	Fried, flesh, with skin:[53]								
	Batter dipped:								
656	Breast, 1/2 breast (5.6 oz with bones)	4.9 oz	140	52	365	35	18	4.9	7.6	4.3
657	Drumstick (3.4 oz with bones)	2.5 oz	72	53	195	16	11	3.0	4.6	2.7
	Flour coated:								
658	Breast, 1/2 breast (4.2 oz with bones)	3.5 oz	98	57	220	31	9	2.4	3.4	1.9
659	Drumstick (2.6 oz with bones)	1.7 oz	49	57	120	13	7	1.8	2.7	1.6
	Roasted, flesh only:								
660	Breast, 1/2 breast (4.2 oz with bones and skin)	3.0 oz	86	65	140	27	3	0.9	1.1	0.7
661	Drumstick, (2.9 oz with bones and skin)	1.6 oz	44	67	75	12	2	0.7	0.8	0.6
662	Stewed, flesh only, light and dark meat, chopped or diced	1 cup	140	67	250	38	9	2.6	3.3	2.2
663	Chicken liver, cooked	1 liver	20	68	30	5	1	0.4	0.3	0.2
664	Duck, roasted, flesh only	1/2 duck	221	64	445	52	25	9.2	8.2	3.2
	Turkey, roasted, flesh only:								
665	Dark meat, piece, 2-1/2 by 1-5/8 by 1/4 in	4 pieces	85	63	160	24	6	2.1	1.4	1.8
666	Light meat, piece, 4 by 2 by 1/4 in	2 pieces	85	66	135	25	3	0.9	0.5	0.7
	Light and dark meat:								
667	Chopped or diced	1 cup	140	65	240	41	7	2.3	1.4	2.0
668	Pieces (1 slice white meat, 4 by 2 by 1/4 in and 2 slices dark meat, 2-1/2 by 1-5/8 by 1/4 in)	3 pieces	85	65	145	25	4	1.4	0.9	1.2
	Poultry food products:								
	Chicken:								
669	Canned, boneless	5 oz	142	69	235	31	11	3.1	4.5	2.5
670	Frankfurter (10 per 1-lb pkg)	1 frankfurter	45	58	115	6	9	2.5	3.8	1.8
671	Roll, light (6 slices per 6 oz pkg)	2 slices	57	69	90	11	4	1.1	1.7	0.9
	Turkey:								
672	Gravy and turkey, frozen	5-oz package	142	85	95	8	4	1.2	1.4	0.7
673	Ham, cured turkey thigh meat (8 slices per 8-oz pkg)	2 slices	57	71	75	11	3	1.0	0.7	0.9
674	Loaf, breast meat (8 slices per 6-oz pkg)	2 slices	42	72	45	10	1	0.2	0.2	0.1
675	Patties, breaded, battered, fried (2.25 oz)	1 patty	64	50	180	9	12	3.0	4.8	3.0
676	Roast, boneless, frozen, sea-soned, light and dark meat, cooked	3 oz	85	68	130	18	5	1.6	1.0	1.4
	Soups, Sauces, and Gravies								
	Soups:								
	Canned, condensed:								
	Prepared with equal volume of milk:								
677	Clam chowder, New England	1 cup	248	85	165	9	7	3.0	2.3	1.1
678	Cream of chicken	1 cup	248	85	190	7	11	4.6	4.5	1.6
679	Cream of mushroom	1 cup	248	85	205	6	14	5.1	3.0	4.6
680	Tomato	1 cup	248	85	160	6	6	2.9	1.6	1.1

[53] Fried in vegetable shortening.

Table A-4 Nutritive Value of the Edible Part of Food *(Continued)*

							Vitamin A value						
Cho-les-terol	Carbo-hydrate	Calcium	Phos-phorus	Iron	Potas-sium	Sodium	(IU)	(RE)	Thiamin	Ribo-flavin	Niacin	Ascorbic acid	Item No
Milli-grams	Grams	Milli-grams	Milli-grams	Milli-grams	Milli-grams	Milli-grams	Inter-national units	Retinol equiva-lents	Milli-grams	Milli-grams	Milli-grams	Milli-grams	
119	13	28	259	1.8	281	385	90	28	0.16	0.20	14.7	0	656
62	6	12	106	1.0	134	194	60	19	0.08	0.15	3.7	0	657
87	2	16	228	1.2	254	74	50	15	0.08	0.13	13.5	0	658
44	1	6	86	0.7	112	44	40	12	0.04	0.11	3.0	0	659
73	0	13	196	0.9	220	64	20	5	0.06	0.10	11.8	0	660
41	0	5	81	0.6	108	42	30	8	0.03	0.10	2.7	0	661
116	0	20	210	1.6	252	98	70	21	0.07	0.23	8.6	0	662
126	Tr	3	62	1.7	28	10	3,270	983	0.03	0.35	0.9	3	663
197	0	27	449	6.0	557	144	170	51	0.57	1.04	11.3	0	664
72	0	27	173	2.0	246	67	0	0	0.05	0.21	3.1	0	665
59	0	16	186	1.1	259	54	0	0	0.05	0.11	5.8	0	666
106	0	35	298	2.5	417	98	0	0	0.09	0.25	7.6	0	667
65	0	21	181	1.5	253	60	0	0	0.05	0.15	4.6	0	668
88	0	20	158	2.2	196	714	170	48	0.02	0.18	9.0	3	669
45	3	43	48	0.9	38	616	60	17	0.03	0.05	1.4	0	670
28	1	24	89	0.6	129	331	50	14	0.04	0.07	3.0	0	671
26	7	20	115	1.3	87	787	60	18	0.03	0.18	2.6	0	672
32	Tr	6	108	1.6	184	565	0	0	0.03	0.14	2.0	0	673
17	0	3	97	0.2	118	608	0	0	0.02	0.05	3.5	[54]0	674
40	10	9	173	1.4	176	512	20	7	0.06	0.12	1.5	0	675
45	3	4	207	1.4	253	578	0	0	0.04	0.14	5.3	0	676
22	17	186	156	1.5	300	992	160	40	0.07	0.24	1.0	3	677
27	15	181	151	0.7	273	1,047	710	94	0.07	0.26	0.9	1	678
20	15	179	156	0.6	270	1,076	150	37	0.08	0.28	0.9	2	679
17	22	159	149	1.8	449	932	850	109	0.13	0.25	1.5	68	680

[54] If sodium ascorbate is added, product contains 11 mg ascorbic acid.

Table A-4 Nutritive Value of the Edible Part of Food *(Continued)*

(Tr indicates nutrient present in trace amount.)

Item No.	Foods, approximate measures, units, and weight (weight of edible portion only)		Grams	Water	Food energy	Protein	Fat	Fatty acids		
								Saturated	Mono-unsaturated	Poly-unsaturated
			Grams	Percent	Calories	Grams	Grams	Grams	Grams	Grams
	Soups, Sauces, and Gravies—Con.									
	Soups:									
	Canned, condensed:									
	Prepared with equal volume of water:									
681	Bean with bacon	1 cup	253	84	170	8	6	1.5	2.2	1.8
682	Beef broth, bouillon, consomme	1 cup	240	98	15	3	1	0.3	0.2	Tr
683	Beef noodle	1 cup	244	92	85	5	3	1.1	1.2	0.5
684	Chicken noodle	1 cup	241	92	75	4	2	0.7	1.1	0.6
685	Chicken rice	1 cup	241	94	60	4	2	0.5	0.9	0.4
686	Clam chowder, Manhattan	1 cup	244	90	80	4	2	0.4	0.4	1.3
687	Cream of chicken	1 cup	244	91	115	3	7	2.1	3.3	1.5
688	Cream of mushroom	1 cup	244	90	130	2	9	2.4	1.7	4.2
689	Minestrone	1 cup	241	91	80	4	3	0.6	0.7	1.1
690	Pea, green	1 cup	250	83	165	9	3	1.4	1.0	0.4
691	Tomato	1 cup	244	90	85	2	2	0.4	0.4	1.0
692	Vegetable beef	1 cup	244	92	80	6	2	0.9	0.8	0.1
693	Vegetarian	1 cup	241	92	70	2	2	0.3	0.8	0.7
	Dehydrated:									
	Unprepared:									
694	Bouillon	1 pkt	6	3	15	1	1	0.3	0.2	Tr
695	Onion	1 pkt	7	4	20	1	Tr	0.1	0.2	Tr
	Prepared with water:									
696	Chicken noodle	1 pkt (6-fl-oz)	188	94	40	2	1	0.2	0.4	0.3
697	Onion	1 pkt (6-fl-oz)	184	96	20	1	Tr	0.1	0.2	0.1
698	Tomato vegetable	1 pkt (6-fl-oz)	189	94	40	1	1	0.3	0.2	0.1
	Sauces:									
	From dry mix:									
699	Cheese, prepared with milk	1 cup	279	77	305	16	17	9.3	5.3	1.6
700	Hollandaise, prepared with water	1 cup	259	84	240	5	20	11.6	5.9	0.9
701	White sauce, prepared with milk	1 cup	264	81	240	10	13	6.4	4.7	1.7
	From home recipe:									
702	White sauce, medium[55]	1 cup	250	73	395	10	30	9.1	11.9	7.2
	Ready to serve:									
703	Barbecue	1 tbsp	16	81	10	Tr	Tr	Tr	0.1	0.1
704	Soy	1 tbsp	18	68	10	2	0	0.0	0.0	0.0
	Gravies:									
	Canned:									
705	Beef	1 cup	233	87	125	9	5	2.7	2.3	0.2
706	Chicken	1 cup	238	85	190	5	14	3.4	6.1	3.6
707	Mushroom	1 cup	238	89	120	3	6	1.0	2.8	2.4
	From dry mix:									
708	Brown	1 cup	261	91	80	3	2	0.9	0.8	0.1
709	Chicken	1 cup	260	91	85	3	2	0.5	0.9	0.4
	Sugars and Sweets									
	Candy:									
710	Caramels, plain or chocolate	1 oz	28	8	115	1	3	2.2	0.3	0.1
	Chocolate:									
711	Milk, plain	1 oz	28	1	145	2	9	5.4	3.0	0.3
712	Milk, with almonds	1 oz	28	2	150	3	10	4.8	4.1	0.7
713	Milk, with peanuts	1 oz	28	1	155	4	11	4.2	3.5	1.5
714	Milk, with rice cereal	1 oz	28	2	140	2	7	4.4	2.5	0.2
715	Semisweet, small pieces (60 per oz)	1 cup or 6 oz	170	1	860	7	61	36.2	19.9	1.9
716	Sweet (dark)	1 oz	28	1	150	1	10	5.9	3.3	0.3
717	Fondant, uncoated (mints, candy corn, other)	1 oz	28	3	105	Tr	0	0.0	0.0	0.0
718	Fudge, chocolate, plain	1 oz	28	8	115	1	3	2.1	1.0	0.1
719	Gum drops	1 oz	28	12	100	Tr	Tr	Tr	Tr	0.1

[55] Made with enriched flour, margarine, and whole milk.

Table A-4 Nutritive Value of the Edible Part of Food *(Continued)*

Cholesterol	Carbohydrate	Calcium	Phosphorus	Iron	Potassium	Sodium	Vitamin A value (IU)	Vitamin A value (RE)	Thiamin	Riboflavin	Niacin	Ascorbic acid	Item No.
Milligrams	Grams	Milligrams	Milligrams	Milligrams	Milligrams	Milligrams	International units	Retinol equivalents	Milligrams	Milligrams	Milligrams	Milligrams	
3	23	81	132	2.0	402	951	890	89	0.09	0.03	0.6	2	681
Tr	Tr	14	31	0.4	130	782	0	0	Tr	0.05	1.9	0	682
5	9	15	46	1.1	100	952	630	63	0.07	0.06	1.1	Tr	683
7	9	17	36	0.8	55	1,106	710	71	0.05	0.06	1.4	Tr	684
7	7	17	22	0.7	101	815	660	66	0.02	0.02	1.1	Tr	685
2	12	34	59	1.9	261	1,808	920	92	0.06	0.05	1.3	3	686
10	9	34	37	0.6	88	986	560	56	0.03	0.06	0.8	Tr	687
2	9	46	49	0.5	100	1,032	0	0	0.05	0.09	0.7	1	688
2	11	34	55	0.9	313	911	2,340	234	0.05	0.04	0.9	1	689
0	27	28	125	2.0	190	988	200	20	0.11	0.07	1.2	2	690
0	17	12	34	1.8	264	871	690	69	0.09	0.05	1.4	66	691
5	10	17	41	1.1	173	956	1,890	189	0.04	0.05	1.0	2	692
0	12	22	34	1.1	210	822	3,010	301	0.05	0.05	0.9	1	693
1	1	4	19	0.1	27	1,019	Tr	Tr	Tr	0.01	0.3	0	694
Tr	4	10	23	0.1	47	627	Tr	Tr	0.02	0.04	0.4	Tr	695
2	6	24	24	0.4	23	957	50	5	0.05	0.04	0.7	Tr	696
0	4	9	22	0.1	48	635	Tr	Tr	0.02	0.04	0.4	Tr	697
0	8	6	23	0.5	78	856	140	14	0.04	0.03	0.6	5	698
53	23	569	438	0.3	552	1,565	390	117	0.15	0.56	0.3	2	699
52	14	124	127	0.9	124	1,564	730	220	0.05	0.18	0.1	Tr	700
34	21	425	256	0.3	444	797	310	92	0.08	0.45	0.5	3	701
32	24	292	238	0.9	381	888	1,190	340	0.15	0.43	0.8	2	702
0	2	3	3	0.1	28	130	140	14	Tr	Tr	0.1	1	703
0	2	3	38	0.5	64	1,029	0	0	0.01	0.02	0.6	0	704
7	11	14	70	1.6	189	117	0	0	0.07	0.08	1.5	0	705
5	13	48	69	1.1	259	1,373	880	264	0.04	0.10	1.1	0	706
0	13	17	36	1.6	252	1,357	0	0	0.08	0.15	1.6	0	707
2	14	66	47	0.2	61	1,147	0	0	0.04	0.09	0.9	0	708
3	14	39	47	0.3	62	1,134	0	0	0.05	0.15	0.8	3	709
1	22	42	35	0.4	54	64	Tr	Tr	0.01	0.05	0.1	Tr	710
6	16	50	61	0.4	96	23	30	10	0.02	0.10	0.1	Tr	711
5	15	65	77	0.5	125	23	30	8	0.02	0.12	0.2	Tr	712
5	13	49	83	0.4	138	19	30	8	0.07	0.07	1.4	Tr	713
6	18	48	57	0.2	100	46	30	8	0.01	0.08	0.1	Tr	714
0	97	51	178	5.8	593	24	30	3	0.10	0.14	0.9	Tr	715
0	16	7	41	0.6	86	5	10	1	0.01	0.04	0.1	Tr	716
0	27	2	Tr	0.1	1	57	0	0	Tr	Tr	Tr	0	717
1	21	22	24	0.3	42	54	Tr	Tr	0.01	0.03	0.1	Tr	718
0	25	2	Tr	0.1	1	10	0	0	0.00	Tr	Tr	0	719

Table A-4 Nutritive Value of the Edible Part of Food (Continued)

(Tr indicates nutrient present in trace amount.)

Item No.	Foods, approximate measures, units, and weight (weight of edible portion only)		Water	Food energy	Protein	Fat	Fatty acids		
							Saturated	Mono-unsaturated	Poly-unsaturated
		Grams	Percent	Calories	Grams	Grams	Grams	Grams	Grams
	Sugars and Sweets—Con.								
	Candy:								
720	Hard---------------------------- 1 oz------------	28	1	110	0	0	0.0	0.0	0.0
721	Jelly beans-------------------- 1 oz------------	28	6	105	Tr	Tr	Tr	Tr	0.1
722	Marshmallows------------------ 1 oz------------	28	17	90	1	0	0.0	0.0	0.0
723	Custard, baked------------------ 1 cup-----------	265	77	305	14	15	6.8	5.4	0.7
724	Gelatin dessert prepared with gelatin dessert powder and water------------------------- 1/2 cup---------	120	84	70	2	0	0.0	0.0	0.0
725	Honey, strained or extracted----- 1 cup-----------	339	17	1,030	1	0	0.0	0.0	0.0
726	1 tbsp----------	21	17	65	Tr	0	0.0	0.0	0.0
727	Jams and preserves-------------- 1 tbsp----------	20	29	55	Tr	Tr	0.0	Tr	Tr
728	1 packet--------	14	29	40	Tr	Tr	0.0	Tr	Tr
729	Jellies------------------------- 1 tbsp---------	18	28	50	Tr	Tr	Tr	Tr	Tr
730	1 packet-------	14	28	40	Tr	Tr	Tr	Tr	Tr
731	Popsicle, 3-fl-oz size----------- 1 popsicle------	95	80	70	0	0	0.0	0.0	0.0
	Puddings:								
	Canned:								
732	Chocolate--------------------- 5-oz can--------	142	68	205	3	11	9.5	0.5	0.1
733	Tapioca---------------------- 5-oz can--------	142	74	160	3	5	4.8	Tr	Tr
734	Vanilla---------------------- 5-oz can--------	142	69	220	2	10	9.5	0.2	0.1
	Dry mix, prepared with whole milk:								
	Chocolate:								
735	Instant------------------- 1/2 cup---------	130	71	155	4	4	2.3	1.1	0.2
736	Regular (cooked)----------- 1/2 cup---------	130	73	150	4	4	2.4	1.1	0.1
737	Rice---------------------- 1/2 cup---------	132	73	155	4	4	2.3	1.1	0.1
738	Tapioca-------------------- 1/2 cup---------	130	75	145	4	4	2.3	1.1	0.1
	Vanilla:								
739	Instant------------------- 1/2 cup---------	130	73	150	4	4	2.2	1.1	0.2
740	Regular (cooked)----------- 1/2 cup---------	130	74	145	4	4	2.3	1.0	0.1
	Sugars:								
741	Brown, pressed down----------- 1 cup-----------	220	2	820	0	0	0.0	0.0	0.0
	White:								
742	Granulated------------------- 1 cup-----------	200	1	770	0	0	0.0	0.0	0.0
743	1 tbsp----------	12	1	45	0	0	0.0	0.0	0.0
744	1 packet--------	6	1	25	0	0	0.0	0.0	0.0
745	Powdered, sifted, spooned into cup----------- 1 cup-----------	100	1	385	0	0	0.0	0.0	0.0
	Syrups:								
	Chocolate-flavored syrup or topping:								
746	Thin type------------------- 2 tbsp----------	38	37	85	1	Tr	0.2	0.1	0.1
747	Fudge type------------------ 2 tbsp----------	38	25	125	2	5	3.1	1.7	0.2
748	Molasses, cane, blackstrap----- 2 tbsp----------	40	24	85	0	0	0.0	0.0	0.0
749	Table syrup (corn and maple)--- 2 tbsp----------	42	25	122	0	0	0.0	0.0	0.0
	Vegetables and Vegetable Products								
750	Alfalfa seeds, sprouted, raw----- 1 cup-----------	33	91	10	1	Tr	Tr	Tr	0.1
751	Artichokes, globe or French, cooked, drained--------------- 1 artichoke-----	120	87	55	3	Tr	Tr	Tr	0.1
	Asparagus, green:								
	Cooked, drained:								
	From raw:								
752	Cuts and tips--------------- 1 cup-----------	180	92	45	5	1	0.1	Tr	0.2
753	Spears, 1/2-in diam. at base-------------------- 4 spears--------	60	92	15	2	Tr	Tr	Tr	0.1
	From frozen:								
754	Cuts and tips--------------- 1 cup-----------	180	91	50	5	1	0.2	Tr	0.3
755	Spears, 1/2-in diam. at base-------------------- 4 spears--------	60	91	15	2	Tr	0.1	Tr	0.1
756	Canned, spears, 1/2-in diam. at base------------------ 4 spears--------	80	95	10	1	Tr	Tr	Tr	0.1
757	Bamboo shoots, canned, drained--- 1 cup-----------	131	94	25	2	1	0.1	Tr	0.2

[56] For regular pack; special dietary pack contains 3 mg sodium.

Table A-4 Nutritive Value of the Edible Part of Food (*Continued*)

							Vitamin A value						
Cho-les-terol	Carbo-hydrate	Calcium	Phos-phorus	Iron	Potas-sium	Sodium	(IU)	(RE)	Thiamin	Ribo-flavin	Niacin	Ascorbic acid	Item No.
Milli-grams	Grams	Milli-grams	Milli-grams	Milli-grams	Milli-grams	Milli-grams	Inter-national units	Retinol equiva-lents	Milli-grams	Milli-grams	Milli-grams	Milli-grams	
0	28	Tr	2	0.1	1	7	0	0	0.10	0.00	0.0	0	720
0	26	1	1	0.3	11	7	0	0	0.00	Tr	Tr	0	721
0	23	1	2	0.5	2	25	0	0	0.00	Tr	Tr	0	722
278	29	297	310	1.1	387	209	530	146	0.11	0.50	0.3	1	723
0	17	2	23	Tr	Tr	55	0	0	0.00	0.00	0.0	0	724
0	279	17	20	1.7	173	17	0	0	0.02	0.14	1.0	3	725
0	17	1	1	0.1	11	1	0	0	Tr	0.01	0.1	Tr	726
0	14	4	2	0.2	18	2	Tr	Tr	Tr	0.01	Tr	Tr	727
0	10	3	1	0.1	12	2	Tr	Tr	Tr	Tr	Tr	Tr	728
0	13	2	Tr	0.1	16	5	Tr	Tr	Tr	0.01	Tr	1	729
0	10	1	Tr	Tr	13	4	Tr	Tr	Tr	Tr	Tr	1	730
0	18	0	0	Tr	4	11	0	0	0.00	0.00	0.0	0	731
1	30	74	117	1.2	254	285	100	31	0.04	0.17	0.6	Tr	732
Tr	28	119	113	0.3	212	252	Tr	Tr	0.03	0.14	0.4	Tr	733
1	33	79	94	0.2	155	305	Tr	Tr	0.03	0.12	0.6	Tr	734
14	27	130	329	0.3	176	440	130	33	0.04	0.18	0.1	1	735
15	25	146	120	0.2	190	167	140	34	0.05	0.20	0.1	1	736
15	27	133	110	0.5	165	140	140	33	0.10	0.18	0.6	1	737
15	25	131	103	0.1	167	152	140	34	0.04	0.18	0.1	1	738
15	27	129	273	0.1	164	375	140	33	0.04	0.17	0.1	1	739
15	25	132	102	0.1	166	178	140	34	0.04	0.18	0.1	1	740
0	212	187	56	4.8	757	97	0	0	0.02	0.07	0.2	0	741
0	199	3	Tr	0.1	7	5	0	0	0.00	0.00	0.0	0	742
0	12	Tr	Tr	Tr	Tr	Tr	0	0	0.00	0.00	0.0	0	743
0	6	Tr	Tr	Tr	Tr	Tr	0	0	0.00	0.00	0.0	0	744
0	100	1	Tr	Tr	4	2	0	0	0.00	0.00	0.0	0	745
0	22	6	49	0.8	85	36	Tr	Tr	Tr	0.02	0.1	0	746
0	21	38	60	0.5	82	42	40	13	0.02	0.08	0.1	0	747
0	22	274	34	10.1	1,171	38	0	0	0.04	0.08	0.8	0	748
0	32	1	4	Tr	7	19	0	0	0.00	0.00	0.0	0	749
0	1	11	23	0.3	26	2	50	5	0.03	0.04	0.2	3	750
0	12	47	72	1.6	316	79	170	17	0.07	0.06	0.7	9	751
0	8	43	110	1.2	558	7	1,490	149	0.18	0.22	1.9	49	752
0	3	14	37	0.4	186	2	500	50	0.06	0.07	0.6	16	753
0	9	41	99	1.2	392	7	1,470	147	0.12	0.19	1.9	44	754
0	3	14	33	0.4	131	2	490	49	0.04	0.06	0.6	15	755
0	2	11	30	0.5	122	[56]278	380	38	0.04	0.07	0.7	13	756
0	4	10	33	0.4	105	9	10	1	0.03	0.03	0.2	1	757

Table A-4 Nutritive Value of the Edible Part of Food (Continued)

(Tr indicates nutrient present in trace amount.)

Item No.	Foods, approximate measures, units, and weight (weight of edible portion only)		Grams	Water Percent	Food energy Cal-ories	Pro-tein Grams	Fat Grams	Fatty acids Satu-rated Grams	Mono-unsatu-rated Grams	Poly-unsatu-rated Grams
	Vegetables and Vegetable Products—Con.									
	Beans:									
	Lima, immature seeds, frozen, cooked, drained:									
758	Thick-seeded types (Ford-hooks)	1 cup	170	74	170	10	1	0.1	Tr	0.3
759	Thin-seeded types (baby limas)	1 cup	180	72	190	12	1	0.1	Tr	0.3
	Snap:									
	Cooked, drained:									
760	From raw (cut and French style)	1 cup	125	89	45	2	Tr	0.1	Tr	0.2
761	From frozen (cut)	1 cup	135	92	35	2	Tr	Tr	Tr	0.1
762	Canned, drained solids (cut)	1 cup	135	93	25	2	Tr	Tr	Tr	0.1
	Beans, mature. See Beans, dry (items 527-535) and Black-eyed peas, dry (item 536).									
	Bean sprouts (mung):									
763	Raw	1 cup	104	90	30	3	Tr	Tr	Tr	0.1
764	Cooked, drained	1 cup	124	93	25	3	Tr	Tr	Tr	Tr
	Beets:									
	Cooked, drained:									
765	Diced or sliced	1 cup	170	91	55	2	Tr	Tr	Tr	Tr
766	Whole beets, 2-in diam.	2 beets	100	91	30	1	Tr	Tr	Tr	Tr
767	Canned, drained solids, diced or sliced	1 cup	170	91	55	2	Tr	Tr	Tr	0.1
768	Beet greens, leaves and stems, cooked, drained	1 cup	144	89	40	4	Tr	Tr	0.1	0.1
	Black-eyed peas, immature seeds, cooked and drained:									
769	From raw	1 cup	165	72	180	13	1	0.3	0.1	0.6
770	From frozen	1 cup	170	66	225	14	1	0.3	0.1	0.5
	Broccoli:									
771	Raw	1 spear	151	91	40	4	1	0.1	Tr	0.3
	Cooked, drained:									
	From raw:									
772	Spear, medium	1 spear	180	90	50	5	1	0.1	Tr	0.2
773	Spears, cut into 1/2-in pieces	1 cup	155	90	45	5	Tr	0.1	Tr	0.2
	From frozen:									
774	Piece, 4-1/2 to 5 in long	1 piece	30	91	10	1	Tr	Tr	Tr	Tr
775	Chopped	1 cup	185	91	50	6	Tr	Tr	Tr	0.1
	Brussels sprouts, cooked, drained:									
776	From raw, 7-8 sprouts, 1-1/4 to 1-1/2-in diam.	1 cup	155	87	60	4	1	0.2	0.1	0.4
777	From frozen	1 cup	155	87	65	6	1	0.1	Tr	0.3
	Cabbage, common varieties:									
778	Raw, coarsely shredded or sliced	1 cup	70	93	15	1	Tr	Tr	Tr	0.1
779	Cooked, drained	1 cup	150	94	30	1	Tr	Tr	Tr	0.2
	Cabbage, Chinese:									
780	Pak-choi, cooked, drained	1 cup	170	96	20	3	Tr	Tr	Tr	0.1
781	Pe-tsai, raw, 1-in pieces	1 cup	76	94	10	1	Tr	Tr	Tr	0.1
782	Cabbage, red, raw, coarsely shredded or sliced	1 cup	70	92	20	1	Tr	Tr	Tr	0.1
783	Cabbage, savoy, raw, coarsely shredded or sliced	1 cup	70	91	20	1	Tr	Tr	Tr	Tr

[57] For green varieties; yellow varieties contain 101 IU or 10 RE.
[58] For green varieties; yellow varieties contain 151 IU or 15 RE.
[59] For regular pack; special dietary pack contains 3 mg sodium.

Table A-4 Nutritive Value of the Edible Part of Food *(Continued)*

							Vitamin A value						
Cho-les-terol	Carbo-hydrate	Calcium	Phos-phorus	Iron	Potas-sium	Sodium	(IU)	(RE)	Thiamin	Ribo-flavin	Niacin	Ascorbic acid	Item No
Milli-grams	Grams	Milli-grams	Milli-grams	Milli-grams	Milli-grams	Milli-grams	Inter-national units	Retinol equiva-lents	Milli-grams	Milli-grams	Milli-grams	Milli-grams	
0	32	37	107	2.3	694	90	320	32	0.13	0.10	1.8	22	758
0	35	50	202	3.5	740	52	300	30	0.13	0.10	1.4	10	759
0	10	58	49	1.6	374	4	[57]830	[57]83	0.09	0.12	0.8	12	760
0	8	61	32	1.1	151	18	[58]710	[58]71	0.06	0.10	0.6	11	761
0	6	35	26	1.2	147	[59]339	[60]470	[60]47	0.02	0.08	0.3	6	762
0	6	14	56	0.9	155	6	20	2	0.09	0.13	0.8	14	763
0	5	15	35	0.8	125	12	20	2	0.06	0.13	1.0	14	764
0	11	19	53	1.1	530	83	20	2	0.05	0.02	0.5	9	765
0	7	11	31	0.6	312	49	10	1	0.03	0.01	0.3	6	766
0	12	26	29	3.1	252	[61]466	20	2	0.02	0.07	0.3	7	767
0	8	164	59	2.7	1,309	347	7,340	734	0.17	0.42	0.7	36	768
0	30	46	196	2.4	693	7	1,050	105	0.11	0.18	1.8	3	769
0	40	39	207	3.6	638	9	130	13	0.44	0.11	1.2	4	770
0	8	72	100	1.3	491	41	2,330	233	0.10	0.18	1.0	141	771
0	10	205	86	2.1	293	20	2,540	254	0.15	0.37	1.4	113	772
0	9	177	74	1.8	253	17	2,180	218	0.13	0.32	1.2	97	773
0	2	15	17	0.2	54	7	570	57	0.02	0.02	0.1	12	774
0	10	94	102	1.1	333	44	3,500	350	0.10	0.15	0.8	74	775
0	13	56	87	1.9	491	33	1,110	111	0.17	0.12	0.9	96	776
0	13	37	84	1.1	504	36	910	91	0.16	0.18	0.8	71	777
0	4	33	16	0.4	172	13	90	9	0.04	0.02	0.2	33	778
0	7	50	38	0.6	308	29	130	13	0.09	0.08	0.3	36	779
0	3	158	49	1.8	631	58	4,370	437	0.05	0.11	0.7	44	780
0	2	59	22	0.2	181	7	910	91	0.03	0.04	0.3	21	781
0	4	36	29	0.3	144	8	30	3	0.04	0.02	0.2	40	782
0	4	25	29	0.3	161	20	700	70	0.05	0.02	0.2	22	783

[60] For green varieties; yellow varieties contain 142 IU or 14 RE.
[61] For regular pack; special dietary pack contains 78 mg sodium.

Table A-4 Nutritive Value of the Edible Part of Food *(Continued)*

(Tr indicates nutrient present in trace amount.)

Item No.	Foods, approximate measures, units, and weight (weight of edible portion only)		Water	Food energy	Pro-tein	Fat	Fatty acids		
							Satu-rated	Mono-unsatu-rated	Poly-unsatu-rated
		Grams	Per-cent	Cal-ories	Grams	Grams	Grams	Grams	Grams

Vegetables and Vegetable Products—Con.

Item No.	Food	Measure	Grams	Water	Cal	Protein	Fat	Sat	Mono	Poly
	Carrots:									
	Raw, without crowns and tips, scraped:									
784	Whole, 7-1/2 by 1-1/8 in, or strips, 2-1/2 to 3 in long	1 carrot or 18 strips	72	88	30	1	Tr	Tr	Tr	0.1
785	Grated	1 cup	110	88	45	1	Tr	Tr	Tr	0.1
	Cooked, sliced, drained:									
786	From raw	1 cup	156	87	70	2	Tr	0.1	Tr	0.1
787	From frozen	1 cup	146	90	55	2	Tr	Tr	Tr	0.1
788	Canned, sliced, drained solids	1 cup	146	93	35	1	Tr	0.1	Tr	0.1
	Cauliflower:									
789	Raw, (flowerets)	1 cup	100	92	25	2	Tr	Tr	Tr	0.1
	Cooked, drained:									
790	From raw (flowerets)	1 cup	125	93	30	2	Tr	Tr	Tr	0.1
791	From frozen (flowerets)	1 cup	180	94	35	3	Tr	0.1	Tr	0.2
	Celery, pascal type, raw:									
792	Stalk, large outer, 8 by 1-1/2 in (at root end)	1 stalk	40	95	5	Tr	Tr	Tr	Tr	Tr
793	Pieces, diced	1 cup	120	95	20	1	Tr	Tr	Tr	0.1
	Collards, cooked, drained:									
794	From raw (leaves without stems)	1 cup	190	96	25	2	Tr	0.1	Tr	0.2
795	From frozen (chopped)	1 cup	170	88	60	5	1	0.1	0.1	0.4
	Corn, sweet:									
	Cooked, drained:									
796	From raw, ear 5 by 1-3/4 in	1 ear	77	70	85	3	1	0.2	0.3	0.5
	From frozen:									
797	Ear, trimmed to about 3-1/2 in long	1 ear	63	73	60	2	Tr	0.1	0.1	0.2
798	Kernels	1 cup	165	76	135	5	Tr	Tr	Tr	0.1
	Canned:									
799	Cream style	1 cup	256	79	185	4	1	0.2	0.3	0.5
800	Whole kernel, vacuum pack	1 cup	210	77	165	5	1	0.2	0.3	0.5
	Cowpeas. See Black-eyed peas, immature (items 769,770), mature (item 536).									
801	Cucumber, with peel, slices, 1/8 in thick (large, 2-1/8-in diam.; small, 1-3/4-in diam.)	6 large or 8 small slices	28	96	5	Tr	Tr	Tr	Tr	Tr
802	Dandelion greens, cooked, drained	1 cup	105	90	35	2	1	0.1	Tr	0.3
803	Eggplant, cooked, steamed	1 cup	96	92	25	1	Tr	Tr	Tr	0.1
804	Endive, curly (including esca-role), raw, small pieces	1 cup	50	94	10	1	Tr	Tr	Tr	Tr
805	Jerusalem-artichoke, raw, sliced	1 cup	150	78	116	3	Tr	0.0	Tr	Tr
	Kale, cooked, drained:									
806	From raw, chopped	1 cup	130	91	40	2	1	0.1	Tr	0.3
807	From frozen, chopped	1 cup	130	91	40	4	1	0.1	Tr	0.3
808	Kohlrabi, thickened bulb-like stems, cooked, drained, diced	1 cup	165	90	50	3	Tr	Tr	Tr	0.1
	Lettuce, raw:									
	Butterhead, as Boston types:									
809	Head, 5-in diam	1 head	163	96	20	2	Tr	Tr	Tr	0.2
810	Leaves	1 outer or 2 inner leaves	15	96	Tr	Tr	Tr	Tr	Tr	Tr
	Crisphead, as iceberg:									
811	Head, 6-in diam	1 head	539	96	70	5	1	0.1	Tr	0.5
812	Wedge, 1/4 of head	1 wedge	135	96	20	1	Tr	Tr	Tr	0.1
813	Pieces, chopped or shredded	1 cup	55	96	5	1	Tr	Tr	Tr	0.1
814	Looseleaf (bunching varieties including romaine or cos), chopped or shredded pieces	1 cup	56	94	10	1	Tr	Tr	Tr	0.1

[62]For regular pack; special dietary pack contains 61 mg sodium.
[63]For yellow varieties; white varieties contain only a trace of vitamin A.

Table A-4 Nutritive Value of the Edible Part of Food (Continued)

Cho-les-terol	Carbo-hydrate	Calcium	Phos-phorus	Iron	Potas-sium	Sodium	Vitamin A value		Thiamin	Ribo-flavin	Niacin	Ascorbic acid	Item No.
							(IU)	(RE)					
Milli-grams	Grams	Milli-grams	Milli-grams	Milli-grams	Milli-grams	Milli-grams	Inter-national units	Retinol equiva-lents	Milli-grams	Milli-grams	Milli-grams	Milli-grams	
0	7	19	32	0.4	233	25	20,250	2,025	0.07	0.04	0.7	7	784
0	11	30	48	0.6	355	39	30,940	3,094	0.11	0.06	1.0	10	785
0	16	48	47	1.0	354	103	38,300	3,830	0.05	0.09	0.8	4	786
0	12	41	38	0.7	231	86	25,850	2,585	0.04	0.05	0.6	4	787
0	8	37	35	0.9	261	[62]352	20,110	2,011	0.03	0.04	0.8	4	788
0	5	29	46	0.6	355	15	20	2	0.08	0.06	0.6	72	789
0	6	34	44	0.5	404	8	20	2	0.08	0.07	0.7	69	790
0	7	31	43	0.7	250	32	40	4	0.07	0.10	0.6	56	791
0	1	14	10	0.2	114	35	50	5	0.01	0.01	0.1	3	792
0	4	43	31	0.6	341	106	150	15	0.04	0.04	0.4	8	793
0	5	148	19	0.8	177	36	4,220	422	0.03	0.08	0.4	19	794
0	12	357	46	1.9	427	85	10,170	1,017	0.08	0.20	1.1	45	795
0	19	2	79	0.5	192	13	[63]170	[63]17	0.17	0.06	1.2	5	796
0	14	2	47	0.4	158	3	[63]130	[63]13	0.11	0.04	1.0	3	797
0	34	3	78	0.5	229	8	[63]410	[63]41	0.11	0.12	2.1	4	798
0	46	8	131	1.0	343	[64]730	[63]250	[63]25	0.06	0.14	2.5	12	799
0	41	11	134	0.9	391	[65]571	[63]510	[63]51	0.09	0.15	2.5	17	800
0	1	4	5	0.1	42	1	10	1	0.01	0.01	0.1	1	801
0	7	147	44	1.9	244	46	12,290	1,229	0.14	0.18	0.5	19	802
0	6	6	21	0.3	238	3	60	6	0.07	0.02	0.6	1	803
0	2	26	14	0.4	157	11	1,030	103	0.04	0.04	0.2	3	804
0	26	21	117	5.1	644	6	30	3	0.30	0.09	2.0	6	805
0	7	94	36	1.2	296	30	9,620	962	0.07	0.09	0.7	53	806
0	7	179	36	1.2	417	20	8,260	826	0.06	0.15	0.9	33	807
0	11	41	74	0.7	561	35	60	6	0.07	0.03	0.6	89	808
0	4	52	38	0.5	419	8	1,580	158	0.10	0.10	0.5	13	809
0	Tr	5	3	Tr	39	1	150	15	0.01	0.01	Tr	1	810
0	11	102	108	2.7	852	49	1,780	178	0.25	0.16	1.0	21	811
0	3	26	27	0.7	213	12	450	45	0.06	0.04	0.3	5	812
0	1	10	11	0.3	87	5	180	18	0.03	0.02	0.1	2	813
0	2	38	14	0.8	148	5	1,060	106	0.03	0.04	0.2	10	814

[64] For regular pack; special dietary pack contains 8 mg sodium.
[65] For regular pack; special dietary pack contains 6 mg sodium.

Table A-4 Nutritive Value of the Edible Part of Food *(Continued)*

(Tr indicates nutrient present in trace amount.)

Item No.	Foods, approximate measures, units, and weight (weight of edible portion only)			Water	Food energy	Pro-tein	Fat	Fatty acids		
								Satu-rated	Mono-unsatu-rated	Poly-unsatu-rated
			Grams	Per-cent	Cal-ories	Grams	Grams	Grams	Grams	Grams
	Vegetables and Vegetable Products—Con.									
	Mushrooms:									
815	Raw, sliced or chopped	1 cup	70	92	20	1	Tr	Tr	Tr	0.1
816	Cooked, drained	1 cup	156	91	40	3	1	0.1	Tr	0.3
817	Canned, drained solids	1 cup	156	91	35	3	Tr	0.1	Tr	0.2
818	Mustard greens, without stems and midribs, cooked, drained	1 cup	140	94	20	3	Tr	Tr	0.2	0.1
819	Okra pods, 3 by 5/8 in, cooked	8 pods	85	90	25	2	Tr	Tr	Tr	Tr
	Onions:									
	Raw:									
820	Chopped	1 cup	160	91	55	2	Tr	0.1	0.1	0.2
821	Sliced	1 cup	115	91	40	1	Tr	0.1	Tr	0.1
822	Cooked (whole or sliced), drained	1 cup	210	92	60	2	Tr	0.1	Tr	0.1
823	Onions, spring, raw, bulb (3/8-in diam.) and white portion of top	6 onions	30	92	10	1	Tr	Tr	Tr	Tr
824	Onion rings, breaded, par-fried, frozen, prepared	2 rings	20	29	80	1	5	1.7	2.2	1.0
	Parsley:									
825	Raw	10 sprigs	10	88	5	Tr	Tr	Tr	Tr	Tr
826	Freeze-dried	1 tbsp	0.4	2	Tr	Tr	Tr	Tr	Tr	Tr
827	Parsnips, cooked (diced or 2 in lengths), drained	1 cup	156	78	125	2	Tr	0.1	0.2	0.1
828	Peas, edible pod, cooked, drained	1 cup	160	89	65	5	Tr	0.1	Tr	0.2
	Peas, green:									
829	Canned, drained solids	1 cup	170	82	115	8	1	0.1	0.1	0.3
830	Frozen, cooked, drained	1 cup	160	80	125	8	Tr	0.1	Tr	0.2
	Peppers:									
831	Hot chili, raw	1 pepper	45	88	20	1	Tr	Tr	Tr	Tr
	Sweet (about 5 per lb, whole), stem and seeds removed:									
832	Raw	1 pepper	74	93	20	1	Tr	Tr	Tr	0.2
833	Cooked, drained	1 pepper	73	95	15	Tr	Tr	Tr	Tr	0.1
	Potatoes, cooked:									
	Baked (about 2 per lb, raw):									
834	With skin	1 potato	202	71	220	5	Tr	0.1	Tr	0.1
835	Flesh only	1 potato	156	75	145	3	Tr	Tr	Tr	0.1
	Boiled (about 3 per lb, raw):									
836	Peeled after boiling	1 potato	136	77	120	3	Tr	Tr	Tr	0.1
837	Peeled before boiling	1 potato	135	77	115	2	Tr	Tr	Tr	0.1
	French fried, strip, 2 to 3-1/2 in long, frozen:									
838	Oven heated	10 strips	50	53	110	2	4	2.1	1.8	0.3
839	Fried in vegetable oil	10 strips	50	38	160	2	8	2.5	1.6	3.8
	Potato products, prepared:									
	Au gratin:									
840	From dry mix	1 cup	245	79	230	6	10	6.3	2.9	0.3
841	From home recipe	1 cup	245	74	325	12	19	11.6	5.3	0.7
842	Hashed brown, from frozen	1 cup	156	56	340	5	18	7.0	8.0	2.1
	Mashed:									
	From home recipe:									
843	Milk added	1 cup	210	78	160	4	1	0.7	0.3	0.1
844	Milk and margarine added	1 cup	210	76	225	4	9	2.2	3.7	2.5
845	From dehydrated flakes (without milk), water, milk, butter, and salt added	1 cup	210	76	235	4	12	7.2	3.3	0.5
846	Potato salad, made with mayonnaise	1 cup	250	76	360	7	21	3.6	6.2	9.3
	Scalloped:									
847	From dry mix	1 cup	245	79	230	5	11	6.5	3.0	0.5
848	From home recipe	1 cup	245	81	210	7	9	5.5	2.5	0.4

[66] For regular pack; special dietary pack contains 3 mg sodium.
[67] For red peppers; green peppers contain 350 IU or 35 RE.
[68] For green peppers; red peppers contain 4,220 IU or 422 RE.

Table A-4 Nutritive Value of the Edible Part of Food (Continued)

Nutrients in Indicated Quantity

Cholesterol	Carbohydrate	Calcium	Phosphorus	Iron	Potassium	Sodium	Vitamin A value (IU)	Vitamin A value (RE)	Thiamin	Riboflavin	Niacin	Ascorbic acid	Item No.
Milligrams	Grams	Milligrams	Milligrams	Milligrams	Milligrams	Milligrams	International units	Retinol equivalents	Milligrams	Milligrams	Milligrams	Milligrams	
0	3	4	73	0.9	259	3	0	0	0.07	0.31	2.9	2	815
0	8	9	136	2.7	555	3	0	0	0.11	0.47	7.0	6	816
0	8	17	103	1.2	201	663	0	0	0.13	0.03	2.5	0	817
0	3	104	57	1.0	283	22	4,240	424	0.06	0.09	0.6	35	818
0	6	54	48	0.4	274	4	490	49	0.11	0.05	0.7	14	819
0	12	40	46	0.6	248	3	0	0	0.10	0.02	0.2	13	820
0	8	29	33	0.4	178	2	0	0	0.07	0.01	0.1	10	821
0	13	57	48	0.4	319	17	0	0	0.09	0.02	0.2	12	822
0	2	18	10	0.6	77	1	1,500	150	0.02	0.04	0.1	14	823
0	8	6	16	0.3	26	75	50	5	0.06	0.03	0.7	Tr	824
0	1	13	4	0.6	54	4	520	52	0.01	0.01	0.1	9	825
0	Tr	1	2	0.2	25	2	250	25	Tr	0.01	Tr	1	826
0	30	58	108	0.9	573	16	0	0	0.13	0.08	1.1	20	827
0	11	67	88	3.2	384	6	210	21	0.20	0.12	0.9	77	828
0	21	34	114	1.6	294	[66]372	1,310	131	0.21	0.13	1.2	16	829
0	23	38	144	2.5	269	139	1,070	107	0.45	0.16	2.4	16	830
0	4	8	21	0.5	153	3	[67]4,840	[67]484	0.04	0.04	0.4	109	831
0	4	4	16	0.9	144	2	[68]390	[68]39	0.06	0.04	0.4	[69]95	832
0	3	3	11	0.6	94	1	[70]280	[70]28	0.04	0.03	0.3	[71]81	833
0	51	20	115	2.7	844	16	0	0	0.22	0.07	3.3	26	834
0	34	8	78	0.5	610	8	0	0	0.16	0.03	2.2	20	835
0	27	7	60	0.4	515	5	0	0	0.14	0.03	2.0	18	836
0	27	11	54	0.4	443	7	0	0	0.13	0.03	1.8	10	837
0	17	5	43	0.7	229	16	0	0	0.06	0.02	1.2	5	838
0	20	10	47	0.4	366	108	0	0	0.09	0.01	1.6	5	839
12	31	203	233	0.8	537	1,076	520	76	0.05	0.20	2.3	8	840
56	28	292	277	1.6	970	1,061	650	93	0.16	0.28	2.4	24	841
0	44	23	112	2.4	680	53	0	0	0.17	0.03	3.8	10	842
4	37	55	101	0.6	628	636	40	12	0.18	0.08	2.3	14	843
4	35	55	97	0.5	607	620	360	42	0.18	0.08	2.3	13	844
29	32	103	118	0.5	489	697	380	44	0.23	0.11	1.4	20	845
170	28	48	130	1.6	635	1,323	520	83	0.19	0.15	2.2	25	846
27	31	88	137	0.9	497	835	360	51	0.05	0.14	2.5	8	847
29	26	140	154	1.4	926	821	330	47	0.17	0.23	2.6	26	848

[69]For green peppers; red peppers contain 141 mg ascorbic acid.
[70]For green peppers; red peppers contain 2,740 IU or 274 RE.
[71]For green peppers; red peppers contain 121 mg ascorbic acid.

Table A-4 Nutritive Value of the Edible Part of Food *(Continued)*

(Tr indicates nutrient present in trace amount.)

Item No.	Foods, approximate measures, units, and weight (weight of edible portion only)		Water	Food energy	Pro-tein	Fat	Fatty acids		
							Satu-rated	Mono-unsatu-rated	Poly-unsatu-rated
	Vegetables and Vegetable Products—Con.	Grams	Per-cent	Cal-ories	Grams	Grams	Grams	Grams	Grams
849	Potato chips---------------------	10 chips--------	20	3	105	1	7	1.8	1.2	3.6
	Pumpkin:									
850	Cooked from raw, mashed--------	1 cup-----------	245	94	50	2	Tr	0.1	Tr	Tr
851	Canned-------------------------	1 cup-----------	245	90	85	3	1	0.4	0.1	Tr
852	Radishes, raw, stem ends, rootlets cut off---------------	4 radishes------	18	95	5	Tr	Tr	Tr	Tr	Tr
853	Sauerkraut, canned, solids and liquid-------------------------	1 cup-----------	236	93	45	2	Tr	0.1	Tr	0.1
	Seaweed:									
854	Kelp, raw---------------------	1 oz------------	28	82	10	Tr	Tr	0.1	Tr	Tr
855	Spirulina, dried---------------	1 oz------------	28	5	80	16	2	0.8	0.2	0.6
	Southern peas. See Black-eyed peas, immature (items 769,770), mature (item 536).									
	Spinach:									
856	Raw, chopped-------------------	1 cup-----------	55	92	10	2	Tr	Tr	Tr	0.1
	Cooked, drained:									
857	From raw---------------------	1 cup-----------	180	91	40	5	Tr	0.1	Tr	0.2
858	From frozen (leaf)-----------	1 cup-----------	190	90	55	6	Tr	0.1	Tr	0.2
859	Canned, drained solids--------	1 cup-----------	214	92	50	6	1	0.2	Tr	0.4
860	Spinach souffle-------------------	1 cup-----------	136	74	220	11	18	7.1	6.8	3.1
	Squash, cooked:									
861	Summer (all varieties), sliced, drained----------------------	1 cup-----------	180	94	35	2	1	0.1	Tr	0.2
862	Winter (all varieties), baked, cubes-----------------------	1 cup-----------	205	89	80	2	1	0.3	0.1	0.5
	Sunchoke. See Jerusalem-arti-choke (item 805).									
	Sweetpotatoes:									
	Cooked (raw, 5 by 2 in; about 2-1/2 per lb):									
863	Baked in skin, peeled--------	1 potato--------	114	73	115	2	Tr	Tr	Tr	0.1
864	Boiled, without skin---------	1 potato--------	151	73	160	2	Tr	0.1	Tr	0.2
865	Candied, 2-1/2 by 2-in piece---	1 piece---------	105	67	145	1	3	1.4	0.7	0.2
	Canned:									
866	Solid pack (mashed)----------	1 cup-----------	255	74	260	5	1	0.1	Tr	0.2
867	Vacuum pack, piece 2-3/4 by 1 in-----------------------	1 piece---------	40	76	35	1	Tr	Tr	Tr	Tr
	Tomatoes:									
868	Raw, 2-3/5-in diam. (3 per 12 oz pkg.)--------------------	1 tomato--------	123	94	25	1	Tr	Tr	Tr	0.1
869	Canned, solids and liquid------	1 cup-----------	240	94	50	2	1	0.1	0.1	0.2
870	Tomato juice, canned-----------	1 cup-----------	244	94	40	2	Tr	Tr	Tr	0.1
	Tomato products, canned:									
871	Paste-------------------------	1 cup-----------	262	74	220	10	2	0.3	0.4	0.9
872	Puree--------------------------	1 cup-----------	250	87	105	4	Tr	Tr	Tr	0.1
873	Sauce--------------------------	1 cup-----------	245	89	75	3	Tr	0.1	0.1	0.2
874	Turnips, cooked, diced----------	1 cup-----------	156	94	30	1	Tr	Tr	Tr	0.1
	Turnip greens, cooked, drained:									
875	From raw (leaves and stems)----	1 cup-----------	144	93	30	2	Tr	0.1	Tr	0.1
876	From frozen (chopped)----------	1 cup-----------	164	90	50	5	1	0.2	Tr	0.3
877	Vegetable juice cocktail, canned	1 cup-----------	242	94	45	2	Tr	Tr	Tr	0.1
	Vegetables, mixed:									
878	Canned, drained solids---------	1 cup-----------	163	87	75	4	Tr	0.1	Tr	0.2
879	Frozen, cooked, drained--------	1 cup-----------	182	83	105	5	Tr	0.1	Tr	0.1
880	Waterchestnuts, canned----------	1 cup-----------	140	86	70	1	Tr	Tr	Tr	Tr

[1] Value not determined.
[72] With added salt; if none is added, sodium content is 58 mg.
[73] For regular pack; special dietary pack contains 31 mg sodium.
[74] With added salt; if none is added, sodium content is 24 mg.

Table A-4 Nutritive Value of the Edible Part of Food *(Continued)*

Nutrients in Indicated Quantity

Cho-les-terol	Carbo-hydrate	Calcium	Phos-phorus	Iron	Potas-sium	Sodium	Vitamin A value		Thiamin	Ribo-flavin	Niacin	Ascorbic acid	Item No
							(IU)	(RE)					
Milli-grams	Grams	Milli-grams	Milli-grams	Milli-grams	Milli-grams	Milli-grams	Inter-national units	Retinol equiva-lents	Milli-grams	Milli-grams	Milli-grams	Milli-grams	
0	10	5	31	0.2	260	94	0	0	0.03	Tr	0.8	8	849
0	12	37	74	1.4	564	2	2,650	265	0.08	0.19	1.0	12	850
0	20	64	86	3.4	505	12	54,040	5,404	0.06	0.13	0.9	10	851
0	1	4	3	0.1	42	4	Tr	Tr	Tr	0.01	0.1	4	852
0	10	71	47	3.5	401	1,560	40	4	0.05	0.05	0.3	35	853
0	3	48	12	0.8	25	66	30	3	0.01	0.04	0.1	(1)	854
0	7	34	33	8.1	386	297	160	16	0.67	1.04	3.6	3	855
0	2	54	27	1.5	307	43	3,690	369	0.04	0.10	0.4	15	856
0	7	245	101	6.4	839	126	14,740	1,474	0.17	0.42	0.9	18	857
0	10	277	91	2.9	566	163	14,790	1,479	0.11	0.32	0.8	23	858
0	7	272	94	4.9	740	[72]683	18,780	1,878	0.03	0.30	0.8	31	859
184	3	230	231	1.3	201	763	3,460	675	0.09	0.30	0.5	3	860
0	8	49	70	0.6	346	2	520	52	0.08	0.07	0.9	10	861
0	18	29	41	0.7	896	2	7,290	729	0.17	0.05	1.4	20	862
0	28	32	63	0.5	397	11	24,880	2,488	0.08	0.14	0.7	28	863
0	37	32	41	0.8	278	20	25,750	2,575	0.08	0.21	1.0	26	864
8	29	27	27	1.2	198	74	4,400	440	0.02	0.04	0.4	7	865
0	59	77	133	3.4	536	191	38,570	3,857	0.07	0.23	2.4	13	866
0	8	9	20	0.4	125	21	3,190	319	0.01	0.02	0.3	11	867
0	5	9	28	0.6	255	10	1,390	139	0.07	0.06	0.7	22	868
0	10	62	46	1.5	530	[73]391	1,450	145	0.11	0.07	1.8	36	869
0	10	22	46	1.4	537	[74]881	1,360	136	0.11	0.08	1.6	45	870
0	49	92	207	7.8	2,442	[75]170	6,470	647	0.41	0.50	8.4	111	871
0	25	38	100	2.3	1,050	[76]50	3,400	340	0.18	0.14	4.3	88	872
0	18	34	78	1.9	909	[77]1,482	2,400	240	0.16	0.14	2.8	32	873
0	8	34	30	0.3	211	78	0	0	0.04	0.04	0.5	18	874
0	6	197	42	1.2	292	42	7,920	792	0.06	0.10	0.6	39	875
0	8	249	56	3.2	367	25	13,080	1,308	0.09	0.12	0.8	36	876
0	11	27	41	1.0	467	883	2,830	283	0.10	0.07	1.8	67	877
0	15	44	68	1.7	474	243	18,990	1,899	0.08	0.08	0.9	8	878
0	24	46	93	1.5	308	64	7,780	778	0.13	0.22	1.5	6	879
0	17	6	27	1.2	165	11	10	1	0.02	0.03	0.5	2	880

[75] With no added salt; if salt is added, sodium content is 2,070 mg.
[76] With no added salt; if salt is added, sodium content is 998 mg.
[77] With salt added.

Table A-4 Nutritive Value of the Edible Part of Food *(Continued)*

(Tr indicates nutrient present in trace amount.)

Item No.	Foods, approximate measures, units, and weight (weight of edible portion only)		Water	Food energy	Pro-tein	Fat	Fatty acids		
							Satu-rated	Mono-unsatu-rated	Poly-unsatu-rated
	Miscellaneous Items	Grams	Per-cent	Cal-ories	Grams	Grams	Grams	Grams	Grams
	Baking powders for home use:								
	Sodium aluminum sulfate:								
881	With monocalcium phosphate monohydrate	1 tsp	3	2	5	Tr	0	0.0	0.0	0.0
882	With monocalcium phosphate monohydrate, calcium sulfate	1 tsp	2.9	1	5	Tr	0	0.0	0.0	0.0
883	Straight phosphate	1 tsp	3.8	2	5	Tr	0	0.0	0.0	0.0
884	Low sodium	1 tsp	4.3	1	5	Tr	0	0.0	0.0	0.0
885	Catsup	1 cup	273	69	290	5	1	0.2	0.2	0.4
886		1 tbsp	15	69	15	Tr	Tr	Tr	Tr	Tr
887	Celery seed	1 tsp	2	6	10	Tr	1	Tr	0.3	0.1
888	Chili powder	1 tsp	2.6	8	10	Tr	Tr	0.1	0.1	0.2
	Chocolate:									
889	Bitter or baking	1 oz	28	2	145	3	15	9.0	4.9	0.5
	Semisweet, see Candy, (item 715).									
890	Cinnamon	1 tsp	2.3	10	5	Tr	Tr	(¹)	(¹)	(¹)
891	Curry powder	1 tsp	2	10	5	Tr	Tr	(¹)	(¹)	(¹)
892	Garlic powder	1 tsp	2.8	6	10	Tr	Tr	Tr	Tr	Tr
893	Gelatin, dry	1 envelope	7	13	25	6	Tr	Tr	Tr	Tr
894	Mustard, prepared, yellow	1 tsp or individual packet	5	80	5	Tr	Tr	Tr	0.2	Tr
	Olives, canned:									
895	Green	4 medium or 3 extra large	13	78	15	Tr	2	0.2	1.2	0.1
896	Ripe, Mission, pitted	3 small or 2 large	9	73	15	Tr	2	0.3	1.3	0.2
897	Onion powder	1 tsp	2.1	5	5	Tr	Tr	Tr	Tr	Tr
898	Oregano	1 tsp	1.5	7	5	Tr	Tr	Tr	Tr	0.1
899	Paprika	1 tsp	2.1	10	5	Tr	Tr	Tr	Tr	0.2
900	Pepper, black	1 tsp	2.1	11	5	Tr	Tr	Tr	Tr	Tr
	Pickles, cucumber:									
901	Dill, medium, whole, 3-3/4 in long, 1-1/4-in diam.	1 pickle	65	93	5	Tr	Tr	Tr	Tr	0.1
902	Fresh-pack, slices 1-1/2-in diam., 1/4 in thick	2 slices	15	79	10	Tr	Tr	Tr	Tr	Tr
903	Sweet, gherkin, small, whole, about 2-1/2 in long, 3/4-in diam.	1 pickle	15	61	20	Tr	Tr	Tr	Tr	Tr
	Popcorn. See Grain Products, (items 497-499).									
904	Relish, finely chopped, sweet	1 tbsp	15	63	20	Tr	Tr	Tr	Tr	Tr
905	Salt	1 tsp	5.5	0	0	0	0	0.0	0.0	0.0
906	Vinegar, cider	1 tbsp	15	94	Tr	Tr	0	0.0	0.0	0.0
	Yeast:									
907	Baker's, dry, active	1 pkg	7	5	20	3	Tr	Tr	0.1	Tr
908	Brewer's, dry	1 tbsp	8	5	25	3	Tr	Tr	Tr	0.0

¹Value not determined.

Table A-4 Nutritive Value of the Edible Part of Food *(Continued)*

Nutrients in Indicated Quantity

Cho-les-terol	Carbo-hydrate	Calcium	Phos-phorus	Iron	Potas-sium	Sodium	Vitamin A value		Thiamin	Ribo-flavin	Niacin	Ascorbic acid	Item No
							(IU)	(RE)					
Milli-grams	Grams	Milli-grams	Milli-grams	Milli-grams	Milli-grams	Milli-grams	Inter-national units	Retinol equiva-lents	Milli-grams	Milli-grams	Milli-grams	Milli-grams	
0	1	58	87	0.0	5	329	0	0	0.00	0.00	0.0	0	881
0	1	183	45	0.0	4	290	0	0	0.00	0.00	0.0	0	882
0	1	239	359	0.0	6	312	0	0	0.00	0.00	0.0	0	883
0	1	207	314	0.0	891	Tr	0	0	0.00	0.00	0.0	0	884
0	69	60	137	2.2	991	2,845	3,820	382	0.25	0.19	4.4	41	885
0	4	3	8	0.1	54	156	210	21	0.01	0.01	0.2	2	886
0	1	35	11	0.9	28	3	Tr	Tr	0.01	0.01	0.1	Tr	887
0	1	7	8	0.4	50	26	910	91	0.01	0.02	0.2	2	888
0	8	22	109	1.9	235	1	10	1	0.01	0.07	0.4	0	889
0	2	28	1	0.9	12	1	10	1	Tr	Tr	Tr	1	890
0	1	10	7	0.6	31	1	20	2	0.01	0.01	0.1	Tr	891
0	2	2	12	0.1	31	1	0	0	0.01	Tr	Tr	Tr	892
0	0	1	0	0.0	2	6	0	0	0.00	0.00	0.0	0	893
0	Tr	4	4	0.1	7	63	0	0	Tr	0.01	Tr	Tr	894
0	Tr	8	2	0.2	7	312	40	4	Tr	Tr	Tr	0	895
0	Tr	10	2	0.2	2	68	10	1	Tr	Tr	Tr	0	896
0	2	8	7	0.1	20	1	Tr	Tr	0.01	Tr	Tr	Tr	897
0	1	24	3	0.7	25	Tr	100	10	0.01	Tr	0.1	1	898
0	1	4	7	0.5	49	1	1,270	127	0.01	0.04	0.3	1	899
0	1	9	4	0.6	26	1	Tr	Tr	Tr	0.01	Tr	0	900
0	1	17	14	0.7	130	928	70	7	Tr	0.01	Tr	4	901
0	3	5	4	0.3	30	101	20	2	Tr	Tr	Tr	1	902
0	5	2	2	0.2	30	107	10	1	Tr	Tr	Tr	1	903
0	5	3	2	0.1	30	107	20	2	Tr	Tr	0.0	1	904
0	0	14	3	Tr	Tr	2,132	0	0	0.00	0.00	0.0	0	905
0	1	1	1	0.1	15	Tr	0	0	0.00	0.00	0.0	0	906
0	3	3	90	1.1	140	4	Tr	Tr	0.16	0.38	2.6	Tr	907
0	3	[78]17	140	1.4	152	10	Tr	Tr	1.25	0.34	3.0	Tr	908

[78]Value may vary from 6 to 60 mg.

(Courtesy of United States Department of Agriculture)

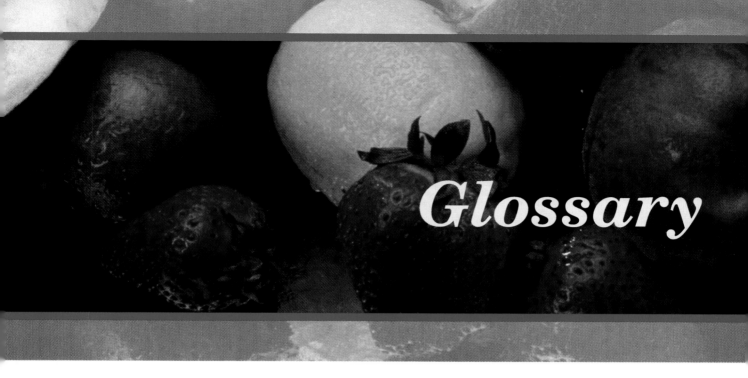

Glossary

A

absorption—taking up of nutrients in the intestines

abstinence—avoidance

acid-base balance—the regulation of hydrogen ions in body fluids

acidosis—condition in which excess acids accumulate or there is a loss of base in the body

acne—pimples

acute—sudden but short-lived

acute renal failure (ARF)—suddenly occurring failure of the kidneys

ADH—antidiuretic hormone, also called vasopressin, excreted by the pituitary gland

adipose tissue—fatty tissue

adolescent—person between the ages of 13 and 20

acquired immune deficiency syndrome (AIDS)—caused by the human immunodeficiency virus (HIV) which weakens the body's immune system leaving it susceptable to fatal infections

albumin—protein that occurs in blood plasma

alcoholism—chronic and excessive use of alcohol

aldosterone—hormone secreted by adrenal glands that triggers kidneys to increase amount of sodium being reabsorbed

alkaline—base; capable of neutralizing acids

alkalosis—condition in which excess base accumulates in, or acids are lost from, the body

allergen—substance-causing allergy

allergic reaction—adverse physical reaction to specific substance(s)

allergy—sensitivity to specific substance(s)

alpha-tocopherol—a form of vitamin E

ambulatory—able to walk

amenorrhea—the stoppage of the monthly menstrual flow

amino acids—nitrogen-containing chemical compounds of which protein is composed

amniocentesis—a test to determine the status of the fetus in utero

amniotic fluid—surrounds fetus in the uterus

amphetamines—drugs intended to inhibit appetite

anabolism—the creation of new compounds during metabolism

analogues—imitations

anemia—condition caused by insufficient number of red blood cells, hemoglobin, or blood volume

anencephaly—absence of the brain

angina pectoris—pain in the heart muscle due to inadequate blood supply

anorexia nervosa—psychologically induced lack of appetite

anthropometric measurements—of height, weight, head, skinfold

antibiotic therapy—use of medications to destroy harmful microbes

antibodies—substances produced by body in reaction to foreign substance; neutralize toxins from foreign bodies

anticoagulant—drug used to thin blood

antioxidant—substance preventing damage from oxygen

anxiety—apprehension

appetite—learned psychological reaction to food caused by pleasant memories of eating

arachidonic acid—one of three fatty acids needed by the body; can be synthesized by the body

arteriosclerosis—generic term for thickened arteries

arthritis—chronic disease involving the joints

ascites—abnormal collection of fluid in the abdomen

ascorbic acid—vitamin C

aspartame—artificial sweetener made from two amino acids; does not require insulin for metabolism

aspirated—inhaled or suctioned

asymptomatic—without symptoms

atherosclerosis—a form of arteriosclerosis affecting the intima (inner lining) of the artery walls

avitaminosis—without vitamins

B

bacteria—microorganism that may or may not cause disease

balanced diet—one that includes all the essential nutrients in appropriate amounts

basal metabolism rate (BMR)—the rate at which energy is needed for body maintenance

beriberi—deficiency disease caused by a lack of vitamin B_1 (thiamin)

bile—secretion of the liver, stored in the gallbladder, essential for the digestion of fats

biochemical tests—involving biology and chemistry

biotin—a B vitamin; necessary for metabolism

bland—mild or soothing

bland diet—diet containing only mild-flavored foods with soft textures

blemish—mark

blood plasma—fluid part of the blood

bolus—food in the mouth that is ready to be swallowed

bonding—emotional attachment

bone marrow—soft tissue in the bone center

botulism—deadliest of food poisonings; caused by the bacteria *Clostridium botulinum*

bouillon—clear soup broth

bran—outer covering of grain kernels

buffer systems—protective systems regulating amounts of hydrogen ions in body fluids

bulimia—condition in which patient alternately binges and purges

buttermilk—milk made from the addition of harmless bacteria to skim milk

C

cachexia—severe malnutrition and body wasting caused by chronic disease

caffeine—stimulant in coffee, tea, and many cola beverages

caliper—mechanical device used to measure percentage of body fat by skinfold measurement

caloric density—energy value; number of kcal in a food

calorie—also known as kcal or kilocalorie; represents the amount of heat needed to raise the temperature of one kilogram of water one degree Celsius (C)

calorimeter—device used to scientifically determine the kcal value of foods

capillaries—tiny blood vessels connecting veins and arteries

carbohydrate—the nutrient providing the major source of energy in the average diet

carboxypeptidase—pancreatic enzyme necessary for protein digestion

carcinogen—cancer-causing substance

cardiac sphincter—the muscle at the base of the esophagus that prevents gastric reflux from moving into the esophagus

cardiovascular—pertaining to the heart and entire circulatory system

cardiovascular disease (CVD)—disease affecting heart and blood vessels

carotene—provitamin A

carotenoids—plant pigments, some of which yield vitamin A

carrier—one who is capable of transmitting an infectious organism

catabolism—the breakdown of compounds during metabolism

catalyst—a substance that causes another substance to react

cataracts—a clouding of the lens of the eye, obstructing sight

celiac sprue—disorder characterized by malabsorption; causes diarrhea, weight loss, and malnutrition; elimination of gluten provides relief

cell membrane—outer covering

cellular edema—swelling of body cells caused by inadequate amount of sodium in extracellular fluid

cellulose—indigestible carbohydrate; provides fiber in the diet

Celsius—metric system of measuring temperature

cerebral hemorrhage—stroke; bleeding in the brain

cerebrospinal fluid—of the brain and spinal cord

cerebrovascular accident (CVA)—either a blockage or bursting of blood vessel leading to the brain

cheilosis—condition caused by riboflavin deficiency; characterized by cracks and sores on the lips

chemical digestion—chemical changes in foods during digestion caused by hydrolysis

chemotherapy—treatment of diseased tissue with chemicals

cholecalciferol—the form of vitamin D that is formed in humans from cholesterol in the skin

cholecystectomy—removal of the gallbladder

cholecystitis—inflammation of the gallbladder

cholelithiasis—gallstones

cholesterol—fatlike substance that is a constituent of body cells; is synthesized in the liver; also found in animal foods

chronic—lasting a long time

chronic renal failure—slow development of kidney failure

chylomicron—largest lipoprotein; transports lipids after digestion into the body

chyme—the food mass as it has been mixed with gastric juices

chymopepsin—pancreatic enzyme necessary for protein digestion

chymotrypsin—pancreatic enzyme necessary for the digestion of proteins

circulation—the body process whereby the blood is moved throughout the body

cirrhosis—generic term for liver disease characterized by cell loss

clear-liquid diet—diet that includes only liquids containing primarily carbohydrates and water; nutritionally inadequate

clinical examination—physical observation

coagulate—to thicken

cobalamin—organic compound known as vitamin B_{12}

coenzyme—an active part of an enzyme

collagen—protein substance that holds body cells together

colostomy—opening from colon to abdomen surface

coma—state of unconsciousness

compensated heart disease—heart disease in which the heart is able to maintain circulation to all body parts

complementary proteins—incomplete proteins that when combined provide all nine essential amino acids

complete proteins—proteins that contain all nine essential amino acids

condiment—"extra" food such as catsup, pickles, relish

congestive heart failure (CHF)—a form of decompensated heart disease

consistency—texture

constipation—difficulty in evacuating feces; characterized by dry, hard stool

constituent—part

consumer—one who makes purchases and uses commercial products

continuous infusion—enteral nutrition administered continuously during a 16- to 24-hour period

convalescent—in a state of recovery

convenience food—food that has been partially prepared commercially and consequently is quickly and easily completed at home

crash diets—fad-type diets intended to reduce weight very quickly; in fact they reduce water, not fat tissue

craving—abnormal intense desire

creatinine—an end (waste) product of protein metabolism

cretinism—stunted physical and mental development

Crohn's disease—a chronic progressive disorder that causes inflammation, ulcers, and thickening of intestinal walls, sometimes causing obstruction

crude fiber—amount of fiber in plant foods after treatment with acids and alkalies in a laboratory; not an accurate measure of actual fiber in food

cultural—relating to one's background

curd—solid part resulting when milk is turned into cheese; liquid part is the whey

cystine—a nonessential amino acid

cysts—growths

daily values—represent percentage per serving of each nutritional item listed on new food labels based on daily intake of 2,000 kcal

D

decaffeinated—having had caffeine removed almost completely

decompensated heart disease—heart disease in which the heart cannot maintain circulation to all body parts

decubitus ulcer—bedsore

deficiency disease—disease caused by the lack of a specific nutrient

dehydrated—having lost large amounts of water

dehydration—loss of water

demineralization—loss of mineral or minerals

density—compactness; the mass of substance per unit of volume

dental caries—decayed areas on teeth; cavities

dentition—arrangement, type, and number of teeth

depression—an indentation; or feelings of extreme sadness

dermatitis—inflammation of the skin

descriptors—terms used to describe something

desensitize—to gradually reduce the body's sensitivity (allergic reaction) to specific items

dextrin—the intermediate product in starch digestion; before it changes to maltose and, ultimately, glucose

dextrose—glucose

diabetes insipidus—caused by damaged pituitary gland

diabetes mellitus—chronic disease in which the body lacks the normal ability to metabolize glucose

diabetic coma—unconsciousness caused by a state of acidosis due to too much sugar or too little insulin

dialysis—mechanical filtration of the blood; used when the kidneys are no longer able to perform normally

diaphragm—thin membrane or partition

diarrhea—loose bowel movement

diastolic pressure—blood pressure measured when the heart is at rest

dietary assessment—evaluation of food habits

dietary fiber—indigestible parts of plants; absorbs water in large intestine, helping to create soft, bulky stool; some is believed to bind cholesterol in the colon, helping to rid cholesterol from the body; some is believed to lower blood glucose levels

dietary laws—rules to be followed in meal planning in some religions

diet therapy—treatment of a disease through diet

digestion—breakdown of food in the body in preparation for absorption

disaccharides—double sugars that are reduced by hydrolysis to monosaccharides; examples are sucrose, maltose, and lactose

diuretics—substances used to increase the amount of urine excreted

diverticulitis—inflammation of the diverticula

diverticulosis—intestinal disorder characterized by little pockets forming in the sides of the intestines; pockets are called diverticula

dried milk—milk with water removed

dumping syndrome—nausea and diarrhea caused by food moving too quickly from the stomach to the small intestine

duodenal ulcer—ulcer occurring in the duodenum

duodenum—first (and smallest) section of the small intestine

durability—strength

dysentery—disease caused by microorganism; characterized by diarrhea

dyspepsia—gastrointestinal discomfort of vague origin

dysphagia—difficulty swallowing

E

eclamptic stage—convulsive stage of toxemia

economic status—status as determined by income

eczema—inflamed and scaly condition of skin

edema—the abnormal retention of fluid by the body

elective surgery—surgery performed at patient's choice

electrolyte—chemical compound that in water breaks up into electrically charged atoms called ions

elemental formulas—those formulas containing products of digestion of proteins, carbohydrates, and fats; also called hydrolyzed formulas

elimination—evacuation of wastes

elimination diet—limited diet in which only certain foods are allowed; intended to find the food allergen causing reaction

embryo—the developing fetus

emotional stress—strain caused by anxiety

emotional trauma—extremely stressful occurrence

emulsified fats—finely divided fat, held in suspension by another liquid

emulsifiers—help maintain emulsions (the combination of oil and water)

endocardium—lining of the heart

endocrine system—the ductless glands

endogenous insulin—insulin produced within the body

endometrium—mucous membrane of uterus

endosperm—the inner part of the kernel of grain; contains the carbohydrate

end stage renal disease (ESRD)—the stage at which the kidneys have lost most or all of their ability to function

energy balance—occurs when the kcal value of food ingested equals the kcal expended

energy imbalance—eating either too much or too little for the amount of energy expended

energy requirement—number of kcal required by the body each day

energy value—the kcal content of specific foods

English system of weights and measures—includes inch, foot, yard, cup, pound, quart, etc., as opposed to the metric system, which is based on the number 10

enriched foods—foods to which nutrients, usually B vitamins and iron, have been added to improve their nutritional value

enteral nutrition—feeding by tube directly into the patient's digestive tract

enterotoxins—toxins affecting mucous membranes

environment—surroundings

enzyme—organic substance that causes changes in other substances

equivalent—equal

ergocalciferol—the form of vitamin D found in plants

erythrocytes—red blood cells

Escherichia coli (E. coli)—species of bacteria found in intestines of animals and humans and in water contaminated by feces

esophagastomy—surgically created opening into esophagus; intended for tube feedings

esophagitis—inflammation of mucosal lining of esophagus

esophagus—tube leading from the mouth to the stomach; part of the gastrointestinal system

essential hypertension—high blood pressure with unknown cause; also called primary hypertension

estrogen—hormone secreted by the ovaries

etiology—cause

evaporated milk—milk that has had 60% of its water removed

exchange lists—lists of foods with interchangeable nutrient and kcal contents; used in specific forms of diet therapy

exogenous insulin—is produced outside the body

extracellular—outside the cell

extracellular fluid—water outside the cells; approximately 35% of total body fluid

F

fad diets—currently popular weight-reducing diets; usually nutritionally inadequate and not useful or permanent methods of weight reduction

fast foods—restaurant food that is ready to serve before orders are taken

fat cell theory—belief that fat cells have a natural drive to regain any weight lost

fats—highest kcal-value nutrient

fat-soluble—can be dissolved in fat

fatty acids—a component of fats that determines the classification of the fat

fecal matter—solid waste from large intestine

feces—solid waste from the large intestine

Federal Food, Drug, and Cosmetic Act—law requiring that food shipped from one state to another be pure, safe to eat, and prepared under sanitary conditions; also requires that ingredients and weight be listed on the label

fermentation—changing of sugars and starches to alcohol

fetal alcohol syndrome (PAS)—subnormal physical and mental development caused by mother's excessive use of alcohol during pregnancy

fetal malformations—physical abnormalities of the fetus

fetus—infant in utero

fever—hypermetabolic state with raised body temperature; commonly due to infection

fiber—indigestible, edible parts of plants

fibrosis—development of tough, stringy tissue

fillet—thin strip of meat or fish

filtrate—the substance to be filtered

flatulence—gas in the intestinal tract

folate-deficiency anemia—form of megaloblastic anemia; characterized by too few red blood cells that are large and immature

folate/folic acid—a form of vitamin B, also called folacin; essential for metabolism

food additives—chemical substances added to foods during processing

food customs—food habits

food deprivation—lack of food

food diary—written record of all food and drink ingested in a specified period

food faddists—people who have certain beliefs about particular foods or diets

Food Guide Pyramid—outline for making food selections based on Dietary Guidelines

food poisoning—foodborne illness

food residue—that part of the food that is indigestible

fortified foods—foods that have had vitamins and minerals added

fructose—the simple sugar (monosaccharide) found in fruit and honey

full-liquid diet—diet consisting of liquids and food that is liquid at body temperature

fundus (of the stomach)—upper part of the stomach

G

galactose—the simple sugar (monosaccharide) to which lactose is broken down during digestion

galactosemia—inherited error in metabolism that prevents normal metabolism of galactose

galactosuria—galactose in the urine

gallbladder—the organ located next to the liver; stores the bile produced by the liver and subsequently releases it as needed for the digestion of fats

gastric bypass—surgical reduction of the stomach

gastric juices—the digestive secretions of the stomach

gastric lipase—enzyme secreted by the stomach to aid in the digestion of fats

gastric ulcer—ulcer in the stomach

gastroesophageal reflux (GER)—backflow of stomach contents into the esophagus

gastrointestinal—pertaining to the stomach and intestines

gastrostomy—opening created by the surgeon directly into the stomach for enteral nutrition

genetic predisposition—inherited tendency

geriatrics—the branch of medicine involved with diseases of the elderly

germ—embryo or tiny life center of each kernel of grain

gerontology—the study of aging

gestational diabetes—diabetes occurring during pregnancy; usually disappears after delivery of the infant

gingivitis—inflammation of the gums

glomerular filtration rate (GFR)—the rate at which the kidneys filter the blood

glomerulonephritis—inflammation of the glomeruli of the kidneys

glomerulus—filtering unit in the kidneys

glossitis—inflammation of the tongue

glucagon—hormone from alpha cells of pancreas; helps cells release energy

glucose—the simple sugar to which carbohydrate must be broken down for absorption; also known as *dextrose*

gluten—protein found in grains

glycerol—a component of fat; derived from a water-soluble carbohydrate

glycogen—glucose as stored in the liver and muscles

glycogen loading—process in which the muscle store of glycogen is maximized; also called carboloading

glycosuria—excess sugar in the urine

goiter—enlarged tissue of the thyroid gland due to a deficiency of iodine

grams—small unit of measurement of weight in the metric system; 30 grams equal one ounce

GRAS list—FDA's list of substances "generally regarded as safe"

gross deficiency—extreme lack of

H

health foods—said by food faddists to have special health-giving characteristics

Heliobacter Pylori—bacteria that can cause peptic ulcer

hematuria—blood in the urine

heme iron—part of hemoglobin molecule in animal foods

hemochromatosis—condition caused by inborn error of metabolism resulting in excessive absorption of iron

hemodialysis—cleansing the blood of wastes by circulating the blood through a machine that contains tubing of semipermeable membranes

hemoglobin—the red coloring matter in the blood

hemolysis—the destruction of red blood cells

hemorrhage—unusually heavy bleeding

hepatitis—inflammation of the liver caused by viruses, drugs, and alcohol

hiatal hernia—condition wherein part of the stomach protrudes through the diaphragm into the chest cavity

high-density lipoproteins (HDLs)—lipoproteins that carry cholesterol from cells to the liver for eventual excretion

homeostasis—state of physical balance; stable condition

homogenized milk—whole milk processed to break fat into small drops that do not separate

hormone—chemical messengers secreted by a variety of glands

human immunodeficiency virus (HIV)—a virus that weakens the body's immune system and ultimately leads to AIDS

hummus—form of serving chickpeas common to Middle Easterners

hunger—physiological need for food

hydrochloric acid—gastric secretion necessary for the digestion of proteins and some minerals

hydrogenation—the combining of fat with hydrogen, thereby making it a saturated fat and solid at room temperature

hydrolysis—the addition of water resulting in the breakdown of the molecule

hydrolyzed formulas—contain products of digestion of proteins, carbohydrates, and fats; also called elemental formulas; used for patients who have difficulty digesting food

hypercholesterolemia—unusually high levels of cholesterol in blood; also known as *high serum cholesterol*

hyperemesis gravidarum—nausea so severe as to be life-threatening

hyperglycemia—excessive amounts of sugar in the blood

hyperkalemia—excessive amounts of potassium in the blood

hyperlipidemia—excessive amounts of fats in the blood

hypermetabolic—higher than normal rate of metabolism

hypersensitivity—abnormally strong sensitivity to certain substance(s)

hypertension—higher than normal blood pressure

hyperthyroidism—condition in which the thyroid gland secretes too much thyroxine and T$_3$; the body's rate of metabolism is unusually high

hypervitaminosis—condition caused by excessive ingestion of one or more vitamins

hypoalbuminemia—abnormally low amounts of protein in the blood

hypocalcemia—abnormally low amount of calcium in the blood

hypoglycemia—subnormal levels of blood sugar

hypoglycemic agents—oral drugs that stimulate the pancreas to produce insulin

hypogonadism—subnormal development of male sex organs

hypokalemia—low level of potassium in the blood

hypoproteinemia—low amounts of protein in the blood

hypothalamus—area at base of brain that regulates appetite and thirst

hypothyroidism—condition in which the thyroid gland secretes too little thyroxine and T$_3$; body metabolism is slower than normal

I

iatrogenic malnutrition—caused by treatment or diagnostic procedures

IDDM—insulin-dependent diabetes mellitus

ileostomy—opening from ileum to abdomen surface

ileum—last part of the small intestine

imitation foods—human-made; intended to resemble natural foods

immerse—dip

immunity—ability to resist certain diseases

inborn errors of metabolism—congenital disabilities preventing normal metabolism

incidental additives—those additives remaining on a food product as a result of farmers' use of fertilizers, pesticides, etc.

incomplete proteins—proteins that do not contain all of the nine essential amino acids

infarct—dead tissue resulting from blocked artery

infectious—contagious; communicable

inflammatory bowel disease—chronic condition causing inflammation in the gastrointestinal tract

ingest—take in orally

insecticide—agent that destroys insects

insomnia—inability to sleep

insulin—secretion of the islets of Langerhans in the pancreas gland; essential for the proper metabolism of glucose

insulin coma—unconsciousness caused by too much insulin or too little food

insulin-dependent diabetes mellitus (type 1 or IDDM)—diabetes occurring suddenly between the ages of 1 and 40; patients secrete little, if any, insulin and require insulin injections and a carefully controlled diet

insulin reaction—hypoglycemia leading to insulin coma caused by too much insulin or too little food

intentional additives—those additives that are added to perform specific functions in food, such as antioxidants to preserve color

International Units (IU)—units of measurement of some vitamins; 5 μg = 200 IU

interstitial fluid—fluid between cells

intima—lining of arteries

intracellular fluid—water within cells; approximately 65% of total body fluid

intracranial hemorrhage—bleeding within the head

intrinsic factor—secretion of stomach mucosa essential for B_{12} absorption

invisible fats—fats that are not immediately noticeable such as those in egg yolk, cheese, cream, and salad dressings

iodized salt—salt that has had the mineral iodine added for the prevention of goiter

ions—electrically charged atoms resulting from chemical reactions

iron—mineral essential to the blood

iron deficiency—intake of iron is adequate, but the body has no extra iron stored

iron-deficiency anemia—condition resulting from inadequate amount of iron in the diet, reducing the amount of oxygen carried by the blood to the cells

iron enhancer—assists in absorption of iron

irradiate—expose to ultraviolet light

irradiated foods—exposed to gamma radiation from cobalt source; to retard spoilage

ischemia—reduced blood flow causing inadequate supply of nutrients and oxygen to, and wastes from, tissues

islets of Langerhans—part of the pancreas from which insulin is secreted

isoleucine—an amino acid

J

jaundice—yellow cast of the skin and eyes

jejunoileal bypass—surgical procedure in which the jejunum of the small intestine is attached to a small section of the ileum in an effort to reduce the amount of absorptive surface

jejunostomy—opening created by the surgeon in the intestine for enteral nutrition

jejunum—the middle section comprising about two-fifths of the small intestine

K

Kaposi's sarcoma—type of cancer common to AIDS patients

kcal—the unit used to measure the fuel value of foods

kcal intake—kcal value of food eaten

kcal requirement—number of kcal required daily to meet energy needs

kcal value—number of kcal in a specific amount of specific food or beverage

Keshan disease—condition causing abnormalities in the heart muscle

ketones—substances to which fatty acids are broken down in the liver

ketonemia—ketones collected in the blood

ketonuria—ketone bodies in the urine

ketosis—condition in which ketones collect in the blood; caused by insufficient glucose available for energy

kilocalorie—*see* kcal

kilojoule—unit used to measure the energy value of food in the metric system; 4.184 kilojoules equal 1 kcal

Krebs cycle—the complete oxidation of carbohydrates, proteins, and fats

kwashiorkor—deficiency disease caused by extreme lack of protein

L

lactase—enzyme secreted by the small intestine for the digestion of lactose

lactation—the period during which the mother is nursing the baby

lacteals—lymphatic vessels in the small intestine that absorb fatty acids and glycerol

lacto-ovo vegetarian—vegetarians who will eat dairy products and eggs but no meat, poultry, or fish

lactose—the sugar in milk; a disaccharide

lactose intolerance—inability to digest lactose because of a lack of the enzyme lactase; causes abdominal cramps and diarrhea

lacto-vegetarians—vegetarians who eat dairy products

lean body mass—percentage of muscle tissue

lecithin—fatty substance found in plant and animal foods; a natural emulsifier that helps transport fats in the bloodstream; used commercially to make food products smooth

legumes—plant food that is grown in a pod; for example, beans and peas

lesions—sores; tissue damage

leucine—an amino acid

leukocytes—white blood cells

linoleic acid—fatty acid essential for humans; cannot be synthesized by the body

linolenic acid—one of three fatty acids needed by the body; cannot be synthesized by the body

lipid—fat

lipoproteins—carriers of fat in the blood

liquid diets—diets that contain foods that are liquid at body temperature

liter—unit of volume measurement in the metric system; the approximate equivalent of one quart in the English system

Lofenalac—commercial infant formula with 95% of phenylalanine removed

longevity—length of life

low-density lipoproteins (LDLs)—carry blood cholesterol to the cells

low-residue diet—diet severely restricted in food residue

lumen—the hollow area in a tube

M

macrosomia—birthweight over 9 pounds

major minerals—those minerals required in amounts greater than 100 mg a day

malignant—life-threatening

malnutrition—poor nutrition

maltase—enzyme secreted by the small intestine essential for the digestion of maltose

maltose—the double sugar (disaccharide) occurring as a result of the digestion of grain

maple syrup urine disease (MSUD)—disease caused by an inborn error of metabolism in which the body cannot metabolize certain amino acids

marasmus—severe wasting caused by lack of protein and all nutrients or faulty absorption; PEM

meat analogues—substances made to imitate meat; usually of soybean origin

mechanical digestion—the part of digestion that requires certain mechanical movement such as chewing, swallowing, and peristalsis

mechanical-soft diet—soft diet for people who cannot chew; all meats are ground and fruits and vegetables are pureed

megadose—extraordinarily large amount

megaloblastic anemia—anemia in which the red blood cells are unusually large and are not completely mature

menadione—synthetic vitamin K

menaquinones—the form of vitamin K found in bacteria, animals, and humans

mental retardation—below normal intellectual capacity

metabolism—the use of the food by the body after digestion which results in energy

metastasize—spread of cancer cells from one organ to another

meter—metric unit of length; 39 inches

metric system—system of measurement based on the number 10

microorganisms—microscopic organisms such as bacteria and viruses

milliequivalent—the concentration of electrolytes in a solution

milling—the grinding of grain

mineral—one of many inorganic substances essential to life and classified generally as minerals

modular formulas—made by combining specific nutrients

mold—is a type of fungus

monosaccharides—simplest carbohydrates; sugars that cannot be further reduced by hydrolysis; examples are glucose, fructose, and galactose

monosodium glutamate (MSG)—a form of spice containing large amounts of sodium

monounsaturated fats—fats that are neither saturated nor polyunsaturated and are thought to play little part in atherosclerosis

morbid—damaging to health

morning sickness—early morning nausea common to some pregnancies

mortality rate—percentage of death in a given population

mucous membrane—lining of body passages that open to the outside such as the gastrointestinal, genitourinary, and respiratory tracts

mutations—changes in the genes

myelin—lipoprotein essential for the protection of nerves

myocardial infarction (MI)—heart attack; caused by the blockage of an artery leading to the heart

myocardium—heart muscle

myoglobin—protein compound in muscle that provides oxygen to cells

myxedema—hypothyroidism

N

nasogastric (NG) tube—tube leading from the nose to the stomach for tube feeding

natural foods—unchanged; contain no additives

nausea—the urge to vomit

necrosis—tissue death due to lack of blood supply

negative nitrogen balance—more nitrogen lost than taken in

neoplasia—abnormal development of cells

neoplasm—abnormal growth of new tissue

nephritis—inflammatory disease of the kidneys

nephrolithiasis—kidney, or renal, stones

nephron—unit of the kidney containing a glomerulus

nephrosclerosis—hardening of renal arteries

neural tube defects—congenital malformation of brain and/or spinal column due to failure of neural tube to close during embryonic development

neuropathy—nerve damage

neurotoxins—toxins affecting the nervous system

niacin—B vitamin

niacin equivalent (NE)—unit of measuring niacin; 1 NE equals 1 mg niacin or 60 mg tryptophan

NIDDM—non-insulin-dependent diabetes mellitus

nitrogen—chemical element found in protein; essential to life

nitrogen balance—when nitrogen intake equals nitrogen excreted

nonheme iron—iron from animal foods that is not part of the hemoglobin molecule; and all iron from plant foods

non-insulin-dependent diabetes mellitus (type 2 or NIDDM)—diabetes occurring after age 40; onset is gradual and production of insulin gradually diminishes; can usually be controlled by diet and exercise

nontropical sprue—a disorder of the gastrointestinal tract characterized by malabsorption; also called gluten sensitivity

norepinephrine—neurotransmitter of vasoconstrictor that helps the body cope with stressful conditions

normal weight—average weight for size and age

nourishing—foods or beverages that provide substantial amounts of essential nutrients

nutrient—chemical substance found in food that is necessary for good health

nutrient-dense foods—foods that contain many nutrients but few kcal

nutrient density—nutrient value of foods compared with number of kcal

nutrient requirement—amount of specific nutrient needed by the body

nutrition—the result of those processes whereby the body takes in and uses food for growth, development, and the maintenance of health

nutritional edema—edema caused by lack of protein in the diet

nutritionally adequate—contains recommended amounts of essential nutrients

nutritional status—one's physical condition as determined by diet

nutritional value—the nutrient content of foods or beverages

nutrition assessment—evaluation of nutritional status

nutritious—foods or beverages containing substantial amounts of essential nutrients

O

obesity—excessive body fat, 20% above average

obstetrician—doctor who cares for the mother during pregnancy and delivery

occlusions—blockages

oliguria—decreased output of urine to less than 500 ml a day

omega-3 fatty acids—polyunsaturated fatty acids found in fish oil; may contribute to reduction of coronary artery disease

oncologist—doctor specializing in the study of cancer

oncology—the study of cancer

on demand—feeding infants as they desire

opaque—neither transparent nor translucent; light cannot pass through

opportunistic infections—caused by microorganisms that are present but that do not normally affect people with healthy immune systems

oral diabetes medications—oral hypoglycemic agents. medications that may be given to type 2 diabetes mellitus patients to lower blood glucose

oral hypoglycemic agents—medications that may be given to NIDDM patients to lower blood glucose

organic foods—grown without synthetic fertilizer and produced without additives

organ meats—liver, kidney, brains, sweetbreads

osmolality—number of particles per kilogram of solution; solutions with high osmolality exert more pressure than do those with fewer particles

osmosis—movement of a substance through a semipermeable membrane

osteomalacia—a condition in which bones become soft, usually in adult women, because of calcium loss

osteoporosis—condition in which bones become brittle because there have been insufficient mineral deposits, especially calcium

ostomy—surgically created opening into an organ of the gastrointestinal tract

overweight—weight 10–20% above average

ovo vegetarian—vegetarians who will eat eggs

oxidation—the process of combining substances with oxygen

P

pallor—paleness of the skin

panacea—supposed cure for all physical problems

pancreas—gland that secretes enzymes essential for digestion and insulin, which is essential for glucose metabolism

pancreatic amylase—the enzyme secreted by the pancreas that is essential for the digestion of starch

pancreatic lipase (steapsin)—the enzyme secreted by the pancreas that is essential for the digestion of fat

pancreatic protease—the enzyme secreted by the pancreas that is essential for the digestion of protein

pancreatitis—inflammation of the pancreas

pantothenic acid—a B vitamin

paralysis—inability to move

parasite—organism that is completely dependent on another organism for its existence

parenteral nutrition—nutrition provided via a vein

pasteurization—process in which harmful microorganisms are killed

pathogens—disease-causing agents

pediatrician—doctor specializing in the health problems of children

peer group—group of people approximately one's own age

peer pressure—pressure of one's friends and colleagues of the same age

pellagra—deficiency disease caused by a lack of niacin

pepsin—an enzyme secreted by the stomach that is essential for the digestion of proteins

peptic ulcers—ulcer of the stomach or duodenum

peptidases—enzymes secreted by the small intestine that are essential for the digestion of protein

perfringens—species of bacterial genus *Clostridium* that can cause food poisoning

pericardium—outer covering of the heart

periodontal disease—disease of the mouth and gums

peripheral vascular disease (PVD)—narrowed arteries some distance from the heart

peripheral vein—a vein that is near the surface of the skin

peristalsis—rhythmical movement of the intestinal tract; moves the chyme along

peritoneal dialysis—removal of waste products from the blood by injecting the flushing solution into the abdomen and using the patient's peritoneum as the semipermeable membrane

pernicious anemia—severe, chronic anemia caused by a deficiency of vitamin B_{12}; usually due to the body's inability to absorb B_{12}

pH—symbol for the degree of acidity or alkalinity of a solution

phenylalanine—amino acid

phenylalanine hydroxylase—liver enzyme necessary to metabolize the amino acid phenylalanine

phenylketonuria (PKU)—condition caused by an inborn error of metabolism in which the infant lacks an enzyme necessary to metabolize the amino acid phenylalanine

phenylpropanolamine—constituent of diet pills; can damage blood vessels

phlebitis—inflammation of a vein

phylloquinone—vitamin K as found in green plants

physical stress—bodily strain

physical trauma—extreme physical stress

physiological—relating to bodily functions

phytochemicals—substances occurring naturally in plant foods

pica—abnormal craving for nonfood substance

pigmentation—coloring matter in the skin

placenta—organ in the uterus that links blood supplies of mother and infant

plaque—fatty deposit on interior of artery walls

plateau period—period in which there is no change

polycystic kidney disease—rare, hereditary kidney disease causing cysts or growths on the kidneys that can ultimately cause kidney failure in middle age

polydipsia—abnormal thirst

polymeric formulas—commercially prepared formulas for tube feedings that contain intact proteins, carbohydrates, and fats that require digestion

polypeptides—ten or more amino acids bonded together

polyphagia—excess hunger

polysaccharides—complex carbohydrates containing combinations of monosaccharides; examples include starch, dextrin, cellulose, and glycogen

polyunsaturated fats—fats whose carbon atoms contain only limited amounts of hydrogen

polyuria—excessive urination

positive nitrogen balance—nitrogen intake exceeds outgo

positive water balance—condition occurring when more water is taken in than is used or excreted

postoperative—after surgery

postprandial—after meals

posture—body position

precursor—something that comes before something else; in vitamins it is also called a provitamin, something from which the body can synthesize the specific vitamin

prefix—first syllable of word

pregnancy-induced hypertension (PIH)—typically occurs during late pregnancy; characterized by high blood pressure, albumin in the urine, and edema

pressure ulcers—bedsores

primary hypertension—high blood pressure resulting from an unknown cause

prohormone—substance that precedes the hormone and from which the body can synthesize the hormone

proteases—enzymes secreted by the pancreas; essential for digestion of proteins

protein energy malnutrition (PEM)—protein energy malnutrition; marasmus

proteins—the only one of six essential nutrients containing nitrogen

proteinuria—protein in the urine

prothrombin—substance that permits clotting of the blood

protozoa—microorganisms that can cause dysentery

provitamin—see precursor

psychological development—development of the psyche

psychosocial development—relating to both psychological and social development

ptyalin—also called salivary amylase; the digestive secretion of the salivary glands

purines—end products of nucleoprotein metabolism

pyloric sphincter—the muscle at the end of the stomach and the beginning of the small intestine that opens and closes to permit chyme to enter the small intestine

pylorus—the end of the stomach nearest the intestine

pyridoxal—one of the three vitamers of vitamin B_6

pyridoxamine—one of the three vitamers of vitamin B_6

pyridoxine—one of the three vitamers of vitamin B_6

R

raw milk—milk that has not been processed in any way; may contain harmful microorganisms

RDAs—recommended dietary allowances as determined by the Food and Nutrition Board of the National Academy of Sciences–National Research Council

REE—resting energy expenditure; the rate at which the body expends energy just for its maintenance; comparable to the basal metabolic rate (BMR)

refined foods—foods that have been processed to remove most or all naturally occurring fiber

registered dietitian—a person who has graduated from a college or university after completing a course of study accredited by the American Dietetic Association (ADA), has completed an internship, and has passed a registration examination; dietitians maintain competency through continuing education

regular diet—normal diet, based on the Food Guide Pyramid

regurgitation—vomiting

renal stones—kidney stones

renal threshold—kidneys' capacity

rennin—enzyme secreted by the stomach necessary for the digestion of proteins in milk

resection—reduction

residue—solid part of feces

resorb—take back; reabsorb

respiration—breathing

retardation—slowing

retinol—the preformed vitamin A

retinol equivalent (RE)—the equivalent of 3.33 IU of vitamin A

retinopathy—damage to small blood vessels in the eyes

riboflavin—the name for vitamin B_2

rickets—deficiency disease caused by the lack of vitamin D; causes malformed bones and pain in infants

S

saccharin—artificial sweetener

saliva—secretion of the salivary glands

salivary amylase—also called *ptyalin;* the enzyme secreted by the salivary glands to act on starch

salmonella—an infection caused by the Salmonella bacteria

sanitation—cleanliness

satiety—feeling of satisfaction; fullness

saturated fats—fats whose carbon atoms contain all of the hydrogen atoms they can; considered a contributory factor in atherosclerosis

scurvy—a deficiency disease caused by a lack of vitamin C

secondary diabetes mellitus—rare disease caused by certain drugs or disease of the pancreas

secondary hypertension—high blood pressure caused by another condition such as kidney disease

secretions—liquid emissions

self-esteem—feelings of self-worth

sepsis—infection of the blood

serum cholesterol—cholesterol in the blood

set point theory—belief that everyone has a natural weight ("set point") at which the body is most comfortable

shellfish—an aquatic invertebrate animal with external shell and no internal bones

skeletal system—body's bone structure

skim milk—milk with fat removed

skin tests—allergy tests using potential allergens on scratches on the skin

sodium chloride—table salt

soft diet—one of the basic hospital diets; contains only foods with soft textures

solute—the substance dissolved in a solution

solvent—liquid part of a solution

somatostatin—hormone produced by delta cells of pancreas and by the hypothalamus

sphygmomanometer—instrument used to measure blood pressure

spina bifida—spinal cord or spinal fluid bulge through the back

spontaneous abortion—occurring naturally; miscarriage

stamina—strength and endurance

standard diets—basic diets used by most hospitals; can be modified in texture, kcal, and nutrient content

Staphylococcus **(staph)**—genus of bacteria causing food poisoning called "staph" or "staphylococcal poisoning"

starch—polysaccharide found in grains and vegetables

stasis—stoppage or slowing

steatorrhea—abnormal amounts of fat in the feces

sterile—free of infectious organisms

stimulant—substance that increases heart rate, such as caffeine

stoma—surgically created opening in the abdominal wall

stomach banding—surgical reduction of stomach, but to lesser degree than bypass

sucrase—enzyme secreted by the small intestine to aid in digestion of sucrose

sucrose—a double sugar or disaccharide; examples are granulated, powdered, and brown sugar

synthesize—to make a substance from other substances

synthetic—human-made

systolic pressure—blood pressure taken as the heart contracts

T

tachycardia—abnormally rapid heartbeat

terminal—situation in which death is certain

tetany—involuntary muscle movement

textured protein—meat analogues; imitation meat products

therapeutic diets—diets used in treatment of disease

thiamin—vitamin B_1

thrombosis—blockage, as a blood clot

thrombus—blood clot

thyroid gland—controls body metabolism; secretes thyroxine and T_3

thyroxine—secretion of the thyroid gland

tocopherols—vitamers of vitamin E

tocotrienols—a form of vitamin E

total parenteral nutrition—*see* TPN

toxic—poisonous

toxicity—state of being poisonous

toxin—poison

TPN—total parenteral nutrition; process of providing all nutrients intravenously

trace minerals—minerals that are essential but only in very small amounts

transferase—a liver enzyme necessary for the metabolism of galactose

trauma—stress to the body

trichinosis—disease caused by the parasitic roundworm *Trichinella spiralis;* can be transmitted through undercooked pork

triglycerides—combinations of fatty acids and glycerol

triiodothyronine (T$_3$)—secretion of the thyroid gland

trimester—3-month period; commonly used to denote periods of pregnancy

trypsin—pancreatic enzyme; helps digest proteins

tryptophan—an amino acid and a precursor of niacin

tube feeding—feeding by tube directly into the stomach or intestine

U

ulcerative colitis—disease characterized by inflammation and ulceration of the colon, rectum, and sometimes entire large intestine

underweight—weight that is 10–15% below average

urea—chief nitrogenous waste product of protein metabolism

uremia—condition in which protein wastes are circulating in the blood

ureters—tubes leading from the kidneys to the bladder

uric acid—one of the nitrogenous waste products of protein metabolism

urticaria—hives; common allergic reaction

V

valine—an amino acid

vascular dilation—expansion of blood vessels

vascular disease—disease of the blood vessels

vascular osmotic pressure—high concentration of electrolytes in the blood; low blood volume or blood pressure

vascular system—circulatory system

vasopressin—antidiuretic hormone; also called ADH

vegans—vegetarians who avoid all animal foods

very-low-density lipoproteins (VLDLs)—lipoproteins made by the liver to transport lipids throughout the body

villi—the tiny, hairlike structures in the small intestines through which nutrients are absorbed

visible fats—fats in foods that are purchased and used as fats, such as butter or margarine

vitamers—different chemical forms of a vitamin that serve the same purpose in the body

vitamins—organic substances necessary for life although they do not, independently, provide energy

vitamin supplements—concentrated forms of vitamins; may be in tablet or liquid form

volume—amount in terms of space consumed

W

water-soluble—can be dissolved in water

weaning—training an infant to drink from the cup instead of the nipple

whole milk—milk with neither fat nor water removed

X

xerophthalmia—serious eye disease characterized by dry mucous membranes of the eye, caused by a deficiency of vitamin A

xerostomia—sore, dry mouth caused by a reduction of salivary secretions; may be caused by radiation for treatment of cancer

Y

yo-yo effect—refers to crash diets; the dieter's weight goes up and down over short periods because these diets do not change eating habits

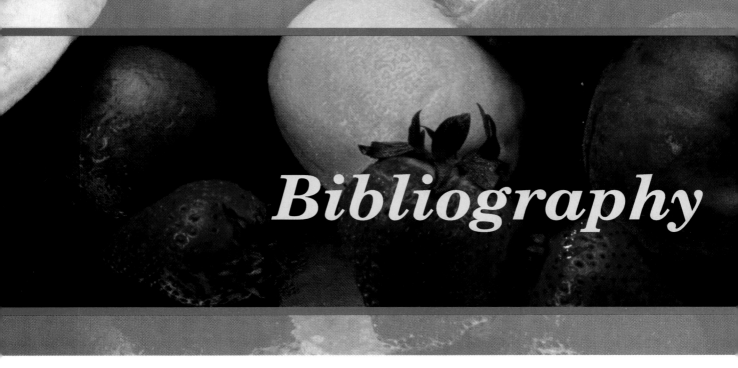

Bibliography

Books

Cataldo, C. B., DeBryne, L. K., & Whitney, E. N. (1995). *Nutrition and diet therapy: Principles & practice* (4th ed.). St. Paul, MN: West.

Davis, J., & Sherer, K. (1994). *Applied nutrition and diet therapy for nurses* (2nd ed.). Philadelphia: Saunders.

Dudek, S. G. (1997). *Nutrition handbook for nursing practice* (3rd ed.). Phildelphia: Lippincott.

Eschleman, M. M. (1996). *Introductory nutrition and nutrition therapy* (3rd ed.). Philadelphia: Lippincott.

Grodner, M., Anderson, S. L., & DeYoung, S. (1996). *Foundations and clinical applications of nutrition: A nursing approach.* St. Louis, MO: Mosby.

Larson, D. E. (Ed.). (1996). *Mayo Clinic family health book* (2nd ed.). New York: Morrow.

Lee, R. D., & Nieman, D. C. (1996). *Nutritional assessment* (2nd ed.). St. Louis, MO: Mosby.

Lutz, C. A., & Rutherford, K. P. (1997). *Nutrition and diet therapy* (2nd ed.). Philadelphia: Davis.

Mahan, L. K., & Escott-Stump, S. (1996). *Krause's food nutrition and diet therapy* (9th ed.). Philadelphia: Saunders.

Mayo Clinic, Rochester Methodist Hospital, & St. Mary's Hospital. (1988). *Mayo clinic diet manual, A handbook of dietary practices* (6th ed.). Philadelphia: Saunders.

Mitchell, M. K. (1997). *Nutrition across the life span.* Philadelphia: Saunders.

Morley, J. E., Glick, Z., & Rubenstein, L. Z. (1995). *Geriatric nutrition* (2nd ed.). New York: Raven Press.

National Research Council Committee on Diet and Health. (1989). *Diet and health implications for reducing chronic disease risk.* Washington, DC: National Academy Press.

National Research Council, National Academy of Sciences. (1989). *Recommended dietary allowances* (10th ed.). Washington, DC: National Academy Press.

Peckenpaugh, N. I., & Poleman, C. M. (1995). *Nutrition essentials and diet therapy* (7th ed.). Philadelphia: Saunders.

Piper, B. (1996). *Diet and nutrition.* London: Chapman & Hall.

Schlenker, E. D. (1998). *Nutrition in aging* (3rd ed.). New York: McGraw-Hill.

Schlenker, E. D.; Pipes, P.; Trahms, C. M.; Worthington-Roberts, B. S.; & Williams, S. R. (Eds.). (1996). *Nutrition throughout the life cycle* (3rd ed.). St. Louis, MO: Mosby.

Shils, M. E., & Young, V. E. (1988). *Modern nutrition in health and disease* (7th ed.). Philadelphia: Lea & Febiger.

Snetselaar, L. G. (1997). *Nutrition counseling skills for medical nutrition therapy.* Gaithersburg, MD: Aspen Publishers.

Stanfield, P. S., & Hui, Y. H. (1997). *Nutrition and diet therapy* (3rd ed.). Boston: Jones & Bartlett.

Stemkard, A. J., & Wadden, T. A. (Eds.). (1996). *Obesity theory and therapy* (2nd ed.). Philadelphia: Lippencott-Raven.

Trahms, C. M. and Pipes P. (1997). *Nutrition in infancy and childhood* (6th ed.). New York: McGraw-Hill.

U.S. Department of Agriculture. (1976). *Composition of foods.* Washington, DC: U.S. Government Printing Office.

Wardlaw, G. M., & Insel, P. M. (1996). *Perspectives in nutrition* (3rd ed.). New York: Mosby-Year Book.

Whitney, E. N., Cataldo, C. B., DeBryne, L. K., & Rolfes, S. R. (1996). *Nutrition for health & health care.* St. Paul, MN: West.

Whitney, E. N., & Rolfes, S. R. (1996). *Understanding nutrition* (7th ed.). St. Paul, MN: West.

Williams, S. R. (1994). *Essentials of nutrition and diet therapy* (6th ed.). St. Louis, MO: Mosby.

Williams, S. R. (1995). *Basic nutrition and diet therapy* (10th ed.). St. Louis, MO: Mosby.

Worthington-Roberts, B. S., & Williams, S. R. (Ed.). (1996). *Nutrition throughout the life cycle.* St. Louis, MO: Mosby.

Zeman, F. J., & Ney, D. M. (1996). *Applications in medical nutrition therapy* (2nd ed.). Upper Saddle River, NJ: Simon & Schuster.

Periodicals and Publications

ADA report: Weight management. (1997). *Journal of the American Dietetic Association, 97*(1), 71–74.

ADA report: Fat replacements. (1991). *Journal of the American Dietetic Association, 91*(10), 1285–1288.

Crance, N. T., Wilson, D. B., Cook, D. A., Lewis, C. J., Yetley, E. A., & Rader, J. I. (1995). Evaluating food fortification options: General principles revisited with folic acid. *American Journal of Public Health, 85*(5), 660–666.

Cuskelly, G. J., McNulty, J., & Scott, J. M. (1996). Effect of increasing dietary folate on red-cell folate: Implications for prevention of neural tube defects. *Lancet, 347,* 657–659.

Enger, S. M., Ross, R. K., Henderson, B., & Bernstein, L. (1997). Breastfeeding history, pregnancy experience and risk of breast cancer. *British Journal of Cancer, 76*(1), 118–123.

Evans, W. J., & Cyr-Campbell, D. (1997). Nutrition, exercise, and healthy aging. *Journal of the American Dietetic Association, 97*(6), 632–638.

Food & Nutrition Board, Institute of Medicine. (1997). *Dietary reference intakes of calcium, phosphorus, magnesium, vitamin D, and fluoride.* Washington, DC: National Academy Press.

Gaull, G. E. (1996). Fortifying policy with science—The case of folate. *Journal of Nutrition, 126,* 749S–750S.

Hankin, J. R. (1994). FAS prevention strategies. *Alcohol Health & Research World, 18*(1), 62–66.

Herwaldt, B. L., Ackers, M., & the Cyclospora Working Group. (1997). An outbreak in 1996 of cyclosporiasis associated with imported raspberries. *The New England Journal of Medicine,* 1548–1556.

Hingley, A. (1997, September–October). Focus on food safety. *FDA Consumer,* 8–11.

Huang, P., Weber, J. T., Sosin, D. M., Griffin, P. M., Long, E. G., Murphy, J. J., Kocka, F., Peters, C., & Kallick, C. (1995). The first reported outbreak of diarrheal illness associated with cyclospora in the United States. *Annals of Internal Medicine, 123,* 409–414.

Hueston, W. J. (1993). Folic acid for the prevention of neural tube defects. *American Family Physician, 47*(5), 1058–1060.

Indiana Prevention Resource Center. (1992). *Factline on marijuana.* Bloomington, IN.

Indiana Prevention Resource Center. (1996). *Factline on methcathinone.* Bloomington, IN.

Indiana Prevention Resource Center. (1991). *Factline on amphetamines.* Bloomington, IN.

Indiana Prevention Resource Center. (1991). *Factline on cocaine.* Bloomington, IN.

Indiana Prevention Resource Center. (1992). *Factline on inhalants.* Bloomington, IN.

Indiana Prevention Resource Center. (1992). *Factline on gateway drugs.* Bloomington, IN.

Jackman, L. A., Millane, S. S., Martin, B. R., Wood, O. B., McCabe, G. P., Peacock, M., & Weaver, C. M. (1997). Calcium retention in relation to calcium intake and postmenarcheal age in adolescent females. *American Journal of Clinical Nutrition, 66,* 327–333.

Kelly, D. G., & Fleming, C. R. (1995). Nutritional considerations in inflammatory bowel diseases. *Gastroenterology Clinics of North America, 24*(3), 597–611.

Kurtzweil, P. (1995, October). Can your kitchen pass the food safety test? *FDA Consumer,* 15–18.

Kurtzweil, P. (1996, September). How folate can help prevent birth defects. *FDA Consumer,* 7–10.

Kurtzweil, P. (1997, March). Fruits & vegetables— Eating your way to 5 a day. *FDA Consumer,* 16–18.

Michels, K. B., Willett, W. C., Rosner, B. A., Manson, J. E., Hunter, D. J., Colditz, G. A., Hankinson, S. E., & Speizer, F. E. (1996). Prospective assessment of breastfeeding and breast cancer incidence among 89,887 women. *Lancet, 347,* 431–436.

National Live Stock and Meat Board. (1992). *A good start: Nutrition during pregnancy.*

National Live Stock and Meat Board. (1992). *A food guide for the first five years.*

National Live Stock and Meat Board. (1994). Safe food backgrounder.

Office of the Federal Register, National Archives and Record Services, General Services Administration. (1993). *Federal Register* (Volume 58, Number 3). Washington, DC.

Owen, A. L., & Owen, G. M. (1997). Twenty years of WIC: A review of some effects of the program. *The Journal of the American Dietetic Association, 97*(7), 777–782.

Papazian, R. (1997, July/August). Bulking up fiber's healthful reputation. *FDA Consumer,* 23–27.

Potter, J. D. (1996). Nutrition and colorectal cancer. *Cancer Causes and Control, 7,* 127–145.

Romano, P. S., Waitzman, N. J., Scheffler, R. M., & Pi, R. D. (1995). Folic acid fortification of grain: An economic analysis. *American Journal of Public Health, 85*(5), 667–676.

Rose, M. C., & Mennuti, M. T. (1995). Periconceptional folic acid supplementation as a social intervention. *Seminars in Perinatology, 19*(4), 243–254.

Stokes, M. A. (1992). Crohn's disease and nutrition. *British Journal of Surgery, 79*(5), 391–394.

Thomas, A. G., Taylor, F., & Miller, V. (1993). Dietary intake and nutritional treatment in childhood Crohn's disease. *Journal of Pediatric Gastroenterol Nutrition, 17*(1), 75–81.

U.S. Department of Agriculture. (1986). *Dietary guidelines and your diet.* (Home & Garden Bulletin No. 232-1-7). Washington, DC: U.S. Government Printing Office.

U.S. Department of Agriculture. (1986). *The sodium content of your food.* (Home & Garden Bulletin No. 233). Washington, DC: U.S. Government Printing Office.

U.S. Department of Agriculture. (1989). *Nutritive value of foods.* (Home & Garden Bulletin No. 72). Washington, DC: U.S. Government Printing Office.

U.S. Department of Agriculture. (1990). *Bacteria that cause foodborne illness.* Food Safety and Inspection Service. Washington, DC: U.S. Government Printing Office.

U.S. Department of Agriculture. (1990). *Dietary guidelines for Americans* (3rd ed.). (Home & Garden Bulletin No. 232). Washington, DC: U.S. Government Printing Office.

U.S. Department of Agriculture. (1990). *Preventing foodborne illness. A guide to safe food handling.* Food Safety and Inspection Service. (Home & Garden Bulletin No. 247). Washington, DC: U.S. Government Printing Office.

U.S. Department of Agriculture. (1990). *A quick consumer guide to safe food handling.* Food Safety and Inspection Service. (Home & Garden Bulletin No. 248). Washington, DC: U.S. Government Printing Office.

Williams, R. D. (1997, July/August). When summertime gets too hot to handle. *FDA Consumer,* 14–16.

Yetley, E. A., & Rader, J. I. (1996). The challenge of regulating health claims and food fortification. American Institute of Nutrition. *Journal of Nutrition, 126,* 765S–772S.

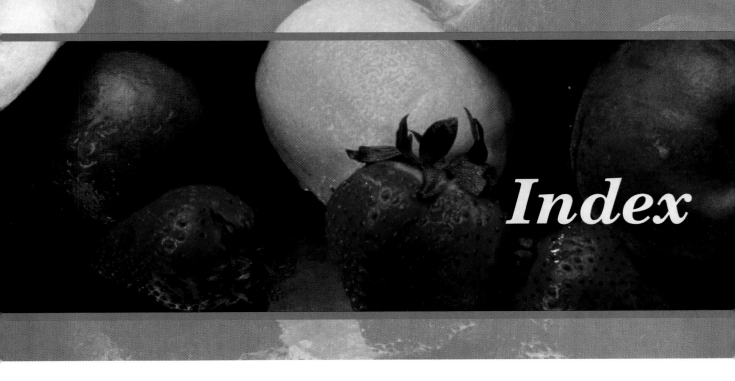

Index